D1416532

Sol S. Zimmerman, M.D.

Associate Professor of Clinical Pediatrics
New York University School of Medicine
Assistant Director of Pediatrics
Director, Pediatric Intensive Care Unit
University Hospital
New York University Medical Center
New York, New York

Indiana University
Library
Northwest

ASSOCIATE EDITOR

Joan Holter Gildea, R.N., B.S., M.A.

Clinical Assistant Director of Nursing
New York University Medical Center
New York, New York

RJ
370
.C747
1985

CRITICAL CARE
PEDIATRICS

1985
W. B. SAUNDERS COMPANY
Philadelphia London Toronto Mexico City Rio de Janeiro Sydney Tokyo Hong Kong

W. B. Saunders Company: West Washington Square
Philadelphia, PA 19105

Indiana University
Library
Northwest

Library of Congress Cataloging in Publication Data

Main entry under title:

Critical care pediatrics.

   1. Pediatric intensive care. I. Zimmerman, Sol S.
II. Gildea, Joan Holter. [DNLM: 1. Critical Care—in
infancy & childhood. WS 366 C93332]
RJ370.C747 1985   618.92′0028   84-10570
ISBN 0-7216-1143-5

Critical Care Pediatrics   ISBN 0-7216-1143-5

© 1985 by W. B. Saunders Company. Copyright under the Uniform Copyright Convention. Simultaneously published in Canada. All rights reserved. This book is protected by copyright. No part of it may be reproduced, stored in a retrieval system, or transmitted in any form or
by any means, electronic, mechanical, photocopying, recording, or otherwise, without written permission
from the publisher. Made in the United States of America. Press of W. B. Saunders Company. Library of Congress catalog card number 84-10570.

Last digit is the print number: 9   8   7   6   5   4   3   2   1

To my mother, for her love and guidance
and
To Diana, Jeffrey, Steven, and Andrew for their love,
encouragement, enthusiasm, and endurance

S.S.Z.

CONTRIBUTORS

LOOL SEGED ABEBE, B.Sc., M.D.

Assistant Professor of Pathology, Albert Einstein College of Medicine, Bronx, New York; Director of Blood Bank, Chief of Hematology Lab, Bronx-Lebanon Hospital Center, Bronx, New York

Component Transfusion Therapy

MARVIN E. AMENT, M.D.

Professor of Pediatrics, Department of Pediatrics, Chief, Division of Pediatric Gastroenterology and Nutrition, Los Angeles, California; Attending, UCLA Medical Center, Cedars-Sinai Medical Center, Long Beach Children's Hospital, and Olive View Medical Center, Los Angeles, California

Upper Gastrointestinal Bleeding; Fulminant Hepatic Necrosis and Hepatic Coma

ROBERT A. BOXER, M.D.

Assistant Professor of Pediatrics, Cornell University Medical College, New York, New York; Physician-in-Charge, Pediatric Intensive Care Unit, Assistant Chief of Pediatric Cardiology and Senior Assistant Attending, Department of Pediatrics, North Shore University Hospital, Manhasset, New York

Application of Echocardiography in the Pediatric Intensive Care Unit; Postoperative Care After Open-Heart Surgery

HARRIS E. BURSTIN, M.D.

Clinical Assistant Professor of Pediatrics, New York University School of Medicine, New York, New York; Assistant Director, Pediatric Intensive Care Unit, University Hospital, New York University Medical Center, New York, New York

Temperature Regulation; Status Asthmaticus; Bronchiolitis; Salicylate Ingestions; Acetaminophen Intoxication

DELORES DANILOWICZ, M.D.

Professor of Pediatrics, New York University Medical Center, New York, New York; Attending Cardiologist, University Hospital, Bellevue Hospital, and Lenox Hill Hospital, Director, Pediatric Cardiac Catheterization Laboratory, University Hospital, New York University Medical Center, New York, New York

Dysrhythmias in Children; Congestive Heart Failure

RAPHAEL DAVID, M.D.

Professor of Pediatrics, New York University School of Medicine, New York, New York; Director, Pediatric Endocrinology, New York University Medical Center and Bellevue Hospital, New York, New York

Adrenal Insufficiency and Steroid Withdrawal; Hyperthyroidism

REGINA R. DE CARLO, M.D.

Clinical Assistant Professor of Pediatrics, New York University School of Medicine, New York, New York; Attending, New York University Medical Center, New York, New York

Hypoxic-Ischemic Encephalopathy; Guillain-Barré Syndrome

FRED J. EPSTEIN, M.D.

Professor of Neurosurgery and Director, Division of Pediatric Neurosurgery, New York University School of Medicine, New York, New York; Attending Neurosurgeon, New York University Hospital, Bellevue Hospital, and St. Vincent's Hospital, New York, New York

Management of Pediatric Head Trauma; Pediatric Spinal Cord Trauma; Postoperative Care Following Intracranial Neurosurgery

BONITA FALKNER, M.D.

Professor of Pediatrics and Director of Pediatric Nephrology and Hypertension, Hahnemann University Hospital, Philadelphia, Pennsylvania

Fluids and Electrolytes

IRVING FISH, M.D.

Director, Pediatric Neurology and Associate Professor of Clinical Neurology, New York University Medical Center, New York, New York; Attending Physician, New York University Medical Center and Bellevue Hospital, New York, New York

Status Epilepticus

FRANCES FLUG, M.D.

Instructor in Pediatrics, New York University School of Medicine, New York, New York; Attending in Pediatrics, Bellevue Hospital and University Hospital, New York, New York

Inherited Disorders of Hemostasis; Acquired Disorders of Hemostasis

MARY ANNE GAZDICH, M.D.

Instructor of Pediatrics, Hahnemann University, Philadelphia, Pennsylvania; Montgomery Hospital, Sacred Heart Hospital, Norristown, Pennsylvania

Fluids and Electrolytes

ANNE A. GERSHON, M.D.

Professor of Pediatrics, New York University School of Medicine, New York, New York; Attending, New York University Medical Center, New York, New York

Encephalitis

JOAN HOLTER GILDEA, R.N., C.M.A.

Clinical Assistant Director of Nursing, Pediatrics, New York University Medical Center, University Hospital, New York, New York

Cardiopulmonary Resuscitation

HOWARD B. GINSBURG, M.D.

Assistant Professor of Surgery and Director of Pediatric Surgery, New York University School of Medicine, New York, New York; Attending Surgeon, University Hospital and Bellevue Hospital, New York, New York

Pancreatitis

JOHN G. GORMAN, M.D.

Director of Blood Transfusion Service, New York University Hospital, and Professor of Clinical Pathology, New York University School of Medicine, New York, New York

Component Transfusion Therapy

MICHAEL GRAFF, M.D.

Assistant Professor of Pediatrics, New York University Medical School, New York, New York; Assistant Attending, Monmouth Medical Center and Co-director, Nursery, Monmouth Medical Center, Long Branch, New Jersey

Noninvasive Respiratory Monitoring; Bronchopulmonary Dysplasia

JONATHAN GREENBERG, M.D., J.D.

Instructor, Division of Neurosurgery, Department of Surgery, University of Maryland School of Medicine, Baltimore, Maryland; Attending Neurosurgeon, Maryland Institute of Emergency Medical Service Systems and the University of Maryland Hospital, Baltimore, Maryland

Pediatric Spinal Cord Trauma

JAY L. GROSFELD, M.D.

Lafayette F. Page Professor of Surgery, Director, Section of Pediatric Surgery, Interim Chairman, Department of Surgery, Indiana University School of Medicine, Indianapolis, Indiana; Surgeon-in-Chief, J.W. Riley Hospital for Children, Indianapolis, Indiana

Multiple Trauma

RICHARD M. HANSON

Clinical Assistant Instructor, Department of Neurology, State University of New York, Downstate Medical Center, Brooklyn, New York

Guillain-Barré Syndrome

LORRAINE HARTNETT, M.D.

Instructor of Pediatrics, New York University School of Medicine, New York, New York; Attending Physician, Emergency Services, Bellevue and University Hospitals, New York, New York

Poisoning

MARGARET KARPATKIN, M.D.

Professor of Pediatrics, New York University School of Medicine, New York, New York; Attending in Pediatrics, Bellevue Hospital and University Hospital, New York, New York

Inherited Disorders of Hemostasis; Acquired Disorders of Hemostasis

KEITH KRASINSKI, M.D.

Assistant Professor of Pediatrics, New York University School of Medicine, New York, New York and Long Island University, New York, New York; Assistant Attending Physician, New York University Medical Center, Assistant Attending Physician, Bellevue Hospital Center, and Assistant Epidemiologist, Bellevue Hospital Center, New York, New York

Infection Control; Bacterial Meningitis Beyond the Neonatal Period; Sepsis

ALAN G. KULBERG, M.D.

Associate Professor of Clinical Pediatrics, New York University School of Medicine, New York, New York; Director, Pediatric Emergency Service and Assistant Director, Emergency Services, Bellevue Hospital Center, New York, New York

Croup and Epiglottitis; Near-Drowning; Poisoning; Hydrocarbon Intoxication

MICHAEL A. LaCORTE, M.D.

Associate Professor of Clinical Pediatrics, Cornell University Medical College, New York, New York; Chief, Division of Pediatric Cardiology and Senior Assistant Attending, Department of Pediatrics, North Shore University Hospital, Manhasset, New York

Application of Echocardiography in the Pediatric Intensive Care Unit; Postoperative Care After Open-Heart Surgery

PHILIP LA RUSSA, M.D.

Instructor in Pediatrics, New York University Medical Center, New York, New York; Assistant Attending Physician, University Hospital, New York University Medical Center, Clinical Assistant Attending Physician, Bellevue Hospital Center, New York, New York

Bacterial Meningitis Beyond the Neonatal Period; Sepsis

HEDI L. LEISTNER, M.D.

Assistant Professor of Pediatrics, New York University School of Medicine, New York, New York; Assistant Attending Physician, New York University Medical Center and Bellevue Hospital Medical Center, New York, New York

Apnea in Infants and Children

LILY LEW, M.D.

Clinical Instructor in Pediatrics, New York University School of Medicine, New York, New York; Physician-in-Charge of Pediatric Endocrinology, Booth Memorial Medical Center, Flushing, New York

Hyperthyroidism; Adrenal Insufficiency and Steroid Withdrawal

DOUGLAS MacGREGOR, M.D.

Clinical Instructor in Pediatrics, New York University Medical Center, New York, New York

Reye's Syndrome

VIJAYALAXMI MALAVADE, M.B.B.S.

Clinical Associate Professor of Pathology, New York University Medical Center, New York, New York; Director, New York Blood Services and Consultant, Blood Bank and Transfusion Services, New York University Medical Center, New York, New York

Component Transfusion Therapy

DANIEL A. NOTTERMAN, M.D.

Assistant Professor of Pediatrics, New York University School of Medicine, New York, New York; Director, Pediatric Intensive Care Unit, Bellevue Hospital, New York, New York

Noninvasive Respiratory Monitoring; Invasive Hemodynamic Monitoring; Clinical Pharmacology in the Critically Ill Child; Hypertension; Status Asthmaticus

MARK S. PERSKY, M.D.

Associate Professor of Clinical Otolaryngology, New York University School of Medicine, New York, New York; Associate Attending, University Hospital, Attending Physician, Bellevue Hospital, Consulting Attending, Manhattan Veterans Administration Hospital, New York, New York

Airway Management and Post-Intubation Sequelae

MONIKA RUTKOWSKI, M.D.

Assistant Professor of Clinical Pediatrics, New York University School of Medicine, New York, New York; Assistant Attending, Bellevue Hospital and New York University Hospital, New York, New York

Common Complications in Infants with Cyanotic Congenital Heart Disease

CLAUDE SANSARICQ, M.D.

Associate Professor of Pediatrics, New York University Medical School, New York, New York; Attending in Pediatrics, New York University Hospital and Bellevue Hospital, New York, New York

Inborn Errors of Metabolism

ROBERT G. SCHACHT, M.D.

Professor of Pediatrics, New York University Medical School, New York, New York; Associate Director of Pediatrics and Director of Pediatric Nephrology, New York University Medical Center, New York, New York

Acute Peritoneal Dialysis; Acute Renal Failure

CHARLES A. SKLAR, M.D.

Assistant Professor, Department of Pediatrics, New York, University Medical School, New York, New York; Assistant Attending, Bellevue Hospital, Assistant Attending, New York University Medical Center, New York, New York

Syndrome of Inappropriate Secretion of ADH; Diabetes Insipidus

SELMA E. SNYDERMAN, M.D.

Professor of Pediatrics, New York University School of Medicine, New York, New York; Attending Physician, Bellevue Hospital, Attending Pediatrician, University Hospital, Director, Metabolic Disease Center, New York University Medical Center, New York, New York

Enteral Alimentation; Total Parenteral Alimentation

JOHN M. STEIN, M.D., F.A.C.S

Clinical Associate Professor of Surgery, University of Arizona, Phoenix; Director, Burn Unit, Maricopa Medical Center, Phoenix, Arizona

Burns

MICHAEL TRAISTER, M.D.

Assistant Professor of Clinical Pediatrics, New York University School of Medicine, New York, New York; Attending Pediatrician, University Hospital, New York, New York

Diabetic Ketoacidosis

STEVEN J. WASSNER, M.D.

Associate Professor of Pediatrics, The Pennsylvania State University, Hershey, Pennsylvania; Chief, Division of Pediatric Nephrology, The Milton S. Hershey Medical Center, Hershey, Pennsylvania

Hemolytic-Uremic Syndrome

THOMAS R. WEBER, M.D.

Associate Professor of Surgery, St. Louis University School of Medicine, Chief of Pediatric Surgery, Cardinal Glennon Hospital, St. Louis, Missouri

Multiple Trauma

FRANK T. WENG, M.D.

Associate Professor of Pediatrics, University of Pittsburgh School of Medicine, Pittsburgh, Pennsylvania; Co-director, Pulmonary Division, Children's Hospital of Pittsburgh, Pittsburgh, Pennsylvania

Assisted Ventilation

KAREN W. WEST, M.D.

Assistant Professor of Surgery, Indiana University School of Medicine, Indianapolis, Indiana; Assistant Professor, Pediatric Surgery, J.W. Riley Hospital for Children, Indianapolis, Indiana

Multiple Trauma

JEFFREY H. WISOFF, M.D.

Instructor, Division of Pediatric Neurosurgery, New York University Medical School, New York, New York; Assistant Attending, New York University Medical Center and Bellevue Hospital, New York, New York

Management of Pediatric Head Trauma; Postoperative Care Following Intracranial Neurosurgery

SOL S. ZIMMERMAN, M.D.

Associate Professor of Clinical Pediatrics, New York University School of Medicine, New York, New York; Assistant Director of Pediatrics, Director, Pediatric Intensive Care Unit, University Hospital, New York University Medical Center, New York, New York

Cardiopulmonary Resuscitation; Shock; Anaphylaxis; Increased Intracranial Pressure; Adult Respiratory Distress Syndrome; Pulmonary Embolism; Reye's Syndrome; Status Epilepticus; Toxic Shock Syndrome; Kawasaki Syndrome; Carbon Monoxide Poisoning

ELAINE ZOBERMAN, M.D.

Clinical Instructor in Pediatrics, New York University School of Medicine, New York, New York

Adult Respiratory Distress Syndrome

PREFACE

Critical care is the field of medicine devoted to the comprehensive care of seriously ill patients who often have multiorgan system failure. It has received recognition in the past 10 to 15 years, but its origins are rooted well in the past. Contributing to this recognition were the advent of intensive care units designed to unify medical, nursing, and technological resources and the development of instrumentation that improved therapeutic and monitoring modalities. The technological advances have resulted in an array of gauges, digital readouts, oscilloscopes, and alarms, which have come to typify critical care. Yet the heart of the intensive care unit is not its instrumentation but rather its medical and nursing staff.

The intensivist, although referred to as a subspecialist, is really a generalist in the most complete sense. He cannot view the complex, critically ill patient from the single organ system vantage point of the traditional subspecialist. In pediatrics, he does not confine his care to a specific age group but treats all patients from infancy through adolescence. With such a diverse patient population, the pediatric intensivist must be expert not only in acute and emergent care, nutrition, and clinical pharmacology but also in the dynamic effects of growth and development on these areas. The intensivist must be able to coordinate a multidisciplinary approach to therapy while maintaining ultimate responsibility for the treatment plan. He must be able to effectively and empathetically explain the clinical condition and management plan to the patient and parents.

Critical care nurses are the mainstay of the intensive care unit, ever present at the patient's bedside. In addition to delivering skilled nursing care and making frequent clinical assessments, they provide the nurturance and emotional support so desperately needed by the child and the family. Since the majority of illnesses resulting in ICU admissions are of an acute onset, patients and their parents have no preparation for their transition into a crisis setting; they are bewildered, anxious, and frightened. All medical, nursing, therapeutic, and ancillary personnel must be sensitive to these feelings, but because of his or her continuous presence at the bedside, the critical care nurse accepts the major share of the responsibility for helping the patient and parents to cope with their emotional stress.

Nowhere in the hospital is the relationship between physician and nurse more of a dynamic partnership than in the intensive care unit. In formulating a management plan, the physician relies upon the nurse's clinical assessment in addition to his own physical examination of the patient, x-ray findings, and data derived from monitoring equipment and the laboratory. The planned therapeutic regimen is communicated to the nurse, who must have a basic understanding of the patient's illness. For conditions commonly seen in a given ICU, this is accomplished by regularly scheduled conferences planned by the intensivist and the nursing leadership. When unusual conditions or newer therapies are encountered, a timely conference should be arranged to familiarize the entire staff accordingly. All ICU medical and nursing personnel must have an excellent grasp of a disease's underlying pathophysiology so as to recognize even subtle changes that may herald a deterioration in a patient's status. Because the clinical conditions of the patients are inherently unstable, treatment plans must frequently be re-evaluated on bedside rounds. The emotional impact upon patients and parents of any major change in therapy must be discussed by the medical-nursing team. The constant exchange of information that characterizes the interaction between the unit's physicians and nurses includes discussion of the staff's own response to the surrounding circumstances. Emotional stress is not limited to children and their families. Members of the staff must routinely support each other.

Critical Care Pediatrics is intended as a reference text for the physicians and nurses who care for seriously ill children. An initial section concerned with general principles and techniques of critical care is followed by a section devoted to specific clinical problems, organized predominantly according to organ systems. The scope of the text includes conditions affecting the entire age range of pediatrics with the exception of entities occurring uniquely in the newborn period. Neonatology is excluded because of the abundance of texts devoted to this subject matter and because neonatal ICUs generally stand apart from pediatric ICUs. Bronchopulmonary dysplasia is included because the chronic nature and sequelae of this disease affect patients well beyond the newborn period.

Chapters concerned with specific clinical conditions are composed of an introductory reference section that addresses etiology, pathophysiology, and treatment. A brief case history follows and then a pertinent medical problem list for that case is presented, as is the practice in the medical chart. The case report is intended to highlight aspects of the clinical presentation and treatment already discussed in the reference section. With each listed problem there is further discussion of management. Case presentations are not included in the chapters on burns and the postoperative management of cardiovascular and neurosurgical patients because the discussion of these cases becomes very lengthy and detracts from, rather than adds to, the reference section. It should be emphasized that the reference sections are complete and independent. The case report format has always been popular with journal readers and is being used here to reinforce points of diagnosis and therapy.

The chapter concludes with a section entitled "Nursing Process for Patient Care." The nursing process is a thought process basic to all nursing activities that includes the traditional components of assessment, planning, implementation, and evaluation but that requires modification when applied to the critical care setting. Two new components, *monitoring* and *anticipation*, are introduced in this text. Assessment, monitoring, and anticipation become the key components representing the dynamic nature of critical care nursing. Planning, implementation, and evaluation of nursing activities follow. The intent of the nursing section is to identify the parameters requiring assessment and monitoring and the problems to be anticipated based upon the patient's medical diagnosis. This is facilitated by the use of a *mind set* that summarizes the relevant parameters and problems. This format is not meant to be an absolute tool; modifications will be required as the patient's clinical circumstances change.

It is our hope that this book will become a valuable, eminently readable reference for physicians and nurses. The use of a combined medical-nursing vantage point reflects our partnership in the care of seriously ill children.

We would like to express our appreciation to Claire Guglielmo and to Diana Zimmerman for their invaluable help in preparing the manuscript.

S. S. ZIMMERMAN
J. H. GILDEA

CONTENTS

SECTION TWO
SYSTEM-SPECIFIC PROBLEMS

Cardiocirculatory

Respiratory

GENERAL PROBLEMS AND TECHNIQUES OF CRITICAL CARE

Cardiopulmonary Resuscitation

JOAN HOLTER GILDEA, R.N.
SOL S. ZIMMERMAN, M.D.

Cardiopulmonary arrest is defined as the cessation of functional ventilation and circulation. The pathophysiologic dynamics that precede this terminal state may be initial respiratory failure and arrest, with subsequent cardiac decompensation or primary cardiac arrest.

In children, most conditions that lead to an arrest are pulmonary in nature and include aspiration, asthma, bronchiolitis, epiglottitis, pneumonia, near-drowning, and both neonatal and adult respiratory distress syndromes. Status epilepticus and drug ingestions, although not intrinsic respiratory diseases, are included in this group because of their adverse effects on ventilation. The heart is essentially healthy and arrests as the hypoxia and acidosis resulting from respiratory failure affect myocardial performance.

Primary cardiac arrest is uncommon in the pediatric population. When it occurs, it is most often in the child with congenital or acquired heart disease. Dysrhythmias are the usual precipitating factors in this type of arrest. Shock, whether hypovolemic, septic, or cardiogenic, is a significant contributing factor.

With the loss of perfusion resulting from cardiac arrest, the tissue needs for glucose and oxygen cannot be met and metabolism changes from aerobic to anaerobic. Metabolic acidosis is the result of the production of lactic acid secondary to this substrate deprivation. Cell membrane permeability is altered, and the cell loses its functional integrity. Potassium shifts out of the cell while sodium and water enter it. The intracellular water and sodium result in lysosomal enzyme release and subsequent cellular death.

Cardiopulmonary resuscitation (CPR) includes those measures used to restore functional ventilation and circulation and to correct metabolic disturbances. Effective pediatric CPR requires a medical team that is knowledgeable in the physiologic and anatomic differences between children and adults.

BASIC LIFE SUPPORT

Basic life support consists of those measures directed toward establishing and maintaining an airway, controlling breathing, and providing adequate circulation. These measures are known as the "ABCs": airway, breathing, and circulation.

The child in need of resuscitation must be quickly recognized and airway patency and adequacy of ventilation and circulation immediately assessed. The status of the central nervous system is evaluated by stimulating the patient by shaking and shouting; absence of response implies inadequate substrate (oxygen and glucose) delivery to the brain.

Airway

Proper positioning is the key to establishing a patent airway. An infant or a small child may have a compromised airway simply from positional narrowing. Airway obstruction can be relieved by gently tilting the head back and, if necessary, lifting the chin forward with the jaw lift or jaw thrust maneuver. The sniffing position is the one of choice. The head is extended, but less so than in the full adult head tilt maneuver. The trachea of the infant and child lacks the firm cartilaginous support of the adolescent or adult, and marked hyperextension will collapse the trachea. The sniffing position is easily achieved in the child who is in a supine position, because a protuberant occiput places the child in the preferred position if the shoulders are properly supported; a rolled towel under the shoulders will suffice. Without adequate shoulder support, the head flexes and the tongue falls back, obstructing the airway.

Following establishment of the airway, it must be cleared of food, mucus, or other debris. This can be accomplished by suctioning or by finger sweep of the oropharynx.

Breathing

Signs of spontaneous respiration are assessed by auscultating the chest, listening for breath sounds over the mouth and nose, or looking for excursion of the chest wall or abdomen. If there are no signs of breathing, artificial ventilation should be initiated.

Mouth-to-nose-and-mouth or mouth-to-mouth breathing is instituted depending upon the size of the child. Four breaths are delivered in rapid succession while chest wall movement is evaluated to determine the adequacy of ventilation. If the patient is a small child, the breaths should be in the form of gentle puffs from the resuscitator's mouth. Forceful blowing can produce pulmonary barotrauma in the infant or young child and may increase the likelihood of gastric distention and emesis. As soon as available, bag and mask ventilation with supplementary oxygen should be substituted for exhaled air breathing.

Breathing must be performed at a rate and volume compatible with the patient's metabolic needs and lung capacity. The recommended rate for infants is 20 to 24 breaths per minute; for children, 16 to 20 breaths per minute; and for adolescents, 12 to 16 breaths per minute.

Circulation

After the airway has been established and ventilation has been initiated, the adequacy of circulation must be assessed by palpating a major peripheral pulse and examining the color of the extremities. In children and adolescents, palpation of the carotid pulse is readily accomplished. Because infants' necks are short, it is difficult to assess the carotid pulse, and brachial and femoral pulses must be evaluated as an alternative. The precordium is not recommended as an assessment site, because precordial activity may reflect ineffective cardiac impulses and not true contractions.

Cardiac compression is initiated when circulation is absent or cardiac output is ineffective. Precordial chest thumps are not used in the resuscitation of children.

In infants and young children, the heart is located higher in the chest than in adults. The proper point for compression, therefore, is midsternum and is located by drawing an imaginary line between the nipples and noting where it intersects the sternum. Care must be taken to prevent the fingers or hand from straying laterally, because rib fractures or separation of the ribs at their cartilaginous articulations may occur, with the potential for perforation of underlying lung, liver, or spleen. The lower third of the sternum is the point of compression in older children and adolescents but is avoided as the site for compression in small children because of the risk of direct hepatic trauma.

Because infants' chests are small, only two fingers are required for cardiac compression. The chest is compressed to a depth of 0.5 to 1 inch at midsternum by the index and middle fingers. The force of compression is that of forearm pressure only. The patient should be placed on a firm surface to maximize the efficacy of the compressions. An alternative method, especially in the absence of a firm surface, is to encircle the infant's chest with both hands and compress the sternum with the thumbs. The location and depth of compression remain the same. If the child is large enough so that the sternum does not readily compress with three fingers, the heel of one hand should be used. The depth of compression must increase to 1 to 1.5 inches. In older children and adolescents, two hands are used, as in adult external cardiac massage. The depth of compression is 1.5 to 2 inches. The rate of compression in infants is 100 per minute; in children, 80 per minute; and in adolescents, 60 per minute. The duration of the compression should be 50 percent of the cycle length, thereby allowing adequate filling time for the heart.

Breathing and compression must be coordinated to maximize the effect of each without adversely influencing the other. The ratio of compression rate to ventilation rate per minute is 5:1 throughout the pediatric age range; 100:20 in infants, 80:16 in children, and 60:12 in adolescents.

ADVANCED LIFE SUPPORT

Advanced life support consists of basic life support with adjunctive equipment, medications, and special techniques for establishing and maintaining effective ventilation and circulation. The key to advanced life support is an organized team approach, with well-defined roles and responsibilities.

Adjunctive Equipment and Special Techniques

Bag–Valve–Mask Devices

Bag and mask ventilation with 100 percent oxygen should be used as soon as practicable. Masks are available in a range of sizes to fit all infants and children. Proper size masks are necessary to obtain the seal required for effective ventilation. Relatively transparent masks are preferred because they allow visualization of secretions and emesis. An oral airway should be inserted, to maintain airway patency, if necessary. Pediatric resuscitation bags are manufactured both with and without pop-off valves to limit the amount of pressure delivered (30 to 40 cm H_2O); bags without valves should be fitted with manometers. To permit delivery of 100 percent oxygen, the resuscitation bags should have gas reservoirs. Bags without the reservoir modification deliver substantially lower concentrations of oxygen and are therefore of limited usefulness in the arrest situation.

Gastric distention occurs as a consequence of artificial ventilation and, if excessive, can interfere with effective ventilation by elevating the diaphragm, thereby reducing lung volume. Distention can be minimized by releasing pressure on the resuscitation bag at the point at which the chest is first observed to rise. This maneuver will often avoid exceeding the esophageal opening pressure. Gentle pressure applied at the level of the cricoid may be effective in reducing gastric distention during bag and mask ventilation. Direct pressure on the abdomen to relieve distention should be avoided because of the danger of vomiting and aspiration. Passage of a nasogastric tube should be performed as soon as possible.

Endotracheal Intubation

Endotracheal intubation should be performed as soon as possible. The presence of an endotracheal tube secures an airway, thereby enhancing the effectiveness of ventilation. In addition, it bypasses any upper airway obstruction, facilitates suctioning of pulmonary secretions, and permits the application of end expiratory pressure.

Knowledge of the airway anatomy of infants and children is essential for endotracheal intubation. Compared with adults, the larynx in infants and children is situated more anteriorly and cephalad; it is funnel shaped rather than cylindrical. The epiglottis is short and U shaped, and the angle formed with the vocal cords is more acute than that in adults. The narrowest portion of the trachea is the subglottic area at the level of the cricoid ring. The soft, vascular gums are easily traumatized by compression, and deciduous teeth, if present, are easily dislodged. Skill commensurate with this knowledge is necessary for successful pediatric intubation.

Intubation also requires familiarity with the necessary equipment. Straight laryngoscope blades are used in infants and children younger than 5 years of age because in this age range, the larynx is situated anteriorly. Physicians prefer to use curved blades in older children. Endotracheal tube and blade sizes are age related (see Chapter 2, Airway Management and Post–Intubation Sequelae). In an acute situation, the size of the tube required is usually estimated using one of the two following methods. The first method recognizes that the diameter of the trachea is approximately equal to the width of the child's fifth finger. The second method involves a simple formula in which the internal diameter (in mm) of the endotracheal tube is determined by adding 16 to the child's age in years and then dividing by

4. Because both methods only approximate the required tube size, tubes one size larger and one size smaller should be prepared and available. Uncuffed tubes are used in young children, but the funnel shape of the larynx permits the use of positive pressure ventilation.

The child is placed in the sniffing position, the cords are visualized, and the tube is inserted. CPR is briefly interrupted for intubation. After the tube has been inserted, proper placement should be checked for immediately, by observing the movement of the chest wall and auscultating for the presence of equal breath sounds throughout both lung fields. Confirmation of tube placement should be obtained by chest x-rays. The tip of the tube should be midway between the level of the clavicles and the carina.

Intravenous Access

Establishing intravenous access is crucial to the resuscitative effort; however, it is frequently difficult and time consuming. Sites that permit placement of central venous catheters are preferable. Two commonly used vessels that can easily be cannulated percutaneously are the external jugular vein and the femoral vein. The femoral vein has the advantage of being out of the direct field of compression and ventilation. The subclavian vein is generally not used because catheter placement does interrupt ongoing CPR and because there is a significant incidence of associated pneumothorax and hemothorax. If a cutdown is necessary, the commonly used vessels are the cephalic or basilic vein in the antecubital fossa and the saphenous vein at the ankle. Intracardiac drug administration should be avoided unless alternate routes are unavailable and cannot be established in an appropriate period of time.

Drugs

Familiarity with commonly used drugs is essential to the appropriate pharmacologic management of a resuscitation. In our Intensive Care Unit, we utilize an Emergency Drug Sheet (Table 1–1), which is filled out upon the patient's admission to the unit. In this way, the high-risk status of these patients is recognized; the preparation and administration of medications during an arrest is facilitated.

Sodium Bicarbonate. Cardiopulmonary arrest results in a mixed respiratory and metabolic acidosis, the respiratory component being the consequence of hypoventilation and CO_2 re-

tention, and the metabolic component originating from inadequate tissue perfusion, with subsequent accumulation of lactic acid. Severe acidosis can depress myocardial contractility and predispose to dysrhythmias. In addition, catecholamines such as epinephrine are less effective in the presence of a low pH.

Respiratory acidosis should be managed by securing the airway and establishing effective ventilation. Successful ventilatory therapy reduces the arterial CO_2 tension, not only correcting the respiratory component of the acidosis but also sometimes compensating, in part, for the metabolic component.

Metabolic acidosis is treated by the administration of sodium bicarbonate. The bicarbonate ion combines with the hydrogen ion to ultimately form carbon dioxide and water. Because carbon dioxide is a product of this acid–base reaction, the use of sodium bicarbonate is predicated on first having provided adequate ventilation. Dosage is determined by measurement of arterial pH; however, during a cardiopulmonary arrest, therapy should not be withheld while awaiting blood gas results. Bicarbonate is given in an initial dose of 1 mEq per kg intravenously. In children younger than 6 months of age, the dose remains the same but the standard concentration of 1 mEq per ml should be diluted 1:1 to minimize the osmotic effects. Subsequent doses should be based upon measurements of base deficit as calculated from the following equation:

$$HCO_3 \text{ (mEq)} = \frac{\text{Base deficit} \times \text{weight (kg)} \times 0.3^*}{2}$$

The product is divided by 2 so that the acidosis is not overcorrected. Excessive administration of sodium bicarbonate should be avoided because of the potential for hypernatremia, hyperosmolarity, and metabolic alkalosis. Additional adverse effects of bicarbonate infusion include inactivation of catecholamines and precipitation of calcium if these agents are given in the same line as the bicarbonate.

Epinephrine. Epinephrine, a catecholamine with both alpha and beta adrenergic activity, remains the primary cardiotonic drug used during CPR. Alpha adrenergic stimulation produces vasoconstriction, with subsequent elevations in systolic and diastolic blood pressure. Beta adrenergic action increases heart rate

---

* 0.3 represents the fraction of body weight in which bicarbonate is distributed.

(chronotropy), improves cardiac contractility (inotropy), and dilates the coronary vessels. Epinephrine is effective in converting fine ventricular fibrillation to the coarse variety, a rhythm that is more susceptible to electrical cardioversion.

Epinephrine, in a concentration of 1:10,000, is infused intravenously in a dose of 0.1 ml per kg. The duration of action is short, and doses may have to be repeated at 5-minute intervals. Continuous drip infusion (see Table 1–1) may be required, with the dose titrated to the patient's response. If intravenous access has not been established, epinephrine, in the same dose as the intravenous bolus, can be instilled directly into the trachea, followed by several positive pressure ventilations to ensure passage into the periphery. The epinephrine will be absorbed at the alveolar–capillary interface. The intracardiac route of administration should be avoided, because it is not more efficacious and is associated with significant morbidity in the forms of hemopericardium, cardiac tamponade, myocardial damage, coronary artery laceration, and pneumothorax.

Atropine. Atropine is a parasympatholytic agent with vagolytic action and resultant increase in discharge from the sinoatrial node and increase in conduction through the atrioventricular node. Atropine is indicated for treatment of bradycardia associated with hypotension, ventricular ectopy, and signs of myocardial ischemia. It may be beneficial in the temporary management of second- and third-degree heart block and slow idioventricular rates. Atropine can precipitate atrial and ventricular tachydysrhythmias and, in low dose, can cause bradycardia. This paradoxical effect is the result of atropine's central action. The dose is 0.01 mg per kg administered intravenously (IV) with a minimum dose of 0.1 mg and a maximum dose of 2.0 mg. Establishment of a minimum dose is designed to avoid the paradoxical central effect. In the absence of secure intravenous access, atropine can be given intratracheally.

Calcium. Calcium increases myocardial contractility, ventricular excitability, and ventricular conduction velocity. It is indicated in the treatment of electromechanical dissociation and ventricular asystole and in circumstances in which additional inotropic action is required. Sinus bradycardia and sustained ventricular contraction with standstill may result from too rapid infusion of calcium. In addition, calcium must be used cautiously in digitalized patients, because it increases the possibility of dysrhythmias. Calcium can be administered in the form of either chloride or gluconate, chloride being the more immediately bioavailable. The dose of calcium chloride is 20 mg per kg, IV; that of calcium gluconate is 30 mg per kg.

Lidocaine. Lidocaine decreases the automaticity of ventricular pacemakers and increases the threshold for fibrillation. It is indicated for the treatment of ventricular ectopy, tachycardia, and fibrillation. The initial dose is 1 mg per kg, IV. Because of its brief duration of action, the initial bolus should be followed by a continuous infusion of 20 to 50 mcg per kg per minute. If intravenous access is unavailable, lidocaine can be administered intratracheally. Lidocaine is metabolized by the liver; consequently, dosage should be modified when there is hepatic dysfunction.

Bretylium. Bretylium has been effective in the management of ventricular tachycardia and fibrillation refractory to other modalities of treatment. Bretylium's mode of action has not been fully established but may be related to sympathetic blockade. The initial dose of bretylium is 5 mg per kg, IV. Subsequent doses can be increased by 5 mg per kg and administered at 15- to 20-minute intervals; the maximum total dose is 30 mg per kg. The most common adverse effect is hypotension.

Naloxone. Naloxone is a competitive narcotic antagonist used to reverse respiratory depression owing to opiate intoxication. It has a rapid onset of action but its effects are transient. A dose of 0.01 mg per kg, IV, is administered, with repeat doses as often as every 3 to 5 minutes if there is a clinical response. Because of the broad dose–response curve, the dose of naloxone may have to be increased up to 0.1 mg per kg. Naloxone itself has no respiratory depressant properties.

Dopamine. Dopamine, a precursor of epinephrine, has dose-dependent alpha- and beta-adrenergic and dopaminergic (delta) activity. When administered in low doses (2 to 6 mcg per kg per minute), the primary action is dopaminergic, with dilatation of renal, splanchnic, coronary, and cerebral vasculature. At moderate doses (7 to 15 mcg per kg per minute), the principal action is beta-adrenergic, with increased myocardial contractility and heart rate; the result is an increase in cardiac output. At high doses (more than 15 mcg per kg per minute), dopamine is an alpha-adrenergic agent, producing a marked increase in peripheral vascular resistance and a decrease in renal blood flow.

Dopamine is indicated in the management of hypotension and decreased renal perfusion when the adequacy of circulating volume has

Table 1–1. Emergency Drugs and Infusions—Pediatric Intensive Care Unit, New York University Medical Center

Name: _____

Weight: _____ (In kilograms 2.2 lb/kg)

Date: _____ Update: _____

Age: _____

ET size: [ ]

Pt. Dose

ml _____ mg

Drug and How Supplied	Dose (mg/kg) × wt (kg)
Atropine 0.4 mg/ml	0.01 mg/kg ×
Na HCO$_3$ 1 mEq/ml	1 mEq/kg ×
CaCl 1 gm/10 ml	20 mg/kg ×
CaGluconate 1 gm/10 ml	30 mg/kg ×
Lidocaine 100 mg/5 ml	1 mg/kg ×
Narcan 0.4 mg/ml	0.01–0.02 mg/kg ×
Epinephrine 1:10,000	<6 mos, 0.5 ml; >6 mos, 1 ml
(Intracardiac)	
Hydralazine 20 mg/ml	0.2–0.5 mg/kg ×
Diazoxide 15 mg/ml	5 mg/kg ×

Defibrillation

2 watt-sec/kg

<2 years 50 watt-sec

2–10 yr 100 watt-sec

>10 yr 200–250 watt-sec

Drip Preparations

Dopamine (200 mg/5 ml) expires 24 hr

*2–15 mcg/kg/min

≤10 kg	>10 kg
50 mg (= 1.25 ml)/250 ml D5W	200 mg/250 ml D5W
200 mcg/min = 60 ml/hr	800 mcg/min = 60 ml/hr
100 mcg/min = 30 ml/hr	400 mcg/min = 30 ml/hr
50 mcg/min = 15 ml/hr	200 mcg/min = 15 ml/hr
25 mcg/min = 7–8 ml/hr	100 mcg/min = 7–8 ml/hr
10 mcg/min = 3 ml/hr	50 mcg/min = 3–4 ml/hr

Begin with rate of _____ ml hr = _____ mcg/kg/min

Dobutamine (250 mg/10 ml) expires 24 hr

*2–15 mcg/kg/min

≤10 kg	>10 kg
50 mg (=2 ml)/250 ml D5W	250 mg/250 ml D5W
200 mcg/min = 60 ml/hr	1000 mcg/min = 60 ml/hr
100 mcg/min = 30 ml/hr	500 mcg/min = 30 ml/hr
50 mcg/min = 15 ml/hr	250 mcg/min = 15 ml/hr
25 mcg/min = 7–8 ml/hr	125 mcg/min = 7–8 ml/hr
10 mcg/min = 3 ml/hr	62.5 mcg/min = 3–4 ml/hr

Begin with rate of _____ ml/hr = _____ mcg/kg/min

Isuprel (expires 8 hr)
2.0 mg/250 ml D5W
*0.1–0.5 mcg/kg/min

8 mcg/min	= 60 ml/hr
4 mcg/min	= 30 ml/hr
2 mcg/min	= 15 ml/hr
1 mcg/min	= 7–8 ml/hr
0.5 mcg/min	= 3–4 ml/hr

Begin with rate of _____ ml/hr = _____ mcg/kg/min

Epinephrine (expires 8 hr)
2.0 mg/250 ml
*0.1 mcg/kg/min (titrate)

8 mcg/min	= 60 ml/hr
4 mcg/min	= 30 ml/hr
2 mcg/min	= 15 ml/hr
1 mcg/min	= 7–8 ml/hr
0.5 mcg/min	= 3–4 ml/hr

Begin with rate of _____ ml/hr = _____ mcg/kg/min

Lidocaine (expires 24 hr)
*20–50 mcg/kg/min

≤ 10 kg		> 10 kg	
1000 mg/500 ml D5W		1000 mg/250 ml D5W	
1000 mcg/min = 30 ml/hr		4 mg/min = 60 ml/hr	
500 mcg/min = 15 ml/hr		2 mg/min = 30 ml/hr	
250 mcg/min = 7–8 ml/hr		1 mg/min = 15 ml/hr	
100 mcg/min = 3–4 ml/hr		0.5 mg/min = 7–8 ml/hr	

Begin with rate of _____ ml/hr = _____ mcg/kg/min

Nitroprusside (expires 24 hr)
*0.5–10 mcg/kg/min

≤10 kg		> 10 kg	
25 mg/250 D5W		50 mg/250 ml D5W	
100 mcg/min = 60 ml/hr		200 mcg/min = 60 ml/hr	
50 mcg/min = 30 ml/hr		100 mcg/min = 30 ml/hr	
25 mcg/min = 15 ml/hr		50 mcg/min = 15 ml/hr	
15 mcg/min = 9 ml/hr		30 mcg/min = 9 ml/hr	
10 mcg/min = 6 ml/hr		20 mcg/min = 6 ml/hr	
5 mcg/min = 3 ml/hr		10 mcg/min = 3 ml/hr	
		5 mcg/min = 1–2 ml/hr	

Begin with rate of _____ ml/hr = _____ mcg/kg/min

*Recommended dose range

been ensured. In addition, it is helpful in improving renal blood flow in patients with congestive heart failure. Adverse effects include tachydysrhythmias, nausea, and vomiting.

Dobutamine. Dobutamine, a synthetic catecholamine, is a selective beta-1 adrenergic agent. It has minimal alpha- and beta-2 adrenergic effects and no dopaminergic activity. Myocardial contractility is increased with minimal tachycardia and peripheral vasoconstriction. Dobutamine is indicated in the management of shock secondary to depressed myocardial contractility. Its use is contraindicated when there is idiopathic hypertrophic subaortic stenosis (IHSS) because of the potential for increasing obstruction. Dobutamine is administered as a continuous infusion, with a dose range of 2 to 20 mcg per kg per minute. Adverse effects include dysrhythmias (premature ventricular contractions), hypertension, headache, nausea, and vomiting.

Isoproterenol. Isoproterenol is a synthetic catecholamine, with almost exclusive beta-adrenergic activity. It increases heart rate, myocardial contractility, and venous return to the heart and causes peripheral vasodilatation. When there is a normal circulating volume, the net effect is to increase blood pressure because the potent inotropic action compensates for the decrease in vascular resistance. Isoproterenol is an adjunct to the treatment of depressed myocardial contractility with digoxin, dopamine, and dobutamine. It is indicated for bradycardia refractory to atropine. It is infused as a continuous drip, with an initial dose of 0.1 mcg per kg per minute. Tachycardia and tachydysrhythmias are common adverse effects. When hypovolemia is evident, the administration of isoproterenol may result in hypotension.

Norepinephrine (Levophed). Norepinephrine, as a potent alpha-adrenergic agonist, produces marked peripheral vasoconstriction, thereby increasing blood pressure. Renal, splanchnic, cerebral, and skeletal muscle blood flow are decreased. Coronary blood flow is enhanced by direct coronary artery vasodilatation and as a consequence of the increased blood pressure. Norepinephrine is infused in a dose of 0.1 mcg per kg per minute and titrated to clinical response. Its potential for impairing organ perfusion has led to a decrease in its use, especially since the discovery of dopamine.

Defibrillation

Ventricular fibrillation is relatively uncommon in the pediatric population. Care must be taken to appropriately identify the rhythm before considering electrical defibrillation. Defibrillation depolarizes a mass of myocardial cells, following which there may be return of a normal sinus rhythm. Acidosis and hypoxia should be corrected to maximize the potential for electrical conversion of the rhythm. Coarse fibrillation is more readily converted than fine fibrillation; epinephrine or calcium can be administered to "coarsen" the rhythm.

Appropriate-sized pediatric electrodes should be selected, with one placed to the right of the sternum below the clavicle and the other placed at the level of the xiphoid in the left mid-clavicular line. The initial dose for defibrillation is 2 watt-seconds per kg. If the first attempt to defibrillate is unsuccessful, the energy dose should be doubled. Failure to defibrillate may be due to bridging of the electrical current across the skin secondary to the large size of the paddles used or to contiguous contact of conductive paste between the paddles. Placement of one of the electrodes over the sternum may result in an unsuccessful attempt to depolarize, because the impedance of bone reduces the dose of energy delivered to the myocardium.

MANAGEMENT OF RESUSCITATION

A successful resuscitation is dependent upon a well-organized approach by a team skilled in all aspects of CPR. Proficiency should be maintained by regularly involving physicians and nurses in a training program that includes both didactic sessions and mock arrest drills. All nurses should be familiar with the nature and location of the drugs and equipment on the mobile emergency cart. This cart should be checked every shift to ensure that it is properly stocked and that all equipment is functional.

The resuscitation team is composed of physicians, nurses, and respiratory therapists. The roles of the team members should be well delineated, although there may be some overlap of responsibilities, depending upon the number of personnel available. Ideally, the team consists of eight members: three physicians, four nurses, and a respiratory therapist. The nurse who initially identifies the arrest victim and the first responding physician perform basic CPR, ensuring ventilation and circulation. The second physician gains intravenous access and obtains arterial blood gases while the third physician interprets the EKG, laboratory data, and clinical response and supervises pharmacologic management. Specific assignments may be rearranged depending upon seniority and expertise of the physicians. While one nurse performs CPR, another nurse is responsible for providing necessary equipment (cutdown trays, thoracentesis trays, chest tubes, and infusion pumps) and drawing up bolus medications. A third nurse prepares medication drips and assists with equipment, while a fourth nurse has a supervisory role, coordinating the activities of the other nurses and recording vital signs, medication, and laboratory data on a flow sheet. The respiratory therapist assists with ventilatory support and sets up the mechanical ventilator.

Resuscitations should be reviewed routinely to assess the sequence of events and the adequacy of the response.

PROLONGED LIFE SUPPORT

Following CPR, attention is directed toward restoration of organ system function, with particular attention to the central nervous system. The goal of therapy during this phase is to maximize cerebral recovery.

Hypotension should be aggressively treated by volume expansion and administration of vasopressors with the goal of therapy being maintenance of a mean arterial pressure of 80 mm Hg or greater. A brief period of mild hypertension has been advocated as a means of producing a cerebral "reflow" phenomenon.

Efforts should be made to reduce intracranial hypertension (see Chapter 12, Increased Intracranial Pressure). If the neurologic state dictates, an intracranial pressure monitoring device should be placed to guide treatment. Therapeutic modalities include hyperventilation, fluid restriction, administration of osmotic and loop diuretics, hypothermia, and barbiturate loading. Although their efficacy in the post-arrest circumstance has not been estab-

lished, corticosteroids may have a beneficial effect upon cerebral edema by stabilizing membranes, and there are relatively few adverse effects with short-term therapy. The head should be elevated 30 degrees to facilitate cerebral venous drainage. Sedation and analgesia may be required prior to tracheal suctioning and chest physiotherapy because these procedures may increase intracranial pressure.

Adequate substrate for cerebral metabolism in the forms of oxygen and glucose must be ensured. Metabolic homeostasis should be reestablished and pH should be maintained within the normal range. Fever should be treated aggressively with cooling blankets and antipyretics in order to minimize cerebral metabolic demand. Anticonvulsants may be required to manage seizures that may arise as a consequence of a hypoxic–ischemic encephalopathy (see Chapter 45, Hypoxic–Ischemic Encephalopathy).

SUGGESTED READING

American Heart Association: Standards for CPR and ECC. JAMA 244 (Suppl):453, 1980.

Auerbach, P.S., and Budassi, S.A.: Cardiac Arrest and CPR: Assessment, Planning, and Intervention. Rockville, Md., Aspen Publications, 1983.

Chameides, L., Melker, R., Raye, J., et al.: Resuscitation of infants and children. *In* Textbook of Advanced Cardiac Life Support. Dallas, Texas, American Heart Association, 1981, pp. XVII–1.

Debard, M.L.: Cardiopulmonary resuscitation: analysis of six years experience and review of the literature. Ann. Emerg. Med. 10: 408, 1981.

Ehrlich, R., Emmitt, S.M., and Rodriguez-Torres, R.: Pediatric cardiac resuscitation team; a six year study. J. Pediatr. 84:152, 1974.

Hodglien, J.E., Foster, G.L., and Nicolay L.I.: Cardiopulmonary resuscitation: development of an organized protocol. Crit. Care Med. 5: 93, 1977.

Orlowski, J.P.: Pediatric cardiopulmonary resuscitation. Emerg. Med. Clin. North Am. 1: 3, 1983.

2

Airway Management and Post-Intubation Sequelae

MARK S. PERSKY, M.D.

Successful management of critically ill pediatric patients in need of ventilatory support requires a fundamental knowledge of proper airway management. This aspect of the patient's care often varies among medical centers, depending upon such factors as the size of the unit, the availability of modern equipment, the level of nursing skill, and whether or not there are physicians with expertise and experience in handling upper airway problems. A logical, well-formulated approach to airway management results from the collaboration of pediatricians with otolaryngologists, anesthesiologists, pediatric general surgeons, cardiothoracic surgeons, respiratory therapists, and physical therapists. A team approach is designed to provide optimal treatment.

It is hoped that knowledge of the various well-established methods of securing control of the airway will result in a decreased incidence of complications for the intubated or tracheotomized child. With the improved rates of survival that have resulted from advances in critical care, physicians are now faced with an increasing number of post-intubation sequelae. Factors that contribute to these complications can often be predicted or avoided during the acute stage of management.

MANAGEMENT OF THE INTUBATED PATIENT

After the decision has been made that intubation is necessary for the respiratory maintenance of a patient, certain steps should be taken to ensure proper tube placement. If the situation is not an acute emergency, time should be taken to engage a physician who has experience in intubating pediatric patients. This physician should be readily available either to perform or to closely supervise the passage of

the endotracheal tube. Appropriate laryngoscopes with well-functioning light sources and a variety of tubes and stylettes should be available. Adequate suctioning apparatus, with aspirating catheters of various sizes, must be at the bedside. A smooth intubation cannot proceed unless knowledgeable personnel and proper equipment are readily accessible.

The patient must be adequately ventilated prior to intubation to allow for the transition time until the tube is properly placed. Correct positioning of the patient greatly facilitates the procedure. Neonates and infants should have a pillow or several folded sheets placed beneath their shoulders to allow for maximum extension of the head and neck. Older children and adolescents may be positioned supine in bed, with the head elevated and extended. An assistant should be ready to apply gentle pressure to the thyroid cartilage, a maneuver that often increases laryngeal exposure for the intubation.

The pharynx is thoroughly suctioned free of secretion or vomitus. If a nasogastric tube has previously been inserted, the stomach should be evacuated. The laryngoscope is inserted smoothly to avoid trauma to the teeth (if present), with the tip usually placed within the vallecula at the base of the tongue. If a straight blade is used, the tip is positioned along the laryngeal surface of the epiglottis. The entire tongue is then lifted anteriorly, avoiding a rotating motion of the laryngoscope. A tube of the appropriate size is then placed gently between the vocal cords and secured to the face with tape. The patient's breath sounds should be checked bilaterally, and an immediate chest x-ray should be obtained to confirm that the tip of the tube is above the carina. The head should be immobilized to prevent undue motion of the endotracheal tube within the airway. The arms of the respirator should also be positioned to avoid tension on the tubing that connects the machine to the endotracheal tube. Sedation may be necessary to prevent the patient from "fighting against" the respirator, and arm restraints may be necessary to avoid self-extubation.

Much has been written about the advantages and disadvantages of nasotracheal and orotracheal intubation. Although orotracheal intubation is faster and requires less technical skill than nasotracheal intubation, the nasotracheal method has certain distinct advantages and is the preferred route of intubation. With nasotracheal intubation, the tube is stented into a secure position in relation to the larynx and trachea, thereby avoiding unnecessary motion and trauma to these structures. Also, accidental extubation by head motion seems to occur less often with this method. Biting of the tube is avoided, and the possibility of "kinking," which would adversely affect ventilatory flow, is reduced. Nasotracheal intubation seems to be better tolerated, with less discomfort than orotracheal intubation, lessening the need for sedation.

The type of endotracheal tube used is important in minimizing intubation sequelae. Many materials have been used in the production of these tubes, with the knowledge that any foreign body in the upper airway will cause trauma that may progress to more severe forms of tracheal and laryngeal complications. In the past, red rubber tubes were poorly tolerated. At present, tubes made of polyvinyl chloride seem to cause the least amount of mucosal change within the upper airway. In addition, with proper nursing care, there is minimal adherence of tracheobronchial secretions to the intraluminal portion of the endotracheal tube.

Proper tube size is an important factor in avoiding unnecessary complications. One should be familiar with tubes that are of the appropriate size for the age of the patient undergoing intubation. The age of the patient is more of a determinant of tube size than his height or weight; the laryngeal and tracheal cross sectional area is relatively constant with age. A cuffless tube should be used when the airway is small enough to allow adequate tidal volume without undue leakage from around the tube. If a cuffed tube is required, the high-volume, low-pressure type is used. The recommended sizes of tubes are listed in Table 2–1. The correct size should be determined at the time of intubation. If there is resistance when inserting the tube at the level of the subglottic larynx, the next smaller size tube should be used. When there is but a minimal leak from around the tube during peak inspi-

Table 2–1. Recommended Sizes of Endotracheal Tubes

Age	Tube Size (ID mm)
Premature	2.5–3.0
0–6 months	3.5
7–11 months	4.0
1–2 years	4.0–4.5
3–4 years	5.0–5.5
5–8 years	5.5–6.0

ratory pressure, one can assume that the tube is of the proper size. One must keep in mind that the tube used in intubating a patient with croup may be 0.5 to 1.0 mm smaller than those listed in Table 2–1. The circumferential subglottic swelling in these patients predisposes them to the development of subglottic stenosis if placement of too large a tube results in significant mucosal injury.

Proper nursing care of the intubated patient is also necessary to prevent complications. Because the normal humidifying function of the upper airway is bypassed by an artificial tube, the inspired gases must be adequately humidified and heated. Frequent instillation of normal saline down the endotracheal tube, followed by atraumatic suctioning, will help prevent mucous plugging and clear the tracheobronchial airway. The cough reflex is attenuated in these patients, and secretions must be eliminated.

METHODS OF EXTUBATION

When assisted ventilation is no longer required, one must prepare for an uncomplicated extubation, which requires several steps. The patient should have tolerated at least 24 hours of unassisted ventilation prior to extubation, with stabilization of arterial blood gases on an FIO_2 of no more than 0.35 to 0.40. When this has been accomplished, extubation may be considered appropriate. Eight hours prior to the proposed extubation, intravenous steroid therapy should be instituted in an attempt to reduce laryngotracheal edema, which is always associated with intubation. Steroids should be continued for 24 hours after extubation. Just prior to the removal of the tube, the nasal cavity, oral cavity, pharynx, and endotracheal tube must thoroughly be suctioned free of secretions. An Ambu bag, with an oxygen concentration of 40 to 50 percent, should assist ventilation for 1 to 2 minutes prior to extubation. The patient's head should then be immobilized while the tube is gently withdrawn. At this time, one must be prepared to reintubate if respiratory distress in the form of persistent stridor ensues after removal of the tube. Occasionally, there is an element of laryngospasm, which should improve after 1 to 2 minutes, especially if the patient is immediately placed in a mist tent or hood that contains racemic epinephrine (0.5 ml in 2.5 ml sterile water and delivered via a nebulizer) and an oxygen concentration of 35 to 40 percent. If the clinical status deteriorates, reintubation should be initiated and extubation should be attempted again in 24 to 48 hours. If there is repeated failure at this time, a tracheostomy should be performed electively, with the patient stabilized and an endotracheal tube in place. Subsequent laryngoscopy and tracheoscopy can be carried out to evaluate the integrity of the upper respiratory tract.

COMPLICATIONS OF ENDOTRACHEAL INTUBATION

The immediate and delayed complications of endotracheal intubation are listed in Table 2–2. An understanding of the following factors, which lead to the development of these complications, enables the physician to identify those patients at risk:

Traumatic intubation
Large endotracheal tube
Duration of intubation
Improper care of intubated patient
Infection
Underlying systemic disease

A traumatic intubation, placement of too large an endotracheal tube, and prolonged duration of intubation predispose the patient to physical trauma of the fragile mucosa. A minor amount of mucosal and submucosal edema is always encountered in the intubated patient but is easily reversible and does not progress to more severe complications. Severe edema and laceration of the mucosa may be followed by local infection leading to vocal cord scarring, webs, or granuloma formation. If perichondritis ensues, the underlying cartilage is prone to exposure, infection, and necrosis, with resulting cicatrix formation and stenosis. The subglottic area is especially prone to this problem, because it is the only site that has a circumferential rigid structure, the cricoid cartilage. Such a process, however, may occur at any point along the upper respiratory tract that the tube traverses (e.g., vocal cords and trachea). If there is documented evidence of infection of the affected area, cultures should be obtained from the infected site and appropriate antibiotic therapy should be initiated. Edema without infection may be managed by steroids (if not otherwise medically contraindicated) to prevent progression of the inflammatory response and resulting scar formation.

Improper care of the intubated patient may also result in complications. Inadequate immobilization of the patient and the tube will result in undue motion and abrasion of mucosa, with resulting consequences. Traumatic suctioning techniques may cause tracheal injury and bleeding. Infrequent suctioning, especially if associated with nonhumidified inspired gases, allows crusting and fissuring of the tracheobronchial tree, with impairment of ciliary function and predisposition to infection. All these complications can be avoided if there is a properly trained staff on hand, following a well-formulated protocol for care of intubated patients.

The severely debilitated patient may be pre-

Table 2–2. Endotracheal Tube Complications

Immediate
Lacerations and abrasions of the pharynx, larynx, and trachea
Introduction of contaminated secretions into the tracheobronchial tree
Bleeding and crusting with improper tube care
Laryngeal edema
Post-extubation dysphagia and aspiration
Tracheoesophageal perforations
Tension pneumothorax
Inadvertent self-extubation
Delayed
Vocal cord granulomas and scarring
Arytenoid ulcerations, chondritis, and fixation
Laryngeal webs
Laryngeal chondritis → stenosis
Tracheal malacia → stenosis

Modified from Freeman, G.R.: A comparative analysis of endotracheal intubation in neonates, children, and adults: complications, prevention, and treatment. Laryngoscope 82:1385, 1972.

disposed to complications of endotracheal intubation, because hypoxia, radiation therapy, poor tissue perfusion, and neutropenia encourage the development of secondary bacterial infections that affect the respiratory tract mucosa. Aggressive treatment of the underlying problem indirectly improves the prognosis for an uncomplicated extubation.

TRACHEOSTOMY

Indications and Techniques

Although much has been written about the indications for a tracheostomy, considerable controversy on this subject still exists. Often, the medical setting of the intensive care unit plays a role in the decision-making process. A tracheostomy is performed more readily when nursing care is less than optimal and when a physician well trained in pediatric intubation is not immediately available. In these circumstances, the accidental extubation of a patient may carry a grave prognosis. In such a setting, a secure airway is more easily accomplished with a tracheostomy. The nursing management of a tracheostomy tube is somewhat easier because of its shorter length and larger lumen compared with the endotracheal tube.

Few physicians argue about the need for an immediate tracheostomy in acute traumatic laryngotracheal damage. The upper airway can be effectively bypassed while ventilation is maintained. The damaged area may then be adequately evaluated by radiographic and endoscopic means without the interference of an endotracheal tube. Surgery, if indicated, may then proceed, with exposure of the airway and repair with insertion of stents, if necessary. If congenital upper airway obstruction cannot immediately be eliminated by endoscopic techniques, a tracheostomy is necessary. Congential webs and stenoses may be immediately resolved by dilatation or laser surgery, but if these pathologic entities are not managed quickly and effectively, the airway must be maintained with a tracheostomy tube. For chronic laryngotracheal problems (e.g., thick stenoses, papillomatosis, severe malacia, iatrogenic scarring, vascular rings, and tumors), long-term respiratory control must also be considered. Such problems are best managed with a tracheostomy.

Anticipation of prolonged endotracheal intubation is a relative indication for tracheostomy. Some reports reveal no increase in morbidity with long-term intubation, but most authors agree that there is a variable time period during which conversion from endotracheal intubation to a tracheostomy is warranted. Even under the best of circumstances, the rate of complications secondary to intubation increases after 10 to 14 days. If respiratory support is foreseen beyond that time, serious consideration must be given to performing a tracheostomy.

Epiglottitis and croup are two conditions about which there is controversy concerning the better mode of establishing an airway. Endotracheal intubation is preferred with epiglottitis, because the supraglottic edema usually subsides within 48 to 72 hours, followed by uneventful extubation. Even if accidental extubation occurs, there is usually a grace period of at least 15 to 20 minutes, at which time the tube can be reinserted. In the case of croup, there is usually an element of subglottic circumferential edema, which an endotracheal tube may predispose toward the development of stenosis, especially in infants. Tracheostomy, if properly performed, prevents trauma to this area and thereby allows for a safe means of respiratory assistance.

Surgical technique in performing a tracheostomy may vary. Unless there is an impending respiratory arrest with unsuccessful attempts at intubation, a tracheostomy should proceed with the security of an endotracheal tube or ventilating bronchoscope in position during the procedure. This ensures adequate respiratory support while the surgery is performed in an orderly manner. The endotracheal tube also provides a certain amount of rigidity to the laryngotracheal complex, which aids in the identification of landmarks and avoids damage to surrounding structures during exposure of the upper trachea. The patient should be positioned with his head midline and slightly extended. Infants and young children, who have more tracheal rings normally positioned above the suprasternal notch than adults, do not require extreme extension for adequate exposure.

Transecting the thyroid isthmus is performed easily and increases tracheal exposure. The site of entrance into the trachea should be at some point between the second and fifth tracheal rings. Damage of the cricoid cartilage or first tracheal ring will predispose to the development of subglottic complications secondary to chondritis of this area. A vertical incision is made at the tracheal midline through two or three rings after prior placement of paramedian traction sutures on each side of the proposed tracheal incision. Portions of tracheal cartilage are not removed, because this might result in future stenosis. A tube of proper size (Table 2–3) is inserted after the endotracheal tube has been carefully withdrawn. The wound is then lightly packed with gauze, which prevents subcutaneous emphysema from air leakage around the tracheal opening into the deep tissues of the neck. This packing can be removed in 48 hours.

A chest x-ray should be obtained immediately to confirm proper placement of the tracheostomy tube with the tip positioned above the carina. The results of this chest film will also help evaluate the possibility of a pneumomediastinum or pneumothorax, which can occur as a complication of the surgery.

The traction sutures extend outside the neck wound and are helpful in identifying the tracheal opening if the tube is accidentally dislodged. These sutures are removed after 1 week, during which time a tracheocutaneous tract has formed. Nursing care of the tracheostomy site must be thorough to prevent infection and skin maceration. There should be frequent dressing changes after removal of all secretions and cleansing with Betadine solution. The tube should be changed only when crusting prevents adequate suctioning or ventilation. There must always be an identical tube at the bedside in case plugging necessitates an immediate change of tubes. The additional precautions described for endotracheal tube care should also be followed.

The choice of proper tube size (see Table 2–3) will prevent tracheal damage and allow, it is hoped, for uncomplicated removal of the tube when there is no longer a need for a tracheostomy. The tubes are made of either Silastic or polyvinyl chloride. Tubes of a smaller size are available without cuffs and provide an adequate seal during positive pressure ventilation. The larger tubes, beginning with a 5-mm inner diameter, have cuffs that should be of the high-volume low-pressure type, minimizing mucosal damage.

When a tracheostomy is no longer necessary, certain steps must be followed for safe extubation. In older patients who require cuffed tubes, the cuff should be deflated for 24 to 48 hours. The patient should be closely observed to identify aspiration of saliva or oral feedings. If aspiration occurs, the cuff should be reinflated and deflation should be attempted again in several days. If deflation is tolerated, a smaller sized, uncuffed tube is inserted. This allows the tracheal stoma to shrink gradually in size and also allows the patient to become reacquainted with the sensation of phonating and breathing through the upper airway. Serially, smaller sized tubes can be introduced until the patient can tolerate a corked tube without difficulty, leading to eventual removal. The wound heals by secondary intention.

Infants and young children with smaller tracheal lumens cannot tolerate the same process of weaning. After the decision has been made to remove the tube, the trachea should be endoscopically examined to determine patency and to remove any granulations. Occasionally, the anterior tracheal wall superior to the level of the stoma may be buckled intraluminally, resulting from a mild chondromalacia. If this is the case, a silicone tracheal T tube can be inserted for 48 hours to act as a stent. After the patency of the trachea has been established, all artificial airways can be removed. The patient should be closely observed.

Complications

As with any type of surgery, tracheostomies are associated with both immediate and delayed complications, which vary in incidence at various medical centers. The most common immediate complications are pneumomediastinum and pneumothorax. Both can be avoided by keeping dissection to a necessary minimum with a midline approach and avoiding entrance into the mediastinal tissues. A postoperative chest x-ray and auscultation will enable the physician to be aware of these problems as well as to verify proper positioning of the tube. Pneumomediastinum will resolve spontaneously over 48 to 72 hours, but a significant pneumothorax must be treated with a chest tube. Additional immediate complications include hemorrhage, aspiration, cardiorespiratory arrest, and iatrogenic tracheoesophageal fistula.

Delayed complications include subglottic stenosis, fused vocal cords, tracheal granulomas and stenosis, mucous plugging, tracheomalacia, and stomal infection. Subglottic stenosis seems to occur more often in patients with previous long-term endotracheal intubation or high

Table 2–3. Recommended Sizes of Tracheostomy Tubes

Age	Tube Size (OD mm)
Premature	4.0
Newborn	4.5–5.0
Up to 1 year	5.5
1–3 years	6.0
3–6 years	7.0
6–12 years	8.0
12–20 years	9.0–10.0

tracheostomies. These factors would obviously expose the subglottic mucosa to increased trauma, with resulting chondritis leading to stenosis.

Age is the most important factor relating to the development of complications. Patients in the younger age groups are more prone to both immediate and delayed complications of tracheostomy; thus, constant attention to the details previously stated is necessary. An additional factor that may lead to possible complications is the underlying disease process, with adverse sequelae developing more frequently in infants with respiratory distress syndrome, croup, and cardiothoracic surgery.

SUGGESTED READING

Aberdeen, E., and Downes, J.J.: Artifical airways in children. Surg. Clin. North Am. 19:311, 1971.

Conner, G.H., and Marsels, M.J.: Orotracheal intubation in the newborn. Laryngoscope 87:87, 1977.

Fearon, B., and Ellis, D.: The management of long-term airway problems in infants and children. Ann. Otol. Rhinol. Laryngol. 80:669, 1971.

Freeman, G.R.: A comparative analysis of endotracheal intubation in neonates, children, and adults: complications, prevention, and treatment. Laryngoscope 82:1385, 1972.

Gaudet, P.T., Peerless, A., Sasaki, C.T., and Kirchner, J.A.: Pediatric tracheostomy and associated complications. Laryngoscope 88:1633, 1978.

Gerson, C.R., Tucker, G.F.: Infant tracheotomy. Ann. Otol. Rhinol. Laryngol. 91:413, 1982.

Gregory, G.A.: Respiratory care of newborn infants. Pediatr. Clin. North Am. 19:311, 1971.

Parkin, J.L., Stevens, M.H., and Jung, A.L.: Acquired and congential subglottic stenosis in the infant. Ann. Otol. Rhinol. Laryngol. 85:573, 1976.

Sasaki, C.T., Horuichi, M., and Koss, N.: Tracheostomy-related subglottic stenosis: bacteriologic pathogenesis. Laryngoscope 89:857, 1979.

Strome, M., and Ferguson, C.F.: Multiple postintubation complications. Ann. Otol. Rhinol. Laryngol. 83:432, 1974.

Strong, R.M., and Passy, V.: Endotracheal intubation—complications in neonates. Arch. Otolarngol. 103:329, 1977.

Zulliger, J.J., Schuller, D.E., Beach, T.P., et al.: Assessment of intubation in croup epiglottis. Ann. Otol. Rhinol. Laryngol. 91:413, 1982.

Assisted Ventilation

FRANK T. WENG, M.D.

BASIC PHYSIOLOGIC PRINCIPLES

The gas exchanging function of the lung can be accomplished by either spontaneous respiration or a mechanical ventilator. The respiratory system is subjected to different physical conditions in these two situations. It is of vital importance that these physiologic differences be understood in order to maximize the benefits while avoiding the potential harmful effects of mechanical ventilation therapy. In this chapter, the basic pulmonary physiology relevant to assisted ventilation is discussed .

PRESSURES OF THE RESPIRATORY SYSTEM

Intrapleural Pressure (Intrathoracic Pressure, Pleural Pressure, Ppl)

Intrapleural pressure (Ppl) is the pressure immediately surrounding the lung (Fig. 3–1). As the elastic recoil pressure of the lung is transmitted to the pleural space, a negative pressure is created in the potential space between the visceral and parietal pleurae. Direct measurement of Ppl cannot be made easily, but overall changes in Ppl can be determined by measuring pressure changes in the esophagus. Ppl is not uniform throughout the pleural cavity. Along the vertical axis in the upright lung, Ppl exhibits a gradient with more negative pressure at the apex than at the base. This pressure gradient influences the size of alveoli in different parts of the lung and, consequently, the distribution of inspired gas. It is important to recognize that Ppl is normally subatmospheric (negative) during the entire cycle of spontaneous breathing, whereas during intermittent positive pressure breathing (IPPB), it becomes intermittently positive. Continuous positive airway pressure and positive end–expiratory pressure (PEEP) also modify the normal res-

piratory cyclic variation of Ppl. The degree to which the Ppl is affected depends upon the airway pressure and the compliance of the lung. The mean Ppl is the principal determinant of venous return and cardiac output and thus is a major concern in the management of patients receiving mechanical ventilation.

Alveolar Pressure (PA), Transpulmonary Pressure (PL)

The alveolar pressure (PA) is always greater than the pressure surrounding the lung. The transpulmonary pressure (PL) is the pressure difference between the alveolar and intrapleural pressures (PA — Ppl; see Fig. 3–1) and is taken to be equal to the transalveolar pressure. Because Ppl is negative during spontaneous breathing and less than PA during mechanical ventilation, PL is always positive and acts as the distending pressure for the lung. At the moments of end-inspiration or end-expiration, when there is no airflow in either direction, PA is equal to the pressure at the airway opening (Pao). During inspiration, the pressure difference between the airway opening and alveoli must overcome the lung resistance in order to produce inflow of air into the lung (Pao > PA); during expiration the pressure relationship is reversed.

Generally, for a patient who is being mechanically ventilated via an endotracheal tube or a tracheostomy, the Pao is the pressure at the mouth (Pm). This pressure can be found on the ventilator dial. The rise and fall of Pm always precedes that of PA. The peak value of Pm represents the driving pressure when the inspiratory flow rate is at its maximum. Its magnitude decreases with decreasing inspiratory flow until it becomes equal to PA when the flow ceases at the end-inspiratory moment. In time- or volume-cycled ventilators, Pm varies with tidal volume, airway resistance, and compliance of the lung.

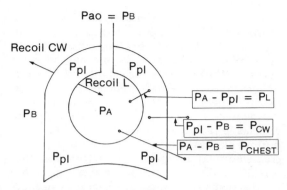

Figure 3–1. Schematic drawing of pressures and transmural pressures of the respiratory system. Pressures within the rectangular boxes are transmural pressures for the lung (P_L), chest wall (P_{CW}) and total chest (P_{CHEST}). At the resting level (FRC), the inward recoil of the lung is exactly counteracted by the outward recoil of the chest wall, producing a negative pressure within the intrapleural space (Ppl). At resting level, there is no air flow. Thus $P_A = Pao = P_B = 0$.

Trans Chest Wall Pressure (P_{CW}), Transthoracic Pressure (P_{CHEST})

The collapsing or distending pressure of the chest wall (depending on the level of lung inflation) is the difference between pressures on opposite sides of the chest wall, or, $Ppl − P_B$, where P_B is the barometric pressure that acts upon the body surface (see Fig. 3–1). Thus,

$$P_{CW} = Ppl − P_B$$

The chest wall tends to spring outward at low lung volumes. The elastic force of the lung tends to reduce its volume. When these two opposing forces are balanced, the chest is said to be at its resting position and the volume it contains is the functional residual capacity (FRC).

MECHANICS OF THE RESPIRATORY SYSTEM

Static Properties

Compliance. The lung is an elastic organ whose characteristics can be defined in terms of the relationship between change in volume and corresponding change in pressure of gas within alveoli. This relationship is termed *compliance of the lung* (C_L).

$$C_L = V/P$$

The compliance describes the distensibility of the organ, which is usually expressed in liters per centimeter of water pressure (L/cm H_2O). The compliance of the lung and the chest wall may be modified by age, posture, anesthetics, or muscle relaxants. Furthermore, even in the normal lung, there are regional differences in lung compliance. Compliance also varies with different levels of lung inflation. At a very high lung volume, lung compliance decreases. When alveoli are overdistended, they become stiffer.

The compliance is a static quantity and can be measured only under static or quasi-static conditions. In clinical conditions, the dynamic compliance is measured by recording the tidal volume and corresponding intraesophageal pressure variation. Under normal conditions, the static and dynamic lung compliances do not differ, but with increasing breathing frequency in pathologic conditions, the latter decreases.

Dynamic Properties

Respiratory Resistance. There are three components to respiratory resistance: inertia of the respiratory system, tissue resistance of the lung and chest wall, and airway resistance to the flow of gas. The airway resistance plus the pulmonary tissue resistance constitutes the total pulmonary resistance. Inertial and tissue frictional resistance are small compared with airway resistance and can be ignored in most clinical conditions. When the flow pattern is laminar, airway resistance is inversely proportional to the fourth power of the radius of the airway. This fact must be taken into consideration when selecting tracheostomy or endotracheal tubes so that the tubes do not unduly increase airway resistance. Laminar flow is the predominant pattern of airflow in peripheral airways. Turbulent flow develops when the direction of airflow suddenly changes at airway branching junctions and when a critical linear velocity is exceeded. During quiet breathing, the flow pattern is turbulent in the trachea and larynx. When the flow is turbulent, the resistance is proportional to the density of the gas and the square of the flow rate and inversely proportional to the fifth power of the radius of the tube. Airway resistance is usually markedly increased in patients with advanced cystic fibrosis, bronchiolitis, or acute asthma, in whom there are reductions in the radii of peripheral airways caused by intramural obstruction resulting from either accumulated secretions or bronchospasm. In patients with cardiac disease and increased pulmonary artery blood flow, airway resistance is higher because of the extrinsic compression of small airways by the increased interstitial pressure. Increased airway resistance can lead to alveolar hypoventilation in patients receiving mechanical ventilation primarily because of the smaller than intended tidal volume delivered within the inspiratory time available. This situation is discussed in more detail under Clinical Aspects.

Time Constant. Alveoli do not fill with inspired gas at the same rate during inspiration, resulting in a nonuniform distribution of inspired air. There are two reasons for the nonuniform ventilation of the lung. First, the magnitude of the Ppl is not uniform across all lung regions. In the normal thorax in the upright position, Ppl is less negative at the bottom of the thorax than it is at the top. This gradient in Ppl affects the size of the alveoli in a predictable way: those at the top are more distended than those at the bottom. Overdistended alveoli are less compliant (i.e., stiffer) than underdistended alveoli. Therefore, when the same magnitude of pressure is applied, the alveoli at the bottom of the lung will be filled with air at a faster rate than those at the top. The second reason for the nonuniform ventilation of the lung is airway resistance. Given an equal compliance, the alveoli with airways of high resistance take longer to fill than those with low resistance. Mathematically, this phenomenon is expressed in terms of time constant (τ). In pulmonary physiology, time constant is the product of compliance and resistance:

$$\tau = C \times R$$

To explain this concept at a practical level: during the inspiratory phase, the alveolus with its particular time constant would be filled to 64 percent of its final tidal volume within one time constant, 87 percent within two time constants, 95 percent within three time constants, and 98 percent within four time constants. The same concept applies to the expiratory phase. The knowledge of overall time constant of the respiratory system is obviously very important in determining the inspiratory and expiratory time limits for assisted ventilation. The average time constant for adults is 0.55 seconds, whereas for infants it is 0.29 seconds.

Mechanical Work Done on the Lung. The total work of breathing cannot be measured directly, because it has not been possible to measure the nonelastic resistance of the chest wall. However, the mechanical work done on the lung can be estimated from the lung volume displacement with its associated intrapleural (intraesophageal) pressure change. A pressure-volume loop thus created during one breath cycle, which consists of the mechanical work necessary to overcome the elastic and nonelastic resistance of the lung, represents this work. During quiet breathing, work done on the lung during inspiration is sufficient to overcome the nonelastic resistance of both the air and lung during expiration. Under conditions of increased airway resistance, expiratory muscular work, in addition to the potential energy stored by the inspiratory muscular work, is needed. On the other hand, when the lung is stiff, more inspiratory work will have to be done to overcome the elastic resistance of the lung.

Distribution of Ventilation

In addition to compliance and airway resistance, the distribution of inspired air is dependent upon the flow rate. Airway resistance has less influence on the passage of air when the flow rate is low but plays the major role in local distribution of inspired air when the inspiratory flow rate is high. Thus, when the inspiratory inflow is low, the distribution of air is compliance dependent; when the inspiratory inflow is high, the distribution of air is dependent upon airway resistance.

Alveolar Ventilation and Minute Ventilation

The levels of oxygen and carbon dioxide tensions in the arterial blood are regulated by alveolar ventilation under the prevailing conditions of barometric pressure, dead space, distribution of ventilation and perfusion, shunting, diffusing capacity, and metabolic activity of the patient. The adequacy of ventilation is reflected in the partial pressure of alveolar CO_2 (PA_{CO_2}), which is approximately equal to the partial pressure of arterial CO_2 (Pa_{CO_2}). PA_{CO_2} is determined solely by alveolar ventilation ($\dot{V}_A$) and the volume of CO_2 ($\dot{V}_{CO_2}$) eliminated per minute.

Partial pressure of arterial oxygen (Pa_{O_2}), on the other hand, is affected by two additional factors: concentration of oxygen in the inspired gas and the degree of venous admixture ($\dot{Q}_{va}$) caused by ventilation/perfusion ($\dot{V}/\dot{Q}$) mismatch or pulmonary shunting.

Although Pa_{CO_2} is approximately equal to PA_{CO_2} under normal conditions, there is usually a certain gradient between PA_{O_2} and Pa_{O_2} that amounts to about 10 mm Hg in young adults and 25 mm Hg in neonates.

Respiratory Dead Space

Physiologic dead space is the volume of the lung that does not take part in gas exchange. The volume of physiologic dead space (V_{Dphys}) is approximately one third of the tidal volume (V_T) ($V_{Dphys}/V_T = 0.3$), which can be calculated by the following formula:

$$(V_{Dphys}) = \frac{Pa_{CO2} - PE_{CO2}}{Pa_{CO2}} \times V_T$$

where PE_{CO2} is the CO_2 tension in the mixed expired air.

In many pathological conditions, V_{Dphys} is increased, the consequence of which is to reduce alveolar ventilation. In order to maintain normal levels of Pa_{CO2} and Pa_{O2}, respiratory minute ventilation must increase when there is increased V_{Dphys}.

V_{Dphys} is composed of anatomic dead space (V_{Danat}) and alveolar dead space (V_{DA}). V_{Danat} is the volume of conducting airways that are not lined by respiratory epithelium. This volume is reduced in tracheotomized or intubated patients.

V_{DA} is that part of the inspired gas that reaches the alveolar level but does not take part in gas exchange and represents the alveolar units that are ventilated but are functionally not perfused. V_{DA} is increased by any mode of mechanical ventilation that tends to reduce either the pulmonary blood flow or the pulmonary vascular pressure. The magnitude of V_{DA} can be estimated by the arterial/end–expiratory P_{CO2} difference. Because of the small size of V_{DA}, in a normal individual the PET_{CO2} (end–tidal CO_2 tension) is identical to PA_{CO2} and there is no difference among PA_{CO2}, Pa_{CO2}, and PET_{CO2}. When V_{DA} increases, PET_{CO2} no longer represents the true alveolar CO_2. In this situation, PET_{CO2} reaches the peak value before the end of spontaneous expiration. This is because the last part of the PE_{CO2} is contributed in part by the low CO_2 tension gas from the V_{DA}.

Pulmonary Perfusion

Total pulmonary blood flow is approximately equal to total systemic blood flow. Although the output of the right and left sides of the heart is approximately the same, pulmonary vascular resistance is markedly lower than systemic vascular resistance. Therefore, the absolute pressure and pressure gradient in the systemic and pulmonary circulations differ greatly. The mean pulmonary artery pressure is about 15 mm Hg, which is about one sixth of the mean aortic pressure (90 mm Hg). The mean left atrial pressure is approximately 5 mm Hg. In clinical situations, the left atrial pressure is approximated by wedging a venous catheter into a distal branch of a pulmonary artery. In the management of critically ill patients who require ventilatory assistance, monitoring of left atrial pressure is very useful. The wedge pressure is used as a guide to estimates of blood volume, pulmonary vascular resistance, and the functional state of the left atrium. This measurement should be taken during the expiratory phase of controlled ventilation. When pulmonary resistance is high, pulmonary artery diastolic pressure is not a reliable guide to left ventricular end–diastolic pressure. By contrast, the wedge pressure is usually a reliable indicator of mean left atrial pressure, except in cases of heart failure or when PEEP is used. The mean right atrial pressure is about 3 mm Hg. The functional state of the right atrium is monitored by a central venous catheter inserted into the superior vena cava. The central venous pressure reflects blood volume, vascular tone, and cardiac function.

The pulmonary vessels can be divided into two groups: the alveolar vessels and the extra-alveolar vessels. The patency of alveolar vessels is determined by the pressure difference between the alveolus and the capillary. When alveolar pressure rises, as during continuous positive pressure breathing, the transmural pressure becomes negative and the alveolar capillary collapses. The nonperfused alveolus then contributes to an increase in physiologic dead space.

The extra-alveolar vessels are subject to the pressure influence of the lung parenchyma. At high volume, the transmural pressure is great because the retractive force of the lung is increased. At low lung volume, the transmural pressure is decreased. Therefore, pulmonary vascular resistance is higher at low lung volume than at high lung volume. Mechanical ventilation with excessive PEEP tends to close down alveolar vessels, reducing pulmonary blood return to the left heart and decreasing cardiac output. This type of treatment is sometimes used in cases of hemodynamic pulmonary edema. Positive pressure breathing is commonly used in treating permeability pulmonary edema. High airway pressure, however, sometimes aggravates pulmonary edema, possibly because of leakage of extra-alveolar vessels.

The blood flow through the lung is determined by the relative magnitude of alveolar pressure (PA), pulmonary arterial pressure (Pa), and pulmonary venous pressure (Pv). As a consequence of these pressure relationships, a vertical gradient of pulmonary perfusion, which essentially is a gravity-dependent phenomenon, exists; pulmonary blood flow is greater at the base of the lung than at the apex. This effect has little application to the infant whose lung is small and whose position is generally recumbent.

Among other clinically significant factors known to influence pulmonary perfusion is alveolar PO_2 (PA_{O_2}). Increases in PA_{O_2} cause pulmonary vasodilation, whereas decreases lead to vasoconstriction. Acidosis contributes to an increase in pulmonary vascular resistance. Carbon dioxide, prostaglandins (PGE_1 and PGA_2), acetylcholine, tolazoline, histamine, and other substances also affect pulmonary vascular tone.

Intrapulmonary Shunt

Normally, a certain amount of venous blood is returned to the left side of the heart without coming in contact with the alveolar gas. The proximal bronchial vein empties into the right and left sides of the heart. Thebesian veins also drain into the left side of the heart. The right-to-left shunts constitute about 2 percent of the cardiac output and account for a 3- to 5-mm Hg alveolar–arterial O_2 tension difference, $(A–a)D_{O_2}$, in older children and adults.

The most common cause of abnormal intrapulmonary right-to-left shunt is perfusion of atelectatic alveoli or alveoli that cannot take part in gas exchange because of alveolar pulmonary edema or consolidation. The magnitude of shunt can be calculated from the shunt equation:

$$\frac{\dot{Q}s}{\dot{Q}t} = \frac{Cc'_{O_2} - Ca_{O_2}}{Cc'_{O_2} - C\bar{v}_{O_2}}$$

where $\dot{Q}$ denotes blood volume; S, shunt blood; t, total blood volume; C, oxygen content; c', alveolar capillary; and $\bar{v}$, mixed venous blood. The oxygen content in volume percent is derived from the following equation:

$$\begin{array}{c} 1.34 \text{ (ml } O_2/\text{gm Hgb)} \\ \times \text{ gm of Hgb} \\ \times \text{ \% saturation} \end{array}$$

The alveolar capillary O_2(Ac_{O_2}) tension is assumed to be equal to alveolar O_2(A_{O_2}) tension. The venous blood in the bronchial vein and the thebesian vein probably has lower PO_2 than $P\bar{v}_{O_2}$; however, this fact is usually ignored; PO_2 is assumed to be equal to $P\bar{v}_{O_2}$. Venous admixture ($\dot{Q}_{va}$) owing to physiologic shunt decreases Pa_{O_2}, but it has relatively little effect on Pa_{CO_2}.

Scatter of Ventilation Perfusion Ratio ($\dot{V}/\dot{Q}$)

The overall alveolar ventilation ($\dot{V}_A$) to pulmonary perfusion ratio ($\dot{V}A/\dot{Q}C$) is 5 L per minute:6 L per minute, or 0.85. $\dot{V}A/\dot{Q}C$ is often abbreviated as $\dot{V}/\dot{Q}$. There is a considerable scatter of $\dot{V}/\dot{Q}$ in the normal upright lung. The $\dot{V}/\dot{Q}$ ratio measured during normal breathing ranges from 1.0 near the level of the third thoracic vertebra to 0.5 near the level of the ninth thoracic vertebra. This $\dot{V}/\dot{Q}$ scatter contributes to the alveolar arterial O_2 tension difference, $(A–a)D_{O_2}$, that is normally present. In pathological states, the $\dot{V}/\dot{Q}$ scatter increases, becoming the major contributing factor to arterial desaturation. Arterialized blood flow leaving areas of very low $\dot{V}/\dot{Q}$ units are approximately equivalent to a right-to-left shunt. The high $\dot{V}/\dot{Q}$ units cannot compensate for the $\dot{Q}_{va}$ effect of low $\dot{V}/\dot{Q}$ areas. The situation becomes worse when PA_{O_2} becomes lower; even the blood leaving the high $\dot{V}/\dot{Q}$ units is less than fully saturated. In contrast, when the PA_{O_2} is high, the effect of $\dot{V}/\dot{Q}$ scatter is minimal, because even the blood leaving the low $\dot{V}/\dot{Q}$ units is almost completely saturated. This principle is used clinically in the oxygen treatment of arterial desaturation, which is mainly caused by scatter of $\dot{V}/\dot{Q}$ ratio.

The intrapulmonary shunt and alveolar dead space represent the two extremes of the $\dot{V}/\dot{Q}$ mismatch; the former represents areas of $\dot{V}/\dot{Q}$ ratio of zero, and the latter represents infinity.

A hyperoxic test is often used to differentiate low Pa_{O_2} caused by an intrapulmonary shunt from that caused by $\dot{Q}_{va}$ of low $\dot{V}/\dot{Q}$ units. However, breathing a high concentration of oxygen invariably leads to absorption collapse of very low $\dot{V}/\dot{Q}$ units, artificially creating an additional intrapulmonary shunt. On the other hand, applying continuous distending pressure, may improve ventilation of low $\dot{V}/\dot{Q}$ units and result in improved Pa_{O_2}.

PATHOPHYSIOLOGY OF ARTERIAL BLOOD GASES

Hypoxemia

Hypoxemia without hypercarbia can occur in unusual circumstances (high altitude, severe physical exercise, and an empty oxygen tank during anesthesia); however, all clinically important hypoxemia occurs in association with hypercarbia. Hypoxemia of pulmonary origin can result from hypoventilation, $\dot{V}/\dot{Q}$ scatter, intrapulmonary shunt, abnormal desaturation of mixed venous blood, and diffusion defect.

Hypoventilation

Alveolar hypoventilation can result from drug intoxication, disease processes involving the medulla, anterior horn cell disease, ineffective bellows mechanism secondary to neuromuscular diseases, and accidental hypoventilation during anesthesia or mechanical ventilation. Hypoxemia is caused by decreased $P_{A_{O_2}}$, which is a result of alveolar hypoventilation. Because Pa_{CO_2} is inversely proportional to $\dot{V}_A$, Pa_{CO_2} always increases. The difference between alveolar and arterial oxygen tensions, $(A–a)D_{O_2}$, is slightly decreased because of a change in position on the oxyhemoglobin dissociation curve. $\dot{Q}s/\dot{Q}t$ is not increased. Adding more oxygen to the inspired gas will correct hypoxemia but not hypercarbia. Increasing minute ventilation by pharmacologic means or mechanical ventilation will correct hypoxemia or hypercarbia.

$\dot{V}/\dot{Q}$ Scatter

This is the most common and clinically most important cause of hypoxemia in the majority of cases. Typically $(A–a)D_{O_2}$ is increased. Increasing $F_{I_{O_2}}$ will minimize the effect of decreased regional $\dot{V}_A$ on Pa_{O_2} by increasing other regional $P_{A_{O_2}}$, resulting in normalization of $(A–a)D_{O_2}$ and improved arterial oxygenation.

Intrapulmonary Shunt

In terms of $\dot{V}/\dot{Q}$ ratio, the shunt represents areas of zero ratio. This means nonventilation of perfused alveoli. Pathologically and radiographically, this situation exists because of atelectatic areas.

Increasing $F_{I_{O_2}}$ does not affect the shunted blood, because it does not come in contact with inspired gas. $(A–a)D_{O_2}$ is increased. The ultimate Pa_{O_2} depends upon the $\dot{Q}s/\dot{Q}T$ ratio. If the $\dot{Q}s/\dot{Q}T$ ratio is greater than 30 percent, breathing even 100 percent oxygen will not correct hypoxemia. Modes of treatment should be aimed at aeration of collapsed air-exchanging units.

Diffusion Defects

Most instances of hypoxemia in pulmonary diseases that previously were thought to be characterized by alveolar–capillary block (and thus decreased diffusing capacity) can be explained on the basis of uneven distribution of inspired gas and $\dot{V}/\dot{Q}$ scatter within the lung. True diffusion defect exists in such clinical entities as granuloma, sarcoidosis, radiation pneumopathy, and pulmonary leukemic infiltration.

Decrease in Mixed Venous P_{O_2} ($P\bar{v}_{O_2}$)

Hypoxemia occurs in the presence of low $P\bar{v}_{O_2}$ because the O_2 pressure gradient between alveolar gas and pulmonary capillary blood increases. Decrease in $P\bar{v}_{O_2}$ may be due to anemia, decreased cardiac output, or increased metabolic activity. $(A–a)D_{O_2}$ may increase if capillary transit time becomes shortened and prevents complete equilibration.

Hypercarbia

Hypoventilation

Any clinical conditions associated with decreased minute ventilation will result in hypercarbia unless there is a significant decrease in V_D/V_T ratio.

Increased Physiologic Dead Space (V_{Dphys})

Hypercarbia can result from an increase in alveolar dead space or an increase in ventilator dead space or both. It can be corrected when there is increased V_{Dphys} by increasing minute ventilation (either by increasing V_T or rate or both), but this mechanism has no effect on Pa_{CO_2} when the V_D/V_T ratio exceeds 0.6. Such patients are almost always in respiratory failure. The appropriate mode of treatment in this situation is mechanical ventilation.

CLINICAL ASPECTS OF ASSISTED VENTILATION

When the ventilatory capacity is impaired to the extent that the lung can no longer function efficiently to supply adequate oxygen and eliminate carbon dioxide, assisted ventilation becomes necessary. Respiratory failure may be due to primary pulmonary parenchymal disease, primary airway disease, abnormal respiratory control mechanism, or dysfunction of ventilatory effectors.

In those patients with primary lung parenchymal disease, hypoxemia is the main feature, resulting from ventilation/perfusion mismatch, intrapulmonary shunts, and alveolar hypoventilation caused mainly by the increase in physiologic dead space. Examples of lung parenchymal disease are: pneumonia, idiopathic pulmonary hemosiderosis, pulmonary fibrosis, pulmonary embolism, and radiation pneumopathy. Each of these clinical conditions has a decreased vital capacity characteristic of restrictive pulmonary disease.

In the initial stage of primary airway disease, the patient is able to prevent alveolar hypoventilation by increasing ventilatory effort. If airway obstruction is severe and unrelieved by bronchodilators, the work of breathing may become so burdensome that normal alveolar ventilation cannot be maintained. Because Pa_{CO_2} is inversely proportional to alveolar ventilation, Pa_{CO_2} increases as alveolar ventilation diminishes. The development of hypoxemia is incidental to alveolar hypoventilation. Common causes of obstructed ventilation in infancy are croup and bronchiolitis. In older children, asthma and cystic fibrosis are the common causes of respiratory failure caused by airway obstruction. Constriction of the trachea resulting from prolonged endotracheal intubation can cause obstructive ventilatory failure at any age, although it is more common in infancy. In some obese children with hypertrophied tonsils, respiratory failure may develop from upper airway obstruction.

The main effector organs of the respiratory system are the diaphragm and the respiratory muscles, whose functions may be impaired in systemic muscular disease or in abnormalities of the nervous system. Respiratory failure as a result of hypodynamic ventilatory failure is seen in such diverse clinical entities as muscular dystrophy, myasthenia gravis, kyphoscoliosis, Reye's syndrome, Guillain-Barré syndrome, and high spinal cord injury. Some obese children not only have restrictive pulmonary abnormalities but also have an ineffectual bellows mechanism and an abnormal respiratory regulatory mechanism during sleep.

In early infancy, congenital cardiac malformations are an important cause of respiratory failure, often requiring assisted ventilation when lung mechanics are altered by abnormal hemodynamics. Pulmonary congestion, pulmonary hypertension, pulmonary edema, or compression of peripheral airways by increased interstitial pressure may lead to respiratory failure.

Spontaneous Breathing and Mechanical Ventilation

During the inspiratory phase of spontaneous breathing, the diaphragm and respiratory muscles contract to expand the thoracic cavity. This action creates a pressure gradient between the intrapleural space and the alveoli, which keeps the latter open by overcoming elastic recoil pressure of the lung. For air to flow through the airways, it is necessary to overcome the resistance of the respiratory system. The pressure difference between the mouth and the alveoli overcomes this resistance during inspiration. At end-inspiration, there is no airflow and the alveolar pressure is equal to the mouth pressure. The transalveolar (i.e., transpulmonary) pressure increases at end-inspiration, because here the intrapleural pressure is more negative than at end-expiration. When expiration begins, the alveolar pressure is the sum of elastic recoil pressure of the lung and the intrapleural pressure, which is now less negative than at the end of expiration. The pressure gradient between the alveolus and the mouth moves air toward the airway opening. At end-expiration, airflow stops and the alveolar pressure drops to atmospheric pressure. The respiratory system assumes its resting state at the end of spontaneous expiration. The volume of gas contained in the lung at the resting position is the FRC.

During mechanical ventilation, the alveoli are kept open by positive pressure applied to the airway opening, not by negative pressure in the intrapleural space. Although the transpulmonary pressure is the same at comparable levels of lung inflation during spontaneous or mechanical ventilation, the absolute pressures in the alveolus and intrapleural space differ. During spontaneous quiet breathing, alveolar pressure at the beginning of inspiration is atmospheric pressure; during the inspiratory phase, it becomes slightly negative (on the order of -1 to -2 cm H_2O; and at the end of inspiration, it returns to atmospheric pressure again. With positive pressure breathing, the alveolar pressure rises to about 14 cm H_2O in the normal lung. At the resting position (FRC), the intrapleural pressure is normally about -5 cm H_2O. During quiet spontaneous breathing, the intrapleural pressure falls to about -8 cm H_2O during inspiration, returning to -5 cm H_2O again at the end of expiration. With positive pressure breathing, the corresponding intrapleural pressure changes are -5 cm H_2O (end-expiration), $+2$ cm H_2O (end-inspiration), and -5 cm H_2O (end-expiration).

Physiologic Effects of Mechanical Ventilation

The Effects on the Cardiovascular Function

SYSTEMIC CIRCULATION

In spontaneous breathing, intrapleural pressure falls during the inspiratory phase, creating a pressure difference between the mouth and the alveolar space, which draws air into the lung. The fall in intrapleural pressure also influences the hemodynamics in such a way that the return of blood from the extrathoracic body segments into the great thoracic vein is facilitated. It is known that Valsalva's maneuver (increase of intrathoracic pressure by forcible exhalation against a closed glottis) raises the intrathoracic pressure and interferes with venous return. The effect of the inspiratory phase of positive pressure breathing is similar to that of Valsalva's maneuver. In normal quiet breathing, intrapleural pressure falls to a value of -8 cm H_2O at the height of inspiratory activity; during the inspiratory phase of positive pressure breathing the corresponding pressure will be approximately $+2$ cm H_2O. At the end of the expiratory phase, the intrapleural pressure is about -5 cm H_2O, both during spontaneous quiet breathing and under positive pressure ventilation. Thus, during spontaneous breathing, the venous return is greater during the inspiratory phase than during the expiratory phase, but the situation is reversed under positive pressure ventilation.

The peak airway pressure itself has no specific effect on the venous return. It is the combination of the magnitude of the inspiratory pressure and the duration of the inspiratory phase that affects the volume of venous return. These two factors are reflected in the mean intrapleural pressure: the higher the mean intrapleural pressure, the lower the venous return. With decreased systemic venous return, cardiac output drops and systemic blood pressure falls. Normally, this adverse effect is offset by a rapid increase in peripheral venous pressure, which restores the pressure gradient necessary for a normal venous return.

PULMONARY CIRCULATION

The alveolar pressure is negative during the inspiratory phase of spontaneous breathing. The action of the diaphragm and the inspiratory muscles creates pressure gradients between the mouth and the respiratory bronchi that draw inspiratory gas into the lung. During the inspiratory phase of positive pressure ventilation, the alveolar pressure is positive, the magnitude and time course of which is dependent upon the time constant of the lung and the mode of positive pressure ventilation. The rise in alveolar pressure relative to the pulmonary capillary pressure tends to impede the blood flow through the lung, adding to physiologic dead space. At the normal level of functional residual capacity, pulmonary vascular resistance is minimal.

The overall effect of positive pressure ventilation on gas exchange is compromised by a decrease in lung compliance resulting from the preferential ventilation of alveolar units, which have low accompanying airway resistances. This negative effect is counteracted by the pulmonary vasodilatation that results from an increase in $P_{A_{O_2}}$. Furthermore, the mechanical effect of opening previously atelectatic alveoli tends to decrease pulmonary vascular resistance. However, when a large tidal volume is used during mechanical ventilation, pulmonary vascular resistance may increase. PEEP may potentially aggravate this situation by preferentially enlarging the more compliant gas exchanging units.

Constant Distending Pressure

Positive End-Expiratory Pressure (PEEP)

Modification of expiratory pressure to produce PEEP has become a popular method of improving oxygenation and facilitating weaning since the 1970's. PEEP is almost a standard mode of ventilatory therapy in pediatric patients in whom arterial oxygen tension is less than 60 mm Hg when oxygen concentration in the inspired gas is equal to or greater than 50 percent. The range of optimal PEEP is usually between 5 and 14 cm H_2O. The PEEP should be adjusted periodically to achieve the maximum benefit while minimizing the deleterious effect. The "best PEEP" coincides with the highest lung compliance. It is also associated with the highest Pa_{O_2} and the greatest oxygen transport. The application of PEEP levels higher than that of "best PEEP" results in diminished available oxygen because of a decrease in cardiac output. Because "best PEEP" involves measurements of cardiac output and oxygen content, it is necessary to place a pulmonary artery catheter. This is not done routinely; therefore, the "best PEEP" must be judged clinically and through frequent determinations of blood gas values.

The undesirable effects of mechanical ventilation on the cardiovascular system can be complicated by PEEP. When PEEP is used in ventilatory therapy, the intrapleural pressure is elevated not only during the inspiratory phase but also during the expiratory phase, aggravating the reduction in venous return. If the cardiac output can be maintained, however, application of PEEP decreases intrapulmonary right-to-left shunting and Pa_{O_2} increases.

The PEEP-induced improvement in oxygen transport is associated with an increase in FRC through recruitment of previously closed gas-exchanging space. This results in redistribution of regional ventilation and perfusion, which tends to decrease venous admixture, improving Pa_{O_2}.

In refractory respiratory insufficiency, high PEEP (super PEEP) has been used with favorable results. This practice has limited use in pediatric practice and probably should be reserved for treatment of children with adult respiratory distress syndrome (ARDS; see Chapter 23). When both very high FI_{O_2} and PEEP (15 to 20 cm H_2O) are used, continuous monitoring of systemic, central venous, pulmonary artery, and capillary wedge pressures becomes mandatory. The subsequent course of ventilatory therapy is guided by measuring cardiac output, $\dot{Q}s/\dot{Q}t$ and V_D/V_T. The use of PEEP, however, increases the incidence of interstitial emphysema and pneumothorax. Signs of barotrauma include sudden deterioration in general condition and intensified cyanosis.

Positive pressure ventilation and PEEP also alter intrarenal hemodynamics. In the presence of increased airway pressure, redistribution of blood from cortical nephrons to juxtamedullary nephrons results in decreased glomerular filtration rate (GFR) and urine flow. Another possible effect is renal vein compression with a resultant decrease in GFR. Continuous positive pressure produces an increase in ADH (antidiuretic hormone) level. Change in urine flow is primarily in the free water clearance. The exact mechanisms of increased ADH and decreased urine flow remain unclear, although they seem to be related to increased airway pressure. Changes in Pa_{O_2} and Pa_{CO_2} may also affect kidney function. High Pa_{O_2} decreases and low Pa_{O_2} increases urine flow in patients with respiratory failure. High Pa_{CO_2} (above 65 mm Hg) depresses renal function.

As can be expected, positive pressure ventilation may interfere with splanchnic blood flow and produce hepatic dysfunction, abnormal gastrointestinal motility, and gastric mucosal ischemia.

Intracranial pressure increases with PEEP. The extent of increase is inversely related to lung compliance and correlates positively with changes in pleural pressure. Increase in intracranial pressure and decrease in systemic arterial pressure reduce cerebral blood flow.

Continuous Positive Airway Pressure (CPAP)

The introduction of CPAP in 1971 changed the perspective of respiratory care. CPAP improves gas exchange by increasing FRC through recruitment of previously closed air–exchanging units by redistributing regional ventilation and perfusion with resultant reduction of V/Q scatter and by decreasing intrapulmonary shunt. Aside from its specific beneficial effects, CPAP also derives merit from the fact that spontaneous breathing is the basic form of ventilation. There are several methods of applying CPAP:

1. Endotracheal tube. This is perhaps the most reliable way of maintaining CPAP. Disadvantages are related to endotracheal intubation itself: vocal cord damage, increased secretions, infection, laryngeal edema, and nasal dilatation. The most common technical error in endotracheal intubation is the misplacement of the tip of the endotracheal tube. Often, the tip lies on the carina, leading to false pressure levels, or it may enter the right mainstem bronchus.

2. Nasal cannula (prongs). Despite difficulty in properly anchoring the nasal cannula, this method is widely accepted for neonates and infants. The baby's head position must be fixed. The positive pressure level attained varies because of leakage, which is unavoidable. The highest pressure attainable is about 15 cm H_2O. Feeding is possible but should be dis-

couraged because of potential distention of the stomach.

3. Face mask and head chamber. With these methods, it is difficult to produce an airtight seal, there is limited accessibility of the baby's facial area for nursing care or nasogastric tube feeding, and the positive pressure levels are inconsistent. There is a significantly higher incidence of intracranial hemorrhage in patients who receive CPAP by face mask.

4. Face chamber. Experience with this type of CPAP is limited. A large mask is held in place by a slight negative pressure. A positive pressure up to 12 cm H_2O is attainable. Trauma to the face area is reported to be uncommon.

5. Garden valve. This is a small unit consisting of a Venturi tube connected to a CPAP device and a pressure manometer. A continuous flow of fresh gas is provided by jet flows through the Venturi tube. Excess flow is vented through a series of radially arranged holes, expiratory port, and reservoir tube. The level of positive pressure developed depends upon the Venturi tube size; the smaller the tube size, the higher the pressure that can be developed.

CLINICAL APPLICATION OF CONTINUOUS DISTENDING PRESSURE (PEEP and CPAP)

Continuous distending pressure (CDP) should be initiated early in any patient who cannot maintain adequate blood oxygenation because of decreased FRC or reduced pulmonary compliance. When initiated early in the course of disease, this mode of therapy significantly reduces the $FI_{O_2} \times$ time index and incidence of chronic pulmonary disease. Some clinical conditions that may benefit from CDP include respiratory distress syndrome, meconium aspiration, and congenital heart disease with increased pulmonary vascularity and decreased lung compliance.

Monitoring During Mechanical Ventilation

After ventilatory support has been initiated, certain vital functions should be carefully monitored.

1. Cardiovascular function. Monitoring of cardiovascular conditions includes heart rate, EKG, systolic and diastolic blood pressures, cardiac filling pressure, and cardiac output. These determinations may require placement of arterial and Swan-Ganz catheters (see Chapter 6, Invasive Monitoring).

Central venous pressure in a critically ill patient receiving assisted ventilation is not a reliable index of circulatory hemodynamics.

2. Respiratory function. Certain indices of pulmonary function, such as spontaneous- or ventilator-delivered tidal volume, minute ventilation, peak inspiratory pressure, esophageal pressure changes (which reflect intrapleural pressure changes), dynamic compliance, and airway resistance, can be obtained with little cooperation, even from pediatric patients. Effectiveness of gas exchange can be monitored by arterial blood gas tension determination, measurement of end–tidal CO_2 tension, transcutaneous P_{O_2}, and ear oximetry.

3. Renal function. Fluid intake and output should be recorded accurately. To assess the adequacy of kidney function, serum osmolality and electrolyte concentrations together with urinary output, specific gravity, and electrolytes should be measured at regular intervals.

Assisted Ventilation and Weaning

Intermittent Mandatory Ventilation (IMV)

In 1977, the concept of combining mechanical and spontaneous ventilation originated in the form of intermittent mandatory ventilation (IMV). With IMV, it is possible to use the selected ventilatory modes that are best for the individual patient. With IMV, the mandatory breaths ensure a certain minute ventilation. The intrapleural pressure is lower than in the case of controlled ventilation; therefore, the undesirable effects of mechanical ventilation on the cardiorespiratory system are minimized. The risk of barotrauma is also lessened. The weaning process is simplified and can be carried out in an orderly manner. Further, trials of spontaneous ventilation can be performed without disconnecting the patient from the breathing circuit.

The IMV system incorporates a gas source that produces sufficient flow to allow the patient to breathe spontaneously without any risk of CO_2 rebreathing. To meet this requirement, the gas flow must be at least twice the patient's minute ventilation. In the newborn infant, an IMV ventilator flow rate of 5 to 10 L per minute should be sufficient. In older children or adults, a demand reservoir system ensures the free flow of ventilatory gas. The mandatory breath is delivered to the patient when the exhalation port is occluded. The tidal breath delivered to the patient is equal to *inspiratory time × duration of exhalation port occlusion* and is a constant volume.

CPAP can be added to the IMV circuit by obstructing the exhalation line of the ventilator. In this way, CPAP can operate either during spontaneous breathing or with the mandatory breath. When IMV was first introduced for pediatric use, it was used primarily for the purpose of weaning infants from controlled or assisted ventilation. Today, IMV with CPAP is the primary mode of assisted ventilation in any patient with respiratory failure. Some ventilators incorporate a mechanism capable of delivering the mandatory tidal volume in synchrony with the patient's inspiratory effort. This mode of IMV is called *synchronized intermittent mandatory ventilation (SIMV)*.

Mandatory Minute Volume (MMV)

This mode of ventilatory therapy was developed primarily to facilitate weaning. The patient breathes from a source fresh gas contained in a concertina bag premeasured for optimal minute volume. The patient receives all the allotted amount of gas for an ensured, adequate minute ventilation. PEEP or CPAP can be added to the ventilator circuit.

General Guidelines for Weaning

Weaning from mechanical ventilation can be attempted when the following requirements have been met:

1. *(A–a)D$_{O_2}$ less than 350 mm Hg with breathing of 100 percent oxygen.* When the patient is weaned from the ventilator, F$_{I_{O_2}}$ is normally increased by 0.1 because a decreased tidal volume during spontaneous breathing may result in alveolar hypoventilation and hypoxemia. If this requirement is not met, the increase in F$_{I_{O_2}}$ required to keep satisfactory arterial blood oxygenation may have to be higher than a 0.1 increment. This increases the risk of oxygen toxicity.

2. *V$_D$/V$_T$ ratio less than 0.6.* When V$_D$/V$_T$ is greater than 0.6, the patient must breathe harder to increase minute ventilation and may become exhausted.

3. *Tidal volume during spontaneous breathing greater than 3 ml per kg.* Tidal volume of less than 3 ml per kg results in CO$_2$ retention and hypoxemia caused by alveolar hypoventilation.

4. *Vital capacity greater than 10 ml per kg or inspiratory capacity greater than 7 ml per kg.* Values below these are associated with ineffective cough, resulting in accumulation of secretions and atelectasis.

5. *Spontaneous breathing rate less than 60 breaths per minute in neonates and less than 45 breaths per minute in older children.* Tachypnea is a sign of decreased lung compliance or increased V$_D$/V$_T$ ratio. It is a sign of increased work of breathing.

After the aforementioned criteria have been met, the next step is to reduce the number of mechanical ventilatory breaths per minute. If there is no deterioration in the blood gas values, F$_{I_{O_2}}$ is reduced to the level that will maintain Pa$_{O_2}$ between 50 and 80 mm Hg in neonates and between 60 and 90 mm Hg in older children. CPAP is then gradually reduced. When the lung mechanics and gas exchange are determined to be satisfactory, the patient is removed from the ventilator and F$_{I_{O_2}}$ is increased by 0.1. CPAP is continued via endotracheal tube or nasal prongs. Finally, the patient is weaned from CPAP.

Nursing Care and Routines

Modern critical care medicine depends upon the excellence of the nursing care. Specially trained nurses play an ever-increasing role in critical care medicine. A critical care unit is only as good as the quality of its nursing staff.

The nursing routines that are directed toward the care of the patient on a mechanical ventilator include:

1. Immobilizing the head with a head roll.

2. Securing endotracheal tube and respirator tubing connections. Stabilizing the endotracheal tube to prevent kinking and excessive tension. Checking skin conditions around the nares or mouth.

3. Using artificial tear/ophthalmic ointment to protect the eyes.

4. Filling a humidifier with sterile water.

5. Maintaining a clear airway. Airway suctioning should be preceded and followed by hyperinflation of the lung with high F$_{I_{O_2}}$ for 1 minute. This minimizes oxygen desaturation caused by a lowered FRC secondary to suctioning gas out of the lung. Hyperinflation also prevents atelectasis and the development of intrapulmonary shunt. Use an infant polyethylene catheter for small infants, a No. 5- or a No. 8-French disposable feeding tube for larger infants, and a No. 14-French oxygen catheter for older children. Care must be taken not to injure the upper airway mucosa. Adherence to sterile technique is essential if nosocomial infection is to be avoided.

6. Changing position frequently to prevent atelectasis.

7. Giving oral hygiene if possible. Changing

the position of the oral airway to prevent pressure necrosis of the oral tissue.

8. Disconnecting the patient from the ventilator once every hour, and maximally ventilating with Ambu bag 8 to 10 times.

9. If the patient has a cuffed endotracheal or tracheostomy tube, maintain cuff pressure at 15 to 20 cm H_2O. Deflate the cuff for 10 minutes every 2 hours to prevent pressure necrosis. (The purposes of inflating the cuffs are to prevent air leakage and to prevent accumulated oropharyngeal secretions from contaminating the lower airways.).

Depending upon the availability of respiratory therapists, the nursing staff may be asked to share responsibility for the following:

1. Checking pressurized gas source, power source, gas cylinders, and regulators. An Ambu bag, a face mask, and an extra endotracheal or tracheostomy tube should be available at bedside.

2. Checking connecting tubings and adaptors.

3. Draining condensed water in the tubings.

4. Checking and recording peak inflation pressure, PEEP, or CPAP levels.

5. Checking F_{IO_2} and, whenever applicable, expired tidal volume per minute volume.

6. Checking the conditions of alarm systems, and evaluating leaks and malfunctioning one-way valves.

Classification of Automatic Ventilators

Basic knowledge of the mechanisms of ventilators is essential for all medical personnel who practice critical care medicine.

The functional characteristics of a ventilator can be described in terms of the basic mechanisms involved in initiating and completing each phase of ventilation. Four variables may be present, either singularly or in combination: time, volume, flow, and pressure. During the inspiratory phase, a ventilator operates either as a pressure generator or a flow generator. During the expiratory phase, most ventilators operate as constant atmospheric pressure generators.

Pressure Generator

In this type of ventilator, the pressure generated during the inspiratory phase may be either constant or variable. The pressure is maintained independent of the resulting flow

into the lungs. The pattern of the pressure generated by the ventilator is not affected by pulmonary resistance or compliance. The flow rate and flow pattern are affected by the mechanical characteristics of the lungs. If the airway resistance (Raw) increases, the flow rate decreases. If the pulmonary compliance (CL) decreases, the delivered tidal volume decreases. Thus, a pressure generator cannot deliver a constant tidal volume when CL and Raw are changing. However, increasing the pressure can compensate for small leaks that may be present in the airways or gas circuit.

Flow Generator

The flow generator produces air flow that is uninfluenced by either pulmonary resistance or compliance. The pressure in the alveoli is determined by the effect of flow on the mechanical characteristics of the lung. If the pulmonary compliance decreases, alveolar pressure increases. If the airway resistance increases, the rate of increase of alveolar pressure decreases and the difference between mouth pressure and alveolar pressure increases.

Ventilator Compliance

When using a ventilator, it is important to consider the fraction of tidal volume that is compressed and never reaches the patient. Volume loss occurs because the gas is compressible and the tubing in the ventilator circuit is distensible. The lost volume can be calculated under specific conditions of flow rate and cycling rate if the compliance of the tubing is known.

$$Cv = \frac{\Delta V}{\Delta P}$$

Cv is the compliance of the ventilator and the tubing. ΔV and ΔP are change in volume and corresponding change in pressure. To measure Cv, the tubing is connected to the ventilator and the distal end (to the patient) is occluded. This compliance value remains a constant if there is no change made in tubing and if the water level of the humidifier is kept at the same level. For example:

Set volume = 100 ml
Occluded peak pressure = 50 cm H_2O
Cv = 100 ml/50 cm H_2O
= 2 ml/cm H_2O

This means that for each cm H_2O pressure developed by the ventilator, 2 ml of air volume is captured in the system. If the ventilator volume is set at 50 ml when the patient is connected and the peak pressure reads 25 cm H_2O, the volume captured is 50 ml (25 × 2). Thus, the patient receives no tidal volume from the ventilator. In order to deliver a tidal volume of 50 ml to the patient, the set volume must be increased. This will result in an increase in peak pressure.

Changeover from Inspiratory Phase to Expiratory Phase

VOLUME CYCLING

In this type of changeover, the cycling mechanism is controlled by a predetermined volume. Changeover takes place when that volume of gas has been delivered, regardless of the time it may take, the pressure needed to deliver it, or the magnitude or pattern of flow.

A volume-cycled flow generator will deliver a correct tidal volume within the normal inspiratory time. With a pressure generator, the time needed to deliver the tidal volume will increase if resistance to airflow increases. If the compliance of the lung decreases, the tidal volume delivered will decrease accordingly and may never reach the pre-set limit. It should be pointed out, however, that the predetermined volume of the ventilator is not the set volume chosen by the operator.

A potential risk may arise from leaks in the system, because the ventilator keeps on cycling rhythmically as though it is delivering the prescribed amount of volume into the patient. An alarm system is necessary to prevent such mishaps from occurring. In volume-cycled ventilators, the inspiratory time/expiratory time (I:E) ratio is affected by the average inspiratory flow rate, the respiratory rate, and the tidal volume. Examples of volume-cycled ventilators are: Barnet Mark II, BOC Pneumotron, and Siemens Elema ventilators.

TIME CYCLING

If a time-cycling mechanism is incorporated into a flow generator, the changeover will be effectively volume-cycled (time × flow = volume). It is incorrect to assume, however, that flow × time is the volume actually delivered to the patient. The actual tidal volume cannot be calculated precisely but can be approximated according to the following equation:

$$V_T = T_i \times \dot{V} - V_c$$

where V_T is the tidal volume, T_i is the inspiratory time, $\dot{V}$ is the inspiratory flow, and V_c is the volume lost to the tubing. The volume lost to the tubing can be calculated if C_V is known (see previous example). This compressed volume will reexpand during expiration and is added to the expired air, which then enters a spirometer. Thus, the spirometer reading of minute volume overestimates the actual minute ventilation of the patient. In time-cycled ventilators, the combination of inspiratory time and expiratory time controls determine the I:E ratio.

If this mechanism is combined with a high-constant pressure generator, the changeover is also equivalent to volume cycling. Therefore, the inspiratory time is controlled and the I:E ratio is fixed. A time-cycled pressure generator will deliver a smaller tidal volume when there is increased pressure. If the pressure remains the same, the volume delivered decreases in proportion to a decrease in lung compliance. Examples of time-cycled ventilators are Cape, Engstrom, and East Radcliffe ventilators.

PRESSURE CYCLING

In pressure-cycled ventilators, the cycling mechanism is controlled by a pre-set pressure. Cycling occurs when the pressure near the mouth reaches the pre-set value. The tidal volume is influenced by both the airway pressure and lung compliance. If resistance increases or compliance decreases, the pre-set pressure limit will be reached before the intended tidal volume is delivered. The I:E ratio is influenced by the rate, inspiratory flow rate, and peak inspiratory pressure. Bird and Blease Pulmoflator ventilators are examples of pressure-cycled ventilators.

FLOW CYCLING

In flow-cycled ventilators, the cycling mechanism is determined by a critical flow rate. When the flow has fallen to the critical level, the inspiratory phase comes to a halt and the expiratory phase begins. Automatic-Vent and Bennett PR-2 ventilators are flow-cycled ventilators.

Expiratory Phase

Most ventilators operate as constant atmospheric pressure generators during the expiratory phase. Some ventilators, however, can generate negative pressure to facilitate expiration (negative end–expiratory pressure, or NEEP). This model is used when end–expiratory pressure is above atmospheric pressure. It should be remembered that NEEP may enhance closure of small airways and therefore may increase air-trapping. It is possible to facilitate expiration without using NEEP, by increasing the diameter or shortening the length of the ventilator tubing or by decreasing the flow rate.

Sometimes expiratory retard is used to prolong the expiratory phase. The purpose is to prevent the collapse of small airways. This effect can be obtained very simply by adding expiratory resistance to a constant atmospheric pressure generator. PEEP can be achieved by incorporating a water-filled column in the expiratory side of the circuit, adding a device to prevent the complete discharge of the exhalation valve, or including a spring-loaded valve. The alveolar pressure remains above the atmospheric pressure at end-expiration. The PEEP mechanism is built into almost all modern ventilators.

Changeover from Expiratory Phase to Inspiratory Phase

In almost all modern ventilators, the changeover from the expiratory phase to the inspiratory phase is time cycled or patient triggered, whichever occurs first.

Negative Pressure Ventilator

The only existing pediatric negative pressure ventilator available commercially is the "Isolette" Respiratory (Airshields Inc., Hatboro, PA). It consists of two plexiglass chambers. The head chamber is maintained at atmospheric pressure at all times, and the body chamber is connected to a vacuum motor. The pressure inside the body chamber is rendered negative to the degree chosen by the operator. During the expiratory phase, the body chamber may either return to the atmospheric pressure or be kept at a residual negative pressure of up to 10 cm H_2O. The advantage of a negative pressure ventilator is that there is no need for an endotracheal tube. Thus, acute and long-term upper airway complications that may arise from endotracheal intubation are avoided. Upper airway function remains intact, and there is no need for frequent airway suctioning, which may be harmful. Infants with RDS (respiratory distress syndrome) who are ventilated with the negative pressure ventilator seem to have a lower incidence of developing bronchopul-

monary dysplasia (BPD) or having abnormal residual chest radiographs. These potential advantages, however, are offset by various technical difficulties. Positioning of the infant must be exact and fixed, a requirement difficult to attain with an infant. Leaks around the neck iris and side ports are common occurrences, causing the infant to rock rhythmically in the direction of the longitudinal axis. This almost certainly has deleterious effects on the distribution of pulmonary and cerebral blood flows. To gain access to the body chamber, the vacuum supply must be turned off and the infant's CDP maintained by face mask. If the body chamber is opened with the vacuum operational, ambient air rushes in, cooling the infant. Another disadvantage is that the infant must be removed from the body chamber during radiographic procedures. Other technical difficulties are that the temperature in the head chamber is difficult to control and often creates temperature gradients between the head and the body, precise Fi_{O_2} is difficult to maintain in the head chamber, and there is no effective mechanism by which the ventilator can function as an assister.

Other Equipment

Patients with crush injury of the thorax, neuromuscular disease, infectious polyneuritis, brain damage, or cervical spinal cord injury may require special equipment during the acute, stabilizing, and rehabilitative phases of respiratory care. The paradoxic movement of the rib cage and diaphragm that is often present in these patients can be stabilized with a chest shell, a pneumatic jacket, or a pneumobelt with pressure sensors. Some patients prefer a rocking bed, which can be used for the same purpose.

High-frequency positive pressure ventilation (HFPPV) at insufflation frequencies of 60 to 100 per minute can maintain lung volumes with a small increase in intrapleural pressure; therefore, the undesirable effects on cardiorespiratory function associated with positive pressure ventilation are minimized. Currently, this technique is undergoing clinical trial.

Assisted Ventilation in the Non-Neonate

Common causes of respiratory insufficiency in preschool children include drug ingestions, hydrocarbon ingestion, and chest/CNS (central nervous system) injuries resulting from traffic accidents. In school-age children, the causes of respiratory insufficiency are more diverse and include status asthmaticus, drug ingestion, nosocomial pulmonary infection in immune deficiency states, Reye's syndrome, muscular dystrophy, other neuromuscular conditions, high spinal cord injury, near-drowning, severe smoke inhalation, crush injury, ARDS, pulmonary edema, CNS diseases, and pickwickian syndrome. Other conditions that occur occasionally include carbon monoxide poisoning, tetanus, and intraoperative or postoperative pulmonary complications.

In older children, the volume–pre-set, assister/controller machines are preferred (Bear, Bennett MA–I, MA–II, Emerson, and Engstrom). The volume–pre-set ventilators will deliver a pre-set volume during the inspiratory phase regardless of changes in resistance and compliance, but the machine does not compensate for volume lost by leaks that may be present in the machine or in the connecting apparatus. It is a common practice to ventilate the patient with tidal volumes that are slightly greater than the normal tidal volume. In most instances, the I:E ratio is set at 1:2 or 1:3. Shorter inspiratory time minimizes the harmful effect of positive pressure ventilation on the cardiovascular system. The use of PEEP is indicated when $(A–a)D_{O_2}$ is great. The range of end-expiratory pressure is usually between 5 and 15 cm H_2O. If PEEP fails to reduce $(A–a)D_{O_2}$, oxygen consumption can be reduced either pharmacologically (morphine sulfate, 0.1 mg per kg IV every 1 to 2 hours, diazepam, 0.2 to 0.5 mg per kg IV every 4 hours, or a muscle relaxant such as pancuronium bromide [Pavulon], 0.1 mg per kg IV every hour) or by the use of hypothermia. Weaning of an older child can be carried out more rationally than the trial and error method often used in weaning an infant. Simple physiologic measurements done at the bedside are valuable guides in determining the patient's readiness to tolerate the weaning process. Before the weaning process is begun, the child should be psychologically prepared. The process is explained to both the patient and his parents. Clinical preparation includes sound nutritional state, positive nitrogen balance, stable cardiovascular state, adequate respiratory muscle strength, normal ventilatory response to CO_2 and hypoxia (in patients with airway obstruction, obesity, and pickwickian syndrome), normal state of electrolyte balance and glucose metabolism, and normal or improved breathing pattern (in patients with high spinal cord injury who initially had paradoxic movement of the abdomen and thoracic cage). Weaning should be withheld until metabolic abnormalities have been corrected. The $F_{I_{O_2}}$ should be less than 0.5, the IMV rate should be less than 4 breaths per minute, and PEEP should be no greater than 10 cm H_2O before the process of weaning can be started.

Weaning can be attempted with a "T-piece," which delivers humidified gas enriched with oxygen to the patient's endotracheal tube. During the time when the patient breathes through the "T-piece," it is customary to increase $F_{I_{O_2}}$ by 0.1. The patient's minute volume should be greater than the sum flow of oxygen and entrained air to ensure the inhalation of prescribed $F_{I_{O_2}}$ without the danger of rebreathing CO_2 from the circuit. Tachypnea and cold sweats are signs of an unsuccessful trial.

SUMMARY

The following example illustrates the principles discussed in this chapter.

A 10-year-old boy is receiving controlled mechanical ventilation because of respiratory failure caused by an accident at a swimming pool. The following data have been collected:

Lung Compliance (C_L) = 0.1 L per cm H_2O
Airway resistance (Raw) = 14.0 cm H_2O per L per second
P_B = 760 mm Hg
$F_{I_{O_2}}$ = 0.5
Set tidal volume = 400 ml
I:E = 1:2
Rate = 15 breaths per minute
PEEP = 10 cm H_2O
Ventilator compliance (C_V) = 3 ml per cm H_2O
Peak pressure = 35 cm H_2O
Alveolar capillary O_2 content (C_{CO_2}) = 20 ml per 100 ml
Arterial O_2 content (C_{aO_2}) = 19 ml per 100 ml
Mixed venous O_2 content ($C_{V_{O_2}}$) = 14 ml per 100 ml
CO_2 tension in expired air ($P_{E_{CO_2}}$) = 36 mm Hg
O_2 tension in expired air ($P_{E_{O_2}}$) = 320 mm Hg
pHa = 7.30
PaO_2 = 80 mm Hg
Pa_{CO_2} = 60 mm Hg
Inspiratory time (Ti) = $1/3 \times 60/15$ = 1.33 seconds

Time constant (τ) (Airway resistance [Raw] × compliance) = 14.0×0.1 = 1.4 seconds
Volume absorbed by the ventilator (Ventilator compliance × Peak pressure) = 3×35 = 105 ml
Estimated tidal volume received by the patient (V_T) = $400 - 105$ ml = 295 ml

Minute ventilation (V_E) = 295 $\times$ 15 = 4.425 L per minute

Physiologic dead space (V_{Dphys}) = $V_T \times (Pa_{CO_2} - PE_{CO_2})/Pa_{CO_2}$ = 295 $\times$ (60 − 36)/ 60 = 118 ml

Alveolar ventilation $(\dot{V}_A)$ = (295 − 118) $\times$ 15 = 2.66 L per minute

V_D/V_T = 118/295 = 0.4

SUGGESTED READING

General

Comroe, J.H.: Physiology of Respiration, 2nd ed. Chicago, Year Book Medical Publishers, Inc., 1974.

Cotes, J.E.: Lung Function, 4th ed. Oxford, Blackwell Scientific Publications, 1979.

Heironimus, and Bageant, : Mechanical Artificial Ventilation, 3rd ed. Springfield, IL, Charles C Thomas, Publisher, 1977.

Murray, J.F.: The Normal Lung. Philadelphia, W.B. Saunders Company, 1976.

Mushin, Rendell-Baker, Thompson, and Mapleson, : Automatic Ventilation of the Lungs, 3rd ed. Oxford, Blackwell Scientific Publications, 1980.

Payne, and Bushman, : Artificial Ventilation. London, Academic Press, Inc., 1980.

Rottenborg, C.C.: Clinical Use of Mechanical Ventilation. Chicago, Year Book Medical Publishers, Inc., 1982.

Skyes, McNicol, and Campbell, : Respiratory Failure, 2nd ed. Oxford, Blackwell Scientific Publications, 1976.

West, J.B.: Respiratory Physiology, 2nd. ed. Baltimore, Williams & Wilkins, 1979.

Selected

Intermittent mandatory ventilation. Int. Anesthesiol. Clin. 18 (2): 1–189, 1980.

Problems with anesthetic and respiratory equipment. Int. Anesthesiol. Clin. 20 (3): 1–247, 1982.

Noninvasive Respiratory Monitoring

DANIEL A. NOTTERMAN, M.D.
MICHAEL A. GRAFF, M.D.

Noninvasive monitoring techniques provide information about organ and system function without disturbing anatomic barriers. These methods permit surveillance with little risk of injury and without pain. These devices are particularly valuable in the neonatal and pediatric intensive care units because of the difficulty and increased risk of establishing invasive monitoring lines in the small vessels of infants and children.

It is important to remember that the senses of the examining physician or nurse are the most highly adapted and, in many respects, are the most productive monitoring system. In a technically oriented era, one occasionally forgets the value of serial measurements of pulse, temperature, and respiratory rate or the perceived color, temperature, and perfusion of the patient's skin. These observations do not require complex or expensive instrumentation and must remain the foundation of patient care. However, in the critically ill patient, appropriate selection and adjustment of therapy may require a greater degree of precision than is afforded by the unaided senses of the examiner. Noninvasive systems can provide this added precision, with little danger or inconvenience to the patient.

In this chapter, methods of noninvasive respiratory monitoring are reviewed. Each method is used to supplant and supplement direct analysis of arterial blood. Included in this discussion are two methods of oxygen (O_2) analysis: transcutaneous oximetry and earlobe oximetry, and two methods of carbon dioxide (CO_2) analysis: transcutaneous CO_2 measurement and expired CO_2 measurement. Other noninvasive systems, such as the Ladd intracranial pressure transducer, pulse oximetry, and oscillometric blood pressure measuring devices, are reviewed elsewhere in this text (see Chapters 6, Invasive Hemodynamic Monitoring, and 12, Increased Intracranial Pressure).

TRANSCUTANEOUS OXIMETRY

Transcutaneous oxygen monitoring has evolved rapidly since its introduction to clinical practice in the past two decades. It is now a significant part of neonatal and pediatric intensive care.

These devices are usually based upon a Clark type polarographic electrode that contains a cathode (gold or platinum) and an anode. The electrode is incorporated into a sensing unit that also contains a heating element and a thermistor. These components are bathed in an electrolyte solution and separated from the skin surface by a thin plastic membrane that is semipermeable to oxygen. The sensing unit is affixed to the patient's skin, which is warmed by the heating element. Heating augments capillary blood flow and promotes diffusion of oxygen from the capillary to the skin surface. Oxygen at the skin surface penetrates the semipermeable membrane, which covers the electrode, enters the electrolyte bath, and is reduced at the cathode. This induces a current between the cathode and the anode. The magnitude of this current is proportional to the surface (or transcutaneous) partial pressure of oxygen. Under ideal circumstances, the partial pressure of transcutaneous oxygen ($P_{Tc}O_2$) is almost the same as the partial pressure of arterial oxygen (Pa_{O_2}).

Typically, the sensing unit is attached to a control/display module by a cable. Although details about products of different manufacturers differ, the essential features are similar. Controls include means for adjusting the zero point and the high O_2 reference point (typically, the ambient Pa_{O_2}). There is always a control for setting the skin-warming temperature and, usually, one for operating an integral alarm system. Most units permit direct digital display of the $P_{T_c}O_2$ as well as a display of the power output (absolute or relative) of the heating element. On most monitors, a strip chart recorder is included and makes a permanent record of the continuously measured $P_{T_c}O_2$.

Accurate measurements require attention to calibration of the electrode, placement of the sensing unit, and selection of an appropriate skin-warming temperature.

Calibration. The electrode must be calibrated before being used. This procedure should be performed with the sensing unit adjusted to the temperature that has been selected for the patient. Usually, calibration involves exposing the electrode to two known partial pressures of O_2 (zero and that of room air) and adjusting the $P_{T_c}O_2$ display to these values. Because details of the calibration procedure differ among the various devices, the procedure is not discussed in detail in this chapter.

Placement. The relationship between $P_{T_c}O_2$ and Pa_{O_2} is affected by the distance between the skin surface and the skin capillaries and by the nature of the intervening integument. The distance is determined by the thickness of the skin. In neonates and young infants, the skin of the abdomen and chest permit ready diffusion of oxygen. Placement of the sensing unit on either of these locations consistently yields a very close correspondence between $P_{T_c}O_2$ and Pa_{O_2} when the patient is hemodynamically stable. In older children, adolescents, and adults, the skin over these areas is thicker, and simultaneously measured Pa_{O_2} and $P_{T_c}O_2$ differ appreciably. Accuracy can be improved by placing the sensing unit on relatively thin areas of the skin (volar aspect of the forearm, inner thigh, forehead, and scrotum) and by using higher warming temperatures. Although these maneuvers improve results, older individuals still do not have the same agreement between $P_{T_c}O_2$ and Pa_{O_2} that is noted in neonates.

In all age groups, the *correlation* between $P_{T_c}O_2$ and Pa_{O_2} is excellent (greater than 0.9 in the "normal" range). However, in neonates, the $P_{T_c}O_2$ is about 95 percent of a simultaneously measured Pa_{O_2}. In adults, this figure is closer to 80 percent, ranging between 60 and 90 percent. In adults in shock, however, the $P_{T_c}O_2$ averages only 10% of the Pa_{O_2}. Thus, in older children, transcutaneous oximetry is not particularly useful as an index of absolute Pa_{O_2}; instead, the method is used to observe trends in the $P_{T_c}O_2$. Among individuals, these trends predict broad changes in Pa_{O_2}.

Temperature. The optimal skin-warming temperature is empirically determined for each patient. Typically, premature infants require a skin temperature of 43° to 43.5°, full-term infants require warming to 44°, and older children and adults require a skin temperature of 44° to 45°. Determining the optimal warming temperature in a particular patient can be somewhat burdensome, because the electrode is temperature sensitive and must be recalibrated whenever the warming temperature is changed. A convenient method of determining the optimal warming temperature is to calibrate the device at the anticipated temperature setting (using the values noted previously). The sensor is placed on the patient's skin, and the $P_{T_c}O_2$ is compared with a directly measured Pa_{O_2}. If there is not an acceptable agreement between these values, that is, if $P_{T_c}O_2$ is appreciably less than Pa_{O_2}, the warming temperature is increased by 0.5°. If the resulting increase in $P_{T_c}O_2$ is more than 10 mm Hg, the monitor should be used at the higher temperature, but it must first be recalibrated at that temperature.

It is important to use the lowest warming temperature that yields an acceptable concordance between $P_{T_c}O_2$ and Pa_{O_2}. This precaution is necessary to avoid burns. The likelihood of thermal injury is increased when excessive temperatures are used, when cutaneous blood perfusion is poor, and when the sensing unit location is not changed every 3 to 4 hours.

Optimal performance of the transcutaneous oximeter requires that the sensing unit surface be cleaned and polished frequently and that the electrode membrane be replaced periodically. The sensing unit should not be permitted to dangle by its cord—these devices are extremely sensitive and cannot tolerate careless treatment.

Clinical Application. Transcutaneous oximetry has become essential to the care of the critically ill newborn. Although its application to pediatric intensive care has lagged, use of these devices in the care of older infants and children is increasing.

In infants, transcutaneous oximetry permits continuous estimation of the Pa_{O_2}. Respiratory therapy can be adjusted as frequently as is needed to produce a constant, safe level of arterial oxygen. Studies at several neonatal centers indicate that apparently stable levels of oxygen are punctuated by periods of hypoxia and hyperoxia that are not detected by intermittent measurements of Pa_{O_2}. These transient changes can be detected by transcutaneous oximetry.

A major advantage is that the frequency of

arterial blood gas sampling can be reduced, thus limiting the volume of blood that is drawn. This may lead to a reduction in transfusion requirements and, potentially, in the incidence of transfusion-related illness.

Continuous measurement of $P_{Tc}O_2$ can improve nursing care. Many procedures such as suctioning the trachea lower Pa_{O_2}. In the past, this complication was not recognized until cyanosis or bradycardia indicated a critical reduction in Pa_{O_2}. Continuous measurement of $P_{Tc}O_2$ during this procedure allows the nurse to alter his or her technique appropriately.

In certain patients, measurement of $P_{Tc}O_2$ presents a more accurate view of baseline or average Pa_{O_2} than does intermittent arterial puncture. This is because arterial puncture is a painful procedure that elicits crying or breath-holding. These responses adversely affect the Pa_{O_2} (Fig. 4–1).

Continuous measurement of $P_{Tc}O_2$ is used to detect apnea. During these episodes, the Pa_{O_2} falls earlier than the heart rate. Thus, a transcutaneous oximeter can signal the occurrence of significant apnea before the event is detected by a heart rate alarm. Indeed, current opinion is that apnea is not harmful and may not warrant therapy if it is not associated with a fall in the Pa_{O_2}. Thus, in apnea of prematurity, continuous measurement of $P_{Tc}O_2$ permits earlier intervention when indicated but forestalls therapy when periodic apnea is not associated with hypoxia.

In older infants and children, the transcutaneous oximeter is also used to refine respiratory therapy and nursing care and to reduce the frequency of blood gas sampling. These systems also serve as back-up respirator alarms and contribute to the surveillance function of the intensive care unit. Even though these devices have been useful in detecting the magnitude and direction of changes in the Pa_{O_2} of individual patients, their use has been impeded by the wide discrepancy between Pa_{O_2} and $P_{Tc}O_2$.

Transcutaneous oximeters have been used to indicate changes in cutaneous perfusion. Perfusion of the skin may be reduced during episodes of shock, hypotension, external cooling, or pressor therapy. This reduction causes the measured $P_{Tc}O_2$ to fall (widened $Pa_{O_2}/P_{Tc}O_2$ difference). In addition, the output of the heating unit decreases because the decreased blood flow reduces the external heat necessary to maintain a particular skin temperature. These changes can be displayed and recorded by the oximeter. Some investigators believe that these perturbations provide insight into the condition of the cutaneous microcirculation and the adequacy of oxygen delivery to peripheral tissues. Although some clinicians report favorably on the usefulness of these indices, further laboratory and clinical investigation is necessary before alterations in $P_{Tc}O_2$ or sensor heating output can be used routinely as a guide to therapy.

In summary, measurement of $P_{Tc}O_2$ in neonates and young infants provides the physician and nurse with a continuous and noninvasive estimate of Pa_{O_2}. In most cases, this estimate is reasonably accurate. This measurement refines respiratory therapy and permits prompt detection of intermittent deviations in Pa_{O_2}. In older infants and children, the $P_{Tc}O_2$ may not indicate Pa_{O_2} accurately. Even so, the correlation between Pa_{O_2} and $P_{Tc}O_2$ is good, and the method

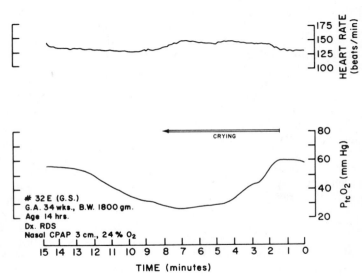

Figure 4–1. Transcutaneous PO_2 recorded simultaneously with heart rate in a crying infant. (Recorded at the Human Infant Physiology Lab, College of Physicians and Surgeons, New York)

can be used to detect trends and to alert critical care staff to abrupt reductions in Pa_{O_2}.

EARLOBE OXIMETERS

Earlobe oximeters determine the oxygen saturation of hemoglobin by measuring the absorption of light as it passes through the earlobe. An earpiece, which contains a light source and a light detector, as well as components that warm the skin and measure skin temperature, is placed over the external ear. Known wavelengths of light originate from the source and pass through the capillaries of the earlobe to the detector. The degree to which different wavelengths of light are absorbed by blood is related to the percentage of hemoglobin occupied by oxygen. The oximeter measures this absorption, makes the appropriate calculations, and derives the hemoglobin oxygen saturation (Sa_{O_2}). This value is displayed on the front panel of the oximeter.

These systems have been available for several years and have been widely used in the pulmonary function laboratory and in adult intensive care units. Until recently, however, the earpieces were cumbersome and bulky. They were uncomfortable during prolonged use and almost impossible to apply to small children or infants. Recently, a new type of oximeter was introduced, and the bulky earpiece of previous configurations was replaced with a small, light-weight earpiece that can be placed on the ear of a small infant (B10X IIA Earlobe Oximeter). Application of the earpiece and calibration of the monitor are simple procedures and require less than 2 minutes.

The earpiece can be moved from patient to patient without elaborate cleaning or application procedures. Unlike transcutaneous oximetry, no stabilization period is needed prior to measurement. Thus, it is possible for a single earlobe oximeter to service several patients in sequence. Alternatively, the device can be used to display and record Sa_{O_2} continuously in a single patient.

In general, earlobe oximeters are quite accurate when compared with spectrophotometric analysis of blood samples. Poor cutaneous perfusion interferes with earlobe oximetry, which may limit the use of these devices in children with shock or severe congestive heart failure. The accuracy of the technique is reduced when carboxyhemoglobin or jaundice is evident and in one study when saturations were less than 65 percent.

Because the earpiece contains a warming ele-

ment, there is a possibility of thermal injury to the sensitive skin of infants. During continuous use with infants, the physician or nurse should examine the earlobe frequently in order to detect hyperemia, if present.

The shape of the hemoglobin oxygen dissociation curve limits the use of these devices in certain patients. When the Pa_{O_2} is greater than 85 mm Hg, the Sa_{O_2} is greater than 95 percent. Further increases in Pa_{O_2} produce minimal additional increases in Sa_{O_2}. Only when the Pa_{O_2} is less than 60 to 70 mm Hg are changes in Pa_{O_2} reflected in substantial changes in Sa_{O_2}. Thus, measurement of Sa_{O_2} is not particularly valuable when the Pa_{O_2} is expected to remain above 75 mm Hg or when detection of hyperoxia is crucial, as in neonates. Earlobe oximeters are valuable for continuous noninvasive monitoring of patients who maintain a Pa_{O_2} of 60 to 70 mm Hg or less, including children with cyanotic congenital heart disease and chronic pulmonary disease. In addition, earlobe oximetry is used to supplement and, in some cases, replace arterial blood gas monitoring during the care of children with acute diseases that may be complicated by hypoxemia. In such cases, measurement of Sa_{O_2} can be used instead of Pa_{O_2} to guide oxygen or ventilator therapy. Like transcutaneous systems, earlobe oximeters provide a means for evaluating the adverse effects of various nursing and medical procedures on oxygen content and serve as a back-up respirator alarm system. It is important to remember that the precise relationship between Pa_{O_2} and Sa_{O_2} is affected by several factors such as blood pH, temperature, and 2,3-DPG content.

Compared with transcutaneous oximeters, earlobe oximeters are easier to set up and apply. Their use requires considerably less technical sophistication and almost no training. In older infants and children, earlobe oximeters are more accurate than transcutaneous monitors. A potential disadvantage is that earlobe oximeters measure Sa_{O_2} rather than Pa_{O_2}. Thus, the technique is relatively insensitive to changes in Pa_{O_2} that occur along the "normal" range. Because detection of hyperoxia is crucial in neonatal care, earlobe devices are not suitable for use with these patients. In older patients, earlobe oximeters may be preferable to transcutaneous devices.

TRANSCUTANEOUS CARBON DIOXIDE MEASUREMENT

In a manner analogous to transcutaneous oximetry, it is possible to measure the partial pressure of CO_2 at the skin surface (Ps_{CO_2}, or $P_{Tc}O_2$). A sensing unit incorporates a pH-sensitive glass electrode and an adjacent silver chloride reference electrode covered with a semi-permeable membrane and attached to a servo-controlled heating unit.

The skin surface is warmed to 44° to 45° to augment skin capillary blood flow. Carbon dioxide diffuses from these capillaries through the membrane and into the electrolyte solution that bathes the electrode. The concentration of hydrogen ions in this solution increases, causing a change in the electrode current. This change is proportional to the logarithm of $P_{Tc}CO_2$.

In theory, the $P_{Tc}CO_2$ is related in a consistent way to the Pa_{CO_2}. In practice, the method of measurement imposes several limitations. For instance, application of heat, which is necessary to ensure adequate capillary blood flow, increases the $P_{Tc}CO_2$. At a skin temperature of 44° to 45°, $P_{Tc}CO_2$ is 1.37 times the Pa_{CO_2} measured at 37°. The manufacturers of these systems have devised methods to reduce the magnitude of this type of error. These methods involve imparting a compensatory error during calibration.

As of this writing, limited clinical studies have been performed using $P_{Tc}CO_2$ monitors. Some investigators have shown poor agreement between $P_{Tc}CO_2$ and Pa_{CO_2} under several frequently occurring clinical events, such as shock and anemia. Other deficiencies include a long response time, relatively high warming temperatures, and cumbersome calibration procedures.

Recently, however, technical improvements in electrode design and in processing of the electrode signal have resulted in a more consistent relationship between $P_{Tc}CO_2$ and Pa_{CO_2}. Of note is that these improved monitors continue to require frequent calibration (at each site change) to preserve this accuracy.

EXPIRED CARBON DIOXIDE ANALYSIS

Expired CO_2 analysis has been available for many years and provides an estimate of Pa_{CO_2}. The underlying principle is that the partial pressure of CO_2 in exhaled gas at the end of exhalation (end–tidal CO_2, PET_{CO_2}) corresponds to the partial pressure of CO_2 in alveolar gas (PA_{CO_2}). Ideally, PA_{CO_2} is equal to the partial pressure of CO_2 in mixed pulmonary venous blood (Pv_{CO_2}), which is closely related to the Pa_{CO_2}. Therefore, measurement of PET_{CO_2} provides an estimate of Pa_{CO_2}. In most cases, this estimate is fairly accurate; usually, the PET_{CO_2}, is about 5 mm Hg greater than the Pa_{CO_2}.

There are several methods of determining PET_{CO_2}. *Capnography* has become the favored method in the intensive care unit and can be applied to patients with or without an endotracheal tube. Several manufacturers produce bedside capnometers, which measure the concentration of CO_2 in the patient's breath by means of infrared spectroscopy. *Sidestream* type analysers sample the patient's respiratory gas by means of a small plastic tube that connects the measurement chamber of the capnograph to the proximal end of the endotracheal tube or to a mouthpiece through which the non-intubated patient is requested to breathe. A pump in the capnometer draws respiratory gases from the patient into the sample chamber. *Mainstream* analysers are placed directly in the path of the respiratory gases, usually at the proximal end of the endotracheal tube.

During inspiration, the concentration of CO_2 in the gas sample falls almost to zero as fresh gas is conveyed to the patient. During exhalation, the concentration of CO_2 rises toward a plateau (not always detected in children) as alveolar gas moves up the tracheobronchial tree and out the mouth or endotracheal tube. Thereafter, the concentration of CO_2 remains at or close to this plateau concentration until inspiration occurs. As fresh gas enters the circuit, the concentration of CO_2 declines. The point of inflection is taken to denote the end of expiration, and the concentration of CO_2 at this point is termed the *end–expiratory,* or *end–tidal CO_2 concentration*. Ideally, the end–tidal CO_2 concentration is equal to the alveolar gas CO_2 concentration. Because alveolar gas is in equilibrium with pulmonary venous blood, or the partial pressure of CO_2 in the alveolar fraction of the expired respiratory gas should correspond to the partial pressure of CO_2 in mixed pulmonary venous blood.

These measurements are made over several respiratory cycles or continuously, if desired. The rise and fall of expiratory CO_2 values inscribes a square wave that can be preserved by a strip chart recorder. This graph is termed a *capnogram* (Fig. 4–2). The PET_{CO_2} is determined by noting the plateau value just prior to the inspiratory decline in CO_2. Monitors that electronically detect the inflection point and compute the PET_{CO_2} are available. This value is displayed on an analogue or digital readout. On some instruments, the CO_2 is displayed as a percent concentration (% CO_2); on others, it is displayed as PET_{CO_2}.

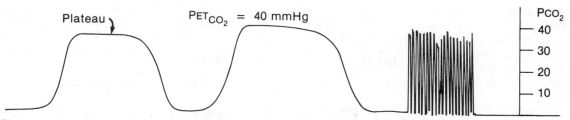

Figure 4.2. Capnogram recorded from a healthy subject breathing room air. The respiratory rate is 19 breaths per minute; Pa_{CO_2} = 35 mmHg. *Left*, chart speed is 25 mm per second, and characteristics of each breath can be analysed. P_{CO_2} of expired air rises to a plateau value and falls as inspiration begins. *Right*, chart speed is 25 mm per minute. The height of the peaks corresponds to the $P_{ET_{CO_2}}$. In this individual, $P_{ET_{CO_2}}$ = 35 to 40 mmHg.

Under some circumstances, the measured end–tidal CO_2 does not correspond to the Pa_{CO_2}. When alveolar ventilation is excessive relative to alveolar capillary blood flow, the PA_{CO_2} is less than the Pa_{CO_2}. In this situation, $P_{ET_{CO_2}}$ will underestimate Pa_{CO_2}. This arises in the case of a pulmonary embolus, when there is a large right-to-left shunt, and when pulmonary blood flow is acutely reduced by a fall in cardiac output.

Extreme reductions in tidal volume may result in the device sensing tracheal gas, even at end-expiration. When this occurs, sampled alveolar gas is diluted and the measured $P_{ET_{CO_2}}$ is lower than the PA_{CO_2} or Pa_{CO_2}. This anomaly is noted when tension pneumothorax impairs ventilation and when ventilator settings are grossly inadequate for the patient's size and medical condition. Indeed, successful reduction of a tension pneumothorax is signified by an increase in $P_{ET_{CO_2}}$ and a corresponding decrease in Pa_{CO_2}.

Technical artifacts may factitiously reduce the $P_{ET_{CO_2}}$. Chief among these is an inappropriately high aspiration flow rate in a small patient when using a sidestream analyser. This causes contamination of alveolar gas with fresh gas. Other technical problems include plugging of the plastic tubing with mucus and other debris and contamination of the measuring cell with condensed water vapor.

Clinical Applications

Capnography lends itself to a variety of applications in the pediatric intensive care unit and is valuable whenever frequent or continuous estimation of the Pa_{CO_2} is desirable.

During Mechanical Ventilation. The monitor is connected to the proximal end of the endotracheal tube, producing a continuous display of $P_{ET_{CO_2}}$. In addition to a digital or an analogue display of $P_{ET_{CO_2}}$, a capnogram is generated. Inspection of this record provides insight into qualitative aspects of ventilation such as sigh frequency, spontaneous breathing frequency, adequacy of muscle paralysis, and alveolar hypoventilation. The $P_{ET_{CO_2}}$ can be used to titrate ventilator therapy, to calculate V_D/V_T (in conjunction with measured Pa_{CO_2}), and to observe the effect of various manipulations (PEEP, fluid loading, and pressor support) on Pa_{CO_2}.

During Spontaneous Breathing. It is often desirable to obtain frequent or continuous estimates of Pa_{CO_2} in spontaneously breathing patients. This category includes patients who have required intubation for airway protection (epiglottitis) and those whose gas exchange is precarious but who have not merited intubation and ventilation (severe status asthmaticus). The technique is invaluable during forced hyperventilation, as during therapy for cerebral edema, when minute-to-minute titration of the Pa_{CO_2} is necessary.

As a Ventilator Monitor/Alarm. Continuous measurement of $P_{ET_{CO_2}}$ facilitates rapid detection of ventilator malfunction, endotracheal tube plugging, or disruption of the ventilator/patient gas circuit.

As a Cardiorespiratory Monitor. As previously noted, changes in $P_{ET_{CO_2}}$ occur during several kinds of disturbance, including pulmonary embolus, tension pneumothorax, acute reductions in cardiac output, and alterations in the ratio of dead space to total ventilation.

SUMMARY

Of the four noninvasive monitoring techniques reviewed in this chapter, at present three are clinically important: transcutaneous oximetry, earlobe oximetry, and expired carbon dioxide analysis. Each of these methods provides accurate information about gas exchange. Because these methods are noninvasive, they are practically risk free. To the extent that these techniques displace invasive blood gas sampling, they will serve the purpose of reducing the chance of iatrogenic injury during critical care.

A second advantage of the methods discussed in this chapter is that each permits continuous evaluation of therapy. One premise of intensive care is that critically ill patients are uniquely susceptible to fluctuations in organ system function. Continuous surveillance holds the promise that these fluctuations can be detected and treated before they induce more serious, secondary disturbances. In some cases, the methods outlined in this chapter can replace invasive monitoring. However, children who are seriously ill will require information that is available only through invasive catheterization and by blood gas analysis. In these individuals, noninvasive systems supplement invasive methods by providing continuous information.

SUGGESTED READING

Chaudhary, B.A., and Burki, N.K.: Ear oximetry in clinical practice. Am. Rev. Respir. Dis. 117:173, 1978.

Hazinski, T., and Severinghaus, J.: Transcutaneous analysis of arterial PCO_2. Med. Instrum. 16:150, 1982.

Huch, A., Huch, R., and Lucey, J.F. (eds.): Continuous Transcutaneous Blood Gas Monitoring, National Foundation of March of Dimes, Birth Defects: Original Article Series, Vol. XV. New York, Alan R. Liss, Inc., 1979.

Kalenda, Z.: Equipment for capnography. Br. J. Clin. Equip. 5:180, 1980.

Rebuck, A.S., Chapman, K.R., and D'Urzo, A.: The accuracy and response characteristics of a simplified ear oximeter. Chest 83:860, 1983.

Application of Echocardiography in the Pediatric Intensive Care Unit

ROBERT A. BOXER, M.D.
MICHAEL A. LaCORTE, M.D.

Echocardiography is a valuable noninvasive test that allows the physician to accurately evaluate cardiac anatomy and the effect of disease states on the cardiac system. This procedure can be performed in a short period of time (15 minutes), with no significant morbidity or interference in the clinical state of the patient. New techniques in echocardiography have centered on the two-dimensional imaging of the cardiac structures. These images are recorded on videotape format and are available for instant replay with stop-frame capability.

This chapter discusses the use of two-dimensional echocardiography in the management of infants and children in the pediatric intensive care unit. The techniques of obtaining a two-dimensional echocardiogram are beyond the scope of this chapter; for this information, the reader is referred to general textbooks on this subject.

In the pediatric intensive care unit, certain clinical situations arise in which the use of echocardiography would significantly aid in the diagnosis and treatment of a patient. The clinical states in which echocardiography have been valuable include the diagnosis of pericardial effusions, the use of contrast echocardiography, and the diagnosis of bacterial endocarditis.

PERICARDIAL EFFUSIONS

One of the first applications of echocardiography was the use of this technique in the diagnosis of pericardial effusions. Normally, the pericardium is adherent to the epicardium of the anterior and posterior surfaces of the heart;

thus, in normal patients, the pericardial space is only a potential space that is not visualized on the echocardiogram. As pericardial fluid accumulates, there is progressive separation of the pericardium from the epicardium. The fluid usually collects first in the posterior pericardial space behind the left ventricle (Fig. 5–1). With progressively larger pericardial effusions, there is also fluid accumulation in the anterior pericardial space, that is, between the anterior chest wall and the right ventricular free wall. Exact quantitation of pericardial fluid is inaccurate. However, in general, with progressively larger pericardial effusions, there is first an effusion posterior to the heart and, as more fluid accumulates, an anterior effusion also develops. When there is posterior pericardial fluid accumulation, it occurs posterior to the left ventricle and usually ends at the level of the left atrial-to-ventricular junction, at which point the pericardium is bound to the left atrial wall by the pulmonary veins. The presence of a large pericardial effusion, that is, anterior and posterior with the heart "swinging" in the pericardial sac, is supportive evidence of the diagnosis of cardiac tamponade. However, the firm diagnosis of this condition is dependent upon the clinical findings of hypotension, pulsus paradoxus, muffled heart tones, and electrocardiographic changes.

In the pediatric intensive care unit, the diagnosis of a pericardial effusion becomes important when a patient presents with a large cardiac silhouette on a chest x-ray examination, diffuse EKG changes suggestive of pericardial disease such as pulsus paradoxus, signs of myocardial dysfunction with cardiomegaly, dif-

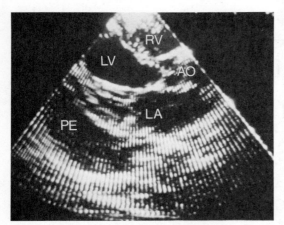

Figure 5–1. A large pericardial effusion is located posterior to the left ventricle. (LV = left ventricle, RV = right ventricle, AO = aorta, LA = left atrium, PE = pericardial effusion)

fuse edema, fever of unexplained origin, muffled heart tones, or unexplained hypotension.

CONTRAST ECHOCARDIOGRAPHY

Contrast echocardiography is a recent application of the echocardiographic technique that permits the visualization of blood flow in the various cardiac chambers. This technique is helpful in diagnosing intracardiac right-to-left shunts and, occasionally, left-to-right shunts. Quantitation of shunts is not accurate by this technique.

This procedure requires the rapid injection in an intravenous site of a small volume (1 to 2 ml) of saline, dextrose solution, or the patient's own blood. While the injection is being made, a simultaneous two-dimensional echocardiogram is obtained. The rapid, forceful injection of solution into the venous system produces dense echos or cavitations in the right heart chambers and pulmonary artery. These cavitations are normally filtered out in the pulmonary capillary bed and, consequently, are not visualized in the left heart structures, that is, the left atrium, the left ventricle, and the aorta. When there is a right-to-left intracardiac shunt, there is movement of blood from the right heart to the left heart either at the atrial, ventricular, or great vessel level, depending upon the pathologic state. If there is a right-to-left intracardiac shunt present, these dense echos or cavitations will be seen to enter the left heart at the site of the anatomic shunt in the heart. For instance, if there is a right-to-left shunt across an atrial communication, the contrast echocardiogram will reveal the movement of echo contrast from the right atrium into the left atrium (Fig. 5–2). If there is a right-to-left shunt through a ventricular septal defect, there will be movement of echo contrast from the right ventricle to the left ventricle through a ventricular septal defect.

Left-to-right intracardiac shunts can sometimes be noted with contrast echocardiography. However, this technique is more invasive, because it requires placement of a left atrial line through which the contrast injections would have to be made.

In the pediatric intensive care unit, contrast echocardiography is helpful when the etiology

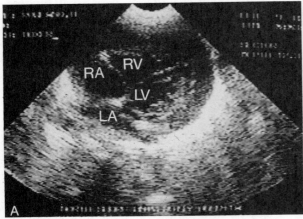
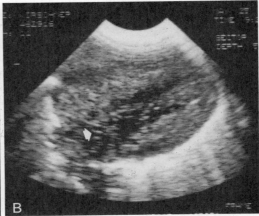

Figure 5–2. *A,* Subxyphoid two-dimensional echocardiogram, revealing all 4 cardiac chambers in this newborn with hypoxemia. (RA = right atrium, LA = left atrium, RV = right ventricle, LV = left ventricle) *B,* Contrast echocardiogram with same view as in *A.* With injection of 1 cc dextrose solution into a peripheral vein, there is appearance of echo contrast in the right atrium with crossing of contrast into the left atrium (*arrow*) through the foramen ovale. Echo contrast is also seen in the right ventricle.

of low arterial PO_2 is unclear, especially when the patient is receiving high inspired oxygen concentrations. In some critically ill patients who require ventilatory assistance, high oxygen administration may be needed to maintain satisfactory arterial blood gases. However, in some instances, even with 100 percent oxygen administration, arterial desaturation may be noted. On these occasions, intracardiac or intrapulmonary shunting may be present and echocardiography can be of great value in assessing the etiology of hypoxemia. Occasionally, in some patients with severe lung disease, high right atrial pressures may result in opening of the foramen ovale with right-to-left atrial shunting through this communication. This shunting can be seen on a contrast echocardiogram. The injection of 1 to 2 ml of saline, dextrose solution, or the patient's own blood into a peripheral IV will result in the presentation of contrast echos in the right atrium. Shunting across the foramen ovale can be demonstrated with the contrast bubbles appearing on the left side of the heart, indicating an intracardiac right-to-left shunt. These studies are particularly useful when there is unexplained arterial hypoxemia or in patients who have undergone open-heart surgery and may have residual defects at the atrial or ventricular levels.

BACTERIAL ENDOCARDITIS

Two-dimensional echocardiography can be of great diagnostic use in localizing vegetations in patients with endocarditis. Vegetations, in general, are highly echogenic, thereby resulting in the appearance of dense, abnormally thickened echos on the cardiac structures involved in the infectious process. In as many as 80 percent of patients with culture-proven endocarditis, a vegetation can be detected and localized with two-dimensional echocardiography.

In patients with cyanotic heart disease, especially tetralogy of fallot, aortic stenosis, ventricular septal defect, or prosthetic heart valves, vegetations are usually readily detectable by echocardiography (Fig. 5–3). However, in cyanotic children with aortic-to-pulmonary shunts, vegetations may not be visualized, because the infectious process often occurs on the pulmonary artery side of the shunt, which is outside the heart in the field of the echocardiographic study.

In the pediatric intensive care unit, echocardiography may play an important role in the evaluation of a child with fever of unknown

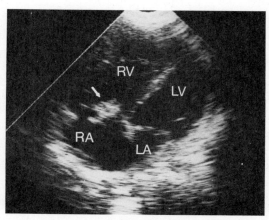

Figure 5–3. Four-chamber two-dimensional echocardiogram of a child with a small ventricular–septal defect, persistent fever, and positive blood culture for *Streptococcus viridans*. There is a prominent vegetation on the tricuspid valve (*arrow*). (RA = right atrium, LA = left atrium, RV = right ventricle, LV = left ventricle)

origin. Bacterial endocarditis must be highly suspected in a child with heart disease and a persistent fever, unexplained anemia, or hematuria. In addition to being useful in diagnosing bacterial endocarditis in patients with congenital or acquired heart disease, the echocardiogram is also of value in patients with fever of unknown origin, in whom indwelling intracardiac catheters have been placed for alimentation. Vegetations related to the indwelling catheters can be localized with two-dimensional echocardiography.

VENTRICULAR FUNCTION

In patients with heart failure owing to primary cardiac disease or in patients with frank cardiogenic shock owing to sepsis or other etiologies, the echocardiogram can provide a rapid noninvasive means of following cardiac function. An M-mode echocardiogram at the level of the left ventricle will provide a shortening fraction of the left ventricle. This fraction is determined by taking the difference in the diastolic and systolic dimension of the left ventricular cavity and dividing by the diastolic diameter.

$$LVID_d - LVID_s/LVID_d$$
$$normal = 0.30-0.36$$

Two dimensional echocardiography provides a more complete view of left ventricular wall motion and can also provide serial data concerning cardiac function.

SUGGESTED READING

Goldberg, S.J., Allen, H.D., and Sahn, D.J.: Pediatric and Adolescent Echocardiography. Chicago, Year Book Medical Publishers, Inc., 1980.

Kavey, R.E., Frank, D.M., Blackman, M.S., et al.: Two-dimensional echocardiographic assessment of bacterial endocarditis in children. 51st Annual Meeting American Academy of Pediatrics, section on Cardiology, October, 1982.

Sahn, D.J., Allen, H.D., George, W., et al.: The utility of contrast echocardiographic techniques in the care of critically ill infants with cardiac and pulmonary disease. Circulation 56:959, 1977.

6

Invasive Hemodynamic Monitoring

DANIEL A. NOTTERMAN, M.D.

Invasive monitoring techniques are used to secure rapid, accurate, and continuous aquisition of physiologic data. These techniques depend upon the introduction of a suitable sensing device into a body space. Although invasive devices thereby produce at least minimal iatrogenic injury, when used cautiously and properly they provide essential information with little risk of serious complication.

Developments in invasive monitoring have lagged in application to pediatric critical care. In part, this reflects the need for miniaturizing, or "scaling-down," equipment that is designed for adult patients. A second factor has been the reluctance of pediatricians to apply these techniques to their critically ill patients. This reluctance usually derives from an unfounded belief that invasive monitoring is "too intrusive" for infants and small children. This prejudice is regrettable, because it may lead to inadequate and substandard care. Instituting hemodynamic monitoring in adults who are critically ill is a routine measure. Yet children who are equally as sick are often managed without the benefit of direct hemodynamic information. The governing principle in critical care must be that the intensity of monitoring escalates with the severity of the illness. Indeed, because the specific physical signs of hemodynamic disturbance become less obvious with decreasing age and size, invasive monitoring may be more likely to provide information that alters therapy in the infant than in the adult.

This chapter reviews currently available invasive techniques, noting their indications and complications. This is not intended as a procedure manual; consequently, the reader should consult one of the suggested readings for information relating to technical aspects of placing these devices in situ. Specific hemodynamic disturbances are not discussed at length in this chapter. The reader should consult the relevant chapters in this book for that information.

ARTERIAL MONITORING

An arterial monitoring system consists of an indwelling arterial catheter attached to fluid-filled tubing. The tubing is interfaced with a transducer from which an electrical signal that is proportionate to the arterial pressure wave is derived. This signal is used to display a pressure waveform on an oscilloscope as well as systolic and diastolic blood pressures.

Types of Catheters

Arterial catheters are composed of soft plastic (usually Teflon). Frequently used configurations include both catheter-over-needle (e.g., Angiocath) and needle-over-catheter sets (e.g., Intracath). Some physicians use the Seldinger technique, in which a guidewire is inserted through a thin-wall needle into the artery. The needle is removed, and the catheter is threaded over the guidewire.

A catheter-over-needle configuration (Angiocath) is most suitable for peripheral sites such as the radial artery. No. 22-gauge (1 to 1.5 inch) catheters are used for infants and small children. No. 20-gauge catheters are used for larger children and adults. Because the rate of arterial thrombus is related to the size of the catheter, it is unwise to use devices larger than 20 gauge in a peripheral artery. Catheters smaller than 22 gauge usually do not yield an adequate pressure waveform.

When it is necessary to place a catheter in a more centrally located artery (femoral or axillary), a needle-over-catheter device (Intracath) or the Seldinger technique is used. The correct size catheter is 19 or 20 gauge. Smaller catheters produce a damped waveform and are prone to occlusion by clot; larger catheters increase the probability of vessel thrombosis.

Monitoring Sites

Several different sites are used for arterial cannulation: radial artery, brachial artery, axillary artery, dorsal pedis or posterior tibeal arteries, superficial temporal artery, and the femoral artery. In neonates, the umbilical arteries are commonly used.

The ideal monitoring site has several characteristics: 1) adequate vessel size to accomodate a 20- or 22-gauge catheter; 2) sufficient collateral blood flow to the limb, in case of thrombosis; 3) proximity to the central circulation so that, in most cases, the measured blood pressure is reasonably close to the central aortic blood pressure; and 4) ease of access. Of the enumerated sites, the radial artery usually satisfies these conditions most closely.

The *radial artery* is accessible, and the limb can be easily and securely immobilized. Collateral blood flow through the ulnar artery is usually adequate to perfuse the entire hand (but should be tested by the Allen test prior to catheterization). The vessel is sufficiently large to accept a 22-gauge catheter, even in a premature infant. In most cases, the blood pressure that is measured in the radial artery is similar to the central aortic pressure. For these reasons, the radial artery is usually the preferred vessel. When there is intense vasoconstriction or critical reduction of blood flow, the radial artery pressure may be lower than the central aortic pressure. Additionally, the risk of catheter-induced ischemia and injury to the hand and forearm is increased. Under these conditions, an alternate site, the femoral or axillary artery, should be selected.

The *dorsalis pedis* and *posterior tibial* arteries satisfy many of the criteria for a monitoring site. However, recent evidence suggests that in some children there may be a serious discrepancy between central aortic blood pressure and that recorded in the foot. Until this issue is resolved, the pedal arteries should be used circumspectly when the indication for catheterization is blood pressure monitoring.

The *brachial artery* should not be catheterized, because collateral blood flow is poor. Occlusion of this vessel can result in catastrophic loss of the forearm and hand.

The *axillary artery* is a large vessel with excellent collateral blood flow. Pressures recorded are generally representative of central aortic pressure. Technical aspects of insertion are somewhat cumbersome, and the site has not gained widespread acceptance in pediatric practice, although it may do so in the future.

The *femoral artery* is frequently used as a monitoring site. The vessel is large, accessible, and proximate to the aorta. Even in infants, it will accept a 19-gauge catheter. A concern in using the femoral artery is the poor collateral blood flow around it; occlusion of the vessel compromises circulation to the leg. There is a danger of contaminating the catheter with perineal flora, and consequently, the rate of infection seems to be somewhat higher at this site. Many authorities mention the possibility of penetrating the hip joint of small children during insertion, thereby inducing septic arthritis or aseptic necrosis of the femoral head. Although this complication has been reported, it is a technical failure and should not occur with properly trained operators.

In many cases, the femoral artery is a satisfactory alternate to the radial artery. It is not generally the vessel of choice; in special circumstances, principally low-flow states with vasoconstriction, it may yield a more accurate blood pressure recording than the radial artery, with a greater margin of safety. Of course, the femoral artery will not provide accurate measurement of blood pressure when coarctation is present.

The *superficial temporal artery* has also been used as a site of catheterization. This artery is easy to palpate, and the scalp is provided with rich collateral blood flow. However, recent evidence indicates that temporal artery catheterization is associated with infarction of the temporal lobe of the brain, probably as a result of retrograde embolization (vide infra). The seriousness of this complication contraindicates use of the temporal artery for monitoring.

To summarize: the radial artery is usually the preferred artery for catheterization. Special circumstances, such as extreme vasoconstriction and reduced arterial perfusion, sometimes dictate the use of a larger, more central vessel, such as the femoral or axillary arteries. In my opinion, catheterization of the brachial or temporal arteries is contraindicated. The dorsalis pedis and posterior tibial arteries provide a safe location, but the reliability of blood pressure measurements made from these vessels has been questioned.

Indications

There are two broad and several specific indications for arterial catheter placement. The broad indications include direct blood pressure monitoring and arterial blood gas measurement.

Direct Blood Pressure Monitoring

It is neither necessary nor desirable to insert an arterial catheter in every patient in whom blood pressure measurement is indicated. Non-invasive instruments, ranging in sophistication from cuff sphygmomanometers to devices that detect blood pressure using oscillometric (Dinamap) or Doppler methods, provide accurate, serial measurements, even in neonates. However, in situations in which there are increases in vascular resistance or decreases in arterial blood flow, these indirect methods are inherently inaccurate. The direction of error is such as to indicate a lower blood pressure than actually exists, and in this context, an arterial catheter is necessary. Other indications include use of pressor agents, vasodilator therapy (afterload reduction), and severe hypertension. A patient in whom the hemodynamic status is rapidly changing or one who is receiving therapy that is likely to induce such changes is a candidate for continuous direct blood pressure recording. Additionally, a continuous display of arterial pressure waveform ensures prompt detection of electrical–mechanical dissociation.

Arterial Blood Gas Measurement

The second major indication for placing an arterial catheter is repeated blood gas analysis. Specific threshhold criteria, in terms of frequency of blood gas determination or concentration of inspired oxygen, are not useful. Any child in whom several measurements must be made in a relatively short period of time will benefit from an indwelling catheter. The physician should definitely insert an arterial catheter in a child who requires acute respiratory support other than a relatively low concentration of oxygen.

Miscellaneous Indications

An indwelling arterial catheter is necessary to aspirate blood samples for cardiac output determination using indocyanine green dye. For most applications, this technique has been supplanted by the thermodilution method. Other indications include insertion of indwelling oxygen and pH electrodes, exchange transfusion, and hemodialysis.

Complications

The complications associated with arterial catheters are predictable. They include bacteremia, thrombosis, embolization, hemorrhage, mechanical injury to contiguous structure, and arterial spasm leading to ischemia.

Infection can be reduced by strict attention to asepsis during insertion. The dressing should be changed daily, and the insertion site should be inspected for evidence of inflammation. Those parts of the transducing system that are in contact with the bloodstream, including all tubing, all connecting devices, the transducing pressure dome, and the flush solution, should be changed daily or at least every 48 hours.

It appears that the incidence of infection increases after the catheter has been in situ for more than 3 days. Therefore, it is prudent to limit the duration of catheterization at any one site to this interval unless there are compelling reasons to do otherwise. This may be particularly important in the case of femoral artery catheters, which are exposed to contamination from the perineum.

The frequency of arterial thrombosis following cannulation is principally related to two factors: the duration that the device is in situ, and the size of the catheter relative to the size of the vessel. Because young children have smaller arteries, it is not surprising that the incidence of thrombosis is greater in those younger than 5 years of age.

Several studies indicate that the frequency of arterial thrombosis increases when the catheters are left in place for more than 3 days. This observation reinforces the previously mentioned "3-day rule" for arterial catheters.

The consequences of arterial thrombosis depend upon the clinical status of the patient. Most often, there is no major unfavorable effect and the thrombosed vessel ultimately recannulates. When there is limited collateral flow or when the arterial circulation is compromised by hypotension or vasoconstriction, distal ischemia may occur. Catastrophic tissue injury results, leading to loss of skin, loss of digits, or loss of an entire extremity. Reflecting the small size of their vessels, infants seem to be more susceptible than older children to tissue loss distal to a thrombosis.

Arterial–arterial embolization results when clots or air are propagated from the catheter site to a more distal location, which can produce distal ischemia and gangrene.

Constant vigilance will reduce the incidence of tissue loss. Any manifestation of ischemia (pallor, diminished pulse, poor capillary refill, pain, or loss of motor or sensory nerve function) *must* entail immediate removal of the catheter. If reperfusion does not occur within 30 minutes, consultation with a surgeon skilled in peripheral vascular surgery is mandatory. The arterial pressure waveform should be continuously monitored. Damping or absence of the pressure curve that does not respond to *gentle* flushing signifies that the catheter or artery is occluded. The device must then be removed.

Other complications can be prevented by careful technique. Disconnection of the tubing will cause exsanguinating hemorrhage. All connections should be made with locking-type interfaces (e.g., Luer-Lok). Hemorrhage and hematoma may occur during insertion if the artery or a contiguous vein is lacerated and after removal if the artery is not compressed for an appropriate length of time. Although coagulopathy and thrombocytopenia do not contraindicate arterial catheterization, they make the procedure somewhat more hazardous. The danger of brachial plexus injury from hematoma makes axillary artery catheterization particularly hazardous in the context of a bleeding diathesis.

Injury to contiguous nerves sometimes occurs during insertion. Efforts to cannulate the axillary artery may damage the brachial plexus, whereas median nerve injury is not rare after inexperienced operators attempt to place a catheter within the radial artery.

It is not commonly recognized that vigorous flushing of an arterial catheter can cause retrograde embolization to the central circulation. Rapid injection of 7 ml of saline into the radial artery of an adult will reach the aortic arch. Serious retrograde embolization might be more likely in children and infants, in whom the distance from the peripheral site of cannulation to the aortic arch is less. Retrograde embolization is reduced by limiting the amount of flush solution injected at any time to 2 ml in adult patients and 0.5 ml in small children. Forceful injection of any amount of fluid is contraindicated.

Maintenance of Arterial Monitoring System

The catheter should be directly connected to a small volume rubber cap with a side extension tubing (Extension Set with "T," Abbott), permitting direct aspiration of blood from the catheter and making the use of a stopcock unnecessary. The "T connector" is attached to low-compliance tubing, which contains a single stopcock and is no longer than 4 feet in length. In order to permit continuous waveform display, a continuous flush device is used (e.g., Intraflow). This system provides a continuous flush of 3 ml per hour, slow enough for the smallest pediatric patient.

Ideally, the solution used for arterial lines is normal saline, because dextrose-containing solutions produce arteriospasm and promote bacterial growth. In practice, 5 percent dextrose or dextrose–electrolyte solutions are frequently used. Heparin is usually added to the infusing solution; concentrations ranging from 0.25 to 4 units per ml have been advocated. The lesser concentration seems preferable, because inadvertent heparinization can occur in small infants if the higher concentrations are used. Injecting any solution other than those mentioned or any medication can produce distal ischemia and necrosis.

Accuracy

Intravascular monitoring devices do not ensure accurate pressure measurement. Some errors are related to hemodynamic factors that are beyond the physician's control. Most of these errors occur because of poor technique in constructing the fluid pathway that connects the catheter to the transducer or because of faulty calibration of the transducer–monitor system. Attention to the waveform display permits recognition of many kinds of error.

Intrinsic properties of the vascular system may factitiously increase or decrease the blood pressure that is measured in peripheral vessels. Poor distal flow such as occurs with arterioconstriction or poor cardiac output causes the peripheral blood pressure to be *lower* than the central aortic pressure. This error is rectified by using large, central arteries to measure pressure. More often, direct arterial pressure measurements are somewhat amplified. This is due to several factors: 1) a slight increase in the arterial pressure pulse wave as it passes from the aorta to the periphery. This is associated with an increase in *systolic,* but not *mean,* blood pressure; 2) conversion of kinetic energy to hydrostatic energy as a result of the use of end–hole catheters; and 3) differences in the elastic properties of central and peripheral arteries. In the aggregate, the error introduced by these factors should be less than 10 mm Hg, assuming that the transduction system is appropriately maintained.

Grossly inaccurate measurements result from improper zeroing and calibration of the monitor. These procedures are described in product information manuals that accompany bedside monitoring systems, as well as in the suggested readings by Civetta and Kaye. The physician responsible for an individual intensive care unit must establish individuals (i.e., nurses, respiratory therapists) who are responsible for setting up and calibrating pressure transduction equipment. Zeroing and calibration must be performed on a routine schedule, according to a written protocol. We suggest zeroing and external calibration to mercury once every 24 hours and zeroing and internal calibration every 8 hours.

Significant error can be introduced by the tubing system that is used to connect the catheter to the transducer. Two phenomena occur: *Damping* is a form of artifact that reduces the amplitude of the pressure wave (Fig. 6–1). The effect is to "round off" the waveform and to artifactually *lower* the measured pressure. This error is produced by air bubbles in the fluid lines (often in stopcocks) and by high-compliance (standard IV) tubing. Warming the flush solution before use will reduce the amount of dissolved air in the solution. Special low-compliance tubing should be used for all pressure monitoring systems. *Resonance* occurs when the arterial pressure waveform has components that match the natural frequency of the fluid pathway. This falsely *increases* the amplitude of these components. This amplification is greatest at parts of the waveform that are associated with most rapid change in pressure, for example, the systolic peak pressure. The result is "systolic overshoot" (or "fling"), which is recognized on the waveform display as a narrow high-systolic peak (see Fig. 6–1). This phenomenon can introduce an error of up to 20 to 30 mm Hg in the systolic pressure. The magnitude of error that is introduced by resonance is determined in part by the length of the fluid pathway. Longer tubing produces more resonance at the frequencies that constitute a blood pressure wave. For this reason, tubing length should be kept as short as pos-

sible, generally no longer than 4 feet. Systolic overshoot is a major problem when the pressure waveform changes rapidly, as it does during hyperdynamic states. When the cardiovascular system is hyperdynamic, the measured systolic blood pressure may be considerably higher than the true systolic blood pressure, even when the tubing has been made as short as possible. Unless the physician takes care to observe the characteristics of the pressure waveform, serious overestimation of the systolic blood pressure results. In such cases, indirect methods of blood pressure measurement may be more accurate.

CENTRAL VENOUS PRESSURE MONITORING

Catheterization of the intrathoracic veins is commonly performed during pediatric critical care. An important indication for this procedure is measurement of the central venous pressure (CVP). Other indications that are not discussed in this chapter include provision of large vessel access for infusion of pressors and hypertonic solution and access to the venous system in conditions in which peripheral veins are collapsed and difficult to cannulate.

Types of Catheters

Central venous catheters are composed of Teflon or a similar plastic. The catheter should be 19 gauge or larger; smaller devices may not permit accurate pressure measurements. Percutaneous insertion rather than venous cutdown is preferred. Needle-over-catheter devices (e.g., Intracath) or the Seldinger technique are used.

Monitoring Sites

Several sites are available, depending upon the age and the condition of the patient and the experience of the operator. Frequently used vessels are the external and internal jugular veins (right side preferred over left); the antecubital or brachial veins; the proximal saphenous and femoral veins; and the subclavian vein. In experienced hands, each of these sites provides rapid and safe access to the central circulation. In children, attempts to cannulate the subclavian vein frequently lead to pneu-

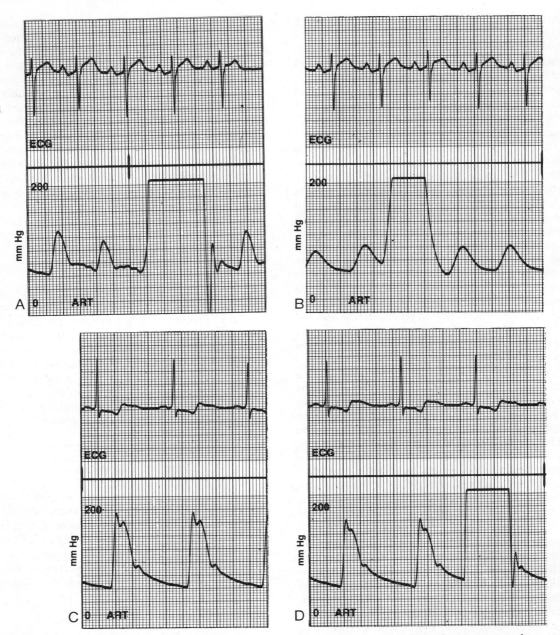

Figure 6–1. Effect of damping (*A* and *B*) and resonance (*C* and *D*) upon arterial blood pressure waveform and measurements. *A*, Normal arterial waveform (ART) with normal square wave response during rapid flushing with continuous flush system. *B*, Damped arterial waveform (ART) with damped square wave response. *C*, Overshoot of apparent systolic pressure (ART) owing to resonance from 72-inch extension tubing. Recorded pressure is 195 mm Hg. *D*, Systolic pressure (ART) recorded with 6-inch extension tubing in same patient as in *C*. The recorded systolic pressure is 175 mm Hg, which correlated with cuff systolic pressure of 170 mm Hg. (From Kaye, W.: Invasive Monitoring Techniques. *In* American Heart Association: Textbook of Advanced Cardiac Life Support, 1981. Used by permission.)

mothorax. This site should be used only by experienced operators. Infection and venous thrombosis seem to be somewhat more frequent with catheterization of the femoral or proximal saphenous veins than with other sites. These vessels should be used for monitoring only when other veins are inaccessible, i.e., during cardiopulmonary resuscitation (CPR).

The jugular and brachial vessels can be approached percutaneously or, when necessary, by cutdown. Indeed, we have been impressed at the rapidity with which even relatively inexperienced operators can learn to place a central catheter via a brachial cutdown.

Indications and Rationale

In the context of normal cardiorespiratory function and anatomy, the mean pressure is approximately the same throughout the intrathoracic veins. The CVP should correspond with both the right and left atrial pressures. Thus, CVP can be used as an index of left ventricular pre-load, a major determinant of cardiac output. Several disorders are characterized by critical reductions in CVP, left ventricular pre-load, and cardiac output in the context of otherwise normal cardiorespiratory function. For the most part, these entities involve disturbances in intravascular volume. Examples include extreme dehydration or hemorrhage, diabetic ketoacidosis, conditions such as elevated intracranial pressure that are managed by iatrogenic fluid depletion, and perhaps, disorders of vascular tone such as anaphylaxis. When these disorders are extreme or complicated by renal dysfunction, abnormal osmoregulation, or raised intracranial pressure, fluid management may be more precise if guided by measurement of the CVP. In such cases, the value of the measurement is that it provides quantitative information regarding the adequacy of the intravascular volume to support the cardiac output. Conversely, there are many conditions, even in previously healthy children, in which cardiorespiratory function is deranged. In such cases, measurement of the CVP predicts neither left ventricular pre-load nor the adequacy of the intravascular volume to support the cardiac output. A more complex method, pulmonary artery catheterization, which is discussed later in this chapter, becomes necessary.

Technique

Techniques for insertion of central venous catheters are not discussed in this chapter. Several of the suggested reading selections contain excellent descriptions of the procedure.

The catheter must terminate in a central, or intrathoracic, vessel. Catheters that inadvertently lie outside of the chest, commonly in the abdominal inferior vena cava or the proximal cephalic vein, should not be used for pressure measurement.

Many physicians continue to use water manometers to measure CVP. Although simple and inexpensive, these devices do *not* produce an accurate recording. This is because the frequency response of the water manometer (2 Hz) is considerably less than that needed to produce a high-fidelity reproduction of the venous waveform (20 Hz). As a rule, the CVP as measured by the water manometer is *greater* than the true CVP. Other limitations of water manometry relate to the absence of a waveform display. Without such a recording, it is difficult to recognize catheter malposition (i.e., in the right ventricle) or occlusion. The central venous catheter should, therefore, interface with the same type of equipment that is used for recording arterial pressures. The system should be configured so as to produce either a continuous or an intermittent pressure waveform display as preferred.

Complications

Many complications can occur during catheter insertion. These may involve injury to contiguous structures, such as the carotid, subclavian, or femoral arteries. Perforation of the trachea has been reported after efforts to cannulate the internal jugular vein. Most such injuries are avoidable and are related to poor technique. Some complications are related to site of insertion; for example, thrombosis appears to be somewhat more common after cannulation of the femoral vein, although thromboembolic phenomena may occur with any central catheter.

A major limitation of central catheters is that they predispose to bacteremia and sepsis. Although strict asepsis during insertion, coupled with fastidious care of the line while it remains in situ, may reduce the incidence of infection, it seems that a major determinant is the duration of catheterization. Several studies have shown that the rate of positive blood cultures rises sharply after the same catheter has been in place more than 72 hours. Therefore, central venous lines should be removed after 3 days (this advice does not apply to catheters that are used exclusively for hyperalimentation). Other precautions include use of an in-line 0.22 micron filter (but not interposed between catheter and transducer); frequent (every 24 to 48 hours) changing of tubing, transducer dome, and flush solution; and minimal use of the central catheter to withdraw blood samples or administer intermittent medications. Dressing changes should occur daily, with inspection of the insertion site. Evidence of local infection or systemic signs of infection (fever, leukocytosis, and hyperglycemia) mandates a blood culture through the catheter and from two peripheral sites, as well as immediate removal of the device.

Rarely, central venous catheters injure intravascular structures. Serious damage to the great veins is not common but can produce hemothorax, as can misadventure during cannulation of the jugular or subclavian veins. Termination of the catheter in the right atrium has been associated with perforation of that chamber, and dysrhythmias have been recorded when the tip of the catheter finds its way into the right ventricle. Air embolus may occur during insertion of the catheter or if the catheter and tubing become disconnected. Use of an infusion pump that does not have an air-in-the-line detector is contraindicated. Thrombosis of the superior vena cava (SVC), with production of an SVC syndrome, has been reported, as has inadvertent placement of the catheter tip through a patent foramen ovale into the left atrium.

PULMONARY ARTERY CATHETERS

Bedside insertion of pulmonary catheters using Swan–Ganz-type flow-directed devices is a routine procedure in many pediatric intensive care units. Catheterization is now feasible in newborns. Pulmonary artery catheters are of value in the management of children in whom cardiorespiratory dysfunction makes the CVP an unreliable predictor of left-sided pressures or in whom measurement of cardiac output or mixed venous oxygen content is desirable.

Description

Most catheterizations are performed with quadrilumen devices that permit measurement of cardiac output by the thermodilution technique. Small children (younger than 10 years of age) require a 5-French, 75-cm catheter. Older children and adults require a 7-French, 110-cm device. Catheters that are smaller than 5-French are available by special request from the manufacturer but have a more restricted range of application.

In the standard 5- or 7-French device, *Lumen 1* is the *distal lumen* and it terminates at the tip of the catheter. During insertion, this port transmits sequentially: right atrial, right ventricular, pulmonary artery, and pulmonary artery occlusion (PAO), or wedge, pressure. Blood samples for determining the mixed venous O_2 content are aspirated through this lumen. *Lumen 2* is the *proximal lumen*. In the standard French catheter, Lumen 2 terminates 30 cm from the catheter tip; in the standard 5-French device, Lumen 2 terminates 15 cm from the catheter tip. (5- and 7-French catheters are available by special order with 20-cm and 10-cm proximal ports, respectively, for use in small individuals). The proximal lumen should terminate in the right atrium or intrathoracic veins. It is used to measure right atrial or central venous pressure and to deliver the injectate necessary to perform cardiac output measurement. *Lumen 3* contains the wires to the thermistor, which is positioned just proximal to the catheter tip. *Lumen 4* is used to inflate and deflate the balloon.

Rationale

The pulmonary artery catheter provides an enormous amount of hemodynamic information. In addition to continuous CVP and pulmonary artery pressure monitoring, during insertion a record is made of right ventricular pressures and when appropriate, blood samples are collected for oximetry. When the catheter is appropriately located, inflation of the balloon allows determination of the PAO, or wedge, pressure. In most cases, the PAO pressure is closely related to the left atrial pressure and left ventricular filling pressure. A major use of the catheter is to measure cardiac output by the thermodilution method. Finally, the distal lumen permits measurement of the mixed venous O_2 content.

These directly measured terms are used to calculate the values of other hemodynamic parameters: stroke volume, systemic and pulmonary vascular resistances, intrapulmonary shunt fraction (Q_{sp}/Q_t), and oxygen consumption ($\dot{V}O_2$). Computer programs that automatically perform these calculations are currently available; the equations are presented in Table 6–1. Normal values are listed in Table 6–2. By relating serial determinations of stroke volume (or cardiac output) to PAO pressure, it is possible to construct a "Starling curve" for individual patients. This permits the physician to select the optimal ventricular pre-load.

Indications

The principle advantage of pulmonary artery catheterization is that it permits estimation of left atrial pressure and cardiac output. As noted

Table 6–1. Equations for Hemodynamic Calculations

$$CI = CO/\text{body surface area}$$
$$SV = CO/\text{cardiac rate}$$
$$SVI = CO \times 1000/\text{body surface area} \times \text{heart rate}$$
$$SVR = (MAP - CVP) \times 80/CO$$
$$PVR = (MPAP - PAO) \times 80/CO$$
$$RVSWI = SVI \times (MPAP - CVP) \times 0.136$$
$$LVSWI = SVI \times (MAP - PAO) \times 0.136$$
$$Q_{sp}/Q_t = (CA_{O_2} - Ca_{O_2})/(CA_{O_2} - C\bar{V}_{O_2})$$

Abbreviations: CO = cardiac output; CI = cardiac index; SV = stroke volume; SVI = stroke volume index; SVR = systemic vascular resistance; PVR = pulmonary vascular resistance; MAP = mean systemic arterial blood pressure; MPAP = mean pulmonary arterial blood pressure; PAO = pulmonary artery occlusion, or wedge, pressure; CVP = central venous pressure; RVSWI = right ventricular stroke work index; LVSWI = left ventricular stroke work index; Q_{sp}/Q_t = intrapulmonary shunt; CA = alveolar oxygen content; Ca = arterial oxygen content; and C$\bar{v}$ = mixed venous oxygen content.

in the section entitled Central Venous Pressure Monitoring, it is not necessary to obtain this information in all patients. Measurement of CVP is sufficient to guide the therapy of children whose illness is due to a disturbance of intravascular volume and for those with normal cardiorespiratory function.

Conversely, there is no disagreement about the need for pulmonary artery monitoring in critically ill children with obvious derangement of cardiac or pulmonary function. This category includes children with congenital or acquired cardiac disease (myocarditis, cardiomyopathy, coronary artery disease, and structural abnormalities) as well as those with severe respiratory embarrassment. Typical respiratory indications include ARDS (diverse etiologies), severe pneumonia, near-drowning, and pulmonary artery hypertension. A large group of candidates for pulmonary artery catheterization is found among children who require ventilation with high peak or end–expiratory pressures, because this kind of therapy reduces cardiac output and causes CVP to be an unreliable index of left-sided pressures.

Optimal management of children with more subtle cardiorespiratory dysfunction, probably the largest group, is less clear. Individuals in this group have no known pre-existing cardiac or pulmonary disease. Although critically ill, often with multisystem dysfunction, high-pressure respiratory support is not necessary. Diseases that fit into this category are Reye's syndrome, septic or hypovolemic shock, severe head trauma, some postoperative states, and serious intoxications. Frequently, placement of a pulmonary artery catheter does not materially affect the therapy of these children. This assertion has been demonstrated in children with Reye's syndrome in whom there is an excellent correlation between CVP and wedge pressure. When children with these conditions have apparently normal cardiac function and enjoy a prompt, predicted response to therapy, insertion of a pulmonary artery catheter is not "routine" and serves only to escalate cost, complexity of care, and risk of complication. When response to therapy is delayed or atypical, it is appropriate to seek the added information that is provided by a pulmonary artery catheter.

Table 6–2. Normal Hemodynamic Values

Cardiac index (CI)	2.5–4.0 L/min/m²
Stroke volume index (SVI)	33–47 ml/beat/m²
Systemic vascular resistance (SVR)	800–1200 dynes/sec/cm⁻⁵
Pulmonary vascular resistance (PVR)	<250 dynes/cm/sec⁻⁵
Right ventricular stroke work index (RVSWI)	4–8 gm/m²/beat
Left ventricular stroke work index (LVSWI)	45–75 gm/m²/beat
Central venous pressure (MEAN)	0–8 mm Hg
Pulmonary artery systolic pressure (PAS)	13–31 mm Hg*
Pulmonary artery diastolic pressure (PAD)	5–17 mm Hg*
Pulmonary artery occlusion (PAO) pressure	0–10 mm Hg*
Intrapulmonary shunt fraction (Q_{sp}/Q_t)	≤ 0.10

*Beyond the neonatal period.

added information that is provided by a pulmonary artery catheter.

The indications for pulmonary artery catheterization are summarized below.

Conditions in which PA catheterization is usually indicated

Critical illness associated with definite myocardial dysfunction (myocarditis, cardiomyopathy, myocardial infarction)

Critical illness associated with severe pulmonary dysfunction (ARDS, severe pneumonitis, pulmonary embolus)

High pressure mechanical ventilation

Condition requiring afterload reducing therapy

Conditions in which PA catheterization is indicated if the response to initial therapy is not satisfactory

Shock (all etiologies)

Intoxications associated with impaired hemodynamic function

Increased intracranial pressure (Reye's syndrome, head trauma, brain tumor)

Multiple trauma

Asphyxia (CO poisoning, near-drowning, strangulation)

Technique of Insertion

The method of insertion is briefly described here. More detailed descriptions are provided in product information and in the suggested reading list at the end of this chapter. Improper use of pulmonary artery catheters can result in lethal complications; therefore, they should be inserted only by individuals who have received appropriate bedside training.

The catheter is inserted in the intensive care unit, usually without fluoroscopy. In small children or those with reduced cardiac output, visualization of the catheter and the cardiac structures is useful and is easily accomplished by echocardiography. Insertion sites are similar to those used for central venous catheters. The device is usually placed percutaneously using the Seldinger technique, although venous cutdown is occasionally necessary.

After the catheter has entered the vein, the distal lumen is attached to a pressure transducer and a waveform is displayed. The catheter is advanced into the right atrium, and the balloon is inflated. Continued insertion is rewarded by, sequentially: a right ventricular, pulmonary artery, and PAO pressure tracing (Fig. 6–2). Once the PAO pressure has been recorded, the balloon is deflated and the catheter is secured to the skin. Anteroposterior (AP) and lateral chest x-ray films are taken to confirm proper location of the catheter tip.

Maintenance of Pulmonary Artery Catheters

The proximal and distal lumens are attached to pressure transducers. The transduction circuit is similar to that described for peripheral arterial lines. Heparin is added to the fluid perfusing the distal lumen, which is connected to a continuous flush device. The distal lumen *must* remain on continuous waveform display; the proximal (CVP) lumen is set to continuous or intermittent pressure monitoring, as preferred.

As the catheter remains in situ it softens, permitting the catheter tip to migrate into more peripheral (and smaller) pulmonary vessels. This predisposes to spontaneous pulmonary artery occlusion (wedging) by the tip. If unrecognized, this can lead to pulmonary infarction and even to rupture of a pulmonary artery. For this reason, the distal lumen waveform *must* be inspected frequently. Spontaneous appearance of wedge tracing indicates that the catheter should be pulled back.

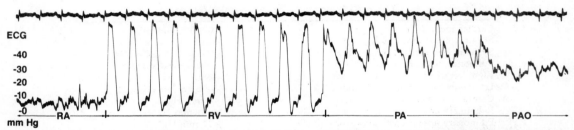

Figure 6–2. Pressure waveform tracing from the distal lumen of the pulmonary artery catheter as the catheter tip is advanced from the right atrium (RA) through the right ventricle (RV) and pulmonary artery (PA) to the pulmonary artery occlusion (PAO) position. (From Kaye, W.: Invasive Monitoring Techniques. *In* American Heart Association: Textbook of Advanced Cardiac Life Support, 1981. Used by permission.)

Measurements

The catheter provides a continuous display of pulmonary artery waveform and pressure. CVP is determined as needed. The mean PAO, or wedge, pressure is measured by inflating the balloon with CO_2 until an occlusion (wedge) tracing appears. It is critical to cease inflation of the balloon as soon as a wedge tracing is noted, because this indicates occlusion of the artery by the balloon. Further inflation can lead to vessel rupture.

High levels of PEEP increase intrathoracic pressure and produce elevations in all *intraluminal* pressures. Generally, if the catheter tip is located *below* the left atrium, the PAO pressure will increase in an amount appropriate to the PEEP-induced increase in left atrial pressure. However, when the catheter resides *above* the left atrium or when it is located far into the periphery, the PAO pressure may reflect *alveolar* rather than left atrial pressure. The catheter then records occlusion pressures that are *higher* than the left atrial pressure. This anomaly is prevented by attention to catheter location on chest x-ray films. Deviations between occlusion pressure and left atrial pressure are greater in volume-depleted states, and when lung compliance is normal.

The effect of PEEP upon catheter measurements is even more complex. When very high levels (greater than 10 to 15 mm Hg) of PEEP are applied, the intraluminal pressures as measured (CVP, PAD (pulmonary artery diastolic), and PAO) may give a misleading view of the true *transmural* vascular-filling pressures. This effect can be compensated for by use of an intraesophageal balloon to estimate intrapleural pressure (transmural pressure = intraluminal pressure − pleural pressure). Several of the suggested readings at the end of this chapter provide information about this procedure.

Cardiac output is measured by injecting a fixed volume of liquid at known temperature into the proximal lumen. At the moment of injection, the cardiac output computer is activated. Two or three determinations are averaged. In order to compensate for variation in body size, the cardiac output is referred to body surface area and is expressed as cardiac index. Several precautions improve accuracy. The computer must be provided with the correct injectate temperature. In several systems, this is now done automatically. Although injectate of any temperature can be used, iced (O°) injections tend to be more accurate. The cardiac output varies during the respiratory cycle. This effect is enhanced during positive pressure ven-

tilation; hence, serial cardiac output determinations should be made during the same phase of the respiratory cycle. Improper location of the catheter tip produces gross errors in output measurement. When intracardiac shunts are present, the thermodilution method tends to overestimate the true left ventricular output. There is no way to reliably compensate for this error or for that which is introduced by valvular incompetence.

Mixed venous blood is aspirated from the pulmonary artery via the distal lumen. The oxygen content of this blood is used to estimate the intrapulmonary shunt fraction (Q_{sp}/Q_t). This term is valuable in determining optimal levels of PEEP.

Equations for estimating pulmonary and systemic vascular resistances and right and left ventricular stroke work are listed in Figure 6–2. Serial measurements of these indices are important in guiding afterload reducing therapy and in finding the optimal relationship between oxygen delivery and myocardial work.

Complications

Many complications are related to the insertion or presence of a catheter in the central venous system. These complications have been discussed in the section entitled Central Venous Pressure Monitoring.

During insertion, the right atrium or right ventricle may be perforated if the guide wire is inserted too far. Dysrhythmias are not uncommon when the catheter tip encounters the right ventricular endocardium. With prompt withdrawal or advancing of the catheter tip, these dysrhythmias usually cease. In small children, the balloon may be sufficiently large to obstruct the pulmonary valve, producing bradycardia, hypoxemia, and hypotension. Other complications that occur during insertion are knotting of the catheter in the right ventricle and damage to the tricuspid or pulmonary valves.

Rupture of the balloon is common (50 percent in a recent study) and can cause air embolization, particularly if efforts to inflate the balloon continue. Small emboli are particularly dangerous in children in whom there is a relatively high incidence of unsuspected right-to-left shunt. For this reason, the manufacturer recommends that the balloon be inflated with CO_2, which is substantially more soluble in blood than air. Other complications related to the balloon are rupture of the pulmonary artery and pulmonary infarction. Infarction occurs when the balloon is inadvertently inflated in a wedge position or when peripheral migration of the catheter tip causes spontaneous wedging. Both events will be detected if proper attention is given to the pressure waveform. Additionally, occlusion pressure should not be measured more often than is necessary. In many patients, the PAD pressure is approximately the same as the PAO pressure. Once the measurement is determined in an individual patient, it is possible to "track" the PAD, rather than risk infarction or balloon rupture by frequent PAO measurements.

Rupture of a pulmonary artery can occur if the balloon is inflated beyond the volume necessary to produce an occlusion-type waveform. Indeed, a reduction in the volume of gas needed to achieve pulmonary artery occlusion signifies that the catheter tip has migrated into a peripheral, smaller pulmonary vessel. The catheter should be pulled back. To reduce the risk of catheter-related sepsis it is advisable to remove the device as soon as it is no longer necessary. It is probably not wise to permit pulmonary artery catheters to remain in situ for more than 72 hours. As with other invasive devices, tubing, transducer dome, and infusate are changed every 24 to 48 hours.

SUMMARY

Invasive hemodynamic monitoring is the foundation of critical care. Without the information provided by these techniques, it is not possible to offer appropriate therapy. Complications are sometimes associated with these devices. Judicious and informed use proscribes insertion on a routine or casual basis. Appropriate patient selection, careful insertion, and meticulous maintenance are rewarded by a highly favorable comparison of risks and benefits.

SUGGESTED READING

Civetta, J.M.: Invasive catheterization. In Shoemaker, W.C. and Thompson, W.L. (eds.): Critical Care—State of the Art, Vol. 1. The Society of Critical Care Medicine, Fullerton, 1980, pp. (B) 1–(B) 47.

Grabencort, W.R.: A cardiopulmonary physiologic profile for use with the Swan–Ganz catheter. Resident and Staff Physician 29:80, 1983.

Kaye, W.: Invasive monitoring techniques. In McIntyre, K.M. and Lewis, A.J. (eds.): Textbook of Advanced Cardiac Life Support. American Heart Association, 1981, pp. (XIII) 1–32.

Pollack, M.M., Reed, T.P., and Holbrook, P.R.: Bedside pulmonary artery catheterization in pediatrics. J. Pediatr. 96:274, 1980.

Weesner, K.M., Rocchini, A.P., and Rosenthal, A.: Use of balloon-tipped catheters in the critically ill child. Clin. Pediatr. 21:146, 1982.

Wetzel, R.C., and Rogers, M.C.: Pediatric hemodynamic monitoring. In Shoemaker, W.C., and Thompson, W.L. (eds.): Critical Care—State of the Art, Vol. 2. The Society of Critical Care Medicine, Fullerton, 1981, pp. (L) 1–(L) 78.

Fluids and Electrolytes

BONITA FALKNER, M.D.
MARY ANNE GAZDICK, M.D.

In this chapter, fluid and electrolyte therapy in relation to the pediatric patient are discussed. The underlying physiology of fluid and electrolyte homeostasis and the principles involved in the determination of maintenance fluids for steady state balance are reviewed. Clinical signs of fluid and electrolyte deficits or dehydration syndromes are discussed and management guidelines are presented.

FLUID COMPARTMENTS AND HOMEOSTASIS

A major portion of the body is composed of water. In lean men, it is approximately 60 percent of the total body weight. Fat tissue contains considerably less water; thus, as adipose tissue increases, the percentage of total body water decreases. Total body water is divided into two major compartments: the fluid within cells, or intracellular fluid (ICF), and all fluid outside the cells, or extracellular fluid (ECF). The cell membrane divides these two compartments. The ECF is further divided into two subcompartments, consisting of the plasma volume (PV) and the interstitial fluid (ISF). As previously noted, total body water is about 60 percent of the total body weight in lean men. It is approximately 55 percent of the total body weight in women, because they have relatively more body fat. In young infants, the fluid compartment distributions are somewhat different. In term infants, total body water is approximately 75 to 80 percent of the total body weight. This higher water content is due to relatively more ECF. During the first few months of postnatal life, there is a decline in the amount of body water and ECF. The rate of shift in relative fluid content of the fluid compartments diminishes in infants after six months of age, and in infants older than 12

months, the fluid distribution values approach those of adults, with 20 to 25 percent of the total body weight being made up of ECF.

The electrolyte composition of the two portions of ECF is essentially similar. The major cation of both the PV and ISF is sodium, with small proportions of potassium, calcium, and magnesium present. The major anion of both spaces is chloride, with lesser amounts of bicarbonate and so-called "undetermined anions" present. The capillary wall or membrane maintains the ISF devoid of the protein present in the plasma volume.

The electrolyte composition of the ICF is different from that of the ECF, with the major cations consisting of potassium and magnesium. The major anions of the ICF appear to be composed of organic phosphates and proteins. The ECF space is the fluid compartment that is clinically accessible. In particular, electrolyte and osmolar determinations are made on the ECF by sampling and analysis of plasma. The ECF is the fluid compartment from which acute volume deficits occur, such as with diarrhea, vomiting, or hemorrhage. The ECF is also the fluid space that is accessible to therapeutic intervention. Either oral or parenteral fluid therapy is delivered to the ECF, with secondary shifts across the cell membranes to restore and to correct the ICF.

FLUID THERAPY

Parenteral fluid therapy is used in a wide variety of clinical situations, ranging from the comatose or surgical patient who requires only maintenance fluids to patients with dehydration or other electrolyte disturbances such as diabetic ketoacidosis, acute renal failure, or syndrome of inappropriate ADH (antidiuretic hormone). Thus, in addition to maintenance requirements, such clinical syndromes will also require parenteral fluid therapy to replace a deficit or to correct an abnormal electrolyte state. Therefore, it is useful to divide management principles of parenteral fluid therapy in children into two steps: the determination of maintenance fluid requirements, and determination of deficit or correction fluids.

Maintenance fluid requirements consist of that amount of water and electrolytes necessary to replace normal insensible fluid losses through respiration, sweat, and stool and to replace urinary water loss. The volume of urinary excretion varies in relation to intrinsic renal regulating mechanisms such as renal blood flow, tubular reabsorption, aldosterone, and antidiuretic hormone. With intact renal function to regulate for modest variation, the quantity of maintenance fluids should maintain the patient in fluid balance with neither net loss nor gain of fluid space volume or electrolyte concentration.

Because of broad variation in body size and hence fluid requirement of pediatric patients, a formula for maintenance fluid requirement based on body weight (i.e., ml per kg) is not feasible. For example, a 70 kg adolescent will require about 35 ml per kg, whereas an infant requires 120 to 140 ml per kg. However, the amount of fluid necessary for maintaining body homeostasis under normal conditions is most closely related to metabolic rate. Table 7–1 provides the usual expenditure of water relative to calories metabolized. The caloric expenditure relative to body size can be estimated on the basis of body weight. With an estimate of caloric expenditure, comparable fluid requirements can be determined. However, because

caloric expenditure is a cumbersome convention for clinical use, this method may be simplified further. The usual fluid requirement is 150 ml of water per 100 calories metabolized or 1500 ml per 1000 calories metabolized. One thousand calories are metabolized per $1m^2$ body surface area. Therefore, a standard of 1500 ml per m^2 body surface area can be used as a simple formula to calculate daily fluid maintenance requirements. Comparable electrolytes are 45 mEq per m^2 sodium and 40 mEq per m^2 potassium.

The range for water requirements may be broadened to 1200 to 1800 ml per m^2 per day, with adjustments indicated according to certain clinical conditions. Based on the underlying concepts in determining fluid requirements, conditions that alter the metabolic state would necessitate adjustment of the maintenance volume. For example, fever, salicylate poisoning, and hyperthyroidism are conditions that increase metabolic rate; thus, the fluid requirements would be higher. On the other hand, hypothermia and hypometabolic states would require a decrease in maintenance volume. Acute CNS (central nervous system) disease such as head trauma or meningitis is a clinical situation in which maintenance fluids would purposely be reduced by one third to one half in an attempt to avoid intracerebral fluid accumulation caused by the intracranial disease process.

With clinical conditions in which fluid and electrolyte losses are in excess of usual expenditure, the potential for development of a deficit state of fluid depletion occurs only when the child can no longer orally replace the excess losses and when the renal capacity to correct the derangement has been exceeded. For example, the child with gastroenteritis who, because of anorexia, malaise, or vomiting, cannot orally replace the excess losses will become dehydrated when the renal capacity to retain fluid and electrolytes by concentration and sodium reabsorption has been exceeded.

The most commonly encountered dehydration state in the pediatric patient is that owing to gastroenteritis. The acute losses of fluid and electrolytes deplete the ECF space. Secondary shifting from the ICF space follows. The infant or small child is particularly vulnerable to acute fluid losses that exceed replacement efforts, because the rapid contraction of ISF by loss of a given amount of ECF reduces this space in a relatively higher proportion. For example, compare an acute fluid loss of 500 ml in a child who weighs 10 kg with the same fluid loss in an adult who weighs 70 kg. A child who weighs

Table 7–1. Expenditure of Water Relative to Calories Metabolized

Water Expenditure per 100 Calories Metabolized	
Skin	28 ml
Sweat	20 ml
Lungs	14 ml
Stool	8 ml
Urine	80 ml
Total	150 ml of water per 100 calories or 1500 ml/1000 calories

Estimated Calorie Expenditure by Body Weight	
Weight (kg)	*Caloric Expenditure*
1–10 kg	100 cal/kg
10–20 kg	1000 calories plus 50 cal/kg for each kg over 10 kg
> 20 kg	1500 calories plus 20 cal/kg for each kg over 20 kg

From Falkner, B.: *Fluid and electrolyte therapy. In* Miller, H.A., Major D.A., and Oaks, W.W. (eds.): ICU Medicine—The Fifty-sixth Hahnemann Symposium. New York, Grune & Stratton, Inc., 1983.

10 kg has an ECF space of approximately 3000 ml versus an ECF space of 14,000 ml in an adult who weighs 70 kg. A 500-ml fluid loss would deplete the ECF space by 17 percent in the child versus only 3 percent in the adult. Therefore, sudden fluid losses that are unreplaced subject the small child to proportionately greater subsequent hemodynamic and metabolic changes resulting from acute fluid depletion.

Evaluation of dehydration includes clinical estimation of the degree of dehydration and determination of the type of dehydration. From these measures, calculations can be made to determine the volume and type of replacement fluids.

Determination of the degree of dehydration is primarily based upon clinical assessment. A clinical estimate of the degree of dehydration, which indicates the percentage of body weight decrease caused by acute water loss, is made. For example, an estimate of 5 percent dehydration indicates that 5 percent of the body weight has been lost as acute fluid loss. Table 7–2 provides guidelines for the clinical signs and symptoms relative to the degree of dehydration. In cases of mild dehydration in which the fluid deficit reduces body weight by up to 5 percent, the clinical signs are usually those of ISF depletion, including decreased skin turgor, sunken fontanels, and dry mucous membranes. These changes are mild and do not reflect major hemodynamic compromise. However, when there are significant ongoing losses,

Table 7–2. Guidelines for Clinical Signs and Symptoms Relative to the Degree of Dehydration

5% Deficit (in body weight owing to fluid loss)
  Clinical signs of interstitial fluid loss
    Poor skin turgor
    Sunken fontanel
    "Hollow-eyed" appearance
    Dry mucous membranes
5–10% Deficit
  Clinical signs of interstitial deficit plus clinical signs of
    intravascular fluid deficit
    Lethargy
    Tachycardia
    Tachypnea
    Low blood pressure
    Decreased urine output
10–15% Deficit
  Clinical signs of interstitial and intravascular fluid
    deficit plus signs of *SHOCK*
    Pallor
    Weak and flaccid
    Rapid, thready pulse
    Hypotension
    Oliguria

From Falkner, B.: *Fluid and electrolyte therapy. In* Miller, H.A., Major D.A., and Oaks, W.W. (eds.): ICU Medicine—The Fifty-sixth Hahnemann Symposium. New York, Grune & Stratton, Inc., 1983.

as with diarrhea, or an inability to take adequate fluid orally, these signs indicate a progressing deficit and warrant intervention with fluid therapy. From 5 to 10 percent dehydration, the clinical signs include those of ISF depletion plus signs that indicate a reduction in intravascular volume. Clinical signs that indicate intravascular volume depletion include tachycardia, tachypnea, lower blood pressure, and a decrease in urine output. Thus, in addition to reduction of the ISF space, these signs reflect significant hemodynamic compromise and indicate the necessity for immediate intervention, with effective fluid therapy. As dehydration exceeds 10 percent and approaches 15 percent, all the signs of ISF and intravascular space depletion are present, in addition to signs of pallor, flaccidity, hypotension, and oliguria, which indicate intravascular collapse and shock. This severity in fluid deficit then requires emergency lifesaving treatment maneuvers.

The type of dehydration is determined by the serum sodium concentration, which indirectly is a reflection of the osmolarity. Determination of the type of dehydration enables one to more accurately calculate replacement electrolyte therapy. Table 7–3 provides the estimated deficits for the different types of dehydration.

Isotonic dehydration occurs with an acute fluid loss in which electrolyte loss is proportional to the ECF concentration. With isotonic dehydration, the serum sodium is 130 to 150 mEq per L. Isotonic dehydration is the most common type of dehydration. Because no osmolar gradients are created between the ICF and ECF, there will be minimal fluid shift and, thus, a low incidence of shock unless the degree of dehydration is very severe. In cases of isotonic dehydration, the estimated fluid deficit can be safely replaced in the first 24 hours of therapy.

Hypotonic dehydration is defined by a serum sodium of less than 130 mEq per L. This type of dehydration occurs in situations in which there is fluid and electrolyte loss, such as gastroenteritis, and replacement consists of only water. Hypotonic dehydration also occurs when sodium losses are in excess of water losses. Therefore, hypotonic dehydration not only can occur in acute gastroenteritis but also can easily develop in children with other types of chronic salt-losing disorders, such as cystic fibrosis, salt-losing adrenogenital syndrome, and salt-losing renal disease. In addition to the absolute loss of fluid from the ECF space, the hypotonicity or hypo-osmolarity of the ECF

Table 7–3. Approximate Deficits in Moderately Severe (10%) Dehydration

Tonicity	H$_2$O ml/kg	Na mEq/kg	K mEq/kg	Cl mEq/kg
Isotonic	100–120	8–10	8–10	8–10
Hypotonic	100–120	10–12	6–10	8–12
Hypertonic	100–120	2–4	0–4	2–6

For estimates of 5% dehydration, one half of these values may be used to determine deficit replacement.

From Falkner, B.: *Fluid and electrolyte therapy. In* Miller, H.A., Major D.A., and Oaks, W.W. (eds.): ICU Medicine—The Fifty-sixth Hahnemann Symposium. New York, Grune & Stratton, Inc., 1983.

space as a result of excess electrolyte loss promotes movement of water from the ECF space to the ICF space. This shift of water results in further contraction of the ECF space and, hence, a greater incidence of shock. With hypotonic dehydration, shock, if present, is treated first, then the deficit is replaced within the first 24 hours of therapy.

Hypertonic dehydration is defined by a serum sodium greater than 150 mEq per L. Hypertonic dehydration occurs when body water losses are in excess of salt losses. More frequently, this type of dehydration occurs in children who have gastroenteritis and are given concentrated salt solutions orally (e.g., boiled skim milk). The hypertonicity or hyperosmolarity of the ECF space results in water movement from the ICF space to the ECF space. The subsequent intracellular dehydration causes a typical doughlike texture to the skin. In severe cases of hypertonic dehydration, the intracellular dehydration and associated severe metabolic acidosis may result in brain damage as a potential sequela. Diabetes insipidus and nephrogenic diabetes insipidus may present with hypertonic dehydration. Therefore, in infants with unexplained hypertonic dehydration, these conditions, should be considered as possible etiologies.

Rapid correction of the hypernatremia in hypertonic dehydration should be avoided. Rapid fluid replenishment can force a rapid reexpansion of cells and often results in seizures during the course of corrective fluid therapy. Shock, if present, should be treated first. When circulation has been restored, the deficit replacement phase of therapy begins. However, unlike other types of dehydration, the deficit in hypertonic dehydration should be replaced slowly and evenly over 48 to 72 hours.

In the first 24 hours, maintenance fluid plus one half the calculated deficit should be given. Hypocalcemia is frequently present in this type of dehydration and is thought to be associated with potassium loss and total body potassium deficit. If serum calcium is 7 mg/dl or less, one ampule of 10 percent calcium gluconate may be added to each 500 ml of infusion fluid. If calcium is added to the infusion fluid, the fluid should not contain bicarbonate, because precipitation of the calcium and bicarbonate would then occur. In such situations, the infusion fluid should have a lactate base. With a bicarbonate base fluid, a separate infusion line for the calcium should be used. Bicarbonate therapy for severe acidosis is frequently necessary. When plasma bicarbonate concentration is less than 10 mEq per L, NaHCO$_3$ (sodium bicarbonate) may be added to the replacement fluid. The sodium given as NaHCO$_3$ should be included in the calculations of sodium replacement. For example, if the total sodium replacement is calculated to be 24 mEq for the first 24 hours and, as a result of acidosis, 10 mEq of NaHCO$_3$ will be given, the amount of sodium given as NaCl will be 14 mEq (i.e., 24 mEq total Na − 10 mEq NaHCO$_3$ = 14 mEq NaCl).

MANAGEMENT

In the management of the child with acute dehydration, the first phase of therapy is to treat shock, if present. Plasma volume must be restored to achieve adequate cardiac output and organ perfusion. Following stabilization of circulation, the second phase in correcting the deficit with concurrent provision of maintenance fluids is begun. The following is a recommended sequence to treatment:

1. Draw blood for electrolytes, BUN (blood urea nitrogen), CBC (complete blood count), blood culture, and other studies clinically indicated, and begin IV fluids.

2. If clinical shock is present or impending, immediately begin infusion of isotonic saline or Ringer's lactate at 20 ml per kg over a period of 1 hour. If shock has not been corrected after 1 hour, repeat the same volume of infusion.

3. Calculate the maintenance fluid requirement and the estimated deficit based on clinical assessment and electrolyte determination. The

sum of the maintenance and deficit will be the total amount of fluid to be infused over the first 24 hours (except in the case of hypertonic dehydration in which the maintenance plus one half the deficit will be given in the first 24 hours).

4. Give one half the total calculated fluids during the first 8 hours, one quarter during the second 8 hours, and one quarter during the third 8 hours. This schedule will help to achieve a more rapid initial restoration. Again, hypertonic dehydration is an exception.

5. Add potassium as KCl (potassium chloride) to the infusion when renal function has been determined to be adequate. Maximum potassium concentration should not exceed 40 mEq per L. Usually, this amount will be considerably less than the calculated potassium deficits. However, complete correction of potassium deficits may be accomplished over a number of days and often occurs when the child resumes an oral intake.

6. Take into account ongoing losses of fluid that may be occurring during therapy. Continuous loss of diarrheal fluid may necessitate augmenting the amounts of fluid that are infused in order to achieve deficit replacement.

7. If acidosis is severe, as indicated by a plasma bicarbonate of less than 10 mEq per L, $NaHCO_3$ should be added to the infusion solution. $NaHCO_3$ at 1 mEq per kg should raise the serum HCO_3 by 2 mEq per L. The sodium given as $NaHCO_3$ should be taken into account in the calculation of the total amount of sodium that is infused.

CASE 1

A boy who weighs 8 kg has had gastroenteritis for 5 days. For 2 days, he has been vomiting and unable to tolerate oral fluids. On physical examination, he is pale and flaccid; BP (blood pressure) = 30/?, P (pulse) = 200/minute, R (respiration) = 55/minute, and T (temperature) = 101°. He has very poor skin turgor; the fontanels are sunken; and the mucous membranes are dry.

Management

1. Electrolytes, CBC, BUN, and blood culture are drawn. An IV is started, and immediate therapy for shock is initiated by infusing 160 ml normal saline (NS) over a period of 60 minutes.
2. Circulation has been restored. Electrolytes have been reported as follows: Na, 122 mEq/L, K, 3.5 mEq/L; Cl, 92 mEq/L; and CO_2, 16 mEq/L.
3. Maintenance fluid is determined: 8 kg approximates a body surface area of 0.4m².

At 1500 ml/m² H_2O =   600 ml

45 mEq/m² Na^+ =   18 mEq
40 mEq/m² K^+ =   16 mEq

4. Deficit is determined for hypotonic dehydration with a 10 percent deficit, which is an appropriate deficit estimate following correction of shock. 8 kg at 10 percent deficit =

100 ml/kg H_2O =   800 ml
10–12 mEq/kg   Na =   90 mEq
6–10 mEq/kg   K =   64 mEq

5. The 24-hour replacement fluid will be the sum of the maintenance plus the deficit.

	H_2O	Na	K
Maintenance	600	18	16
Deficit	800	90	64
Total	1400 ml	108 mEq	80 mEq

6. In the first 8 hours, the child will receive one half the total fluid, or 700 ml H_2O with 54 mEq NaCl. A standard solution of ½ NS in 5 percent dextrose water (D5W) will provide 50mEq of Na in 700 ml of fluid and can be used.
7. During the second 8 hours, the child will receive 350 ml H_2O and 27 mEq NaCl or 350 ml ½ NS with D5W and added KCl. This solution will be given again in the third 8 hours.
8. When adequate renal function has been established, KCl will be added to the infusion solution at a maximum concentration of 40 mEq/L.

CASE 2

A 2-month-old male infant has had diarrhea for 5 days. He has been taking oral fluids in limited amounts until the day of admission, when he became lethargic and flaccid. His weight is 5 kg. On physical examination, his BP = 70/30, P = 120/minute, R = 32/minute, and T = 101°. The child is very lethargic, the fontanels are sunken, eyeball turgor is soft, his skin turgor is "doughy." His lungs are clear to auscultation, the results of cardiac examination are normal.

Management

1. Electrolytes, CBC, BUN, and blood culture are drawn and an IV is started. Although the child is extremely lethargic, there are no other hemodynamic signs indicating circulatory collapse; therefore, fluid restoration will consist of deficit plus maintenance.
2. The electrolytes are reported as follows: Na, 165 mEq/L; K, 5.0 mEq/L; Cl, 118 mEq/L; and HCO_3, 7 mEq/L. (Note: If signs of clinical shock were present in a case of hypertonic dehydration, immediate therapy with an isotonic solution such as NS would be necessary for volume expansion and circulatory restoration before deficit and electrolyte correction could be begun.)

3. Maintenance fluid is determined: 5 kg approximates a body surface of 0.3m².

At 1500 ml/m²	H_2O =	450 ml
45 mEq/m²	Na =	14 mEq
40 mEq/m²	K =	12 mEq

4. Deficit is determined for hypertonic dehydration with a 10 percent deficit. 5 kg at 10 percent deficit =

100 ml/kg	H_2O =	500 ml
2–4 mEq/kg	Na =	15 mEq
0–4 mEq/kg	K =	10 mEq

5. The 24-hour replacement fluid will be the sum of the maintenance plus ½ the deficit, because in the case of hypertonic dehydration, the deficit will be replaced evenly over a period of 48 hours.

	H_2O	Na	K
Maintenance	450	14	12
½ Deficit	250	7	5
	700	21	17

6. The child is quite acidotic with a serum bicarbonate of 7 mEq/L. $NaHCO_3$ will be added to the infusion fluid in a dose sufficient to raise the serum bicarbonate to 15 mEq/L. Using the formula 1 mEq/kg $NaHCO_3$ will raise the plasma bicarbonate by 2 mEq, then 4 mEq × 5 kg = 20 mEq $NaHCO_3$ will be added to the infusion fluid.

7. In this case, the restoration fluid for the first 24 hours will consist of 700 ml of D5W with 20 mEq $NaHCO_3$, because the calculated deficit and maintenance Na equal the amount of Na given as $NaHCO_3$. When adequate renal function has been established, 17 mEq KCl will be added to the infusion fluid. In this case, the rate of infusion will be uniform at 30 ml/hour for the 24-hour period.

8. During the second 24-hour period, assuming that the acidosis has been partially corrected and the plasma bicarbonate is 15 mEq/L or greater, no further bicarbonate will be given and the replacement fluid will be 700 ml D5W with 21 mEq NaCl and 17 mEq KCl. A stock solution of ¼ NS in D5W with 17 mEq KCl added will closely approximate this requirement.

During the first day of therapy, clinical signs should be monitored. Chemical and metabolic abnormalities should be checked to document continued improvement. If improvement is not evident, the situation must be reassessed and the possibility of contributing disorders should be considered.

Fluid and electrolyte therapy is used to correct a variety of conditions beyond simple dehydration resulting from gastroenteritis. Fluid management should be individualized to meet the needs of each patient in his or her specific clinical state. This may be accomplished with an understanding of the normal fluid and electrolyte volumes, the usual fluid and electrolyte requirements for homeostasis relative to body size, and the effect imposed by the disease process in each patient. Thus, in management of the child with diabetic ketoacidosis, the clinician must account for dehydration, hyperglycemia, acidosis, large potassium deficits, and possibly an underlying triggering event. Management will involve correction of hyperglycemia and acidosis plus restoration of large fluid and electrolyte deficits. Another situation that requires a different approach is the syndrome of inappropriate ADH (S–IADH). In S–IADH, the patient has a relative fluid excess, with hyponatremia and inappropriate sodium excretion caused by excess ADH. In this case, management will involve providing limited volumes of fluid with high sodium content. If the hyponatremia results in seizures or a high seizure risk range of hyponatremia, rapid correction of plasma osmolarity with hypertonic NaCl may be indicated.

CASE 3

A 7-month-old female infant presented with extreme irritability and a seizure. The diagnosis of *Hemophilus influenza* meningitis was made, and antibiotic therapy was instituted. On the third day of therapy, she had another generalized seizure, which was controlled with intravenous anticonvulsants. On physical examination, the child appeared clinically well hydrated.

Management

1. The following laboratory studies were obtained: Blood glucose, 112 mg/dl; Ca, 9.6 mg/dl; Na, 118 mEq/L; K, 3.0 mEq/L; CO_2, 18 mEq/L; Cl, 92 mEq/L; urine Na, 164 mEq/L; and urine osmolarity, 570 mEq/L.

2. Laboratory values confirm the diagnosis of S–IADH. Because of the presence of seizures, the serum sodium level will be rapidly increased to take the child out of the seizure-risk range of hyponatremia. NaCl as a hypertonic solution (usually 3 percent) will be infused over a period of 30 to 60 minutes. The amount to be infused is calculated by the following formula:

$$(Na_{desired} - Na_{patient}) \times wt \ (kg) \times 0.6$$

$$= mEq \ Na \ to \ infuse$$

Complete correction of the serum Na is neither necessary nor desirable. Increasing the serum sodium from 118 to 128 mEq/L will remove the patient from immediate risk of seizure. Based upon the formula just given:

$$(128 - 118 \ mEq) \times 8 \ kg \times 0.6 = 48 \ mEq$$

If 3 percent NaCl is the hypertonic NaCl solution to be given, 94ml would be infused over a 60-minute period.

3. Following the partial correction of S–IADH-induced hyponatremia, fluids should be adjusted to further control S–IADH when CNS (central nervous

Table 7–4. Clinical Syndromes Requiring Different Fluid and Electrolyte Management

Conditions Requiring Maintenance Fluids
  Surgical cases
  Comatose patient
  Repiratory disorders precluding oral intake
Conditions Requiring Maintenance Fluids Plus Deficit Replacement
  Dehydration
  Salicylate toxicity
  Salt-wasting renal disease
  Diabetic ketoacidosis
  Pyloric stenosis
  Other continuous gastrointestinal (GI) losses (e.g., nasogastric drainage, ileostomy)
Conditions Requiring *Adjusted* Maintenance Plus Correction of Electrolyte Status
  Acute renal failure
  Syndrome of inappropriate ADH (S–IADH)
  Increased intracranial pressure
  Nephrotic syndrome

current state of fluid and electrolyte balance, evaluation of the underlying disease process, development of a management plan to correct an abnormal state of fluid and/or electrolyte balance, and ongoing monitoring to ensure progressive correction. If monitoring indicates that the corrective course is not progressing satisfactorily, the patient's status should be reevaluated and adjustments in the management should be made.

SUGGESTED READING

Darrow, D.C.: The physiologic basis for estimating requirements for parenteral fluid therapy. Ped. Clin. North Am. 6:29, 1959.
Dell, R.B.: The pathophysiology of dehydration in the body fluids in pediatrics. Winters, R.W. (ed.): The Body Fluids in Pediatrics: Medical, Surgical, and Neonatal Disorders of Acid–Base Status, Hydration and Oxygenation. Boston, Little, Brown, and Co., 1975, pp. 134–154.
Gruskin, A.B.: Fluid therapy in children. Urol. Clin. North Am. 3:277, 1976.
Holliday, M.A., and Segar, W.E.: Maintenance need for water in parenteral fluid therapy. Pediatrics 19:823, 1957.
Rowe, M.I., and Arango, A.: The choice of intravenous fluid in shock resuscitation. Pediatr. Clin. North Am. 22:269, 1975.
Winters, R.W.: Maintenance fluid therapy in the body fluids in pediatrics. Ed. Winters, R.W. (ed.): The Body Fluids in Pediatrics: Medical, Surgical, and Neonatal Disorders of Acid–Base Status, Hydration and Oxygenation. Boston, Little, Brown and Co., 1975, pp. 113–133.

system) disease is present. The child should have her maintenance fluids reduced to 2/3 total calulated maintenance per 24-hour period, and this volume should be given as NS.

A categorization of some of the clinical conditions that require different fluid and electrolyte therapy management in children is provided in Table 7–4. The general guidelines that are applicable in all clinical conditions include assessment of the patient's

Enteral Alimentation

SELMA E. SNYDERMAN, M.D.

Whenever a pediatric patient is unable to ingest enough formula or food to maintain an adequate nutritional state, some form of intervention is indicated. If the gastrointestinal tract is intact and functional, its use is preferable to intravenous alimentation. Intervention via the gastrointestinal tract is usually initiated by the insertion of a feeding tube into the stomach or through the pylorus into the jejunum. There are both advantages and disadvantages to each of these techniques. There is a much greater risk of aspiration using the gastric site, particularly in weak patients with poor sucking and swallowing reflexes, as well as in those with depressed central nervous systems. Filling of the stomach may result in some aggravation of respiratory embarassment in those with pulmonary pathology. On the other hand, it may be difficult to get the tube through the pylorus to the duodenum or jejunum.

The effect of bypassing the digestive processes that normally take place in the stomach is not known, and a greater growth of intestinal bacteria has been reported when this route is used. Trauma to the mucosa with some bleeding may occur at either location, and there is a greater possibility of perforation of the small intestine than of the stomach, although this is a rare complication.

Food may be administered at either site by bolus or constant drip. The latter, when placed in the stomach, has a definite advantage in those situations in which gastric dilatation may compromise pulmonary or cardiac function. When used in the jejunum, it prevents the dumping syndrome, improves absorption, and prevents diarrhea, symptoms that frequently accompany bolus feeding at this site.

CHOICE OF FEEDING

The formula used for tube feeding depends upon the age and the medical condition of the patient. Premature infants can be given one of the special formulas designed for this group or a mixture of human milk and formula. Older infants can be given standard formulas or formulas specially constructed to treat specific gastrointestinal disturbances. Lactose-free, hydrolyzed protein and medium-chain triglyceride–containing infant formulas are available commercially.

There are numerous products on the market that can be used for older patients with ingestion problems. If the problem is simply the inability to ingest enough food, feedings that are not predigested and that do not omit any specific dietary component can be used. If the patient can use the oral route, the diet can be supplemented with fats and carbohydrates to increase the caloric intake or one of the whole formula products can be used. These products are made in several different flavors to increase palatability; often, their use makes it possible to avoid tube feeding.

If the problem is gastrointestinal in origin, the choice of feeding will depend upon the functional deficiency. After a severe episode of diarrhea or if there is any significant degree of malnutrition, a diet free of lactose is preferred, because lactose is the enzyme that is most vulnerable to any untoward influence on the gastrointestinal tract. In several feedings that are available, the protein component has been modified; this may consist of either hydrolysates or a mixture of pure amino acids. Hydrolysates in which there is a mixture of amino acids and small peptides are preferred, because such a mixture is better absorbed than are amino acids. Formulas that contain medium-chain triglycerides (MCT) can be used in those situations in which there is impaired fat absorption.

COMPONENTS OF FORMULAS FOR ENTERAL ALIMENTATION

In Table 8–1, the major types of formulations are listed.

When administered as supplied or in the rec-

Table 8-1. Enteral Alimentation Components

Protein	Carbohydrate	Fat
Whole protein	Lactose Lactose-free	Milk Vegetable and Medium-chain triglycerides (MCT)
Hydrolyzed protein	Lactose-free	Vegetable and MCT
Small peptide + free amino acids	Lactose-free	Vegetable, or vegetable and MCT
Free amino acids	Lactose-free	Vegetable

ommended dilution, the caloric density of these formulas varies between 1 and 2 cal per ml. The caloric distribution varies in the same manner as a usual mixed diet: protein, 9 to 24 percent; fat, 9 to 36 percent; and carbohydrate, 48 to 70 percent. Several products have a very low fat content, approximately 1 percent of the total calories necessary to provide essential fatty acids. A whole protein and a crystalline amino acid mixture are in this category. There is a wide range, 300 to 850 mOsm per kg of water, in the osmolality of these preparations. All these preparations contain all the known vitamins and most trace minerals. Low-sodium-content mixtures are also available among the approximately 25 preparations now on the American market.

INITIATING ENTERAL ALIMENTATION

If the gastrointestinal tract has not been used for some time or if there is a marked degree of malnutrition, the osmolality of the formula is of great importance. It is usually expedient to choose a formula of low osmolality and dilute it by half. It should be noted that the feedings that contain crystalline amino acids have the highest osmolality. The volume to be administered depends upon the age and size of the patient, but initiating the feeding with 1/3 to 1/2 the total required volume is usually tolerated. The rate and concentration may then be advanced in a stepwise manner until fluid and caloric requirements are met. This advancement can be accomplished either by alternating volume and concentration increments or by delaying the increasing of the concentration until at least 75 percent of the fluid volume has been met. The latter method seems to be associated with fewer untoward symptoms. Any gastric residual or the appearance of glucosuria is an indication that one should not advance the

feeding but should go back one step before proceeding further.

COMPLICATIONS AND MONITORING

There are fewer complications with the enteral route than with the parenteral route. However, some complications do occur with the enteral route; therefore a certain degree of monitoring is necessary. The mechanical complications have been enumerated under the section entitled Choice of Feeding. Metabolic complications have included fluid overload, hypernatremia, hyperkalemia, hypoglycemia, hyperglycemia, hypophosphatemia, and hypozincemia. Serum electrolyte, glucose, and phosphate levels should be monitored daily during the first week and then one or two times weekly. There should be a similar schedule for urinalyses.

Elevated transaminases have been reported in children on enteral alimentation who were receiving mixtures of crystalline amino acids. There have been no other signs of liver involvement.

NUTRITIONAL MANAGEMENT OF ORGAN FAILURE

Liver Disease

The nutritional management of hepatic failure should be directed toward providing sufficient protein and calories to meet requirements. Although the cause of hepatic encephalopathy is not precisely known, it is possible to alleviate the biochemical abnormalities and improve the clinical condition with nutritional management. Elevation of plasma ammonia level should be managed with reduction of the protein intake while the caloric intake is maintained. This can be accomplished by dietary manipulation if the patient is able to take food orally. If a formula feeding is being used, it must be reduced to meet the need for protein restriction but must also be supplemented with fat and carbohydrate to supply caloric requirements.

A change in plasma amino acid pattern often accompanies hepatic encephalopathy. This change involves an elevation of the levels of the aromatic amino acids, phenylalanine, tyrosine, and tryptophan and a depression of the levels of the branched chain amino acids, leucine, isoleucine, and valine. There is a preparation available in which the amino acids are distributed in a manner designed to alter the plasma amino acids (high-branched chain and low-aromatic amino acids). This preparation should not be used as a preventative measure; it should be used only after quantitative determination of plasma amino acids has shown that these changes have occurred. If this preparation constitutes the major source of nutrition, it must be supplemented with vitamins and minerals, because these elements are not included in the formula.

Renal Failure

In end-stage renal disease, the use of a mixture of essential amino acids has been shown to postpone the need for dialysis, or, if dialysis has been initiated, it has been shown to prolong the interval between dialyses. Two preparations are available: one contains adequate calories, very low amounts of sodium, potassium, calcium, and magnesium, and no vitamins or trace minerals. The absence of phosphorus and the low quantities of other minerals make it possible to manipulate these components according to the patient's requirements. A tablet that contains only essential amino acids is also available. This might be used with a diet low in protein but adequate in all other ways. It might also be useful in situations in which extra nitrogen is required, for example, to offset the amino acid losses of continuous peritoneal dialysis.

SPECIAL FEEDINGS FOR INHERITED METABOLIC DISORDERS

This is a very specialized area and should be undertaken only by those with experience in the field and with the necessary laboratory back-up. Children with these disorders are often first diagnosed when admitted to the ICU (intensive care unit), especially in the newborn period. Proper therapy, of course, depends upon the fact that the specific diagnosis has been made, but there are certain alterations of dietary intake that may be helpful until a diagnosis is confirmed. Thus, if an anomaly of amino acid metabolism, one of the organic acidurias, or one of the defects in the urea cycle is suspected, it is wiser to reduce the protein intake (the amount depends upon the patient's age, but should not be more than 1 gm per kg in the newborn period) while maintaining the caloric intake by the addition of fat and carbohydrate. Maintenance of caloric intake is especially important to reduce tissue catabolism, which would aggravate the situation. The possibility of an error in fructose or galactose metabolism is handled by the use of one of the formulas free of these sugars. (Note: Galactose is a component of lactose, and fructose is a component of sucrose). As soon as the diagnosis has been confirmed, specific therapy should be initiated.

SUGGESTED READING

Greene, H.L., McCabe, D.R., and Merenstein, G.B.: Protracted diarrhea and malnutrition in infancy: changes in intestinal morphology and disaccharidase activities during treatment with total intravenous nutrition or oral elemental diets. J. Pediatr. 87:695, 1975.

McIntire, B., and Wright, R.A.: Enteral alimentation—an update on new products. Nutritional Support Services 1:7, 1981.

Panel Report on nutritional support of pediatric patients. J. Clin. Nutr. 34:1223, 1981.

Total Parenteral Alimentation

SELMA E. SNYDERMAN, M.D.

The need for maintenance of a good nutritional state to prevent infection, to reduce morbidity, and to withstand the many procedures that may be required in an intensive care unit cannot be overemphasized. Excellent nutritional support can be provided by use of either the gastrointestinal or the intravenous route. It should be stressed, however, that if the gastrointestinal tract is functional, it is the preferred route for nutrition and that there is no advantage to the use of the intravenous route. The possibility that there are still unidentified nutritional factors, the uncertainty about exact intravenous requirements, and the numerous complications that can occur during total intravenous nutrition all emphasize the need for caution in initiating the intravenous route.

There are, however, several situations in which the use of total parenteral nutrition can be lifesaving, including low-birthweight infants whose nutritional requirements cannot be met by the gastrointestinal route; infants with severe respiratory problems are such an example. Neonates with surgical problems of the gastrointestinal tract, such as congenital obstructive lesions of the small intestine, omphalocele, tracheoesophageal fistulae, necrotizing enterocolitis, and various short bowel syndromes, can benefit greatly from this procedure. Children with severe chronic diarrhea may be candidates for intravenous alimentation. Certain patients with inflammatory bowel disease who do not respond to oral alimentation will improve with this therapy, and fistulae that complicate these disorders respond very well to intravenous nutritional support. It can be very helpful in the management of children with malignancies and enteritis as a result of their therapy, and it has been used to advantage in acute renal failure.

An exact knowledge of both the qualitative and quantitative requirements is necessary for optimal nutrition by the intravenous route. It should be noted that we still do not know all

that there is to know about the requirements for use of the oral route. When the intravenous route is used, the modifications of the oral requirements are not completely known. An important site of nutrient regulation is lost when the gastrointestinal tract is bypassed; the effects of delivery directly to the liver are still under investigation. In addition, there is little available information about the effects of such variables as fever, stress, and trauma on the requirements of children at different ages.

The currently known nutritional requirements are listed in Table 9–1.

COMPOSITION OF THE INFUSATE

Protein

Protein may be provided by either a protein hydrolysate or a mixture of amino acids. Hydrolysates are rarely used at the present time because of the variable degree of hydrolysis, which results in small peptides that are not usable by the intravenous route; also, appreciable amounts of ammonia may remain in the hydrolysate. Mixtures of amino acids are preferred, because the exact amounts in the infusate are known. There are now five amino acid mixtures available on the American market. Two have been developed for pediatric use, and these have a better distribution of amino acids than the others. Their administration has not resulted in the elevation of plasma amino acid levels that occurred with the earlier mixtures. These new products have addressed the deficiency of cystine and tyrosine in other mixtures, which is due to the relative insolubility of these two amino acids. Although cystine and tyrosine are not usually considered to be essential, they may be required by premature and some full-term infants who have not fully developed the capacity to synthesize these amino acids. One of the new pediatric mixtures contains tyrosine in the acetyl form, which is sol-

Table 9–1. Nutritional Requirements

Protein or amino acids
Calories
Minerals
  Macro—sodium, chlorine, potassium, calcium, magnesium, phosphorus, sulfur
  Micro (trace)—iron, zinc, copper, iodine, fluorine, chromium, silicon, cobalt, manganese, molybdenum, selenium, nickel (?), vanadium (?)
Vitamins
  Fat-soluble—A, D, E, K
  Water-soluble
    B vitamins—thiamine, riboflavin, niacin, pyridoxine, pantothenic acid, folic acid, biotin, cyanocobalamin
    Vitamin C
Essential fatty acids
Other factors—carnitine, inositol ?, choline ?

uble, and also provides cysteine to be added just before administration. The other mixture, which contains cysteine but is tyrosine-deficient, has been temporarily withdrawn from the market because of unexpected reactions with certain additives.

Carbohydrate

Carbohydrate is supplied as glucose. The solution may be as concentrated as 10 percent for the peripheral route and 20 percent for the central route. It may be initiated as a 5 percent solution and increased by daily increments of 5 percent except for preterm infants. A lower concentration, usually 2.5 percent, is tried initially in the premature infant and gradually the concentration is increased while the infant's tolerance is observed.

Fat

Intravenous fat is used for two purposes: to supply calories, and to supply essential fatty acids. There are two available preparations: one is an emulsion of soy bean oil, and the other is made from safflower oil. Both are prepared in 10 and 20 percent concentrations, thereby supplying a large quantity of calories in a small volume. Both supply adequate amounts of linoleic acid, the fatty acid known to be essential to man. The safflower oil preparation is deficient in linolenic acid; this fatty acid has not yet been shown to be essential for man, yet it is known to be essential for several animal species, including primates. There is the very real possibility that long-term intravenous alimentation, especially in small premature infants,

may produce a deficiency of this nutrient. Very few untoward reactions to intravenous fat have been encountered when the infusion is given at a slow enough rate. Fat overload is avoided by ascertaining that the fat has been cleared before the next dose is administered. The criteria for clearing have been subject to some discussion. Observation of the plasma for turbidity is commonly used but is not as reliable as nephelometry. Determination of serum triglyceride, cholesterol, and free fatty acid levels is the most reliable criterion in determining that fat overloading is not occurring.

There are possible untoward effects of intravenous fat in premature infants. Minor changes in oxygen diffusion that may be of importance if impairment of oxygenation has developed for other reasons have been reported. It should be noted, however, that these occurred only when the recommended rate of infusion was exceeded. Lipid deposits in the pulmonary arterial walls have been observed at post mortem examination of premature infants who received fat infusions but only in those who had vascular damage resulting from pulmonary hypertension. Intravenous fat is not recommended for neonates who have any appreciable degree of jaundice, because its hydrolysis to free fatty acids may displace bilirubin bound to albumin, thus increasing the risk of kernicterus. It should be emphasized, however, that premature infants are those most susceptible to the development of essential fatty acid deficiency; hence, the advantages of intravenous fat should be carefully weighed against any possible risks. Slow administration over a period of 20 to 24 hours and precautions to ensure clearing before the next dose is administered should make intravenous fat safe for premature infants.

Vitamins

A vitamin mixture specially formulated for pediatric patients is now available. It contains all known essential vitamins in recommended amounts for this age group (Table 9–2). It is stable and does not contain propylene glycol, which may cause lactic acidosis in infants. The dose for infants who weigh less than 3 kg is 65 percent of the content of the vial; one vial daily is recommended for patients up to 11 years of age. The adult vitamin mixture may be used for older children; it is supplied in two vials that contain all the vitamins with the exception of vitamin K, which should be provided weekly as a separate injection.

Table 9–2. Composition of Pediatric Vitamin Mixture

Each vial contains:

Vitamin A	0.7 mg (2300 U)
Vitamin D	10 μg (400 U)
Vitamin E	7 mg (7 U)
Vitamin C	80 mg
Thiamin	1.2 mg
Riboflavin	1.4 mg
Niacinamide	17.0 mg
Pyridoxine	1.0 mg
Dexpanthenol	5.0 mg
Biotin	20 μg
Folic acid	140 μg
Vitamin B$_{12}$	1 μg
Vitamin K$_1$	200 μg

Minerals

The requirement for minerals through the parenteral route is usually less than that through the enteral route. Phosphate is frequently not required during the first week of life, and the plasma level should be determined before it is administered. To provide the total requirement of both calcium and phosphate, it is advisable to prepare the solution in two bottles, one containing calcium, and the other phosphate, in order to prevent the precipitation of calcium phosphate. A maximum of 10 mM of phosphate is recommended.

Trace Minerals

Trace minerals are available either individually or as a mixture of zinc, copper, chromium, and manganese. Selenium, molybdenum, and iodine are also supplied as individual solutions by one manufacturer. At present, there are no commercial sources for any of the other trace minerals. It should be emphasized that there are large gaps in our knowledge of trace mineral requirements and that all recommendations can be considered only as tentative.

Other Factors

Intravenous preparations of carnitine, choline, and inositol are not yet available.

It is recommended that whole blood or plasma be given weekly to provide trace factors and unknown nutrients.

CATHETER PLACEMENT AND CARE

The choice of a central or a peripheral vein for alimentation depends upon the length of time that it will be used, the caloric requirement, and the availability of veins. All nutrients can be given by either route; however, the glucose concentration is limited to 10 percent when given peripherally. The number of calories that can be supplied by this route may be increased by giving more fat, the upper limit usually being 4 gm per kg, or increasing the total fluid volume to more than the usually recommended 150 ml per kg. If one administers 150 ml per kg and 4 gm of fat per kg, the highest caloric intake will be 104 cal per kg; with the use of a central line and 20 percent glucose, as much as 164 cal per kg can be provided (Table 9–3).

The usual site for central catheter placement in infants and young children is through the external or internal jugular vein to the superior vena cava. In older and larger children, it is possible to approach the superior vena cava by threading the catheter through the subclavian vein. The proximal end of the catheter is tunneled subcutaneously to exit at a distance from the point of insertion to help reduce the incidence of infection. A membrane filter is inserted between the catheter and the filter, and an infusion pump is used to ensure a constant rate of delivery. Intravenous fat is administered distal to the filter, close to the insertion site, with its own pump, so that the emulsion is not affected.

The catheter must receive meticulous care so that infection is avoided. It should not be used for other purposes, such as blood sampling or drug injection. The exit site should be dressed at least three times weekly with aseptic technique, the skin should be cleansed, and antiseptic ointment and a new dressing should be applied. If sepsis is suspected, a culture through the catheter is indicated. If the catheter is removed, the tip should also be cultured. If a central line with hypertonic glucose infusion must be removed, a peripheral line to infuse glucose should be inserted to prevent a reactive hypoglycemia.

MONITORING

Adequate monitoring is necessary to avoid the many possible complications and to ensure that the nutritional intake is adequate. The problems in monitoring the lipids have been noted previously. Trace mineral levels are not included in Table 9–4, because they are not readily available. However, weekly determinations would be desirable. Table 9–4 lists suggested parameters to be monitored during the

Table 9–3. Specific Recommendations for Composition of Infusate

Infants to 1 yr or 10 kg
  Protein: 2 gm/kg/day
  Calories: 100–110 cal/kg/day
  Fat: initiate with 1 gm/kg/day and increase with
    proper precautions to 4 gm/kg/day
  Minerals: kg/day
    Sodium: 2–3 mEq
    Potassium: 2–3 mEq
    Chloride: 2–3 mEq
    Calcium: 1–2 mEq
    Phosphorus: 2 mM
    Zinc: 100 μg
    Chromium: 0.14–0.20 μg
    Copper: 20 μg
    Manganese: 2–10 μg
  Vitamins: Pediatric vitamin mixture: 65% of vial un-
    der 3 kg; entire vial over 3 kg
  Whole blood or plasma weekly
Preterm Infants
  Protein: 2.5 gm/kg/day
  Calories: 100–125 cal/kg/day
  Fat, vitamins, minerals: same as for the full-term in-
    fants except zinc 300 μg/kg/day
Children 1–5 yr or 10–20 kg
  Protein: 1.5 gm/kg/day
  Calories: 80 cal/kg/day
  Other constituents: same as for full-term infants
Children 5–10 yr or 20–40 kg
  Protein: 1 gm/kg/day
  Calories: 55 cal/kg/day
  Other constituents: same as for full-term infants
Older Children
  Protein
    11–14 yr: 1 gm/kg/day
    15–18 yr: 0.8 gm/kg/day
    18+ yr: 0.7 gm/kg/day
  Calories*
    Males: 2500/day
    Females: 2000/day
  Minerals: per day
    Calcium: 200–400 mg
    Phosphorus: 10 mM
    Magnesium: 8–20 mEq
    Zinc: 2.4–4.0 mg
    Copper: 0.5–1.5 mg
    Manganese: 0.15–0.8 mg
    Chromium: 10–15 μg
  Vitamins: 5 ml of each of 2 vials of adult vitamin
    preparation
    Vitamin K, 1 mg weekly

*These are average figures; the caloric requirement varies widely and the intake must be adjusted to changes in weight.

Table 9–4. Monitoring During Intravenous Alimentation

	First Week (per wk)	Later Weeks (per wk)
Growth		
Weight	7	7
Length	1	1
Head circumference	1	1
Biochemical		
Blood		
Acid-base status	7	3
CBC, platelets, reticu-locytes	2	2
Electrolytes	7	3
BUN	7	3
Creatinine	2	2
Calcium, phosphorus, magnesium	2	2
Glucose	7	7
Transaminases, bilirubin	2	1
Alkaline phosphatase	2	1
Total protein, A/G (albumin–globulin)	2	1
Ammonia	—	1
Osmolarity	7	2
Prothrombin time	1	1
Urine		
Glucose	4–6 $\times$ daily	1–2 $\times$ daily
Specific gravity	2–4 $\times$ daily	7
Osmolarity	3	1

first week or until the patient becomes stabilized and also during later weeks.

COMPLICATIONS

Even with the most meticulous care and monitoring, various untoward effects may be encountered with total perenteral alimentation.

Table 9–5 lists some of these complications and the possible precipitating causes.

RETURN TO ENTERAL FEEDING

The ease or difficulty of reinstating enteral feeding is related to the condition for which intravenous alimentation was initiated and the length of time that the gastrointestinal tract was not used. It is usually advantageous to start with small amounts of lactose-free feedings of low osmolality. During this period, intravenous alimentation is maintained but is gradually decreased as more enteral feeding is tolerated. Many patients have diarrhea that may persist for a week or 10 days after significant quantities of feedings are taken. This is not an indication to stop feeding but is a sign to continue it. Many atrophic changes occur in the gastrointestinal tract when it is not utilized; however, these changes reverse after food is introduced. Numerous animal studies have shown a reduction in weight and protein content, as well as a depression in enzyme activity when parenteral feeding is substituted for oral feed-

Table 9–5. Complications of Intravenous Alimentation

Abnormality	Possible Cause
Metabolic	
Hyperglycemia, glucosuria	Too much or too rapid glucose infusion, especially in preterm infants; sepsis, stress, chromium deficiency
Hyper- or hyponatremia	Inappropriate sodium intake in relation to water intake, especially with unusual loss
Hyperkalemia	Excessive potassium intake
Hypokalemia	Deficient potassium intake, especially with protein anabolism
Metabolic acidosis	Excessive cationic amino acids in mixture
Hyperammonemia	Free ammonia in hydrolysates; amino acid imbalance or excess; deficient arginine
Anemia	Blood loss; folic acid; B_{12}; iron or copper deficiency
Elevation of transaminases and/or hyperbilirubinemia	Hepatotoxic effect of one or more components in infusate; interruption of enterohepatic circulation; decreased bile acid production; sepsis, carnitine deficiency, nonspecific response to refeeding
Bone demineralization, rickets	Inadequate phosphorus, calcium, or vitamin D intake
Azotemia	Excessive nitrogen administration, especially with caloric deficit
Low BUN	Inadequate nitrogen intake
Skin rash	Essential fatty acid, zinc, or biotin deficiency
Technical	
Catheter dislocation	—
Pneumothorax, hemothorax	Site of catheter tip not confirmed
Sepsis	Inadequate catheter care
Venous thrombosis	—
Perforation	—
Phlebitis	Peripheral alimentation

ing, even when a good nutritional state is maintained.

SUGGESTED READING

Heird, W.C., and Winters, R.W.: Total parenteral nutrition: the state of the art. J. Pediatr. 86:2, 1975.

Statement by an Expert Panel: Guidelines for essential trace element preparations for parenteral use. JAMA 241:2051, 1979.

Statement by the Nutrition Advisory Group: Multivitamin preparations for parenteral use. J. Parent. Ent. Nutr. 3:258, 1979.

Wilmore, D.M., and Dudrick, S.J.: Growth and development of an infant receiving all nutrients by vein. JAMA 203:860, 1968.

Shock

SOL S. ZIMMERMAN, M.D.

Shock denotes the clinical syndrome resulting from the failure of circulation to meet the metabolic demand of the tissues. Although shock is classically thought of in terms of its cardiovascular changes, diagnostically it is prudent to consider its biochemical manifestations, because these often precede the alterations in vital signs. The earlier in its progression that shock is identified, the sooner treatment can be begun and the better the prognosis.

Inadequacy of tissue circulation is the consequence of either hypovolemia, absolute or relative, or pump failure. Hypovolemia is absolute when there is true loss of intravascular fluid such as in hemorrhage, burns, gastroenteritis, diabetes, and "third-space" sequestrations. Relative hypovolemia exists in the presence of an acute decrease in vascular tone such as in sepsis, drug intoxications, spinal cord trauma, and anaphylaxis. The decreased tone results in an increased vascular compartment, for which the previous volume becomes relatively inadequate. The clinical syndromes associated with relative hypovolemia are frequently labeled by their etiology: *septic shock, neurogenic shock,* and *anaphylactic shock.*

Because shock is a reflection of circulatory failure, it can only be fully understood by first considering the parameters involved in controlling normal circulatory physiology.

Adequacy of circulation is dependent upon characteristics of myocardial contractility reflected in the Frank–Starling curves, neural influences over cardiac rate and vascular tone, and endocrine influences over cardiac rate and contractility and vascular volume and tone. Specific distribution of blood flow is influenced by both central neural and local autoregulatory mechanisms.

Cardiac output is determined by the stroke volume per contraction multiplied by the number of contractions per minute. Parameters influencing stroke volume are myocardial contractility, ventricular filling during diastole

(preload), and the resistance against which the ventricle contracts during systole (afterload). The primary determinant of preload is venous return, whereas that of afterload is systemic vascular resistance. Increases in heart rate are mediated by epinephrine and norepinephrine; decreases are mediated by the vagus nerve.

Vascular tone and volume are significantly influenced by several hormones. The catecholamines, epinephrine and norepinephrine, not only influence cardiac rate and contractility but also produce systemic and pulmonary vasoconstriction. Decreases in circulating volume to the kidneys bring into play the renin-angiotensin axis. Angiotensin II is a potent vasoconstrictor. As one of the mediators of sodium and potassium balance, aldosterone influences water retention and maintenance of an adequate vascular volume.

HYPOVOLEMIC SHOCK SYNDROMES

Absolute Hypovolemia

This is the most common etiology for shock in the pediatric patient. Circulatory failure from absolute hypovolemia results from an acute intravascular depletion, generally in the range of 15 to 25 percent of the circulating blood volume. Usual etiologies include hemorrhage, burns, gastroenteritis, both diabetes mellitus and insipidus, and third-space losses such as those in pancreatitis and peritonitis.

Venous return to the heart declines with resultant decreases in central venous pressure and stroke volume. Heart rate increases in an attempt to preserve cardiac output. Systolic blood pressure declines as a consequence of the lower stroke volume, whereas diastolic pressure remains unchanged or increases slightly secondary to peripheral vasoconstriction; pulse pressure decreases. Peripheral vasoconstriction initially occurs in a preferential manner so as to spare the brain and myocardium. As tissue perfusion progressively declines, metabolic acidosis supervenes. Increased oxygen extraction by the tissues is indicated by a greater than normal difference between arterial and venous oxygen contents.

Interstitial fluid is mobilized into both the intravascular and intracellular spaces. The fluid shift into the vascular compartments causes a decline in hematocrit. The fluid shift into the cells is a consequence of sodium pump dysfunction secondary to ischemia. In volume replacement, therefore, consideration has to be given to reconstitution of all fluid compartments. The required replacement is often significantly larger than would be anticipated from estimating exogenous losses alone.

The clinical presentation is easily understood by considering the pathophysiology. The tachycardia is an attempt to compensate for a decreased stroke volume. Decreased urine output and pale or gray, cold, clammy skin and extremities are the result of vasoconstriction. This vasoconstriction may initially maintain a normal systolic pressure even in the presence of a reduced stroke volume, but if hypovolemia goes uncorrected, systolic hypotension eventually occurs. A decreased systolic pressure and narrow pulse pressure account for the classic description of a poorly palpable, "thready" pulse. As the shock syndrome progresses, preservation of normal cerebral perfusion may no longer be possible, and anxiety, confusion, lethargy, and stupor occur in sequence. In the presence of severe tissue underperfusion, vasomotor nephropathy, "shock lung," ischemic bowel disease, and disseminated intravascular coagulation may occur as complications.

Relative Hypovolemia

Septic Shock

In the presence of infection, caused primarily by gram-negative organisms, circulatory failure may result from acute vasodilatation and extravasation of fluid from a "leaky" capillary bed. The alteration in vascular tone and permeability is the consequence of bacterial endotoxin as mediated through vasoactive substances such as the kinins. The septic shock syndrome has an early, hyperdynamic phase in which cardiac output remains normal or increases and a late, hypodynamic phase in which cardiac output drops.

The initial clinical picture is often termed *warm shock*, because the vasodilatation results in warm, erythematous skin and extremities. Systolic blood pressure in this stage is generally normal, whereas the diastolic pressure may decrease secondary to the vasodilatation. Pulse pressure, therefore, increases. Tachypnea may be marked and is often the finding that draws attention to the patient. This increase in respiratory rate is most likely the result of an increase in lung water from capillary leak. Primary, rather than compensatory, respiratory alkalosis results. Tachycardia may be disproportionate to the magnitude of fever that is present and should alert the clinician to the events that are transpiring. Leukopenia frequently occurs in this phase. There is a modest decline in urine output.

In the hypodynamic phase, cardiac output can no longer be maintained, vasoconstriction occurs, and the clinical picture is that of "classic" shock. Metabolic acidosis becomes evident; urine output declines markedly; and disseminated intravascular coagulation may occur.

Neurogenic Shock

In spinal cord trauma, loss of sympathetic autonomic innervation results in peripheral vasodilatation. The skin and extremities have the clinical appearance of warm shock.

Shock in the presence of head trauma should not automatically be attributed to that injury, because most often it is not the etiology. The patient should be carefully examined for other possible causes of shock.

Anaphylactic Shock

Anaphylactic shock is discussed in Chapter 11.

PUMP FAILURE OR CARDIOGENIC SHOCK

Pump failure as an etiology of the shock syndrome is uncommon in pediatric patients. It is even more infrequent if the neonatal period is excluded. It is during that period that hypoplasia of the ventricles, severe valvular stenosis, and large left-to-right shunts present. Differential diagnostic considerations include myocarditis, cardiomyopathies, myocardial ischemia, and collagen–vascular disease. Dysrhythmias, severe electrolyte disturbances, acidosis, hypoxia, and hypoglycemia all negatively influence myocardial function. Entities that impede venous return to the heart or egress from the ventricle, such as pericardial effusion and tension pneumothorax, may cause pump failure. In this overall group of infrequent conditions, one of the most common circumstances is the postoperative cardiac patient who has undergone ventriculotomy.

Evaluation and Treatment

Absolute Hypovolemia

Adequacy of volume replacement and control of ongoing losses are critical. As estimates of volume necessary for reconstitution are complicated by fluid shifts, a central venous catheter should be passed either percutaneously or by venous cutdown. In children, central venous pressure (CVP) generally correlates well with left atrial pressure and is usually the only invasive hemodynamic parameter required for successful fluid resuscitation of the patient. Measurements made by transducer are often more accurate than water manometry. A single measurement does not determine the adequacy of circulating volume, because CVP may be preserved in the normal range by a vasomotor decrease in venous capacitance. Relative changes in CVP determined by continuous monitoring will reflect adequacy of fluid administration.

Most often the CVP is low initially. If a measurement of 15 cm or more of H_2O is found initially in a patient with clinical shock, pump failure, pulmonary embolus, pericardial tamponade, hemothorax, pneumothorax, or pneumomediastinum should be considered. A chest x-ray should be obtained immediately.

In addition to the routine continuous measurement of heart rate, respiratory rate, and blood pressure, other parameters that must be monitored include urine output, arterial blood gases, hematocrit, coagulation profile, and serum BUN, creatinine, and electrolytes. Urine output is determined by insertion of a drainage catheter; "bagging" the patient is inadequate, because it does not give the continuous monitoring that is required. The periodic comparison of arterial and venous oxygen contents may be helpful as an indicator of tissue perfusion.

Selection of replacement fluid will vary depending upon the type of loss and the availability of blood and fresh frozen plasma. An initial "push" of 20 ml per kg of crystalloid (Ringer's lactate or normal saline) or 10 ml per kg of colloid (blood, fresh frozen plasma, or 5 percent salt-poor albumin) is administered intravenously over a 20-minute period. These "pushes" are repeated until vital signs are normalized, the CVP increases to 5 cm or more of H_2O, skin perfusion improves, and urine output exceeds 1 ml per kg per hour. Hematocrit and electrolytes are corrected as circumstances dictate. Transfusion of large volumes of citrated blood may require the administration of calcium (10 mg per kg of calcium chloride) to avoid hypocalcemia.

As in any resuscitation, appropriate airway and ventilation must be ensured. One of the most common errors is the delay in administering oxygen to the patient in shock who continues to breathe spontaneously, Although the patient may have profound tissue hypoxia, the clinical presentation is more often pallor than cyanosis and the need for oxygen therapy is overlooked. In the patient who requires intubation, high-peak inspiratory and end-expiratory pressures should be avoided, because they may compromise pulmonary blood flow. Hypoxia and hypercarbia should be corrected. Severe metabolic acidosis will require the administration of sodium bicarbonate, but this is a temporizing measure; maintenance of a normal pH requires restoration of adequate perfusion.

Because shock represents a state in which perfusion is inadequate to meet the needs of tissues, an effort should be made to minimize metabolic demands. Both hypothermia and hyperthermia increase metabolic demand; therefore, efforts should be made to keep the patient in the thermoneutral zone.

Relative Hypovolemia

In the syndromes of relative hypovolemic shock, the increased capacity of the vascular compartment will require infusions of large volumes. The principles and guidelines for fluid administration are the same as previously described.

Septic Shock

In septic shock, appropriate antibiotic therapy must be instituted and indicated drainage procedures performed (see Chapter 53, Sepsis). In the early, hyperdynamic phase, the mainstay of therapy is fluid infusion to ensure adequate expansion of circulating volume rather than attempting to induce peripheral vasoconstriction. As septic shock moves into the hypodynamic phase, peripheral vasoconstriction and a decreased cardiac output dominate the picture. Adequacy of circulating volume must be ensured and CVP should be followed closely. If in the presence of an adequate volume the syndrome of low cardiac output and increased systemic vascular resistance persists, pharmacologic agents should be introduced to improve tissue perfusion (Table 10–1). The placement of a pulmonary artery (Swan–Ganz) catheter in this circumstance is extremely valuable, because it enables cardiac output to be monitored while the drugs are being administered (Chapter 6, Invasive Hemodynamic Monitoring). These agents should be infused through a secure intravenous catheter, and these infusions should not be interrupted for other medications or fluids. Isoproterenol is the drug of choice, because it both reduces arteriolar resistance and increases myocardial contractility. Nitroprusside, a smooth muscle relaxant, is an alterna-

tive, but this form of afterload reduction carries the risk of sudden, severe hypotension. Inotropic agents such as dopamine or vasoconstrictors such as norepinephrine or phenylephrine should be immediately available for use in conjunction with the nitroprusside if hypotension occurs.

Although their efficacy is unproven, steroids in high doses are commonly used in the management of septic shock. Solu–Medrol, 40 mg per kg IV, as an initial dose, and 10 mg per kg IV are given every 6 hours thereafter for 24 to 48 hours; an alternative is Dexamethasone, 5 mg per kg IV, initially and 1.0 mg per kg every 6 hours thereafter for 24 to 48 hours.

Because the incidence of disseminated intravascular coagulation is greater in septic shock than in some of the other forms of circulatory failure, close attention to coagulation profiles is required.

Table 10–1. Cardiotonic and Vasoactive Drugs for The Management of Shock in Children

Drug	Mode of Action* and Effects	Dose	Comments/Warnings

Epinephrine	Alpha- and beta-adrenergic action
	Increases:
	  Heart rate
	  Myocardial contractility
	  Systemic vascular resistance
	  Pulmonary vascular resistance
	  Myocardial oxygen consumption
	Decreases:
	  Airway resistance
		IV push:
		  (1:10,000) 0.1 ml/kg
		IV drip:
		  2 mg/250 ml D5W (8 mcg/ml)
		Begin at a rate of 0.1 mcg/kg/min and titrate
			Do not administer with isoproterenol, because serious dysrhythmias may result.
			At low doses (0.1 mcg/kg/min), epinephrine is primarily a beta agonist.
			At doses of ≥0.5 mcg/kg/min, effect is primarily alpha-adrenergic.

Isoproterenol (Isuprel)	Beta-adrenergic action
	Increases:
	  Heart rate
	  Myocardial contractility
	  Myocardial oxygen consumption
	Decreases:
	  Systemic vascular resistance
	  Pulmonary vascular resistance
	  Airway resistance
		IV drip:
		  2 mg/250 ml D5W (8 mcg/ml)
		Begin at a rate of 0.1 mcg/kg/min and titrate
			Tachycardia may be striking.
			Do not exceed rates of 180–200/min, because risk of dysrhythmia increases.
			In the presence of hypovolemia, peripheral vasodilatation may result in hypotension.
			Do not administer with epinephrine, because serious dysrhythmias may result.

Dopamine (Intropin)	Dopaminergic at low doses
	Beta-adrenergic at moderate doses
	Alpha-adrenergic at high doses
	Low–moderate doses:
	  Increases:
	    Myocardial contractility
	    Renal, splanchnic, coronary blood flow
	    Cardiac output
	  Decreases:
	    Systemic vascular resistance
		IV drip:
		  200 mg/250 ml D5W (800 mcg/ml)
		Low dose: 2–6 mcg/kg/min
		Moderate dose:
		  7–15 mcg/kg/min
		High dose:
		  >15 mcg/kg/min
			In the presence of hypovolemia, low-dose therapy may cause hypotension.

*See footnote on next page.

Table continued on following page.

Table 10–1. Cardiotonic and Vasoactive Drugs for The Management of Shock in Children *Continued*

Drug	Mode of Action* and Effects	Dose	Comments/Warnings
Dopamine (Intropin) (cont.)	Low–moderate doses: Decreases: Pulmonary vascular resistance High doses: Increases: Systemic vascular resistance		
Dobutamine	Beta-adrenergic action primarily Increases: Myocardial contractility	250 mg/250 ml D5W (1,000 mcg/ml) Begin at a rate of 2 mcg/kg/min and titrate Usual range: 2–20 mcg/kg/min	Occasionally causes tachycardia. Can produce PVCs. Contraindicated in idiopathic hypertrophic subaortic stenosis, because obstruction may be increased.
Phenylephrine (Neo-Synephrine)	Alpha-adrenergic Increases: Systemic vascular resistance Decreases: Renal and splanchnic blood flow	0.1 mg/kg IM	Rare usage in neurogenic shock. May be required to overcome hypotension secondary to afterload reduction by nitroprusside.
Nitroprusside (Nipride)	Smooth muscle relaxant Decreases: Systemic vascular resistance Pulmonary vascular resistance	IV drip: 50 mg/250 ml D5W (200 mcg/ml) Begin at a rate of 0.5 mcg/kg/min and titrate Usual range: 0.5–10 mcg/kg/min	For use in syndrome of low cardiac output and high systemic vascular resistance in the presence of an adequate circulating volume. Onset and termination of action are almost immediate. May cause severe, abrupt hypotension. Must be protected from light. End product of metabolism is thiocyanate. Monitor levels and do not allow them to exceed 10 mg/dl.

*Alpha-adrenergic: Cutaneous, coronary, splanchnic, and renal vasoconstriction
Beta-adrenergic:
    Beta–1   Increased cardiac rate (chronotropic); increased myocardial contractility (inotropic)
    Beta–2   Skeletal muscle vasodilatation; bronchodilatation
Dopaminergic: Splanchnic and renal vasodilatation

Neurogenic Shock

Volume expansion with restoration of a normal CVP is the only circulatory support required to counter the loss of vascular tone in spinal cord trauma. In the rare circumstance in which this is inadequate, vasoconstriction can be induced by an alpha-adrenergic agent such as phenylephrine (see Table 10–1).

Anaphylactic Shock

Anaphylactic shock is discussed in Chapter 11.

Cardiogenic Shock

As in all shock syndromes, circulating volume must be adequate. If the CVP is low, fluids should be infused; if the CVP is high, diuretic therapy should be instituted. Hypoxia and imbalances of acid–base and electrolytes should be corrected to improve myocardial performance. One or more inotropic agents (see Table 10–1) such as digoxin, epinephrine, isoproterenol, dopamine, and dobutamine may be required to increase cardiac contractility. Optimal management of cardiogenic shock will require measurement of right and left ventricular-filling pressures, cardiac output, and systemic vascular resistance. This will necessitate the placement of a Swan–Ganz catheter so that direct determinations and appropriate calculations can be made. (See Chapter 6, Invasive Hemodynamic Monitoring.) These measurements will be particularly valuable if pharmacologic afterload reduction is required. (See Chapter 19, Congestive Heart Failure.)

SUGGESTED READING

Crone, R.K.: Acute circulatory failure in children. Pediatr. Clin. North Am. 27:525, 1980.

Lefer, A.M., and Spath, J.A.: Pharmacologic basis of the treatment of circulatory shock. *In* Antonaccio, M. (ed.): Cardiovascular Pharmacology. New York, Raven Press, 1977, pp. 377–428.

Perkin, R.M., and Levin, D.L.: Shock in the pediatric patient, Part I—definition, etiology and pathophysiology. J. Pediatr. 101:163, 1982.

Perkin, R.M., and Levin, D.L.: Shock in the pediatric patient, Part II—therapy. J. Pediatr. 101:319, 1982.

Shoemaker, W.C.: Pathophysiology, monitoring, and therapy of shock syndromes. *In* Shoemaker, W.C., and Thompson, W.L. (eds.): Critical Care—State of the Art. Fullerton, CA, Society of Critical Care Medicine, 1980, pp. I (D) 1–63.

Tarazi, R.C.: Sympathomimetic agents in the treatment of shock. Ann. Intern. Med. 31:364, 1974.

Weil, M.H., Shubin, H., and Carlson, R.W.: Sympathomimetic and related vasoactive agents for treatment of circulatory shock. *In* Weil, M.H., and Shubin, H. (eds.). Critical Care Medicine—Current Principles and Practices. New York, Harper and Row, Publishers, 1976, pp. 99–108.

11

Anaphylaxis

SOL S. ZIMMERMAN, M.D.

Anaphylaxis is the acute clinical syndrome resulting from the interaction of an allergen and a patient who is hypersensitive to it. The syndrome may be immediate in onset, is often life threatening, and frequently involves multiple organ systems. The most commonly affected systems are cardiovascular, respiratory, gastrointestinal, and cutaneous (Table 11–1). Because anaphylaxis is sudden and often unpredictable, it poses a challenge that requires quick diagnosis and rapid institution of therapy.

Exposure to the allergen can be by ingestion, inhalation, or injection. Common offending substances include antibiotics, local anesthetics, analgesics, radiographic contrast materials, foods, and insect stings (Table 11–2). Clinical circumstances often associated with anaphylaxis are parenteral administration of penicillin and other antibiotics, intravenous infusion of contrast material for radiologic studies, and injection of allergenic extracts for desensitization.

The initial immunologic reaction occurs between the allergen and pre-existing specific immunoglobulin E (IgE). This antigen–antibody interaction results in the release of chemical mediators, which, in turn, influence target organ systems. Histamine, the primary mediator, induces vasodilatation, bronchoconstriction, and increased capillary permeability. Other mediators of these reactions include slow-reacting substance of anaphylaxis (SRS-A) and the kinins.

The onset of clinical symptoms usually occurs within minutes of exposure to the offending allergen. There seems to be a correlation between the time of onset of symptoms and the severity of the clinical syndrome; the sooner the onset, the more severe the reaction. One or more of the symptoms listed in Table 11–1 may be clinically evident in the anaphylactic reaction. Laryngeal edema, with its acute upper airway obstruction, and relative hypovolemic shock (Chapter 10) are presentations that carry a more ominous prognosis. Shock results from mediator-induced vasodilatation and the sudden inadequacy of the circulating volume to meet the metabolic demands of the tissues. This relative hypovolemic state is further complicated by increased capillary permeability and true loss of volume into the interstitial space.

TREATMENT

Successful outcome depends upon rapid recognition of the anaphylactic reaction and immediate institution of treatment.

Epinephrine, 1:1000, at doses of 0.1 to 0.5 ml (0.01 mg per kg), should be given subcutaneously and repeated at 20- to 30-minute intervals as necessary. The subcutaneous route of administration is adequate, and epinephrine should not be withheld pending the establishment of an intravenous (IV) route. If an IV is inserted at the time of reaction, epinephrine 1:10,000, at a dose of 0.1 mg per kg, should be given intravenously.

If the allergen can be identified, further exposure should be terminated or minimized. This can be accomplished by discontinuing intravenous drug, blood, or contrast material infusions or by placement of a tourniquet proximal to the site of an injection. An additional dose of epinephrine, 1:1000, 0.1 to 0.2 ml, may be given subcutaneously at the site of allergen injection to decrease the rate of absorption.

In severe reactions, an intravenous line must be established for administration of fluids and additional medication. In the presence of relative hypovolemia and hypotension, crystalloid, at 20 ml per kg, or colloid, at 10 ml per kg, should be given as a "push" over a period of 20 minutes, with repetition until the central venous pressure (CVP) returns to normal and tissue perfusion improves. Alpha-adrenergic agents (epinephrine, norepinephrine, and

Table 11–1. Symptoms of Anaphylaxis

Cardiovascular
Tachycardia
Dysrhythmias
Hypotension (fainting)
"Relative hypovolemic" shock (Chapter 10)
Respiratory
Rhinitis (sneezing, nasal itching, rhinorrhea)
Laryngeal edema (stridor)
Bronchospasm (cough, wheezing)
Gastrointestinal
Nausea and vomiting
Abdominal pain
Diarrhea
Skin
Diffuse flush ppearance
Urticaria
Angioedema (periorbital and perioral)

Table 11–2. Common Allergens Associated with Anaphylaxis

Drugs
Antibiotics
Penicillin, cephalosporins, tetracycline, streptomycin
Local anesthetics
Lidocaine, procaine
Analgesics/anti-inflammatory agents
Aspirin, indomethacin, phenylbutazone
Biologics
Allergen extracts, gamma globulin, antitoxins (diphtheria and tetanus), blood, snake antivenin, antilymphocytic serum
Diagnostic Agents
Iodinated contrast material, Bromsulphalein dye (BSP)
Foods
Eggs, fish, shellfish, chocolate, milk, and nuts
Venoms
Hymenoptera, snake

phenylephrine) may be required to maintain blood pressure by producing vasoconstriction.

An airway must be ensured, and adequate oxygenation must be provided. Endotracheal intubation and even tracheostomy may be required. In the presence of bronchospasm that persists after the administration of epinephrine, aminophylline, 6 mg per kg, should be given intravenously as a loading dose, followed by a continuous aminophylline drip (see Chapter 24).

Diphenhydramine hydrochloride (Benadryl), 1.0 to 1.5 mg per kg P.O. or IV, may be given at 6-hour intervals. Although such an antihistamine will not counter the effect of histamine already released, it has a therapeutic role when exposure to allergen may continue. In addition, it may relieve any significant pruritus.

Steroids do not have a role in the management of the usual acute anaphylactic reaction, and their use is not indicated. If the reaction is severe or if the clinical course is anticipated to be long, steroids may be helpful.

PREVENTION

Attempts should be made to minimize the incidence of anaphylaxis by identifying individuals who have had significant hypersensi-

tivity reactions in the past. These patients should wear or carry the commercially available bracelets, tags, and cards that warn of specific sensitivities. Thorough histories of patients should be taken before medication is administered.

In circumstances in which the incidence of reaction is increased, such as desensitization therapy ("allergy shots"), the patient should be observed for at least 15 minutes following injection of the allergen extract. Emergency equipment, oxygen, and medication should be available in this setting as well as in radiology suites where contrast material is infused.

When exposure to the allergen may be unavoidable, as with insect stings, and the reaction may be severe, desensitization therapy should be considered. Commercially prepared insect sting kits are available, but their use must be carefully explained as well as rehearsed.

SUGGESTED READING

Austen, K.F.: Systemic anaphylaxis in the human being. N. Engl. J. Med. 291:661, 1974.
Corbascio, A.N.: Countermeasures for anaphylactic reactions. Drug Ther. 6:101, 1976.
Kelly, J.F., and Patterson, R.: Anaphylaxis. JAMA 227:1431, 1974.

Increased Intracranial Pressure

SOL S. ZIMMERMAN, M.D.

The cranial cavity is a relatively rigid structure that contains three incompressible substances: brain tissue, cerebrospinal fluid (CSF), and cerebral blood volume. Intracranial pressure (ICP) is a dynamic measurement that fluctuates as the volume of these components varies. If the ICP is to remain relatively constant, an increase in the volume of one component requires reciprocal volume changes in one or both of the other components. If a pathologic component (tumor, hematoma, or abscess) is added to the cranial cavity, there must be a reduction in the volume of the remaining contents. Increases in ICP are the consequence of increases in the volume of one or more of these components that exceed the capacity of compensatory mechanisms. These mechanisms initially include displacement of CSF into the spinal sac and reduction of cerebral venous capacity. A minimal increase in volume can be accommodated while maintaining the ICP within the normal upper limit of 15 mm Hg, but as volume increases, the pressure rises rapidly. When the buffering capacity is exhausted, the pressure–volume relationship becomes nonlinear; small increments in volume result in progressively greater rises in intracranial pressure (Fig. 12–1). Causes of increased ICP can best be appreciated by considering the individual intracranial components and the processes that affect them.

Although the volume of neurons and glia remains relatively constant, the volume of brain tissue can be affected by diffuse or local edema. Cerebral edema may be conceptually divided into vasogenic and cytotoxic. Vasogenic edema is the interstitial accumulation of fluid that results from alteration in capillary permeability secondary to such processes as head trauma, brain tumors, infection, and hypoxia. Cytotoxic edema is the increase in ICF that results from metabolic derangements such as hypoxia, water intoxication, and the effect of toxins. Local edema is most often seen surrounding a space-occupying lesion.

In the usual circumstance, production and reabsorption of CSF are in equilibrium. If the normal dynamic is altered by obstruction of flow or impairment of absorption, the volume of CSF increases. Such alterations can be the consequence of congenital anomalies, infection, trauma, or masses and may result in either communicating or noncommunicating hydrocephalus and an increase in ICP.

Cerebral blood volume is affected by the interrelationship between cerebral blood flow (CBF), cerebral perfusion pressure (CPP), and cerebral vascular resistance (CVR).

$$CBF = \frac{CPP}{CVR}$$

CPP is equal to the difference between mean systemic arterial pressure (MAP) and intracranial pressure (ICP).

$$CPP = MAP - ICP$$

CBF is maintained at a relatively constant level over a wide range of blood pressures; this ability is termed *autoregulation*. Constancy of flow is achieved by either increasing or decreasing CVR at the arteriolar level. In the absence of normal autoregulation, CBF varies directly with CPP.

CBF is also affected by changes in arterial oxygen and carbon dioxide tensions. The influence of arterial oxygen tension occurs only at hypoxic levels ($Pa_{O_2} < 50$ mm Hg), where the effect is to increase CBF. The influence of arterial carbon dioxide tensions, however, is over a wide range of levels with an almost linear relationship; increases in Pa_{CO_2} increase CBF, decreases in Pa_{CO_2} decrease CBF. The effect of Pa_{CO_2} on cerebral arteriolar tone is mediated by the resulting change in the pH of CNS interstitial fluid. Maximal cerebral vasoconstriction occurs as Pa_{CO_2} approaches 20 mm Hg, at which point tissue ischemia may result.

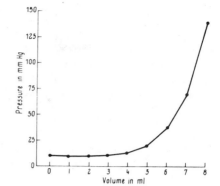

Figure 12–1. Intracranial pressure vs. volume response curve. (From Hahn, J.F.: Cerebral edema and neurointensive care. Pediatr. Clin. North Am., 27:588, 1980. Used by permission.) From Langfitt, T.W., et al.: Vascular factors in head injury. *In* Caveness, W.F., and Walker, A.E. (eds.): Head Injury Proceedings. Philadelphia, J.B. Lippincott Co., 1966, pp. 172–194.

The ensuing local acidosis will then cause an increase in CBF.

CBV may increase as a consequence of obstruction to venous return from the head. The venous obstruction may result from conditions such as superior vena cava syndrome or sagittal sinus thrombosis.

CLINICAL PRESENTATION

The clinical syndrome resulting from an acute increase in ICP consists of headache, vomiting, and lethargy. Subacute increases in ICP are often associated with personality change and memory deficits, in addition to the other complaints. Papilledema may be present on physical examination, but its absence does not rule out an increase in ICP. Sixth-nerve palsy may be a physical finding. The long intracranial course of the sixth cranial nerve and its path across the petrous portion of the temporal bone make it susceptible to injury from diffuse increases in ICP. Pressure gradients can cause herniation of brain tissue across such structures as the falx cerebri, tentorium, or foramen magnum. Transtentorial herniation may result in third-nerve palsy. Alterations in state of consciousness and vital signs become evident as ICP becomes markedly elevated. Loss of consciousness, bradycardia, hypertension, and slowing of respiration result from compression or distortion of the brain stem. The presence of these signs denotes a life-threatening emergency that requires rapid intervention to lower ICP.

MONITORING

Management of increased ICP is dependent upon the recognition of the clinical setting in which it occurs and monitoring the amplitude of pressure increase. Clinical monitoring requires frequent reassessment of vital signs, pattern of respiration, level of consciousness, corneal response, pupillary size and response, extraocular movement, oculocephalic or oculovestibular reflex, and motor response. Continuous measurement of ICP can be accomplished by using devices such as the intraventricular catheter, subarachnoid screw, or epidural monitor. These monitoring techniques do not replace the need for frequent clinical evaluation of the patient.

The intraventricular catheter provides accurate measurements and is the only monitoring modality that can also be used therapeutically to decrease ICP by removing CSF. It can also be used to determine the patient's ability to tolerate further increases in intracranial volume by measuring the ventricular pressure response. A small volume (1 ml) is injected into the ventricle, and the corresponding change in pressure is measured. If the pressure increase is greater than 4 mm Hg, little tolerance remains and the patient is on the steep portion of the ventricular-pressure response curve. The disadvantages of the intraventricular catheter are the necessity to pass through brain substance and a 3 to 5 percent risk of infection. In the presence of diffuse cerebral edema where the ventricles may be slitlike, placement of a ventricular catheter may be a very difficult procedure. If the ventricles are very small or if a large volume of CSF is removed therapeutically, maintenance of catheter patency may pose a problem.

The subarachnoid screw requires opening of the dura and arachnoid, but it does not enter brain tissue. It consists of a hollow stainless steel "bolt," which is anchored by "threading" into the skull. It cannot be used therapeutically, because no CSF can be drained, and it does have a risk of infection, although the risk is less than that associated with the intraventricular catheter.

The epidural monitor is the least invasive of the techniques and is easy to place. Its position must be directly flush with the dura to obtain accurate ICP measurements. The necessity of a precise interface between dura and monitor has limited the usefulness of this technique. The potential for alteration of this interface with changing intracranial dynamics has cast doubt on the reliability of its measurements. There is very little risk of infection.

The choice of technique to be used may be dictated by the clinical circumstances. Most neurosurgeons, however, have a preference for one of the techniques, and the ICU staff should become comfortable with its set-up and use and recognize its advantages and limitations.

The monitoring device is connected to a calibrated transducer, and measurements are displayed on an oscilloscope or strip recorder. Normal ICP is defined as less than 15 mm Hg. Various wave forms have been described, and attempts are being made to correlate them with the clinical state.

TREATMENT

The goals of therapy are to decrease ICP to normal levels or at least to less than 20 mm Hg and to maintain CPP greater than 50 mm Hg.

The most rapid and effective mode of treatment is hyperventilation. This can be accomplished by bag and mask method or by intubation and use of a mechanical ventilator. When using a positive pressure ventilator, tidal volume should be set relatively high and ventilatory rate and inspiratory and end-expiratory pressure should be set relatively low in order to minimize the effect of intrathoracic pressure on venous return from the head. If the patient has spontaneous respirations that are out of phase with the ventilator, the resulting increased intrathoracic pressure will raise intracranial pressure. Sedation (diazepam, barbiturate) and muscle paralysis (pancuronium) may be required to permit optimal ventilatory management. Arterial carbon dioxide tension should be brought down to the 25- to 30-mm Hg range.

If a ventricular catheter is in place, CSF can be removed as another rapid therapeutic modality. Excessive withdrawal of CSF, however, can result in ventricular collapse and catheter occlusion. This can be avoided by establishing a minimum pressure (10 to 15 mm Hg) against which drainage occurs.

Reduction in brain water can be accomplished by decreasing fluid intake to two thirds of maintenance requirements and by use of osmotic or loop diuretics. The osmotic agents include mannitol, which is the most widely used medication, urea, and glycerol. When first administered, the osmotic agents expand the intravascular volume, and in the absence of normal autoregulation, a brief increase in ICP may result. A 20 percent solution of mannitol, in a dose of 1 gm per kg, is administered intravenously over a 30-minute period and is repeated at 4- to 6-hour intervals. Urea, as a 30 percent solution, is infused intravenously over a 30-minute period in a dose of 0.5 to 1.0 gm per kg every 4 to 6 hours. Glycerol can be given either orally or intravenously. Orally, the dose is 0.5 to 2.0 gm per kg administered by nasogastric tube. The intravenous preparation is a 10 percent solution, whigh is infused in a dose of 1.0 gm per kg over a 30-minute period. Intravenously, glycerol has been associated with hemolysis. When using any of these agents, serum osmolality should be closely followed and not allowed to exceed 320 mOsm.

A loop diuretic, furosemide or ethacrynic acid, may be given intravenously at a dose of 1 mg per kg. A vigorous diuresis results, requiring that fluid and electrolyte status be closely monitored. Fluid restriction and diuresis can easily result in hypotension. This must be avoided because of the adverse effect upon cerebral perfusion pressure.

Steroids are used in the treatment of increased ICP because of their ability to stabilize cell membranes and reduce cerebral edema. Although commonly used for treatment of cerebral edema secondary to head trauma, their efficacy has not been demonstrated. Dexamethasone is given in a dose of 1.0 to 1.5 mg per kg intravenously, with repeat doses at 6-hour intervals. An alternative is methylprednisolone in a dose of 4 to 6 mg per kg every 6 hours.

Cooling blankets and antipyretics are used to aggressively treat fever, because elevated body temperature increases cerebral metabolic demand and cerebral blood flow. Hypothermia, itself, may be a useful adjunct in the management of increased ICP. Using hypothermia blankets, the body temperature is decreased to 30 to 32°C.

Barbiturate-induced coma is used if the other therapeutic modalities fail to lower the ICP to the desired level. High-dose barbiturates decrease cerebral metabolic demand, increase CVR, and reduce cerebral blood flow. In addition, the ability of barbiturates to scavenge free radicals may help protect cellular integrity. High-dose barbiturates have a significant effect upon circulatory dynamics in that they reduce systemic vascular resistance. In the patient who is hypovolemic as a consequence of fluid restriction and diuretic therapy, this action can result in profound hypotension. Volume expansion and pressor therapy may be required. Systemic and pulmonary artery catheters are essential in the management of these patients because of the absolute need to monitor systemic arterial pressure, pulmonary capillary wedge pressure, and cardiac output.

Pentobarbital is given intravenously in an initial dose of 3 to 5 mg per kg. The end point of therapy is an EEG pattern of burst suppression. The patient is maintained in this state by a steady infusion of pentobarbital at a dose of 1 to 2 mg per kg per hour. Serum levels should be followed, the target level being in the range of 3 to 4 mg/dl.

There are several general principles in the care of patients with increased ICP. The head should be kept in a neutral position and elevated to 30 degrees to facilitate venous return from the head. All procedures such as suctioning, turning, and chest physiotherapy should be preceded by sedation (with either short-acting barbiturates or diazepam) and, if necessary, analgesia to avoid increases in ICP. This premedication is necessary even in the patient receiving curare or pancuronium for muscle paralysis, because agitation can cause a rise in ICP. Similarly, EEG evidence of seizure activity in the paralyzed patient must be vigorously treated, because even in the absence of a visible motor response, seizures can increase ICP. Stool softeners should be given to avoid the need for a Valsalva maneuver. As always, care must be taken to ensure adequate substrate (glucose and oxygen) for cerebral metabolism.

The various therapeutic modalities are withdrawn in a gradual, stepwise manner after ICP has been maintained in the desired range for 24 hours. The interval between sequential changes in therapy should be at least 6 to 8 hours. The first measure to be withdrawn is that which is most invasive or associated with the greatest adverse effects. Barbiturate coma, therefore, would be withdrawn first, followed by hypothermia. The hypothermic patient is allowed to rewarm slowly, at a rate of 0.5°C per hour.

SUGGESTED READING

Bruce, D.A., Berman, W.A., and Schut, L.: Cerebrospinal fluid monitoring in children; physiology, pathology, and clinical usefulness. Adv. Pediatr. 24:233, 1977.

Cottrell, J.E., Robustell, A., Post, K., and Turndorf, H.: Furosemide- and mannitol-induced changes in intracranial pressure and serum osmolality and electrolytes. Anesthesiology 47:28, 1977.

Miller, J.D.: Barbiturates and raised intracranial pressure. Ann. Neurol. 6:189, 1979.

Sullivan, H.G., and Becker, D.P.: Intracranial pressure monitoring and interpretation. In Cottrell, J.E., and Turndorf, H. (eds.): Anesthesia and Neurosurgery. St. Louis, The C.V. Mosby Co., 1980, pp. 58–88.

Zierski, J.: Extradural, ventricular, and subdural pressure recording: comparative clinical study. In Schulman, K., Marmarov, A., Miller, J.D., et al. (eds.): Intracranial Pressure IV. Berlin, Springer–Verlag, 1980, pp. 371–376.

Temperature Regulation

HARRIS E. BURSTIN, M.D.

Problems with temperature regulation are common in the critically ill child, both as a symptom and as a reason for admission. This chapter addresses the pathophysiology of temperature regulation and its consequences in the critically ill, as well as heat illness, malignant hyperthermia, and accidental hypothermia.

MECHANISMS OF THERMOREGULATION

Mammals are endothermic. Body temperature is regulated by adjustment of heat gain and loss, not by the environment. The thermoregulatory center is located in the hypothalamus and controls body temperature through a complex biofeedback system. The *thermostat* is the body's temperature sensor. It directly measures the temperature of blood entering the brain as well as receiving information from distal temperature sensors in the skin, deep tissues, spinal cord, and other parts of the brain. The *set point area* of the hypothalamus maintains euthermia by stimulating the *heat gain center* or the *heat loss center*. Heat is gained by increasing the metabolic rate, inducing peripheral vasoconstriction, and increasing muscle tone. Heat is lost by inducing peripheral vasodilatation and decreasing heat production.

The core body temperature varies from person to person as well as according to the time of day. Rectal temperatures between 36° and 38°C (97° and 100°F) are considered within the range of normal. Fever is defined as an increase in body temperature above 38°C (100.4°F) as a result of an organized response by the body to an insult or disease. Hyperthermia implies an abnormal elevation of body temperature in spite of the body's attempt to lower it.

Infections, malignancies, and collagen diseases produce fever by increasing the hypothalamic set point, an increase that is mediated by endogenous pyrogens and certain prostaglandins. Core temperature elevation may be caused by abnormal heat production (i.e., ma-

lignant hyperthermia), defective heat loss, or elevated environmental temperature (i.e., heat stroke). Central fever is seen in neurologically impaired patients with a damaged thermoregulatory apparatus.

FEVER IN THE CRITICALLY ILL CHILD

Temperature elevation in the critically ill child with compromised cardiopulmonary or neurologic status has serious consequences. The metabolic rate increases as core body temperature increases so that at a temperature of 43°C (110°F), there is a 100 percent increase. This increases oxygen consumption, carbon dioxide and organic acid production, insensible water losses, and caloric requirements.

Heart rate increases 10 beats per minute for every 1°F elevation of temperature. Cardiac work and the metabolic needs of the heart increase. Systemic blood pressure decreases as a result of peripheral vasodilatation. Respiratory rate increases 2 breaths per minute for every 1°F elevation of temperature. Vasoconstriction of pulmonary arterioles occurs. This, coupled with systemic hypotension, can increase intrapulmonary and/or intracardiac shunting. Fever also shifts the oxyhemoglobin dissociation curve to the right.

Fever increases intracranial pressure and the oxygen requirement of the brain. Coupled with systemic hypotension, this may result in cerebral hypoxia and decreased cerebral blood flow. Fever is known to lower the seizure threshhold, and irreversible brain damage is reported with temperatures above 42°C (108°F).

Despite its possible theoretical beneficial effects, fever in the critically ill child should be treated aggressively. The etiology of fevers must be investigated, and indicated specific therapy must be instituted (i.e., antibiotics).

Fever should be treated with aspirin or acetaminophen and external cooling with a hypothermia blanket. Aspirin and acetaminophen lower temperature by their antiprostaglandin effect. The usual dosage of each is 10 to 15 mg per kg P.O. or per rectum every 4 hours. The use of aspirin may be limited in postoperative cases because of its effect upon platelet aggregation and its potential for gastric irritation. Acetaminophen should be used with caution in patients with liver disease.

HEAT ILLNESS

The most benign form of heat illness is heat cramps, which consist of muscle pain probably caused by sodium loss and which are treated with oral electrolyte replacement solutions.

Heat exhaustion or prostration is more severe and presents with increasing lassitude, headache, vomiting, tachycardia, hypotension, and hypovolemia as a result of water depletion. Treatment consists of rehydration and rest.

Heat stroke is the most severe form of heat illness, with a 7 to 70 percent reported mortality rate depending upon length of exposure and age. It is defined as a rise in core body temperature with a decreased heat dissipation caused by high ambient temperature. In children, environmental temperature rather than physical activity is the most important factor. Children with cystic fibrosis, ectodermal dysplasia, familial dysautonomia, birth injuries, and fluid deprivation are predisposed. Heat stroke has been reported in infants left in locked cars for short periods of time in the summer. Mortality in children younger than 1 year of age is very high.

The three cardinal signs of heat stroke are hot, dry skin following initial sweating, hyperthermia, and central nervous system (CNS) changes. Pathophysiologically, initial sweating and water loss lead to decreased blood volume and then to peripheral vasoconstriction. This, plus high ambient temperature, decreases heat dissipation and increases core temperature.

CNS-related symptoms include headache, dizziness, and confusion progressing to loss of consciousness, stupor, and coma as the duration of exposure increases. Convulsions are also seen. Multiorgan system effects include electrocardiogram changes of cardiac strain, hepatic abnormalities, hemolysis, fibrinolysis, disseminated intravascular coagulation, and renal damage caused by myoglobinuria and thermal injury.

Treatment is directed at cooling and circulatory support. Cooling is obtained by removing all clothing, vigorous massage to increase vasodilatation, and immersion or sponging with cool water. Iced intravenous fluids, enemas, and/or gastric lavage may be necessary to reduce the temperature below 39°C (103°F).

Intravenous fluids are given quickly to establish and maintain adequate urine output. Electrolytes and bicarbonate are given as indicated. Cardiotonic medications may also be required. Beta-sympathomimetic agonists such as isoproterenol are preferred, because they increase cardiac output and also induce vasodilatation. Atropine or other anticholinergic drugs should be avoided, because they decrease sweating. Alpha-sympathomimetic agonists are also avoided, because they increase vasoconstriction. Phenothiazines are used to decrease shivering. Anticonvulsants such as phenobarbital may be required.

MALIGNANT HYPERTHERMIA

Severe hyperthermia with profound metabolic derangements and muscle rigidity associated with general anesthesia is now a well-described syndrome of malignant hyperthermia.

Malignant hyperthermia seems to be due to complex alterations in calcium control, resulting in an exaggerated response of skeletal muscle exposed to an appropriate stimulus. Increased muscle metabolism produces lactic acid, carbon dioxide, and heat. The calcium derangement also has multiorgan system effects suggestive of a generalized alteration in membrane permeability. Unstable blood pressures resulting from capillary leakage and third spacing of fluids are also seen. Pulmonary edema may be present. Peripheral vasoconstriction, in the body's attempt to correct hypovolemia, interferes with heat dissipation and aggravates the hyperthermia. Untreated, malignant hyperthermia carries a 50 to 80 percent mortality rate.

The incidence of malignant hyperthermia seems to be between 1:15,000 and 1:50,000 among patients to whom anesthesia is administered. Patients with myopathies and neuropathies are predisposed. Young males with undescended testis, spinal and pectus deformities, mandibular hypoplasia, antimongolian palpebral fissures, ptosis, low-set ears, and webbed neck have been described at increased risk.

The occurrence of muscle rigidity following administration of an appropriate dose of succinylcholine is highly suggestive of malignant hyperthermia. This factor plus evidence of hypermetabolism, including tachycardia, tachypnea, and dysrhythmia, mottling of skin or cyanosis, and elevated temperatures to as high as 44°C (111°F), establishes the diagnosis. Myoglobinuria and elevated creatine phosphokinase (CPK) are confirmatory factors in the diagnosis but are not required.

After malignant hyperthermia has been recognized, the first therapeutic measure should be to cease delivery of anesthetic agents. The metabolic acidosis, respiratory acidosis, and unstable blood pressures are treated vigorously with bicarbonate, hyperventilation with 100 percent O_2, and fluid resuscitation. Hyperthermia should be aggressively treated, with ice packs, iced gastric and/or peritoneal lavage, and iced intravenous solutions, if the temperature is above 40.6°C (105°F). Rarely, cooling via pump bypass is necessary (if available).

Urine output must be maintained to prevent damage to the kidneys from myoglobinuria. Dysrhythmias are treated appropriately to maintain cardiac output. Pulmonary edema, if present, may require prolonged positive pressure ventilation. Potassium levels must be followed closely, because the hyperkalemia that can be seen in the early stages can, with fluid and bicarbonate therapy, quickly change to hypokalemia.

Dantrolene is the only known specific therapeutic agent for malignant hyperthermia. It is a direct acting skeletal muscle relaxant that has been shown to be effective if given within 24 hours (preferably as soon as diagnosis is made). One mg per kg is given intravenously every 3 to 5 minutes up to a total of 10 mg per kg or until the muscle rigidity stops. An average of 4 to 7 mg per kg is usually required.

Although dantrolene and the previously outlined therapy have greatly reduced the mortality of malignant hyperthermia, prevention is the goal. A detailed history and physical examination are required for evidence of clinical or subclinical muscle weakness and recognition of described syndromes. A family history of malignant hyperthermia is suggestive of susceptibility. The exact genetics of malignant hyperthermia are unclear. A preoperative elevation of CPK is about 70 percent reliable in predicting those at risk. Muscle biopsy is indicated in known susceptible individuals with normal CPK's. Histologic and chemical testing of the muscle specimen is more than 90 percent accurate in establishing the diagnosis.

ACCIDENTAL HYPOTHERMIA

Accidental hypothermia is defined as a core body temperature below 35°C (95°F) caused by prolonged exposure to cold. Because standard thermometers read only to 34°C (94°F), glass thermometers that read to 24°C (75°C) must be used. Iatrogenically induced hypothermia will not be discussed here.

Accidental hypothermia can be seen in winter months, resulting from inadequate housing, cold water immersions, prolonged exposure after automobile accidents, and intoxications with alcohol or drugs. Patients with diabetes, mental illness, and CNS or endocrine disorders are at higher risk. Infants are predisposed as a result of poor thermoregulatory control and a large surface area relative to body volume.

The body's intitial response to a core temperature of 35°C (95°F) is to maximize the metabolic rate and increase peripheral vasoconstriction by increased release of catecholamines. Shivering is induced by the hypothalamus to increase heat production.

At core temperatures of 32°C (90°F), the metabolic rate falls. There are decreases in respiratory effort, cardiac dynamics, and systemic blood pressure. A combined metabolic and respiratory acidosis is present secondary to anaerobic metabolism and hypercapnea. Blood viscosity increases, and shivering is replaced by rigidity. Neurologic status deteriorates as the core temperature falls.

At core temperatures of 24° to 25°C (75° to 77°F), respiration ceases and the myocardium becomes extremely irritable. At core temperatures below 15°C (59°F), cardiac standstill occurs.

A profound state of hypothermia is indistinguishable from death. The patient appears cold, rigid, apneic, pulseless, areflexic, and unresponsive with fixed and dilated pupils. Death is confirmed only when near normal temperatures are achieved and the patient is still unresponsive to cardiopulmonary resuscitation.

A full minute or longer may be required to detect vital signs. The cold bradycardiac heart is extremely irritable. Aggressive resuscitation should be avoided if the heart is beating. The patient should be handled gently; vigorous rewarming without the ability to monitor cardiac electrical activity is dangerous.

Wet clothing should be removed, and the patient should be covered with blankets to decrease heat loss. Alcohol is contraindicated in hypothermia, because induced peripheral vasodilatation will increase heat loss. If available, warm, humidified oxygen and intravenous fluids can be given en route to the hospital.

Rewarming should be performed in an intensive care unit to provide optimal monitoring of cardiovascular, respiratory, and renal function. A rectal or esophageal probe is required to monitor core body temperature continuously.

Patients with core temperatures above 32°C

(90°F) usually have stable vital signs and can be passively rewarmed slowly with warmed blankets. With core temperatures between 29° and 32°C (85° and 90°F) and stable cardiovascular function, patients are rewarmed more actively with hyperthermic blankets, warmed intravenous fluids, and heated, humidified oxygen. Warm water immersion is reserved for only short-term hypothermia. Monitoring is difficult in water. The recommended rewarming rate is no greater than 1°C (1 to 2°F) per hour.

For patients with core temperatures below 29°C (85°F), active core rewarming is required. Peripheral rewarming can be harmful, because it can cause peripheral vasodilatation and allow cold acidotic blood into the vascular space. This can further decrease core temperature and increase acidosis. Heated oxygen, intravenous fluids, and gastric and/or peritoneal lavage are required. Oxygen and fluids given should be heated to 40°C (104°F). Hemodialysis, extracorporeal blood rewarming, or even mediastinal lavage may be required for the persistent fibrillating or asystolic heart.

Supportive therapy for vital systems is crucial. Ventricular fibrillation is common in prolonged hypothermia. Most antidysrhythmic drugs are not helpful until core temperature is near normothermic and until acidosis is corrected. Defibrillation may be effective above 29°C (85°F); (see chapter on Dysrhythmias).

Most patients are dehydrated and should be rehydrated with normal saline and glucose pending electrolytes. Renal function and input and output must be closely monitored. Bicarbonate may be given after intravascular volume and systemic pressure are restored and hypercapnia is corrected.

Most patients with prolonged hypothermia require ventilator support. Core temperatures must be reported to the laboratory so that accurate blood gas results can be obtained.

Steroids have little beneficial effect. Thyroid hormone should be used only in patients who are hypothyroid. Indiscriminate use will only aggravate cardiac irritability. Antibiotics are used only for a specific infection, not prophylactically.

Reported mortality rates range from 21 to 87 percent, depending upon length of exposure. Death is usually a result of cardiac or pulmonary complications.

SUGGESTED READING

Abramowicz, M. (ed.): Treatment of hypothermia. Med. Lett. 25:9, 1983.

Clowes, G.H.A., and O'Donnell, T.F.J.: Heat stroke. N. Engl. J. Med. 291:564, 1974.

Gronert, G.A.: Malignant hyperthermia. Anesthesiology 53(5):395, 1980.

Kolb, M.E., et al. Dantrolene in human malignant hyperthermia. Anesthesiology 56:254, 1982.

Lorin, M.J.: The Febrile Child. New York, John Wiley & Sons, Inc., 1982.

Stern, R.C.: Pathophysiologic basis for sympatomatic treatment of fever. Pediatrics 59:92, 1977.

Stine, R.S.: Accidental hypothermia. J. Am. Coll. Emerg. Phys. 6(9):413, 1977.

Waldington, W.B., et al.: Heat stroke in infancy. Am. J. Dis. Child. 130:1250, 1976.

14

Clinical Pharmacology in the Critically Ill Child

DANIEL A. NOTTERMAN, M.D.

Healthy children manifest age-related differences in their response to drugs. In critically ill children, these age-related changes are compounded by the effects of multisystem dysfunction and by multiple drug exposure. Age, illness, and drug interaction affect response to therapy. Accordingly, drug treatment of critically ill children is often not optimal. Chances of a successful therapeutic outcome are increased when the physician is informed about the basic principles of pharmacology and is sensitive to the fact that each patient's response to therapy is unique.

The human may be described as an organism to which an input is applied—a specific drug—and from which an output is derived—a pharmacologic response. For the "average" patient, this simple paradigm may suffice, and in this patient, a standard amount of drug will yield a predictable response. When the response is not the expected one, a more complete description is required. The simple paradigm is divided into two fundamental and complementary relationships. On the one side is the pharmaco*kinetic* description, which makes the relationship between drug regimen and plasma drug concentration explicit. On the other side is the pharmaco*dynamic* description, which specifies the relationship between concentration and effect.

Based upon this understanding, atypical responses to therapy are attributed to deviations in either kinetic or dynamic properties of a drug. Unfortunately, such alterations are common in the critically ill child. Through knowledge of these potential disturbances, the physician is able to predict and forestall harmful deviations in response.

THE THERAPEUTIC RANGE

When a drug has relatively predictable pharmacodynamic properties, it may be possible to define a range of desirable plasma concentrations. This range of concentrations is delimited at one extreme by a minimum effective concentration and at the other extreme by a concentration associated with an unacceptable frequency of toxicity. The *therapeutic range* varies with different drugs, and sometimes, with different indications for the same drug. It is often possible to devise and adjust drug regimens by measuring the concentration of drug in the patient's plasma or serum. This procedure is termed *therapeutic drug monitoring*; it is practical when the following* conditions have been met.

No readily observable physiologic index of drug activity

Substantial pharmacokinetic variation

Minimal pharmacodynamic variation

Narrow therapeutic range

Plasma concentration of drug is related to therapeutic and toxic activity

Accurate, prompt laboratory assay available

Age–appropriate therapeutic range is described

Some drugs for which concentration monitoring is useful are listed in Table 14–1. For these drugs, dosage regimens are adjusted to keep the drug concentration within the therapeutic range, and maintaining the drug concentration within this range of concentrations becomes an

---

*Adapted from Sheiner, L.B., and Tozer, T.N.: Clinical pharmacokinetics: the use of plasma concentrations of drugs. *In* Melmon, K.L., and Morelli, H.F. (eds.): Clinical Pharmacology, 2nd ed., Macmillan Publishing Co., 1978.

Table 14–1. Drugs for Which Concentration Monitoring Is Useful

Antidysrhythmics
Lidocaine
Procainamide (and N-acetyl procainamide)
Quinidine
Antibiotics
Aminoglycosides
Chloramphenicol
Vancomycin
Anticonvulsants
Carbamazepine
Ethosuximide
Pentobarbital (when used to induce coma)
Phenobarbital
Phenytoin
Valproic acid
Cardiac Glycosides
Miscellaneous
Caffeine
Ethanol
Lithium
Salicylate
Theophylline
Tricyclic antidepressants

"intermediate goal of therapy" (Scheiner and Tozer). This method of individualizing drug treatment has been termed a *target concentration strategy*. The therapeutic range is a guideline to drug therapy and should not be slavishly applied or conceived as rigid and inflexible. Thus, even if one is following a target concentration strategy, a drug concentration measurement that is not precisely within the customary therapeutic range does not reflexively prompt a change in drug regimen if the patient's response has been satisfactory.

A *target effect strategy* is the traditional and still more usual approach to pharmacotherapy. It is appropriate for agents that produce an easily quantitated, clinically relevant response that is closely related to the ultimate goal of therapy. Included in this group are pressors, antihypertensives, diuretics, anticoagulants, hypoglycemics, tranquilizers, and analgesics. With such drugs, dosage adjustment is based upon direct measurement or observation of the relevant physiologic variable (e.g., blood pressure, urine flow, and serum glucose.) Dosage adjustment does not depend upon direct measurement of drug concentrations. Even so, there is usually (but not always) a relationship between the drug concentration and the intensity and quality of response. Thus, an understanding of kinetic and dynamic factors must also govern the use of these drugs.

VARIATIONS IN THERAPEUTIC RESPONSE

Unusual therapeutic responses result from either pharmacokinetic or pharmacodynamic alterations. Although deviations in kinetic properties are described most often, changes in pharmacodynamics, when present, can have profound therapeutic effects. Age-related pharmacodynamic differences, particularly as they pertain to children, have not been widely studied. They constitute a major area for future investigation.

Pharmacodynamic Variation

Frequently, pharmacodynamic variation leads to an attenuated, excessive, or otherwise unexpected drug response. These alterations may be genetically determined, or they may be related to concurrent drug therapy, to the patient's age, or to coexisting medical conditions.

For example, the myocardium in newborn infants may be less sensitive to the inotropic effects of digoxin than the myocardium in older children. This means that a comparable improvement in cardiac function may require a higher plasma digoxin concentration in neonates than in older children. This change in the concentration–response relationship is one type of pharmacodynamic alteration.

Examples of genetically transmitted alterations in pharmacodynamics that may lead to an untoward pharmacologic response include malignant hyperthermia during general anesthesia, fulminant hemolysis after exposure of a G-6-PD (glucose-6-phosphate dehydrogenase) deficient patient to primaquine, and hereditary resistance to the anticoagulant effect of Coumadin. Many other similar examples have been described.

Coexisting medical conditions have a profound effect upon drug response. Hypokalemia alters the sensitivity of the myocardium to the cardiac glycosides, and, in this context, cardiac toxicity may occur at a plasma digoxin concentration that would otherwise be well tolerated. When hypokalemia is secondary to concurrent diuretic therapy, the situation becomes one of an adverse drug interaction in which one drug alters the dynamic properties of a second drug. Other examples include the observations that acidemia and hypoxemia render the myocardium abnormally sensitive to the dysrhythmogenic effects of pressor amines and methylxanthines and that severe acidemia seems to blunt the inotropic response to these agents. When exposed to inhibitors of prostaglandin synthesis (i.e., aspirin, indomethacin), patients with pre-existing renal insufficiency or poor renal perfusion seem to be particularly likely to develop abrupt worsening of renal function. This deterioration occurs because prostaglandins seem to subserve an important function in maintaining renal function in the marginally adequate kidney.

There are many *drug interactions* that produce a change in the dynamic properties of one or more of the coadministered drugs. These interactions can be beneficial, as when naloxone is used to reverse narcotic overdosage, or harmful, as when ethanol acts synergistically with pentobarbital to produce respiratory arrest or when an aminoglycoside antibiotic and a loop diuretic interact to impair hearing.

As mentioned previously, dynamic variation can be age related. The inotropic effect of moderate dosages of dobutamine seems to be less in infants than in older children and adults. This may be related to the relative insensitivity of the immature myocardium to β-1 stimulation and to differences in the relationship between pre-load and stroke volume in infants compared with older patients. The tetracyclines are a classic example of an age-related toxic effect. When administered to children younger than 7 years of age, this group of antibiotics sometimes produces permanent discoloration of the teeth and may injure bone. This unpleasant side effect has not been noted in older children or adults. Thus, the clinician must be alert to variation in the pharmacodynamic properties of a drug. A quantitative approach to this problem is not available. For this reason, the careful physician will consult current product information whenever a drug regimen is instituted in a critically ill child.

KINETIC VARIATION—BASIC PHARMACOKINETIC CONCEPTS

Unfortunately, the relationship between drug dosage and resulting plasma drug concentration is frequently unpredictable. Sources of pharmacokinetic variation include alterations in: 1) the rate of administration (R for continuous infusions; dosage/interval, D/T, for intermittent schedules) and the extent and rapidity of absorption; 2) the space into which the drug is distributed (volume of distribution, V_d); and 3) the rate of elimination (E).

Single Dose Kinetics

Several concepts can be illustrated by the following clinical case. A child weighing 10 kg receives a 60-mg IV injection of theophylline. The plasma concentration of theophylline is measured at several intervals thereafter. Figure 14–1 is a time concentration curve based upon these measurements. The concentration of the drug reaches a maximum, or *peak*, immediately after the injection. Assuming a one compartment model, the concentration then declines monoexponentially such that $dC/dt = -(k)c$, where dC/dt is the fall in concentration during interval c and k is a rate constant (vide infra). Exponential decline in drug concentration is characteristic of a *first order* kinetic process, in which a *constant fraction* of drug is eliminated per unit time. An important characteristic of such a process is the velocity with which it occurs. The drug *half-life* ($t_{1/2}$) is that interval during which one half the drug is eliminated.

The data may be replotted on semilogarithmic paper. As can be seen in Figure 14–2, the relationship between time and concentration now defines a straight line. The slope of this line is related to k_{el}, the elimination rate constant ($k_{el} = 2.3 \times$ slope). This term has units of reciprocal time (hr^{-1}, or 1/hr) and specifies the fractional rate of elimination. When $k_{el} = 0.25\ hr^{-1}$, 25 percent of the drug is eliminated each hour. The elimination rate constant, k_{el}, is determined by calculating the slope of the linear portion of the time concentration curve, as displayed on semilogarithmic paper. After k_{el} is known, $t_{1/2}$ is calculated:

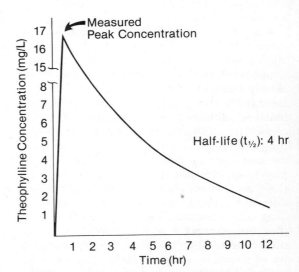

Figure 14–1. Time concentration curve following single IV dose.

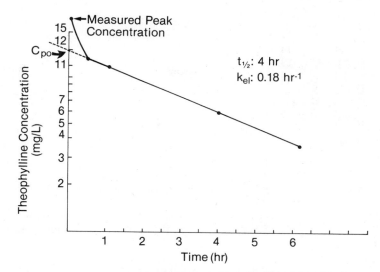

Figure 14–2. Semi-log time concentration curve following single IV dose.

$$t_{1/2} = \frac{0.7}{k_{el}} \qquad (14.1)$$

Alternatively, one can *estimate* $t_{1/2}$ by noting the interval required for the plasma concentration to decline by 50 percent. In Figure 14–2, $k_{el} = 0.18 \text{ hr}^{-1}$ and $t_{1/2} = 4.0$ hr.

The volume of distribution, (V_d), is the *hypothetical* space into which a drug would be distributed if its concentration were uniform throughout the body. Even though this is not the case, the term has considerable utility. An analogy may be helpful. Consider a beaker that contains an *unknown* volume of water. A *known* amount of theophylline (i.e., 60 mg) is added. After allowing a sufficient interval for the drug to distribute uniformly, an aliquot of the solution is removed and analyzed for theophylline concentration. Suppose that the concentration is found to be 10 mg per L. Because concentration (C) =

$$\frac{\text{amount of theophylline in the beaker (A)}}{\text{volume of the beaker (V)}}$$

it follows that:

$$V = \frac{A}{C}$$

In the present example,

$$V = \frac{60 \text{ mg}}{10 \text{ mg/L}} = 6 \text{ L}$$

The apparent volume of distribution (V_d) of a drug in the body can be estimated by a similar procedure. The relevant equation is:

$$V_d = \frac{\text{amount of drug in the body at } t_n \text{ (Ab)}}{\text{plasma concentration of drug at } t_n \text{ (C)}}$$

The numerator, (Ab), is derived by recognizing that immediately after an IV injection the amount of drug in the body (Ab) is equal to the dosage (D), which is known. However, the denominator, (C), is difficult to specify, because the *measured* concentration of drug that occurs immediately following injection (when Ab=D) will be spuriously high as a result of incomplete drug distribution from the vascular space. This problem is resolved by use of the semilogarithmic time concentration plot (Fig. 14–2). The linear portion of the time concentration curve is extrapolated back to time zero, the moment of injection. The point of intersection with the y-axis is the plasma drug concentration, which would result if distribution from the vascular space to the rest of the body were instantaneous. This concentration is abbreviated C_{pO}. The equation for volume of distribution becomes:

$$V_d = \frac{D}{C_{pO}} \qquad (14.2)$$

In the example (Fig. 14–2), C_{pO} is 12 mg per L. Because the dosage (D) was 60 mg, it follows that V_d is 5 L. In order to permit intersubject comparison, V_d is usually expressed as L per kg. In this example of a 10-kg child, V_d of theophylline is 0.5 L per kg, a typical value. This method of estimating V_d is inherently inaccurate (overestimates) but is sufficient for clinical application.

In clinical practice, the semilogarithmic curve is constructed using two concentration mea-

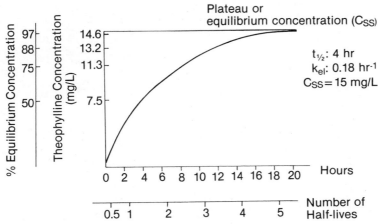

Figure 14–3. Concentration of theophylline during continous IV administration.

surements separated by an interval greater than the estimated half-life. When the rates of administration and distribution are rapid relative to elimination, as is the case with IV injection of many drugs, a *measured* peak concentration drawn 15 to 30 minutes after the dose and a *trough* concentration measured just prior to the next dose permit construction of the time concentration curve and estimation of half-life and volume of distribution. This method is less useful and may produce erroneous information when applied to a drug with a very slow rate of distribution (i.e., digoxin).

This procedure is valid when applied to the first dose of a medication. After the first dose, modification is necessary to account for residual drug from previous doses. Although more complete descriptions are occasionally necessary to account for multiple compartment kinetics, the foregoing is sufficiently accurate for most clinical applications.

The *volume of distribution, V_d,* is a hypothetical term, not an actual or physical space; indeed, it is often larger than the total body volume. Nonetheless, V_d is an important index of drug dispersal. The aminoglycoside antibiotics have relatively low volumes of distribution (0.2 to 0.3 L/kg) and are principally confined to the extracellular water. Theophylline and vancomycin have somewhat higher volumes of distribution (0.5 to 0.6 L/kg) and are distributed throughout the total body water. Agents that are widely dispersed (high tissue binding) have very high volumes of distribution. For digoxin, V_d is 10 L per kg, for chlorpromazine, V_d is 22 L per kg.

The volume of distribution (V_d) is a valuable term because it relates the *amount* of a single dose to the resulting plasma *concentration.* Knowledge of the V_d enables the physician to determine the required amount of drug to pro-

duce a desired concentration with a single dose. When the dosage is already known, as it may be after a poisoning, the V_d permits the physician to estimate a peak plasma level.

Continuous Dose Kinetics

The discussion in this chapter has been concerned with the events after a single IV dose of a drug. However, most often, patients either receive repeated doses or are placed on a continuous IV infusion. During continuous or repeated administration of a drug, an individual enters *equilibrium* with respect to that drug. Once equilibrium is achieved, the concentration of drug (C) remains constant unless R (rate of administration), E (rate of elimination), or Vd (volume of distribution) changes. Consider an individual who has not previously been exposed to theophylline. At time zero, a continuous IV infusion is started at rate R (mg/hr). At several time intervals thereafter, blood is withdrawn from the patient and the concentration of theophylline is determined. These data are displayed in Figure 14–3. Note that the plasma concentration of theophylline rises asymptotically to a *plateau*, denoting drug equilibrium. At the plateau, the rate of administration is equal to the rate of elimination (R = E). No further change in concentration will occur unless a kinetic variable is altered.

An interval elapses between the start of a continuous infusion and the time at which the plateau or equilibrium concentration (C_{ss}) is achieved. The duration of this interval is determined *only* by the half-life of the drug. In an interval equal to one half-life, the concentration will be 50 percent of the equilibrium concentration; in two half-lives, the concentration will be 75 percent of the equilibrium concentration; in 3.3 half-lives, it will be 90 percent; and in five half-lives, it will be 97 percent of the plateau level.

Dosage recommendations for continuous infusions are designed to produce appropriate plasma concentrations at equilibrium. The phenomenon just described, which is often termed *drug accumulation,* entails a delay in achieving this concentration. The magnitude of the delay is related to the half-life of the drug, whereas the ultimate concentration is determined by the V_d, the half-life, and the rate of administration.

Plasma Drug Clearance

The plasma clearance (Cl) of a drug is of primary importance in appreciating the relationship between rate of drug administration and consequent drug concentration. Drug clearance, like creatinine or inulin clearances, is determined by relating the rate of elimination (E) to the plasma concentration at equilibrium (C_{ss}):

$$Cl = \frac{E}{C_{ss}}$$

At equilibrium, E = R. Thus,

$$Cl = \frac{R}{C_{ss}}$$

or, with rearrangement,

$$C_{ss} = \frac{R}{Cl} \qquad (14.3)$$

$$R = Cl \times C_{ss} \qquad (14.3A)$$

where R = rate of administration.

Equation 14.3A emphasizes that it is drug clearance, rather than half-life, which determines the rate of administration (R) or dosage per interval (D/T) necessary to achieve a specific concentration. Ultimately, clearance is related to half-life and volume of distribution:

$$Cl = \frac{0.7 \times V_d \times Wt.}{t_{1/2}}$$

when V_d is expressed in L/kg, half-life ($t_{1/2}$) in hours, and clearance (Cl) in L/hr.
With substitution into equation 14.3, this becomes:

$$C_{ss} = \frac{R \times t_{1/2}}{0.7 \times V_d \times Wt.} \qquad (14.4)$$

where R is expressed in mg/hr and C_{ss} is expressed in mg/L.

Equation 14.4 indicates that equilibrium drug concentration is related to three variables: half-life ($t_{1/2}$), volume of distribution (V_d), and rate of administration (R, or D/T). Thus, doubling V_d has the same effect upon steady state concentration as halving $t_{1/2}$. Either alteration will lead to a 50 percent reduction in drug concentration that can be exactly offset by doubling the dosage.

Multiple Dose Kinetics

The reader has been introduced to the phenomenon of drug accumulation as it occurs during continuous infusion. Drug accumulation also occurs with intermittent dosage schedules.

Consider a drug that is given by intermittent IV injection. When the first dose is given, the concentration of drug is zero. Immediately after the dose, a peak concentration is recorded. The concentration then declines at a rate determined by the drug's half-life. If the next dose is given before the concentration has once again reached zero, the second peak will be higher than the first. As this process continues, the peak (C_{max}) and trough (C_{min}) levels rise toward plateau values, as will the average concentration, C_{ave}. This process is illustrated in Figure 14–4. Drug accumulation occurs during intermittent administration when a second, or nth, dose is administered before all the previous dose has been eliminated. For most clinical purposes, this condition is satisfied when the dosing interval is less than twice the half-life of the drug. As with continuous infusions, 50 percent of a plateau concentration is achieved in one half-life; 97 percent is achieved after five half-lives.

C_{ave} is analogous to the equilibrium concentration (C_{ss}) that develops during continuous infusion. Thus, its value is determined only by the relationship between clearance (Cl) and rate of administration (R; see Equation 14.3). The peak (C_{max}) and trough (C_{min}) concentrations fluctuate around the C_{ave} in a manner that is determined by the size of the dose and the length of the dosing interval. For example, theophylline may be administered by intermittent IV injection. In an adult, a standard regimen calls for 300 mg every 6 hours (1200

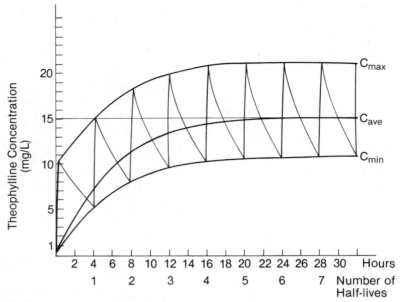

Figure 14–4. Concentration of theophylline during intermittent IV administration. Note that C_{max}, C_{min}, and C_{ave} increase to equilibrium values. $C_{ave} = C_{ss}$ that obtains during continuous administration if the total daily dosages are identical.

mg/day). Alternatively, one may administer 150 mg every 3 hours (1200 mg/day). Finally, some physicians administer a continuous infusion of 50 mg/hr (1200 mg/day). Both intermittent regimens produce the same (C_{ave}), which is equal to the C_{ss} during the continuous infusion. This does not mean that the regimens are equivalent. The 6-hour schedule produces much greater fluctuation around C_{ave} than the 3-hour schedule. With the 3-hour regimen, the peaks and troughs lie closer to C_{ave}. This increases the likelihood of remaining within the therapeutic range throughout the dosing interval (Fig. 14–5).

In this regard, the half-life of a drug is a watershed. When a drug is given at an interval that is equal to its half-life (T = $t_{1/2}$), C_{max}/C_{min} is approximately 2. During more frequent administration (T < $t_{1/2}$), C_{max}/C_{min} is less than 2, and during less frequent administration (T > $t_{1/2}$), C_{max}/C_{min} is greater than 2.

Thus, drugs with a long half-life, such as digoxin or phenobarbital, are often given once daily, because even with this schedule, T is less than $t_{1/2}$ and the plasma concentration remains within the relatively narrow therapeutic range of these agents. Conversely, theophylline and quinidine have relatively short half-lives (3 to 6 hours in children). When conventional formulations of these agents are administered, they require relatively frequent dosing (every 3 to 6 hours) if the plasma concentration is to remain within the respective therapeutic ranges throughout the dosing interval.

Nonlinear Kinetics

To this point, the discussion has concerned *first-order* kinetic behavior in which a *fixed proportion* of drug is eliminated per unit time. *Zero-order* kinetics occurs under some conditions, notably when plasma drug concentrations are rel-

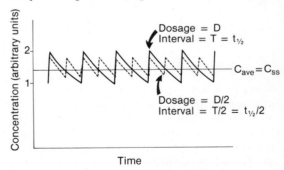

Figure 14–5. Effect of varying both dosage and dose interval upon peak (C_{max}) and trough (C_{min}) concentrations during steady state. The solid saw tooth line indicates the time concentration curve that results with intermittent IV administration of dosage D at an interval T equal to the drug $t_{1/2}$. Note that $C_{max}/C_{min} = 2$. The interrupted line indicates the curve that results when dosage (D/2) and interval (T/2) are halved. $C_{max}/C_{min} = 1.5$. The straight solid line indicates C_{ave}, which is the same during both conditions, and is equal to C_{ss}, which results when the same total daily dosage is administered by continuous IV infusion.

atively large. With zero order or nonlinear kinetics, a fixed *amount* of drug is eliminated per unit time. Ethanol is an extreme example, because the usual dosage is large (gm amounts) relative to other drugs (mg amounts). Within the usual range of blood ethanol concentrations, humans eliminate about 120 mg per kg per hr of the substance. Because the volume of distribution of ethanol is about 0.5 L per kg, blood ethanol levels decline at a fixed rate of 20 to 25 mg/dl per hr. The rate of elimination does not change with increases in concentration. Consequently, increments in dosage produce much greater changes in concentration than would be the case for a drug eliminated in accordance with first-order kinetics.

Many substances follow a first-order model at low plasma concentrations but a zero-order model at higher concentrations. When the transition from first- to zero-order elimination occurs at concentrations appreciably higher than the usual therapeutic range, the pharmacokinetic treatment of the drug is uncomplicated and a first-order kinetic model will be sufficiently accurate for most clinical purposes.

Unfortunately, a few commonly used drugs, such as phenytoin and salicylate, exhibit this transition at concentrations within the therapeutic range.

A change from first- to zero-order kinetics as concentration increases is typical of an enzyme-mediated process. This change is due to saturation of the enzyme system that is responsible for metabolic transformation of the drug. There is a limited amount of enzyme at the metabolic site; therefore, there is a maximum rate at which transformation can occur (V_{max}). At concentrations that are low relative to V_{max}, first-order behavior predominates. As concentration increases, V_{max} is approached. After V_{max} has been achieved, further increases in concentration cannot augment the metabolic rate. Thus, a fixed amount of drug is metabolized per unit time. This amount, of course, is equal to V_{max}. Mathematically, this process is described by the Michaelis–Menton equation:

$$E = \frac{V_{max} \times C}{K_m + C} \qquad (14.5)$$

where E is the rate of elimination or metabolism; V_{max} is the maximum rate of metabolism; K_m is the Michaelis–Menton constant, which defines the affinity of the enzyme for the drug; and C is plasma drug concentration.

Note that when C is much less than K_m, E varies directly with C. This resembles a first-order process. When C is greater than K_m, E

approaches V_{max}, and zero-order behavior occurs.

There are two important consequences of this kinetic behavior. The first is that an increase in dosage produces an *exponential*, rather than a linear rise in concentration. This occurs very often when treating patients with phenytoin (Fig. 14–6); on occasion, this phenomenon is recognized during treatment with theophylline. It requires that dosage adjustments must be made cautiously and in small amounts. The second major consequence of Michaelis–Menton kinetics is that the *apparent* plasma half-life increases with the plasma concentration. The greater the plasma concentration, the slower is the relative rate of elimination. Using representative values of K_m and V_{max} for phenytoin, one can estimate that at a concentration of 10 mg per L, the apparent $t_{1/2}$ of phenytoin is 24 hours; at a concentration of 25 mg per L, the apparent $t_{1/2}$ is 42 hours. This means: 1) increases in dosage cause lengthening of the apparent $t_{1/2}$ (thus, Michaelis–Menton kinetics is sometimes referred to as *dose dependent* kinetics), 2) small increments in dosage can produce huge increases in drug concentration, and 3) intoxication with phenytoin will be prolonged, because, at high concentrations, elimination is extremely slow relative to the amount of drug in the body.

MAINTENANCE DOSE

The maintenance dose (MD) is the amount of drug (R for continuous infusion, D/T for an intermittent schedule) that is administered during equilibrium. Thus, from Equation 14.3A, maintenance dose, MD, is equal to the product of clearance, Cl, and desired steady state plasma concentration, C_{ss}, (MD = Cl × C_{ss}). The maintenance dose is often determined by consulting standard reference material. In patients

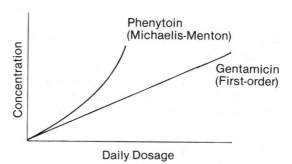

Figure 14–6. Effect of dosage upon plasma concentration for drugs following first-order vs. Michaelis-Menton kinetics.

with abnormal drug disposition, better individualization of therapy is achieved if one appreciates the relationship between changes in Cl and consequent changes in C_{ss}. Knowledge of a patient's Cl can be used to calculate dosage requirements. This procedure is described in the case study at the conclusion of this chapter.

It is not always appropriate to *initiate* therapy with the maintenance dose. Both continuous and intermittent schedules produce a gradual rise from the initial (usually zero) to the equilibrium concentration. Recall that 75 percent of the plateau is reached in two half-lives, and 97 percent is reached in five half-lives. Thus, for drugs that have a long half-life, there will be a substantial delay in acquisition of the plateau concentration. Because the plateau concentration may be close to the minimum effective concentration, this delay may be unacceptable in acutely ill patients. For example, an asthmatic who is simply placed on a theophylline infusion will not begin to experience relief for about 8 hours.

LOADING DOSE

The solution to the problem of delay in achieving adequate levels is to administer a loading dose (LD). The loading dose is the amount of drug that will rapidly produce a therapeutic plasma concentration.

If one is emphasizing a target concentration strategy, calculating the loading dose is simple, because the loading dose and the desired concentration (C_{ss}) are related through the volume of distribution (see Equation 14.2). With appropriate modifications, this expression becomes:

$$LD = V_d(L/kg) \times Wt(kg) \times C_{ss}(mg/L)$$

$$(14.6)$$

where C_{ss} is the desired equilibrium concentration. Thus, for a child weighing 10 kg in whom one wishes to achieve a plasma theophylline ($V_d = 0.5$ L/kg) concentration of 12 mg per L, the correct loading dose is 60 mg. This amount of drug should be administered slowly, over about a 15-minute period. Immediately thereafter, the appropriate maintenance dose is initiated. The effect of a loading dose is shown in Figure 14–7.

If one is using an empirically derived maintenance dose and is not attempting to achieve a specific drug concentration (target effect strategy), the problem is less straightforward. In such cases, it is probably best to consult

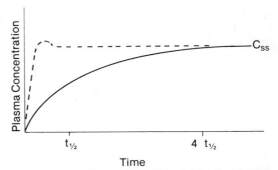

Figure 14–7. Administration of an appropriate loading dose eliminates the delay ($4t_{1/2}$) in achieving equilibrium concentration, C_{ss}. Solid line-infusion alone, beginning at T = 0. Interrupted line—loading dose at T = 0, followed by continuous infusion.

individual product information when designing the loading dose. Readers interested in a theoretical approach to this issue should consult the suggested reading by Rowland and Tozer.

When intravenous therapy is indicated, the loading dose is often given as a single relatively brief infusion. In the case of a drug with a narrow therapeutic range or a prolonged phase of distribution, the physician may choose to divide the loading dose, as is commonly done with digoxin. In general, a loading dose is not indicated when the half-life is much less than the dosing interval (i.e., drug accumulation does not occur) or when the therapeutic range is wide. Thus, penicillin therapy does not begin with a loading dose. Of course, a loading dose is not indicated when there is no urgency in achieving the equilibrium drug concentration. There is also no point in administering a loading dose when the half-life of a drug is very short, as with most pressor agents, because equilibrium conditions are reached in a matter of minutes during continuous maintenance infusion.

The foregoing kinetic description applies to intravenous administration. Following intramuscular or oral administration one must extend the analysis by taking into account the rate and extent of absorption. Drugs that are completely and efficiently absorbed after intramuscular injection should maintain a similar C_{ave}, although peak and trough levels may lie closer to C_{ave} (lower peak, higher trough). After oral administration, many drugs either are not completely absorbed from the gastrointestinal tract or once absorbed are efficiently extracted and then biotransformed on the first pass through the liver. This process effectively reduces the dosage of drug that reaches the systemic circulation. Equations 14.2 through 14.4 are modified by multiplying the dosage administered (R, or D/T) by f_{oral}, the fraction of orally administered drug that reaches the systemic circulation. Several of the suggested readings contain a table of representative f_{oral} values.

KINETIC VARIATION—CLINICAL APPLICATION

In the foregoing discussion, three variables that affect the plasma drug concentration have been identified: 1) the rate of administration (R, or D/T), 2) the volume of distribution (V_d), and 3) the half-life ($t_{1/2}$). These three variables are related to one another through Equation 14.4. Of these, only the rate of administration is under the physician's control. Thus, the art of pharmacokinetics consists of altering this parameter in order to compensate for individual differences in elimination or distribution.

Altered Distribution

Critical illness and the age of the patient affect the distribution of many drugs. Several mechanisms may be involved, including changes in the content or distribution of body water, alterations in plasma protein binding, perturbations in regional blood flow, and differences in body fat content.

AGE–RELATED CHANGES

The water content of the body changes dramatically with age. At 28 weeks gestation, the water content of the body is 85 percent. This figure decreases to 70 percent at term and to 60 percent in adults. There is a concurrent increase in the amount of body fat from 1 percent of body weight at 28 weeks to 15 percent at term, as well as altered binding to protein. Disease (tachypnea, dehydration), the environment in which the infant is nursed, and the volume and composition of administered fluids produce fluctuations in body water. Thus, it is anticipated that drugs that are distributed mainly in the body water have a different, usually greater, volume of distribution (V_d) in infants and young children than in adults. Table 14–2 lists several drugs for which the V_d is known to differ between newborn infants and adults. This information provides the rationale for many empirically determined dosage modifications. A larger V_d does not necessarily involve a larger dosage. The actual determinant of the maintenance dosage requirement is clear-

Table 14–2. Selected Drugs With Altered Volume of Distribution (V_d) in Neonates and Children

Drug	Effect on V_d
Diazepam	↓ N
Digoxin	↑ N, ↑ C
Furosemide	↑ N,
Gentamicin	↑ N, ↑ C
Lidocaine	↑ N
Phenobarbital	↑ N
Phenytoin	↑ N
Theophylline	↑ N

↑ = V_d larger; ↓ = V_d smaller; N = neonate; and C = children older than 1 month. The effect of changes in V_d may be modified by alterations in protein binding and elimination rate.

ance. Clearance (Cl) is related to both V_d and half-life. In infants, drug half-life may be prolonged (vide infra), and this may offset the increase in V_d (recall that $Cl = 0.7 \times V_d/t_{1/2}$). The net effect is frequently a *reduced* dosage requirement or an increased loading dose, followed by a reduced maintenance dose.

DISEASE–RELATED CHANGES

Several processes affect V_d by altering body water content, body fat content, or the degree of protein binding. Notable examples are uremia, chronic liver disease, and congestive heart failure.

In uremia, the water content of the body is frequently greater than normal. This factor, together with disturbed protein binding, causes the volume of distribution (V_d) of several drugs to increase (e.g., gentamicin) or decrease (e.g., digoxin). As in newborns, the larger V_d is frequently accompanied by prolongation of drug half-life.

Chronic liver disease is associated with decreased levels of plasma proteins and with fluid accumulation. Thus, it is not surprising that the V_d of several drugs increases in the presence of cirrhosis. Other conditions associated with extracellular fluid expansion also increase the distribution of certain drugs; for example, aminoglycoside antibiotics distribute into ascitic fluid. Thus, in the presence of ascites, the V_d of these agents may be substantially increased. In cystic fibrosis, the V_d of several of the aminoglycosides seems to be higher than average. Unless daily dosage is increased, this may lead to subtherapeutic drug concentrations.

Abnormalities of regional or global blood flow may reduce distribution by limiting perfusion to sites of uptake. In patients with low-output states (congestive heart failure, CHF; shock), the *rate* of distribution is likely to be slower than normal. Thus, it is a wise precaution to administer all IV drugs slowly to these patients, avoiding transiently excessive plasma concentrations.

It is important to recognize the effect of body composition upon drug distribution. Fat is essentially anhydrous. Drugs that distribute principally in body water do not partition well into fat. With these drugs, obese patients have a lower V_d than lean patients; as a consequence, obese patients may require smaller per kilogram dosages. This effect is of major importance when prescribing theophylline to obese patients.

The net effect of a change in V_d upon clearance cannot be predicted without reference to other kinetic variables. It is imprudent to alter therapy solely on the basis of a suspected change in distribution. Before a new regimen can be planned, the physician must be aware of the effect of the age and disease upon other factors.

Altered Elimination

Elimination occurs by two processes: excretion and metabolism (biotransformation). *Excretion* of unchanged drug or of drug metabolites is primarily accomplished by the kidney but also, to an important extent, by the lungs, skin, and gastrointestinal tract. *Metabolism,* or biotransformation, occurs chiefly in the liver and, for some drugs, in the skin, lungs, kidneys, and even plasma.

Alterations in either excretion or biotransformation change the elimination rate constant and therefore the half-life. This will affect clearance if there is no reciprocal change in V_d.

ALTERED EXCRETION

Changes in rate of excretion are most frequently caused by renal function that differs from that in the healthy individual. These changes are either age related or the result of disease. For many drugs, most of a dose is excreted unchanged. When this happens, there is usually a direct (not necessarily linear) relationship between elimination rate and glomerular filtration rate (GFR). Although other factors, such as urine flow, urine pH, tubular secretion, and resorption, may cause this relationship to be modified, for these drugs, a decrease in GFR is accompanied by a decrease in clearance and usually by a prolongation of half-life. Some drugs that require reduced dosage during renal function impairment are listed in Table 14–3.

Dosage modification is not always necessary when there is reduced renal function, even when the kidney is the primary means of elimination. When the therapeutic range is wide, as with penicillin, or when the kidney is responsible for eliminating mainly inactive metabolites (chloramphenicol), dosage adjustment may not be needed.

Some agents, particularly the aminoglycoside antibiotics, have narrow therapeutic ranges and are exclusively eliminated by the kidney. They must be administered in reduced dosages when even mild degrees of renal impairment exist.

Even in healthy people, the elimination of drugs excreted by the kidney is greatly affected by age. This is not surprising, because the GFR is lower in normal infants than in older children or young adults. In addition to a reduced filtration rate, neonates are also likely to have impaired tubular function relative to older children. Thus, the dosage of drugs eliminated by the kidney must be related to the infant's maturity and extrauterine age. Several of the suggested readings contain dosage schedules for neonates and older infants with normal renal function. Such information is particularly important for drugs with a narrow therapeutic range in which renal excretion is the principal route of elimination. The aminoglycoside antibiotics are perhaps the best known example.

Without a valid estimate of GFR at the outset of therapy, initiation of treatment in children with renal dysfunction is problematic. In this context, it is important to recognize that the "normal" values of serum creatinine do not have the same meaning at the extremes of life (the newborn, the elderly) that they have in older children and young adults, because infants and elderly patients have a reduced muscle mass compared with young healthy adults. Thus, in infants, the rate of production of creatinine is less than in adults. Consequently, an apparently normal plasma creatinine of 1.2 mg/dl in a 3-week-old infant (or an 80-year-old woman) denotes a serious reduction in renal function and requires a considerable reduction in the dosage of aminoglycoside antibiotics.

Recently, Schwartz and Feld devised a general equation for estimating the GFR in infants and children:

$$GFR = k \times (\text{length in cm})/\text{serum creatinine}.$$

For premature infants, $k = 0.4$; for full-term infants, $k = 0.45$; and for children older than 1 year, $k = 0.55$ when creatinine is measured by an automatic analyzer. If validated by drug clearance studies, these equations will be helpful in determining appropriate dosage sched-

Table 14–3. Selected Drugs That May Require Dosage Reduction During Renal Insufficiency

Drug	Degree of Renal Insufficiency			
	Mild	**Moderate**	**Severe**	**Comment**
Antibiotics				
Aminoglycosides	+	+	+	nephrotoxic
Ampicillin	0	0/+	+	
Carbenicillin	+	+	+	
Cefamandole	0	+	+	?nephrotoxic
Cefotaxime	0	0	?	?nephrotoxic
Cephalothin	0	0	+	?nephrotoxic
Methicillin	0	0	+	nephrotoxic
Moxalactam	0/+	+	+	?nephrotoxic
Penicillin G	0	0/+	+	
Pentamidine	0	0/+	+	nephrotoxic
Piperacillin	0	0/+	+	
Quinine	0	0/+	+	
Sulfamethoxazole/				
Trimethoprim	0	+	+	
Vancomycin	+	+	+	nephrotoxic
Non-Antibiotics				
Allopurinol	0	0	+	active metabolite
Cimetidine	0	+	+	
Digitoxin	0	0	+	
Digoxin	0	+	+	
Insulin	0	+	+	titrate to glucose
Lithium carbonate	0	avoid	avoid	
Meperidine	0/+	avoid	avoid	active metabolite
Methyldopa	0	+	+	active metabolite
Pancuronium	0	0	+	
Primidone	0	0/+	+	
Procainamide	0	+	+	active metabolite
Spironolactone	0/+	+	avoid	hyperkalemia
Thiazides	0	0	avoid	

0 = no change in dosage; + = change in dosage usually necessary.

ules for patients with renal functional impairment. These equations (and similar methods for use in adults) assume that the patient is in a steady state with respect to creatinine elimination. Thus, the equations are of value in chronic but not in acute renal insufficiency.

It is not always necessary to know, or to estimate, the GFR before beginning drug therapy in patients with abnormal renal function. This is particularly true when renal function is changing rapidly. If the clinical laboratory personnel are cooperative, an excellent solution to the problem is to use drug concentration data from the individual patient. A usual, or "full," initial dose is administered. At several (peak, midpoint, and trough) intervals, the plasma is analyzed for drug concentration. The data is graphed on semilogarithmic paper (see Figure 14–2), and the half-life ($t_{1/2}$) is estimated. Using this half-life in renal failure ($t_{1/2r}$) and the usual age-appropriate half-life ($t_{1/2n}$) and dosing interval, (T_n), one may *estimate* the corrected dosing interval (T_r):

$$T_r = \frac{t_{1/2r} \times T_n}{t_{1/2n}} \qquad (14.7)$$

Subsequently, full doses are administered at T_r(vide infra), with follow-up determinations of drug concentration.

If the creatinine clearance or GFR is known or can be estimated prior to the first dose, a second method is applicable. Using this value, one calculates K_f, the fraction of remaining renal function:

$$K_f = \frac{\text{creatinine clearance of patient}}{\text{age-appropriate creatinine clearance}}$$

The rate of administration (D/T for intermittent regimens, R for continuous infusion) is determined by:

$$(D/T)_r = (D/T)_{normal} \times 1 - [f(1 - K_f]$$

where f is the fraction of drug eliminated by the kidney (Table 14–4). For example, the dose of gentamicin (f = 0.98) for a child who weighs 10 kg with normal renal function (creatinine clearance 100 ml/min/1.73 m²) is 17 mg every 8 hours. To find the correct regimen after clearance falls to 30 ml/min/1.73 m², use the following equation:

Table 14–4. Approximate Half-Lives and Fraction Excreted Unchanged by the Kidney(s) of Selected Drugs in Adults

Drug	t½ (hr)	f
Amikacin	2	0.98
Ampicillin	0.8	0.88
Carbenicillin	1.1	0.9
Cephalexin	1.0	0.95
Chloramphenicol	2.3	0
Cimetidine	2	0.77
Digitoxin	170	0.3
Digoxin	40	0.71
Gentamicin	2	0.98
Isoniazid		
Fast acetylators	1.5	0.3
Slow acetylators	3	0.5
Kanamycin	2	0.97
Lithium	22	0.95
Methicillin	0.5	0.88
Oxacillin	0.5	0.8
Penicillin G	0.5	0.9
Streptomycin	3	0.96
Sulfamethoxazole	9	0.3
Tetracycline	8–9	0.50
Tobramycin	2	0.99
Trimethoprim	10–12	0.7
Vancomycin	6	0.98

Modified from Dettli, L.: Drug dosage in renal disease. Clin. Pharmacokinet. 1: 126, 1976, and Rowland, M., and Tozer, T.N.: Clinical Pharmacokinetics: Concepts and Ap-

$$K_f = \frac{30 \text{ ml/min}}{100 \text{ ml/min}} = 0.33$$

$$(D/T)_r = 17 \text{ mg/8 hr} \times$$

$$1 - [0.98(1 - 0.33)] = 6 \text{ mg/8 hr}$$

Thus, the child should receive an altered dosage of 6 mg at the customary interval of 8 hours. Alternatively, one can administer the usual dosage, 17 mg, at the altered interval of 22.6 hours (i.e., once a day), because 6 mg/8 hr = 17 mg/22.6 hr. Which regimen, altered *dosage* or altered *interval*, is preferable? The average gentamicin concentration (C_{ave}) will be the same with both schedules. If the amount of each dose is reduced and the interval is held constant, fluctuations about C_{ave} will *decrease* and the peak will be *lower* and the trough will be *higher* than in the patient with normal renal function who is receiving the customary dosage. Conversely, when the interval is lengthened and the amount of each dose is unchanged, the peak, trough, and average concentrations will have normal values. This *apparent* similarity to the standard pattern re-

sults in many physicians favoring this approach. However, the similarity extends only to the peak, trough, and mean concentrations. The *time course* of drug exposure is very different than with the usual schedule. For example, a renal patient may receive the usual amount of gentamicin every 16 hours to compensate for a 50 percent reduction in clearance. With this adjustment, the time spent below C_{ave} is twice as long as in the patient with normal renal function who receives the drug every 8 hours. This situation places the patient at risk of prolonged exposure to subtherapeutic concentrations of gentamicin. In this circumstance, a better solution might be to alter the dosage rather than the interval. Probably, the most desirable approach is a compromise: alter both dosage and interval in equal proportion. Thus, for the preceding example, one could administer 12 mg every 16 hours.

Several other methods for altering drug regimens in the context of renal insufficiency are available. This type of information is helpful with moderate to severe reductions in renal function. The material presented here is not designed for the functionally anephric patient or for patients undergoing dialysis.

In addition to disturbances in renal function that are associated with changes in creatinine clearance, functional perturbations are frequent and are related to altered hemodynamics, to the effect of fluid and diuretic regimens upon urine flow and pH, and to concurrent drug regimens. This type of drug interaction is not rare; the classic example is probenecid, which greatly prolongs the half-life of penicillin by impeding tubular secretion.

Diminished renal blood flow (RBF) is common in shock or CHF and has been found to delay excretion of some drugs. For example, in severe CHF, renal clearance of digoxin is reduced. This is attributed to lower than normal RBF and is reversed by administration of afterloading reducing agents, which improve RBF.

Changes in hydration also affect renal tubular function. Lithium is actively resorbed in the proximal tubule; dehydration and salt restriction tend to augment this process. Hence, volume depletion of a patient who is receiving lithium may produce intoxication with that drug.

Many drugs undergo non-ionic back diffusion, in which previously filtered drug leaves the tubular fluid and ultimately re-enters the plasma. The importance of this process depends upon whether or not the drug is ionized at the pH of the urine, because only non-ionized forms readily permeate the tubular epithelium. Weak acids (pK 3–7.5) are non-ionized in an acid urine. Thus, elimination of these drugs is retarded in an acid urine and augmented in an alkaline urine. Aspirin and phenobarbital are so affected. In intoxications involving these agents, it is useful to alkalinize the urine. The opposite effect is noted with drugs that are weak bases (pK 6–12), such as quinine and quinidine. For these drugs, renal elimination is enhanced by acidifying the urine.

The physician must recall that the kidneys serve to excrete many products of drug *metabolism*. These metabolites may possess pharmacologic activity. During renal failure, these active metabolites accumulate, sometimes producing a toxic effect. At least 20 such drugs have been identified. For example, normeperidine, a metabolite of meperidine, accumulates during renal failure and can produce CNS (central nervous system) excitation, including convulsions. N-acetylprocainamide (NAPA), an active metabolite of procainamide, accumulates in the serum of patients with poor renal function.

It is important to note that, for some drugs, uremia indirectly affects hepatic drug metabolism by inhibiting enzymes that control oxidation, acetylation, and hydrolysis.

The net effect of these various processes upon drug elimination is difficult to predict in an individual patient. The likelihood of an adverse effect is reduced when the physician is sensitive to the possibility of alterations in renal function. This sensitivity is manifested by conservative drug regimens, by attention to potential drug interactions, and by use of therapeutic drug monitoring when appropriate.

ALTERED METABOLISM

Biotransformation, or metabolism, represents a second major route of elimination. It occurs mainly in the liver. A reduced rate of biotransformation is usually associated with decreased drug clearance. Hepatic drug metabolism is altered by: 1) age, 2) parenchymal liver disease (hepatitis, cirrhosis), 3) altered hepatic blood flow, 4) enzyme induction, 5) enzyme inhibition, 6) protein binding, and 7) coexisting medical conditions such as uremia.

Age. Pediatricians are familiar with the effect of age upon the metabolic rate of drugs. In neonates, the capacity for biotransformation of many drugs is markedly reduced, thereby impeding elimination. This impairment is related to depressed activity of several enzyme systems, including those that mediate both Phase I (i.e., oxidation, reduction) and Phase II reactions (conjugation). Chloramphenicol is the best known example. When newborns receive the same per kilogram dosage as older children, a toxic concentration of the drug accumulates, leading to cardiovascular collapse, the gray baby syndrome. Before this phenomenon was recognized and before newborn dosage schedules were revised, many deaths occurred.

Conversely, some drugs are metabolized more rapidly by young patients. The clearance of theophylline is approximately 30 percent greater in 7-year-old children than in healthy adults. Infants, however, metabolize theophylline less rapidly than older children; the typical 7-year-old child has clearance that is almost four times as great as the typical neonate.

Clinicians should assume that the metabolic fate of any drug is different in neonates and young children than in healthy adults unless there is convincing information to the contrary. Because there is no way to predict the extent of age-related alteration, the physician *must* consult individual drug information before administering any substance to a child. Selected drugs for which there is altered hepatic metabolism in infants and children include

Acetaminophen
Chloramphenicol
Diazepam
Indomethicin
Meperidine
Phenobarbital
Phenytoin
Salicylates
Theophylline

Immaturity also affects the *end products* of biotransformation. In newborn infants, but not in older persons, theophylline is methylated to caffeine. Caffeine shares many of the pharmacologic properties of theophylline; this is an example of a pharmacologically active metabolite. Thus, the plasma caffeine concentration as well as the theophylline concentration must be considered when adjusting theophylline dosage in neonates.

Parenchymal Liver Disease. Intuitively, one anticipates that liver disease may impede biotransformation of drugs that are metabolized by the liver. Although this is often true, there are frequent exceptions. The theoretic treatment of this issue is complex and controversial. Factors such as the intrinsic hepatic clearance of the drug (extraction ratio), protein binding, type of liver disease (cirrhosis, viral hepatitis, portal hypertension), and the effect of these processes upon liver blood flow interact and make generalization and prediction difficult. Table 14–5 summarizes the effect of hepatic disease upon selected drugs. However, the fact that the metabolism of a particular drug is affected by liver disease does not mean that there must be a change in dosage, because reductions in elimination may be offset by alterations in other pharmacokinetic or pharmacodynamic factors.

The complexity of the problem becomes greater when one considers that there is no direct measurement of hepatic functional impairment, as there is for the kidney. Thus, it is virtually impossible for the clinician to accurately predict the degree to which biotransformation is impaired in an individual patient. Although standard "liver function tests" (particularly, tests of coagulation function) provide a clue as to the severity of liver disease, there is no simple quantitative approach to the problem of dosage adjustment. The suggested reading by Chernow and Lake provides a clinical approach to drug therapy in patients with hepatic dysfunction.

Hepatic Blood Flow. The following drugs have a high intrinsic hepatic clearance.

Lidocaine
Meperidine
Morphine
Pentazocin
Propranolol
Verapamil

A high intrinsic hepatic clearance means that most of the drug presented to the liver is re-

Table 14–5. Selected Drugs That May Require Dosage Reduction in Hepatic Disease

Antidysrhythmics
Lidocaine
Propranolol
Quinidine
Verapamil
Antibiotics
Cefoperazone
Chloramphenicol
Clindamycin*
Erythromycin
Isoniazid*
Nafcillin
Rifampin*
Anticonvulsants
Diazepam
Phenobarbital*
Phenytoin
Valproic acid
Miscellaneous
Cimetidine*
Theophylline

*Decrease dosage with severe disease

moved during a single pass through that organ. For these agents, the rate of metabolism is sensitive to changes in hepatic blood flow. Conditions that affect blood flow to the liver (CHF, shock, intrinsic liver disease) or cause blood to bypass the liver (portasystemic shunting) may sharply decrease clearance. For example, there is a direct relationship between cardiac output and lidocaine clearance. This relationship is clinically relevant; patients with CHF will develop evidence of toxicity if the dosage of lidocaine is not reduced. For each of the drugs in the preceding list, one should consider a reduction in dosage when treating patients with poor liver perfusion. In addition, agents with high intrinsic hepatic clearance may manifest greater *oral bioavailability* in the context of disturbed hepatic blood flow or function. This phenomenon may require a reduction in oral dosage but is of little practical importance in the critically ill patient.

In addition to reduced cardiac output, other factors, including certain drugs, may influence hepatic blood flow (Table 14–6). Recently, it was shown that propranolol, partly through causing a reduction in liver blood flow, impairs elimination of lidocaine. Cimetidine is commonly administered to critically ill patients and has been shown to cause a decrease in liver blood flow. Based upon this finding, one can predict that cimetidine will affect the elimination rate of efficiently cleared drugs.

Enzyme Induction. Many drugs and chemicals increase the activity of hepatic enzyme systems, which may result in a faster rate of metabolism for drugs that are transformed by these systems. In part, the effect upon clearance will depend upon whether the drug is efficiently extracted by the liver. Enzyme induction has little effect upon the clearance of those drugs with high hepatic clearance, because metabolism of these substances is very efficient prior to induction of the enzyme. For drugs with low hepatic clearance, enzyme induction increases clearance and, therefore, reduces drug concentration. Clinically important drug interactions are regularly associated with enzyme induction. For example, phenobarbital induces metabolism of many drugs, including phenytoin, tricyclic antidepressants, warfarin, digitoxin, and chloramphenicol. This may reduce plasma concentration and efficacy. It is well known that people addicted to cigarette smoking have an accelerated theophylline clearance and require a higher than average dosage. Over two hundred such interactions have appeared in the medical literature. Although not all such interactions may be clinically important, en-

Table 14–6. Factors That Alter Hepatic Blood Flow*

	Increase Flow	Decrease Flow
Physiologic/Pathologic	Supine posture	Upright posture
		Exercise
		Volume depletion
		CHF
		Shock
		Renovascular hypertension
		Cirrhosis
Drugs	Glucagon	Propranolol
	Isoproterenol	Norepinephrine
	Phenobarbital	Antihistamines (H_1, H_2)
		Indomethicin
		Cimetidine

*Effects upon hepatic drug metabolism have not been demonstrated for each factor.
Modified from Williams, R.L., and Benet, L.Z.: Hepatic function and pharmacokinetics. *In* Zakim, D., and Boyer, T.D. (eds.): Hepatology. Philadelphia, W.B. Saunders Company, 1982, pp. 230–246.

zyme induction is a rich source of therapeutic mischief.

A different pattern of induction occurs when a second drug induces formation of a toxic metabolite of a first drug. For instance, combined use of rifampin and isoniazid (INH) is associated with an increase in the frequency of hepatotoxicity. Evidence indicates that this results from rifampin-enhanced conversion of INH to a toxic metabolite.

Enzyme Inhibition. An increasing number of drugs are known to *reduce* the metabolism of other drugs. When these agents are used concurrently, the plasma concentration of the inhibited drug may increase, thereby producing a toxic response. Erythromycin reduces theophylline clearance. Serious theophylline toxicity has been reported when the two drugs were administered simultaneously without a reduction in theophylline dosage. Phenytoin appears to reduce biotransformation of chloramphenicol, necessitating a 25 percent reduction in the dosage of the antibiotic. Conversely, both INH and methylphenidate have been implicated in reduced phenytoin clearance. Cimetidine, by virtue of its interaction with cytochrome P450, reduces the rate of oxidative biotransformation (Phase I) of many drugs transformed by this enzyme system. Indeed, the potential for interaction is so great that the physician should assume that cimetidine will prolong the elimination of any co-administered drug that undergoes appreciable P450-dependent metabolism unless there is evidence to the contrary. As the discussion suggests, the number of known interactions of this type is quite large. Undoubtedly, the other instances of enzyme inhibition await description. Therefore, one must be vigilant in anticipating this problem in patients.

Whether inhibition or induction occurs does not contraindicate co-treatment with the agents in question; it merely indicates to the physician that he should undertake the appropriate adjustments in dosage. This is particularly important when treatment with an inducer or inhibitor is initiated or terminated.

Altered Protein Binding

Deviations in protein binding are common. Conditions that are known to affect binding of drugs to plasma proteins (albumin, alpha-1-acid glycoprotein) include uremia, hepatic disease (cirrhosis, hyperbilirubinemia), hypoalbuminemia (malnutrition, nephrotic syndrome), immaturity (term and preterm infants), and concurrent drug therapy (Table 14–7). Each of these disturbances may occur in the critically ill child. Although a detailed analysis is beyond the scope of this chapter, some generalizations can be made. Basically, changes in binding have clinical relevance only for drugs with a narrow

Table 14–7. Effect of Hepatic or Renal Disease Upon Protein Binding of Selected Drugs

Drug	Effect
Diazepam	↓ Urem ↓ Cirr
Dicloxacillin	↓ Urem
Furosemide	↓ Urem
Phenytoin	↓ Urem ↓ AVH ↓ Cirr
Propranolol	↓ AVH ↓ Cirr
Salicylate	↓ Urem
Sulfonamides	↓ Urem
Valproic acid	↓ Urem ↓ Cirr
Warfarin	↓ Urem

Urem = Uremia; Cirr = Cirrhosis; and AVH = Viral hepatitis.

theraputic range that are more than 80 percent bound.

Interpretation of drug concentration data (therapeutic drug monitoring) may be affected by disturbances in protein binding. For example, the anticonvulsant phenytoin is highly bound to albumin. The unbound (or free), but not the bound, fraction is pharmacologically active. However, routine laboratory methods measure the *total* (bound and unbound) plasma phenytoin concentration. This is not a problem in normal people in whom there is a predictable relationship between bound, unbound, and total phenytoin concentrations. In such people, the therapeutic range lies between 10 and 20 mg per L (total phenytoin concentration). If the affinity of albumin for phenytoin is reduced by half (unbound fraction doubles), as it is in patients with uremia, the unbound *active* concentration of phenytoin *doubles*, with no corresponding increase in the measured *total* concentration. Thus, a *total* concentration of 15 mg per L in uremic patients provides the same *unbound* concentration as a *total* concentration of 30 mg per L in normal people. Phrased in a different way, in uremic patients, a (total) phenytoin concentration of 15 mg per L will produce the same pharmacologic response as a total concentration of 30 mg per L in normal people. This concentration may be associated with appreciable toxicity. In patients with uremia, the range of desirable total phenytoin concentrations is reduced in proportion to the degree of renal failure and frequently lies between 5 and 10 mg per L.

This analysis also applies to other drugs that are highly albumin bound. For these drugs, the usual therapeutic range may require revision in the context of abnormal protein binding. Because a common cause of this abnormality is uremia, it is useful to know that this illness tends to affect the binding of acidic drugs more than that of basic drugs. This phenomenon appears to be of major importance with phenytoin and valproic acid. For both of these drugs, the therapeutic range decreases as the serum creatinine increases.

In addition to occasionally affecting interpretation of drug concentration data, changes in protein binding may alter drug kinetic behavior. Agents with low intrinsic hepatic clearance (e.g., phenytoin) or that are principally eliminated by glomerular filtration rather than tubular secretion undergo an *increase* in total drug clearance when protein binding is reduced because more free drug is available to the size of disposition. Because clearance is increased, *total* drug concentration is decreased. However, the decrease in total drug concentration is offset by an increase in the unbound, or free drug *fraction*. The free drug *concentration* remains the same, and there is no net change in pharmacologic effect. In kinetic terms, total clearance, total volume of distribution, and free drug fraction are increased; half-life and free drug concentration are unchanged; and total drug concentration is reduced. *The usual dosage produces the normal effect, albeit at a lower total drug concentration.* With phenytoin or valproic acid, it is inappropriate to "compensate" for lower than usual total concentrations by increasing the dosage, which may produce toxicity. In summary: The usual maintenance dosage of phenytoin administered to patients with uremia is likely to produce the expected pharmacologic effect. The measured total phenytoin concentration is apt to fall between 5 and 10 mg per L, and the physician must understand that this apparently subtherapeutic concentration does not usually require an increase in dosage.

A few drugs are both efficiently extracted by the liver and highly protein bound. For such drugs (e.g., lidocaine), reduced binding does not increase clearance because extraction is already maximal. However, the unbound fraction rises, thereby increasing the intensity of response to any given total drug concentration. Hence, the usual dosage produces the normal total drug concentration, but a supranormal effect. In the context of reduced protein binding, one may wish to reduce the maintenance dosage of this category of drug.

Concurrently administered drugs can influence each other's binding to plasma proteins. Highly bound acidic drugs compete for albumin-binding sites. Such competition may result in one drug being displaced from its binding site. This displacement increases the free *fraction* of that drug; it has the same effect upon free fraction as does a reduction in the affinity of albumin for that drug. For poorly extracted drugs, the free *concentration* transiently rises, thereby augmenting hepatic clearance or glomerular filtration of that drug. Because clearance increases, the total drug concentration eventually decreases. The end result is that there is no net change in pharmacologic effect, because the increase in free drug fraction is offset by a decrease in total drug concentration. The free concentration is not altered.

The best studied example of this type of interaction concerns the anticoagulant warfarin. When phenylbutazone is started in a patient receiving warfarin, the anticoagulant is displaced from its binding site, thereby increasing the free concentration. As clearance increases, the free concentration decreases toward its previous value. Until this action occurs, however, excessive hypoprothrombinemia results. The correct approach is to reduce the dose of warfarin when phenylbutazone (or another displacing drug) is initiated. The prothrombin time is measured serially, and the dosage is titrated accordingly. Eventually, the patient again requires the initial warfarin dosage. In the past, the importance of protein-binding interactions was greatly overstated. It is now recognized to affect therapy with only a few drugs.

The effect of age upon protein binding deserves special comment. Many drugs show a decrease in protein binding in neonates compared with that in older children and adults. Selected drugs with reduced protein binding in neonates include

Ampicillin
Chloramphenicol
Diazepam
Digoxin
Lidocaine
Nafcillin
Phenobarbital
Phenytoin
Salicylate
Sulfisoxazole
Theophylline

The effect of this disparity has not been widely studied, and the effect upon dosage requirement may be modified by other factors. Seizures have been observed following administration of standard doses of lidocaine to neonates, possibly because a reduced concentration of the binding protein, alpha-1-acid glycoprotein, leads to higher than customary free drug concentrations. For phenytoin, reduced binding to the albumin of neonates may involve adjusting the usual therapeutic range.

Displacement of unconjugated bilirubin from its albumin binding site occurs during therapy with several agents and can be of major importance. It was seen when infants who were treated with sulfonamide antibiotics developed kernicterus. This issue has been extensively reviewed but is not discussed in this chapter.

PRACTICAL APPLICATION

In previous sections, methods for calculating dosage adjustments in renal failure have been explained. The same principles apply in hepatic disease, although attempts to establish a quantitative linkage between indices of liver function and rate of metabolism have not proved successful. Thus, the clinical approach to dosage modification is largely empiric. For drugs whose metabolism is affected by liver disease (see Table 14–5), the usual loading or initial dose is administered unless altered distribution or protein binding indicates that there should be a change. When appropriate, direct measurement of plasma drug concentration permits estimation of kinetic parameters. Therapy is then adapted according to this information. When such measurements are not appropriate or feasible or when subsequent doses must be administered before one receives this data, the physician must make an informed judgment. For selected drugs, estimates of clearance or half-life in liver disease either have been published or are indicated on product literature. Using this information, the physician begins therapy. If this information is not available, the physician should reduce the maintenance dose by at least 25 to 50 percent when the drug's clearance is known to be significantly reduced by liver dysfunction. After therapy has begun, the regimen can be adjusted according to the patient's response or drug concentration data.

Case Study

An 18-month-old child weighing 10 kg with cirrhosis develops asthma and is placed on theophylline. Assuming a normal V_d (this assumption may not be valid in cirrhosis), the loading dose is computed in the usual manner (Equation 14.6) and is found to be 75 mg. A maintenance infusion is calculated by assuming that the average clearance of theophylline in an 18-month-old child is 80 ml per kg per hour. Anticipating reduced hepatic function, this is revised to 40 ml per kg per hour. The desired equilibrium concentration is 15 mg per L. Using equation 14.3A the dosage is calculated

$$MD = 40 \text{ ml/kg/hr} \times 10 \text{ kg} \times 15 \text{ mg/L}$$

$$= 6.0 \text{ mg/hr}$$

The loading dose is given and the maintenance infusion is started. After 24 hours of therapy, the child has not improved. The theophylline concentration is 8 mg per L. In order to rapidly increase the concentration to about 15 mg per L, a second loading dose is given. The desired change in concentration (C^*) is 15 mg per L — 8 mg per L or 7 mg per L. The second loading dose (LD') is calculated by a modification of Equation 14.6.

$$LD' = C^* \times V_d \times k_g$$

or

$$LD' = 7 \text{ mg/L} \times 0.5 \text{ L/kg} \times 10 \text{ kg}$$

$$= 35 \text{ mg}$$

At the conclusion of the second loading dose, the theophylline concentration should be 15 mg per L. In order to maintain the concentration at this level, it will be necessary to increase the maintenance infusion. Because the initial rate of administration (MD) and concentration (C) are both known, it is possible to calculate the actual clearance using Equation 14.3. In this case, it is 75 ml per kg per hour. When the actual clearance is known, one can calculate the new maintenance rate using Equation 14.3A. Alternatively, the arithmetic can be simplified by establishing the proportionality.

$$\frac{MD_{(initial)}}{C_{ss(initial)}} = \frac{MD_{(revised)}}{C_{ss(desired)}}$$

The proportionality reflects the central assumption of first order kinetics: increases in rate of administration produce proportionate increases in concentration. In the case study,

$$\frac{6.0 \text{ mg/hr}}{8 \text{ mg/L}} = \frac{MD_{(revised)}}{15 \text{ mg/L}}$$

$$MD_{(revised)} = 11.3 \text{ mg/hr}$$

the child receives an additional loading dose of 35 mg, and the infusion is increased to 11.3 mg per hour. After 24 hours, the theophylline level is 17 mg per L, quite close to the desired value. Suppose that the child is given a drug that reduces theophylline clearance. After a day or two, the child becomes tachycardic and vomits; the theophylline concentration is 32 mg per L. Obviously, the infusion must be stopped, but for how long? At what rate should it be restarted? The problem is solved by using Equation 14.4, together with the assumed V_d, to *estimate* the half-life. In this case, $t_{1/2}$ is approximately 9.9 hours. If the infusion is interrupted for 10 hours, the concentration will decline by about 50 percent to 16 mg per L. At this time, the maintenance infusion is restarted, at a new, lower rate. This new rate should be 5.3 mg per hour.

DOSAGE ADJUSTMENT

These examples illustrate the general approach to dosage adjustment of continuous infusion when therapeutic drug monitoring is available. As a rule, the rate of infusion is increased in proportion to the desired increase in concentration. The same approach is used to achieve a target C_{ave} during intermittent therapy, although the problem is made more complex by the need to consider peak (C_{max}) and trough (C_{min}) concentrations and by the fact that adjustments are made in dose interval as well as in the amount of dose. This multiplicity of factors makes the mathematical description of dosage adjustment for intermittent therapy somewhat more complex than it is for continuous infusions. Again, however, the main principle is that increases in amount per dose produce proportionate increases in C_{max} and C_{min}.

Thus, if a patient is receiving 100 mg of theophylline every 6 hours and the trough concentration is 5 mg per L with a peak concentration of 10 mg per L, doubling the dosage to 200 mg every 6 hours will yield (after equilibrium is achieved at the new dosage) a trough concentration of 10 mg per L and a peak concentration of 20 mg per L. If the peak concentration were somewhat higher, 15 mg per L, before the dosage was adjusted, simply doubling the amount per dose would have caused the peak to increase to 30 mg per L, a concentration substantially exceeding the therapeutic range. In that circumstance, the appropriate adjustment would have been to decrease the interval between doses, rather than the amount at each dose.

The following guidelines are suggested: 1) When the trough and peak concentrations are both below the therapeutic range, *increase* the amount given per dose in proportion to the desired increase in peak and trough concentrations. 2) If the peak is acceptable but the trough is too low, decrease the interval between doses. Both the peak and trough will increase, and it may be necessary to decrease the amount given with each dose. 3) If the peak is too high but the trough is appropriate, decrease the amount given with each dose. If subsequent measurements indicate that the new trough is too low, it may be necessary to reduce the interval between doses.

With some categories of drugs (e.g., the aminoglycoside antibiotics and vancomycin), it is probably important to monitor both peak and trough concentrations because, the peak and trough have *different* therapeutic ranges. For many drugs, however, monitoring trough drug concentrations is sufficient. This simplifies application of therapeutic drug monitoring, because the time of the trough concentration is always known (just before a dose), but the time of the peak concentration is subject to biologic and technical variability. Use of trough concentration data alone will be most useful with drugs that have a relatively long half-life, such as digoxin, phenobarbital, phenytoin, and sustained release preparations of oral theophylline.

Inappropriate use of the quantitative methods discussed in this chapter can produce precision without accuracy. These tools must be used in the context of individual drug information. In individual patients, disturbances in protein binding, distribution, elimination, and pharmacodynamics may coexist and interact in unpredictable ways. The art of therapeutics, in part, consists in knowing when it is safe to assume that one variable is stable while another changes. Optimal therapy of critically ill patients demands attention to kinetic detail; it also requires a sound factual knowledge of individual drugs and a conservative approach to therapy.

SUGGESTED READINGS

Anderson, R.J.: Drug prescribing for patients in renal failure: Hosp. Pract. 18:145, 1983.

Chernow, B., and Lake, C.R. (eds.): The Pharmacologic Approach to the Critically Ill Patient. Baltimore, Williams & Wilkins, 1983.

Hansten, P.D.: Drug Interactions, 4th ed. Philadelphia, Lea & Febiger, 1979.

Kock–Weser, J., and Sellers, E.M.: Binding of drugs to serum albumin. N. Engl. J. Med. 294:311–316 and 526–531, 1976.

Reidenberg, M.M., and Drayer, D.E.: Drug therapy in renal failure. Ann. Rev. Pharmacol. Toxicol. 20:45, 1980.

Rowland, M.: Drug administration and regimens. In Melmon, K.L., and Morelli, H.F. (eds.) Clinical Pharmacology, 2nd ed. New York, Macmillan Publishing Co., Inc., 1978, pp. 25–70.

Rowland, M., and Tozer, T.N.: Clinical Pharmacokinetics. Philadelphia, Lea & Febiger, 1980.

Schwartz G.J., Feld L.G., and Langford O.J.: A simple estimate of glomerular filtration rate in full-term infants during the first year of life. J. Pediat. 104:845–854, 1984.

Sheiner, L.B., and Tozer, T.N.: Clinical pharmacokinetics: the use of plasma concentrations of drugs. In Melmon, K.L., and Morelli, H.F. (eds.): Clinical Pharmacology, 2nd ed. New York, Macmillan Publishing Co., Inc., 1978, pp. 71–109.

Thompson, W.L.: Dosage optimization in critical care: use and abuse of drug analysis and computers. In Shoemaker W.C., and Thompson, W.L. (eds.): Critical Care—State of the Art, Vol. 2. Fullerton, Society of Critical Care Medicine, 1982, pp. (G) 1–(G) 102.

Williams, R.L., and Benet, L.Z.: Hepatic function and pharmacokinetics. In Zakim, D., and Boyer, T.D. (eds.): Hepatology. Philadelphia, W.B. Saunders Company, 1982, pp. 230–246.

Yaffe, S.J.: Pediatric Pharmacology. New York, Grune & Stratton, Inc., 1980.

Acute Peritoneal Dialysis

ROBERT G. SCHACHT, M.D.

. . . should the kidneys fail . . . neither bone, muscle, gland, nor brain could carry on . . .
Homer W. Smith

When a disease process results in the accumulation of metabolic waste products, in severe fluid and electrolyte imbalance, or in drug intoxication, efficient maneuvers should be promptly initiated to detoxify or eliminate them from the body. Dialysis is an effective therapeutic modality that may assist the physician in the restoration of normal body homeostasis. Two types of dialysis are available: peritoneal dialysis and hemodialysis.

Although hemodialysis is the more efficient method for rapid removal of solute and water, two technical problems limit its use in infants and young children. The size of the patient's blood vessels is of primary importance in the establishment of vascular access; thus its use is markedly restricted in patients who weigh less than 20 kg. Of less importance is the amount of the patient's circulating blood volume "lost" to the extracorporeal system. Thus, peritoneal dialysis is the preferred method for children. This procedure consists of the placement of a sterile glucose and electrolyte solution (dialysate) into the peritoneal cavity through a trocath or surgically implanted catheter. Water, electrolytes, and toxins are passively transferred from the capillaries of the peritoneum into the dialysis fluid, which is then drained from the body.

THEORY

Six decades ago, Gantner reported the removal of toxins in humans with uremia via the peritoneal route. His therapeutic accomplishment was based on the fact that the peritoneum is a semipermeable membrane that by processes of diffusion and ultrafiltration permits the passive movement of water, electrolytes, and small crystalloids from the peritoneal capillaries into the dialysate solution. In infants, the area of this exchange membrane that lines the abdominal cavity and covers all of its viscera is approximately two times that of the adult. Although the surface area available for net movement of solute and water is not the only factor to be considered, in newborn animals and in infants, it has been shown that peritoneal dialysis is twice as effective as that in older subjects.

Recent evidence suggests that molecules somewhat smaller than albumin, after being delivered to the peritoneal exchange site, cross into the peritoneal cavity through endothelial and mesothelial pores. Thus, similar to the anatomic barrier of the glomerular capillary loop, the peritoneum offers a resistance to the passage of molecules in the form of pores and a basement membrane. Similar to the glomerulus, the peritoneum requires an adequate blood flow (provided primarily by the superior mesenteric aretery) to be an efficient dialyzing membrane. Further impediment to passage of solutes is offered by the interstitial fluid and interperitoneal fluid films. In summary, the efficacy of peritoneal dialysis depends upon splanchnic blood flow, concentration gradients, surface area and pore size available for diffusion of solute, the physical characteristics of the molecule to be dialyzed, the resistances offered by the membrane, and finally, the dialysate itself.

Studies in adult humans indicate that equilibrium between the peritoneal capillaries and the dialysate is most efficient for smaller molecules (under 600 daltons) between 30 and 60 minutes and when the volume of the dialysate is approximately 3.5 L. Urea clearances approximating 25 to 30 ml per minute can be achieved using a 2-L volume and a dwell time of 30 to 60 minutes. Obviously, these volumes cannot be achieved in children and I prefer a volume of 30 to 40 ml per kg with dwell times of 20 to 30 minutes. Additional information will be given in the methods section.

FACTORS AFFECTING PERITONEAL TRANSPORT

Factors that might increase peritoneal dialysis efficiency for all size solutes include increased peritoneal blood flow, increased volume, adequate dwell time, hypertonic dialysate, and prewarmed solutions. Conversely, decreased splanchnic blood flow, decreased pore size or surface area available for diffusion, prolonged dwell times, small volumes, and cold dialysate impede the dialytic process.

Clinically, patients in shock who are receiving vasoconstrictor agents that adversely affect mesenteric flow or who have peritoneal adhesions or paralytic ileus will have decreased areas for diffusion. It has also been shown that prewarming of the dialysate increases the efficiency of dialysis compared with that of solutions administered at room temperature (cooler solutions will effect a significant lowering of the patient's body temperature). Rapid flow rates and hypertonic solutions improve the passage of larger molecules. It is theorized that these maneuvers limit or abolish the resistance afforded by the interstitial fluid and the peritoneal fluid film, thereby favoring the process of ultrafiltration. As mentioned previously, small molecules enter the dialysate primarily by diffusion. The removal of these particles may be augmented by the addition of vasodilatory substances into the peritoneal fluid or into the systemic circulation.

INDICATIONS AND CONTRAINDICATIONS

By far, the most common indication for acute peritoneal dialysis is acute renal failure. However, any clinical event that results in: 1) intravascular volume overload as it occurs in intractable congestive heart failure (CHF), 2) severe electrolyte imbalance (e.g., hypercalcemia or salt poisoning), 3) severe disturbance of acid–base balance, 4) drug intoxication, or 5) accumulation of metabolic waste products may be ameliorated by peritoneal dialysis. This form of therapy is useful in delivering antibiotics to and lavaging the peritoneal cavity when bowel perforation has caused peritonitis. In patients with inborn errors of metabolism, such as maple syrup urine disease, congenital lactic acidosis, or hyperammonemia, peritoneal dialysis may be lifesaving. The efficacy of dialysis in the therapeutic regimen for Reye's syndrome is questionable.

The current trend is to intervene with dialytic therapy at an early phase rather than wait for specific signs and symptoms to emerge or for predetermined levels of toxins to be reached. Obviously, one should be aware of the natural or expected duration of the insult and the patient's ability to cope with the disturbance in homeostasis. For example, a patient in acute renal failure whose course will be complicated by catabolic processes and who requires large volumes of fluids to provide calories, antibiotics, or vasoactive drugs will require dialysis much sooner and more frequently than a patient with a less complicated course.

Contraindications to peritoneal dialysis are relatively few and are related to complications that might occur. The risk of bowel perforation in infants with necrotizing enterocolitis and in older patients with inflammatory lesions of the bowel might prompt the pediatrician or the nephrologist to use more stringent medical therapies or hemodialysis before initiating peritoneal dialysis. The risk of infecting an area in which a recent vascular procedure has been carried out or of restarting an intra-abdominal bleeding diathesis should also prompt one to try all other forms of therapy before resorting to peritoneal dialysis. Relative contraindications include known diffuse peritoneal adhesions, respiratory insufficiency that would be further compromised by impairing diaphragmatic movement, and recent abdominal surgery. It should be kept in mind that when no other form of therapy is possible, peritoneal dialysis should be expertly initiated.

TECHNICAL CONSIDERATIONS

Although peritoneal dialysis is technically easier to perform than hemodialysis, it should not be thought of as a simple procedure that anyone can initiate. In practice, if untrained personnel or areas that are not specified or equipped for dialysis are used, complications that further compromise the patient's course may result.

Placement

To safely place the catheter, certain precautions should be taken. If the patient is conscious, he should be sedated with meperidine (Demerol) and promethazine (Phenergan) intramuscularly or diazepam (Valium) intravenously (IV). Care should be taken to empty the bladder by crede or catheter so that it is not perforated by the trocath. It is my preference to restrain the patient during placement of the peritoneal catheter and throughout dialysis. The restraints offer the patient limited movement but not enough to dislodge the trocath. Rarely does a patient require continuous sedation throughout dialysis.

Two sites are commonly used for catheter placement: The most common site is midline, one third the distance between the umbilicus and the pubic symphysis; the other is in the left anterior axillary line between the last rib and the iliac crest. (I favor the latter site for small infants who have umbilical lines in place.) The site is widely prepped with Betadine and infiltrated with a local anesthetic. A large bore angiocath is placed into the peritoneal cavity, and 20 to 30 ml per kg of dialysate is introduced into the peritoneal cavity. This amount of fluid should distend the abdomen, decreasing the risk of bowel perforation. When surgically implanting the catheter, this maneuver may be omitted.

For easier manual introduction of the trocath, a small 0.5-cm-skin incision is made at the site of insertion and the area is dissected bluntly to the linea alba (midline) or muscle facia (laterally). The trocath, which consists of a metal stylet inside the dialysis catheter, is inserted through the incision in a perpendicular direction. I have found that firm pressure directed downward and clockwise facilitates insertion. As the peritoneum is perforated, a loud pop is heard and/or felt by the operator. At that point, downward pressure is eased and the stylet is withdrawn approximately 2 inches inside the catheter. The catheter is then directed inferiorly and laterally to the right paracolic gutter. The stylet is removed, and at this point, I usually cut the excess portion of the catheter 2 inches above the abdominal exit. A shorter extra-abdominal segment of catheter should initiate less intra-abdominal catheter movement, thereby lessening the possibility of intra-abdominal trauma. The catheter is connected to the administration tubing. The dialysate, which was introduced for insertion, is now emptied and 30 to 50 ml per kg of dialysate is rapidly (2 to 5 min) infused into the abdomen. This infusion is continued until the abdomen is distended.

Several observations should be made at this time. If cardiorespiratory embarrassment is observed, the reservoir is too large and subsequent infusions should be decreased until they are tolerated by the patient. The inflow and egress of fluid should be rapid; if not, the catheter should be repositioned. If leakage occurs, a pursestring suture is placed around the catheter and tightened. A sterile dressing is applied either with or without an antiseptic ointment. The dressing is changed, and the insertion site is cleansed daily. It is not uncommon for the first few exchanges to be blood tinged. If this continues, local pressure or deeper sutures may be applied. It may be reassuring to determine serial hematocrits on the waste dialysate.

The patient is now ready to be dialyzed. Each exchange or run should have a minimal volume of 30 to 50 ml per kg in infants and 50 to 100 ml per kg in older patients, provided that no cardiorespiratory embarrassment occurs. For controlled dialysis, each exchange of continually warmed dialysate should last approximately 1 hour. The fluid should be infused and drained as rapidly as possible, thus defining the dwell time. If there is an urgent need to remove toxins or fluid, more rapid exchanges (q 30 min) should be made until a more stable dialysis can be affected. A prolonged (1 hr) dwell time actually decreases the efficiency for removal of small solutes; therefore, dwell times of under 30 minutes are preferred. Most patients require 48 to 72 hours of dialysis per week; if dialysis is to be interrupted, the catheter may be removed and a Dean's prosthesis may be inserted.

Dialysate

The dialysate consists of a solution of 1.5 percent glucose and electrolytes whose osmolality (350 mOsm/L) is slightly higher than normal serum osmolality (280 to 290). The electrolyte constituents are slightly hypotonic when compared with normal serum. They contain no potassium, and acetate is substituted for bicarbonate so calcium can be added. The hyperosmolar dialysate solution initiates a water flux from the peritoneal capillaries into the dialysate while electrolytes and small solutes diffuse down a gradient from the blood to the peritoneal fluid. Larger molecules and more water can be removed by increasing the osmolality of the dialysate (ultrafiltration). Commercially available solutions contain either 1.5 percent (350 mOsm/L) or 4.25 per cent (480 mOsm/L), which can be mixed by the pharmacy or administered alternately. Because there is no potassium in the dialysate, one should remember to add it either to the initial dialysate if the patient does not present with hyperkalemia or to subsequent volumes when the hyperkalemic patient has been adequately treated by dialytic therapy. Heparin should be added to the first few exchanges (1000 U/2L) to prevent blockage of the catheter by fibrin or clots. If the effluent continues to be bloody or if protein exudation occurs, I use heparin in all exchanges. The dialysate is commercially available in 2-L bottles, which are adequate for one exchange in larger patients but might last for 24 hours in infants. It may be more convenient to ask the hospital pharmacist to divide the solutions into sterile 500-ml aliquots.

COMPLICATIONS

Complications encountered during acute peritoneal dialysis are predictable and can usually be managed without interruption of dialysis. The more common problems, including abdominal pain, bloody effluent, inadequate dialysis flow, leakage of dialysate either into subcutaneous tissue or to the exterior, respiratory embarrassment, and viscus perforation, are mechanical in nature and manifest themselves within the first 24 hours of therapy. The patient may experience abdominal discomfort caused by the trauma of catheter insertion, by malposition of the catheter, by abdominal distention, by chemical or infectious irritation of the peritoneum, or by viscus perforation. Relief is obtained either by repositioning of the catheter or by decreasing the volume or composition of the dialysate.

As described previously, a bloody effluent may result from perforation of blood vessels within the abdominal wall, of peritoneal vessels, or of the bowel itself. With minor trauma, the effluent usually clears within several runs. During this period, heparin, 500 U per L is added to the dialysate so that clots do not block the catheter. The use of pursestring sutures or pressure dressings may be beneficial. Inadequate drainage, although sometimes secondary to fibrin clots or peritoneal adhesions, is most often due to poor positioning of the catheter. When effluent flow decreases, the patient may be repositioned by elevating the head of the bed, flexing the knees, and turning the patient onto his side. The catheter should then be flushed rapidly with dialysate and drainage should be attempted. As a last resort, it may be necessary to reposition or replace the catheter.

Respiratory efforts may be hampered by the volume of the dialysate impairing diaphragmatic excursion, by accumulation of dialysate in the pleural space, or by diminished pulmonary toiletry, a sequel of the patient's supine position. After it has been recognized, this problem may be ameliorated by diminishing the volume of dialysate, by deep breathing exercises, and by repositioning of the patient. It is uncommon for pleural collections to accumulate to the extent that dialysis must be interrupted. Although opinions vary on therapy for hydrothorax, that is, cessation of dialysis or thorocentesis, the nature of the patient's requirement for dialytic therapy will dictate the course to be followed.

Subcutaneous dissection of dialysate into the abdominal wall, genitalia, and other dependent areas may be managed by the placement of a pursestring suture, by elevation of the dependent edematous sites, or by temporary interruption of dialysis. A more common and more worrisome occurrence is the onset of edema observed in very young patients who require dialysis. The generalized edema that develops is a natural sequel to the relative and perhaps absolute hypoproteinemia of the infant in the setting of a large saline (dialysate) load. This clinical event usually becomes manifest during the second to fourth days of dialysis and may require no specific therapy other than the planned cessation of dialysis.

When a viscus is perforated during catheter placement, the patient presents with decreased dialysis effluent, which is often bloody, and watery bowel movement (bowel perforation) or a sudden and marked increase in urine output (bladder perforation). The catheter should be removed and repositioned, and the patient should be monitored for signs of peritonitis.

As the dialysis continues, the patient may experience metabolic disturbances. The most common metabolic disturbances are hypoproteinemia, hyperglycemia, and hypernatremia. Protein metabolism may be markedly affected by the primary illness, by dietary restriction, or by peritoneal loss of protein. It is estimated that approximately 0.50 gm of protein is lost with each liter of effluent. This amount is magnified if the technique of ultrafiltration (by hyperosmolar dialysis) is used or if peritonitis develops. Obviously, high biologically active protein should be administered and catabolism should be stopped.

The patient's blood glucose level is frequently elevated during dialytic therapy. Modest elevation to levels of 180 to 250 mg/dl rarely requires alteration of the therapeutic regimen. However, when these levels are exceeded, the complication that results from the peritoneal absorption of glucose from the dialysate may prove to be fatal. Severe hyperglycemia that is observed particularly when dialyzing with frequent hypertonic exchanges (4.25 percent = 4250 mg/dl) may be managed by the parenteral or peritoneal administration of insulin. I prefer the addition of insulin to the dialysate while the patient's blood levels are carefully monitored, because there may be a delay in peritoneal absorption of insulin. Admixing of the 1.5 and 4.25 percent solutions still offers ultrafiltration while decreasing the peritoneal load of glucose.

A related hyperosmolar complication is the development of hypernatremia. As the glucose in the dialysate osmotically draws water across the membrane, the patient's serum constituents may become concentrated. After this has been recognized by blood sampling, water intake should be increased or the osmolality of the dialysate should be decreased. When observed, hypokalemia and hypocalcemia should be treated by the addition of these electrolytes to the dialysate for maintenance. It may be necessary to administer them parenterally if an acute correction is required.

The most serious complication is peritonitis. Emphasis should be placed on prevention rather than on recognition and cure. Dialysis should be initiated and performed by experienced personnel. Aseptic and closed techniques should be assiduously followed. The dressing and dialysate tubing should be changed, and routine surveillance cultures should be obtained every 24 hours. If symptoms of peritonitis develop, if the effluent becomes cloudy, or if the dialysis suddenly proves to be less effective, the effluent should be collected for culture and the centrifuged sediment should be stained for bacterial and fungal identification. At this juncture, the rapidity of peritoneal exchanges is increased for lavage purposes and specific (if the offending invader has been identified) or broad-spectrum antibiotics are added to the dialysate. The lavaging procedure, which also provides dialytic therapy, is continued for 48 to 72 hours. Within this period of time, symptoms should abate, cultures should be negative, and the peritoneal cell count should markedly diminish. Antibiotics are continued for 10 to 14 days. The most common antimicrobials that are used and their dosages for peritoneal administration are gentamicin, 5 to 10 mg per L of dialysate; cephalothin, 25 to 50 mg per L; carbenicillin, 50 to 75 mg per L; and tobramycin, 5 to 10 mg per L. It is recommended that a systemic loading dose of these antibiotics be administered and that serial serum concentrations be followed. For fungal candidal peritonitis, amphotericin B, 1 mg per L, can be administered twice a day or 5-fluorocytosine, 5 mg per L, can be administered in each run.

Because the most common cause of peritonitis is the entry of organisms through or around the catheter, it is imperative that this site be kept sterile and that the system remain closed. Recent data emphasize the importance of prevention rather than cure of this serious complication, which occurs in most acute peritoneal dialysis patients younger than 2 years of age and in almost one third of those older than 2 years.

Rapid changes in intravascular volume may occur as dialysis progresses; therefore, careful monitoring of the patient's cardiovascular status must be continuous both by dialysis personnel and by monitoring equipment. Prompt attention to changes in weight and in fluid balance should guide therapy in correcting errors of underhydration or overhydration. Dysrythmias secondary to the patient's primary disease, to electrolyte imbalance, to circulating toxins, or to reflex changes in vagal tone may develop during dialysis. When a morbid cardiac event occurs, it is imperative that the abdomen be emptied by dialysis before other corrective or supportive therapies are instituted.

TAILORING OF DIALYSIS FOR SPECIFIC DISORDERS

The most common clinical situation in which peritoneal dialysis is used is acute renal failure. After the clinician has determined that dialysis must be instituted, a standard dialysis solution of 1.5 percent without additives is used. This solution, exchanged every 30 minutes to 1 hour, should effectively remove urea and small molecules and restore biochemical balance within 48 to 72 hours. If an additional objective of dialysis is the rapid correction of intravascular overload, a 4.25 percent solution can be infused intraperitoneally. I have issued several caveats regarding the use of this effective solution, which results in hyperosmolar syndrome, pain, and so on; therefore, sterile admixing of 1.5 and 4.25 percent solutions by the hospital pharmacist may be preferred. I have found that several exchanges with a hypertonic solution are required before a significant change in water balance occurs. Obviously, this form of therapy, hyperosmolar dialysis, would be offered to patients who present in intractable congestive heart failure (CHF). Such patients are often in delicate electrolyte balance, and there is no need to withhold potassium from the onset of dialysis. Less frequently but more dramatically encountered in the dialysis unit are patients with inborn errors of metabolism whose incomplete metabolites overwhelm the body's homeostatic mechanisms, resulting in maple syrup urine disease, urea cycle deficiencies, and so on. Rapid diagnosis and institution of dialysis using a standard 1.5 percent solution and 30-minute runs results in dramatic reversal of the insult within hours. This form of dialysis is also used when, secondary to acute gastrointestinal disease, the patient cannot be maintained on his special diet and toxins cannot be effectively removed by medical management.

The removal of sodium from the patient who is salt poisoned may be effected by the use of a dialysate consisting primarily of 5 to 8 percent glucose solution. One should eliminate sodium chloride from the dialysate and maintain vascular volume by intravenous administration of free water.

Patients with inborn errors of acetate metabolism who present with lactic acidosis should be dialyzed with a solution that contains bicarbonate rather than acetate. Obviously, calcium cannot be added to the dialysate in this particular situation. Finally, in patients who present in renal failure with severe metabolic alkalosis, a presentation frequently encountered in post–open-heart renal failure patients, dialysis with a low–acetate, high-chloride solution may be beneficial.

PHARMACOLOGIC AGENTS AND PERITONEAL DIALYSIS

The peritoneal membrane may allow the transport of certain pharmacologic agents either into the dialysate or into the patient's circulation. The dialyzability of these drugs is increased when their characteristics include being extravascularly distributed, lipid insoluble, and poorly bound to protein and having a small molecular size. It is therefore incumbent upon the physicians who take care of dialyzed patients to be familiar with those agents whose bioavailability is affected by dialysis. The agents that are removed by peritoneal dialysis are listed at the end of this section. Their administration should be altered either by addition of that agent to the dialysate in a concentration approaching the desired blood level or by increasing the systemic administration of the drug.

When dialysis is used in the therapy of an overdose, the addition of certain substances may facilitate the removal of the toxin. When placed in the dialysate, albumin and lipids might increase the transport of protein-bound or lipid-soluble products; bicarbonate may alleviate lactic acidosis; acidifying agents would facilitate the movement of ammonia; and so on. The technique of ultrafiltration by hypertonic dialysate may allow the removal of large-sized molecules.

Antimicrobial agents frequently administered to pediatric patients whose concentrations are affected by dialysis include amikacin, cephalothin, colistin, erythromycin, 5-fluorocytosine, gentamicin, isoniazid, kanamycin, sulfonamides, ticarcillin, and tobramycin. Other agents that may be used are aspirin, procainamide, nitroprusside, methyldopa, phenobarbital, and diphenylhydantoin.

SUMMARY

Peritoneal dialysis is an efficient therapeutic modality, particularly suited to pediatric patients whose renal function cannot maintain body homeostasis. The rational use of this procedure by personnel knowledgeable in the physiologic and pharmacologic manipulations that affect peritoneal transport and of those complications that are inherent to dialysis is an important adjuvant to the care of patients in pediatric intensive care units.

SUGGESTED READING

Boen, S.T.: Peritoneal Dialysis in Clinical Medicine. Springfield, Illinois, Charles C Thomas, Publisher, 1964.

Day, R.E. and White, R.H.: Peritoneal dialysis in children. Review of 8 years' experience. Arch. Dis. Child. 52:56, 1977.

Fine, R.N.: Peritoneal dialysis update. J. Pediatr. 100:1, 1982.

Maher, J.F., Hirszel, P., and Lasvick, M.: An experimental model for study of pharmacologic and hormonal influences on peritoneal dialysis. Contrib. Nephrol. 17:131, 1979.

16

Component Transfusion Therapy

VIJAYALAXMI MALAVADE, M.D.
JOHN G. GORMAN, M.D.
LOOL SEGED ABEBE, M.D.

Steady advances in blood banking have enabled blood bankers to cope with increasing demands. Since the 1950's, the advent of plastic bags has enabled blood bankers to make components that are more potent and reduced in volume. Recent advances in anticogulants and more modern plastic bags have extended the storage life of blood to 49 days and platelets to 7 days.

The invention of blood–cell separators has made it possible to supply large quantities of platelets and granulocytes from a single donor. These cell separators also have the capacity to perform therapeutic plasmapheresis and cytapheresis, as well as total or partial exchange transfusions, with relative ease and safety.

Cryopreservation techniques have made it possible to store rare types of blood for prolonged periods in order to meet the specific needs of sensitized patients with unusual antibodies. Frozen deglycerolized red cells are relatively leukocyte-free and have been used extensively in hypertransfusion regimens and in patients who need repeated transfusions, thus limiting leukocyte sensitization.

Selective harvesting of neocytes, the younger population of red cells, is also possible with combined apheresis and freezing techniques. Such preferentially harvested neocytes survive longer in vivo, thus decreasing the transfusion requirements. Cryopreservation for later transfusion of autologous platelets from patients is currently being investigated and has promising results.

Tissue-typing technology has opened new horizons in transplantation and provided a method of treating patients who are otherwise refractory to regular components.

Optimal transfusion therapy requires that the specific needs of a patient be matched to the appropriate blood component, which requires thorough understanding of each blood component. The risk/benefit ratio must be carefully considered before embarking on transfusion therapy. Because of allosensitization, with each transfusion there is the risk that future transfusions will not be effective. One must also consider the risks of immediate and delayed transfusion reactions and disease transmission.

Blood components are prepared from a unit of whole blood by differential centrifugation and separation. Blood derivatives are manufactured by chemical fractionation and purification processes that are not available in most blood banks.

ANTICOAGULANTS AND STORAGE LESIONS

The anticoagulant most widely used for collection and storage of blood is citrate phosphate dextrose (CPD), with or without added adenine. The widely used CPD–A1 preserves the red cell viability and oxygen unloading capacity for 35 days. Approximately 450 ml of blood is collected from a donor and mixed with the anticoagulant, yielding a final volume of 510 ml, with a hematocrit of 35 to 40 percent as a result of dilution.

There are few metabolic changes in the first week of storage, but the pH of the blood drops to below 7.0. Thereafter, metabolites accumulate gradually, with increasing concentrations of free hemoglobin, potassium, and lactic acid in the stored blood. The 2,3-DPG of the red cells, which reflects the O_2-unloading capacity, is maintained at adequate levels in the first week with CPD blood and up to 12 to 14 days with CPD–A1 blood. Based upon these findings, fresh blood may be defined as anything less than 5 days old.

A unit of whole blood must be fractionated within 4 to 6 hours of collection. The platelet yield is optimal when separated from whole blood maintained at room temperature for less than 6 hours. There is no appreciable loss of Factors V and VIII when fresh frozen plasma (FFP) is prepared within 4 hours.

WHOLE BLOOD

In the early days of blood transfusion, all transfusions consisted of whole blood because glass bottles did not lend themselves to fractionation or closed separation. Now that component therapy is available, it is thought that whole blood transfusions are unjustified in most settings except perhaps for exchange transfusions. Valuable elements of whole blood are wasted when given to patients who do not need them.

The virtue of whole blood lies in its capacity to simultaneously correct hypovolemia, oxygen transport deficit, and, with some limitation, bleeding disorders.

Whole blood is available in most blood banks as (1) unmodified whole blood, (2) modified whole blood from which platelets and/or cryoprecipitate are removed, and (3) reconstituted whole blood (red cell concentrate plus FFP).

Platelets are viable in whole blood only during the first 24 to 48 hours.

Indications

Rapid blood loss with hypovolemia and reduced O₂-carrying capacity associated with shock is best treated with whole blood. Even though similar results can be achieved with component therapy, the resultant delay, added cost, and increased exposure to more than the minimal number of donors makes the latter a less attractive option. In situations of massive transfusion, optimally 1 of 4 units should be relatively fresh.

All red cell transfusions require a clotted sample for compatibility testing. Meticulous attention must be paid to the identification of the patient and the specimen; errors can result in fatality. For surgical procedures that rarely require blood transfusion, a type and screen (ABO, Rh grouping, and screening for unexpected antibodies), rather than a type and crossmatch request, should be made. This maximizes blood inventory, yet allows prompt and safe availability if blood is needed.

RED CELL CONCENTRATES

All red cell concentrates are prepared by centrifugation of whole blood with removal of most of the plasma and/or other constituents. Certain special products such as washed red cells or frozen thawed red cells (frozen deglycerolized red cells) are pure red cell suspensions in protein-free media. These concentrates have very few white cells and can be manipulated to adjust the hematocrit (Hct) to any desired level. Usually, the hematocrit of a unit of red cells is 75 percent. Leukocyte-poor red cells are prepared by removing the buffy coats, and 75 percent of the original leucocytes are removed.

A list of the commonly available red cell concentrates and general guidelines for their use are shown in Table 16–1.

Indications

Red cell transfusions are indicated whenever there is a need to supply oxygen transport capacity when there is no attendant hypovolemia.

Massive Transfusions. In the management of hypovolemia, there is substantial evidence supporting the effectiveness of crystalloids as the primary resuscitation fluid, aided by whole blood and red cell concentrates as necessary.

At one time it was thought that abnormal bleeding following massive transfusion in trauma patients was the result of dilution of platelets and coagulation factors that were deficient in the stored blood. The existence of such a "washout phenomenon" could not be substantiated, because there was no correlation between the amount of blood transfused and the tendency for bleeding. Abnormal coagulation tests and fibrinolytic activity are commonly seen in trauma patients as a result of shock, tissue damage, and infection. Therefore, empirical component therapy is not advocated in the absence of active bleeding. Supportive platelet transfusion is deemed unnecessary unless the platelet count is less than 50,000 per μL and surgical intervention is anticipated or if the platelet count is less than 20,000 per μL in postoperative bleeding. Similarly, unless the prothrombin and partial thromboplastin times are elevated to more than one and a half times normal, administration of FFP is not necessary.

Table 16–1. Products Used for Red Blood Cell Content

Blood Component	Clinical Indications	RBC	Plasma	WBC	Shelf Life
		Approximate Composition			
Whole blood	Exchange transfusion or massive transfusion	155–270 ml	180–305 ml	25×10^8	35 days*
Red blood cells	Chronic anemia, surgical blood loss, or hemorrhage	155–270 ml	40–115 ml	25×10^8	35 days*
Leukocyte-poor red blood cells	Repeated febrile transfusion reactions and anemia, surgical blood loss, or hemorrhage	125–215 ml	30–90 ml	5×10^8	35 days*
Saline-washed red blood cells	Febrile transfusion reactions or IgA deficiency with antibody and anemia, surgical blood loss, or hemorrhage	140–240 ml	—	1×10^8	24 hours
Deglycerolized red blood cells	Autologous transfusion, rare donor blood, IgA deficiency with antibody, bone marrow transplant candidates, or febrile transfusion reactions	140–240 ml	—	0.5×10^8	24 hours

Reprinted from Kennedy M., Adkins, S., and Wansky, J.: Safe transfusion. AABB publication, 1981.
*Forty-nine days when collected in Optimal Additive Solution.

In unusual situations in which fibrinogen levels have dropped below 100 mg/dl, it may be necessary to administer cryoprecipitate. In addition to raising the fibrinogen level, cryoprecipitate is also thought to supply the opsonization protein fibronectin.

When component therapy must be administered on an empirical basis, 1 unit of FFP and 2 units of platelets may be used for every 6 units of stored whole blood or red cell concentrates.

The same guidelines should be followed for massive transfusion in cardiac surgery, with special consideration for functional platelet defects caused by the pump-oxygenator.

Anemia. When prompt correction of anemia is necessary before specific therapy can be instituted, as in severe iron deficiency anemia with cardiac decompensation, red cell transfusions are indicated.

Preparation for Surgery or Anesthesia. In elderly patients with decreased cardiac reserve, low hemoglobin is known to predispose the patient to cardiac dysrhythmias under general anesthesia. However, it is not advisable to raise the hemoglobin to a minimum of 10 gm per dl in children, because a shift in the oxygen dissociation curve by the transfusion of stored 2,3-DPG depleted blood may nullify any benefit.

Insidious Blood Loss without Hypovolemia. Operative or other bleeding when red cell replacement is needed is a sign that red cell transfusions are necessary.

Renal Transplant Candidates. It is a well-known fact that graft survival is better in patients receiving transfusions than in those who are not; patients receiving red cell concentrates or whole blood transfusions have better graft survival than those receiving leukocyte-poor red cells or frozen red cell transfusions. There is evidence that a protocol involving donor-specific transfusions prolong graft survival.

Universal Donor Mode. When transfusions are given in the universal donor mode, red cell concentrates are the product of choice. This limits the amount of infused plasma containing anti-A and anti-B antibodies.

In the following situations, the components of choice are *leukocyte-depleted red cells* prepared by buffy coat removal, washing with saline, or freeze-thawing:

1. Supportive therapy for patients awaiting bone marrow recovery, patients receiving chemotherapy, and patients who have aplastic or hypoplastic anemia. Frozen deglycerolized red cells or leukocyte-poor red cells minimize sensitization to other components.

2. IgA-deficient patients with anti-IgA antibodies requiring blood transfusions. Because these patients have serious reactions to any component that contains IgA, they must receive components that are free of plasma. Frozen, deglycerolized red cells or washed red cells are well tolerated.

3. Patients who have repeated febrile transfusion reactions to red cell concentrate. Microaggregate filters are used, because they are known to reduce the white cell debris from the stored blood and prevent febrile reactions.

4. Bone marrow transplant candidates. Avoid transfusions from family members who may be future donors for transplant. When transplant is being contemplated, avoid transfusions, when possible, because graft survival is better in untransfused patients.

5. Sickle cell anemia patients undergoing sur-

gery. It is necessary to raise the level of the adult hemoglobin (Hb) to 60 percent in order to minimize complications of anesthesia. This may be best accomplished by partial exchange transfusion with frozen red cell concentrates, because these cells have better 2,3-DPG levels. The volume of exchange may be calculated by using the following formula:

Volume of exchange

$$= \frac{Wt \; (kg) \times 75 \; ml/kg \times desired \; rise \; in \; Hb}{22 \; gm/dl - Hbw}$$

Where,

$$Hbw = \frac{Initial \; Hb + desired \; Hb}{2}$$

The Hb content of frozen deglycerolized red cells is 22 gm per dl.

Dose Calculation and Administration

For red cell replacement therapy, 10 to 15 ml per kg will raise the Hb by 3 gm per dl in children.

All whole blood and red cell transfusions must be administered through a standard blood administration set with a filter.

Warming of blood is not necessary except in massive transfusions. Only an in-line blood warmer with proper visual and audible alarms may be used.

It is not advisable to use microaggregate filters in massive transfusions, because they limit the blood flow and may diminish the effectiveness of the components that are simultaneously being administered.

Blood may be administered at the rate of 10 to 15 ml per kg per hour in the absence of hemorrhage or cardiac decompensation. The flow rate should be adjusted accordingly for the aforementioned conditions. The patient should be observed closely for the first 15 minutes. If no adverse effects are noted, flow rate may be increased.

GRANULOCYTE TRANSFUSIONS

Granulocyte transfusions have proved to be a lifesaving measure in severely neutropenic children with gram-negative or fungal sepsis.

Buffy coats prepared from donations of whole blood as leukocyte concentrates are less effective than single donor leukocytes obtained by cell separators. There are several machines that use either continuous flow centrifugation or intermittent flow centrifugation to separate the various cell components from whole blood and return the undesired components to the donor. It is possible to collect adult therapeutic doses of leukocytes in this manner from a single donor. The final yield from such a procedure depends upon whether the donor has been prestimulated by steroids or has received a sedimenting agent such as hydroxyethyl starch (HES) during the collection procedure. Combined usage of prestimulation and HES provides the best yield. The risk of using this agent is unknown, and the compound is known to remain in the recipient's body for several months. It is for this reason that many donor centers will not recruit granulocyte donors and depend upon physicians to recruit donors from family members and friends.

Granulocytes obtained by filtration leukapheresis seem to have diminished functional capability, abnormal morphology, decreased post-transfusion recovery, and short intravascular half-life, even when autotransfused in normal donors. However, they are capable of migrating to a skin window in infected neutropenic patients.

Even though human leukocyte antigen (HLA)-compatible donor transfusions result in better post-transfusion increments and are associated with fewer side effects, use of ABO-compatible unrelated donor leukocytes is quite effective. ABO (and preferably Rh) compatibility is essential, because granulocyte concentrates are heavily contaminated with red cells, hence the need for compatibility testing. If it is necessary to transfuse Rh positive components for Rh negative recipients, prophylaxis with Rh immune globulin must be used.

The yield from various methods of collection has a mean of 0.5 to 1.5×10^{10} granulocytes without steroid stimulation and 1.5 to 4×10^{10} with steroids. It takes 2 to 3 hours to process 3 to 8 L of blood on the machine. The final product has a volume of 350 to 700 ml, with 35 to 50 ml of red cells and a large number of lymphocytes and platelets.

A buffy coat prepared from a whole blood unit has approximately 2×10^9 granulocytes. Therefore, several units must be pooled to obtain enough leukocytes. Each buffy coat has a volume of 35 to 50 ml with 15 to 25 ml of red cells; therefore, it must be compatible with recipient plasma.

Indications

Granulocytes should be administered to febrile patients who have a neutrophil count of less than 300 to 500 per μL and proven gram-negative or fungal sepsis and who have not responded to appropriate antibiotic therapy after 48 hours of treatment. Prophylactic treatment for neutropenia without infection is not recommended. Granulocyte transfusions should be continued for a minimum of 4 days; they may be continued for up to 14 days or until the infection subsides or marrow recovery occurs. An increase of leukocytes in peripheral blood is rare and is not an index of therapeutic effectiveness.

Dose Calculation and Administration

The most commonly recommended dose is 0.5×10^{10} granulocytes per m² body surface per day. If the transfused volume is excessive for the child, removal of as much plasma as possible may be considered. However, centrifugation of granulocytes is not recommended. Occasionally in cases of Rh or ABO incompatibility, it may be necessary to remove red cells. This may be achieved by sedimentation when the original collection is made with HES. If possible, granulocytes should be transfused soon after collection; however, they must be transfused within 24 hours. If necessary, the concentrate can be divided into 4 aliquots and transfused every 6 hours. The concentrate should be administered through a standard blood administration set with a filter.

Common side effects associated with granulocyte transfusion are the same as those seen with red cell transfusions, although fever and chills are more common with granulocyte transfusion. In general, children tolerate granulocyte transfusions well; discontinuation of transfusion is rarely necessary.

PLATELET CONCENTRATES

Platelet concentrates are available in two forms: The first form is composed of random donor–batched units prepared by centrifugation of whole blood with subsequent separation of platelets. These units contain a minimum of 5.5×10^{10} platelets. The second form includes therapeutic quantities of platelets collected from a single donor with a cell-separator machine. Approximate compositions are given in Table 16–2.

Donor selection is important for both methods, because aspirin ingestion and other nonsteroid anti-inflammatory agents can affect the function of the harvested platelets. Aspirin, however, is less important than other anti-inflammatory agents in random donor pools, because a minimum of 20 percent of the pool must be affected before the function of the transfused platelets is changed.

The recommended storage temperature for platelets is 22°C, because mean post-transfusion survival and function are better main-

Table 16–2. Platelet, Leukocyte, and Plasma Components

Blood Component	Clinical Indications	Approximate Composition		Shelf Life Storage Temperatu
		Plasma	*Platelets*	
Random donor platelet	Thrombocytopenia with hemorrhage, severe thrombocytopenia, or functional platelet disorders with hemorrhage	30 ml (4°C) 50 ml (20–24°C)	> 5.5×10^{10}	48 hr at 4°C 72 hr at 20–
Single donor platelet concentrate by apheresis	Refractory to random donor platelet concentrate and severe thrombocytopenia or hemorrhage with thrombocytopenia or functional disorder	300–500 ml	$3–8 \times 10^{11}$	24 hr at 20–
Leukocyte concentrate by apheresis	Severe neutropenia, fever, and infection unresponsive to antibiotics	300–700 ml	$3–8 \times 10^{11}$ (Granulocytes = 1×10^{10})	24 hr at 4°C 20–24°C
Fresh frozen plasma (FFP)	Multiple coagulation deficiencies	200–275 ml	—	1 yr at 18°C 24 hr at 4°C
Single donor plasma	Plasma expansion	200–275 ml	—	5 yr at 18°C 24 hr at 4°C
Cryoprecipitate	Factor VIII deficiency, Factor XIII deficiency, von Willebrand's factor, or hypofibrinogenemia	10–15 ml	—	1 yr at 18°C 6 hr at 20–

Reprinted from Kennedy, M., Adkins, S., and Wansky, J.: Safe transfusion. AABB publication, 1981, p. 5.

tained at this temperature. The pH of the storage medium is important, because the post-transfusion survival rate will decrease if the storage pH drops below 6.0. Therefore, there must be enough plasma left behind in the platelet preparation for proper pH to be maintained. New plastic bags allow oxygen and CO_2 transfer and thus maintain viability for 5 days. Random donor platelets have a volume of 50 ml per unit. This volume can be reduced to 35 ml if the platelets are to be stored at 1 to 6°C for 24 to 48 hours. The amount of plasma in these concentrates also provides some coagulation factors. Platelet preparations are also heavily contaminated with lymphocytes and a small volume of red cells (0.5–4.0 ml/concentrate).

Batched platelet concentrates are usually pooled for transfusion. After the concentrates have been pooled, storage time is limited to 6 hours because the oxygen requirement cannot be maintained and there is the possibility of contamination.

Single donor platelet units contain 3 to 5 $\times$ 10^{11} platelets. Because this method of collection is considered an "open" system, the storage limit is only 24 hours. Although the platelets share the ABO antigens, this is not a significant factor in post-transfusion survival. However, because of the plasma, platelet concentrate should preferably be compatible with the red cells of the recipient. Platelets do not share the Rh antigens. When Rh positive platelets are used for Rh negative patients, the red cell contamination should be covered with Rh immunoglobulin prophylaxis. Graft vs. host reaction is a known complication when platelets are given to immunocompromised patients because of the lymphocyte contamination. Irradiation of the platelet concentrate with 1500 to 5000 rads will selectively destroy their ability to proliferate without affecting platelet function.

HLA-matched single donor platelets provide better increments and survive longer in patients who are alloimmunized to platelets. When a matched single donor is not available, family members or siblings are the best choice. Exact matching for all the antigens is not required; one can take advantage of cross-reactive antigens and "blank" antigens. This practice also increases the available donor pool per patient.

Indications

Platelet concentrates are indicated for thrombocytopenic patients who have associated hemorrhage, who are prone to bleeding because of low platelet count (usually under 20,000 per μL), and who have abnormalities in platelet function.

The decision to transfuse platelets depends upon the clinical state of the patient, the future needs of the patient, and laboratory data. Differentiation between destructive thrombocytopenia and decreased platelet production is necessary in determining the therapeutic role of the platelet transfusion. Post-transfusion recovery of less than 30 percent at 24 hours signifies increased destruction. Destructive thrombocytopenia seldom responds to platelet transfusion. If there is active bleeding, hemostasis may be achieved by transfusing large amounts of platelets. Prophylactic therapy will not be helpful.

Other factors that hinder post-transfusion recovery are fever, splenomegaly, sepsis, bleeding, alloimmunization, and medication. In disorders of decreased production, the effects of transfusion are excellent until alloimmunization becomes a problem.

Dose Calculation and Administration

One unit of platelet concentrate per 5 to 6 kg of body weight or per m² of body surface area is expected to increase the count by approximately 50,000 to 75,000 per μL in neonates and by 12,000 to 15,000 per μL in older children. This increase reflects initial splenic sequestration of approximately 30 percent of the transfused platelets.

The desired level for achieving surgical hemostasis is 50,000 to 100,000 per μL, and for nonsurgical hemostasis, the desired level is 20,000 per μL. However, at much lower counts, bleeding may not necessarily occur when there are large numbers of young giant platelets in circulation.

The daily drop in post-transfusion platelet count is expected to be approximately 10 percent per day in nondestructive thrombocytopenia. The most widely used indicators of post-transfusion recovery are the 1-hour post-transfusion count and the 18- to 24-hour post-transfusion count. In the absence of other causes of poor recovery, lack of expected increment 1-hour post-transfusion reflects the degree of refractivity as a result of alloimmunization.

Single donor platelet concentrates contain more platelets than the required pediatric dose and therefore may be divided in half and transfused on two consecutive days within the 24-hour dating period. They should be administered through a component filter (platelet, cryoprecipitate) or a standard blood filter.

All the complications associated with red cell transfusion may be seen after platelet transfusion.

FRESH FROZEN PLASMA

Fresh frozen plasma (FFP) is a source for several blood constituents, including albumin, immunoglobulins, all the coagulation factors, complement, fibronectin, and trace elements. Plasma is frozen within 6 hours of collection and stored at −30°C for up to 1 year. The volume of FFP ranges from 200 to 275 ml and contains approximately 200 U of all the clotting factors and 400 mg of fibrinogen.

Indications

Active bleeding associated with multiple clotting factor deficiencies are implicated, such as in disseminated intravascular coagulation, after massive transfusion of stored blood, in liver disease, or vitamin K deficiency, is an indication for FFP. In the latter two instances, use of FFP is justified when there is insufficient time to correct the deficiency with vitamin K administration.

FFP is the only blood component source for Factors V and XI. In congenital Factor V deficiency and in liver disease when vitamin K administration does not correct the coagulation abnormality, FFP is the component of choice.

When abnormal coagulation does not reveal any specific deficiency, FFP is indicated.

Dose Calculation and Administration

For coagulation factor replacement, transfusing 15 to 20 ml per kg of FFP will achieve hemostasis. The plasma must be ABO compatible with the red cells of the recipient, because the plasma contains ABO agglutinins. See Table 16–3 for the exact dosage.

CRYOPRECIPITATE

The method of preparation for cryoprecipitates was devised by Pool and Shannon in 1965. FFP, when thawed at 1 to 6°C over a 14- to 18-hour period, forms a white gelatinous precipitate that is separated, refrozen, and stored between −20 and −30°C for up to 1 year. Cryoprecipitate contains Factor VIII (antihemophilic factor, AHF), von Willebrand's factor, fibrinogen, fibronectin, and Factor XIII. The volume varies between 15 and 25 ml per bag and contains 80 to 100 I.U. of AHF and approximately 300 mg of fibrinogen.

Indications

Cryoprecipitate is indicated in the following situations:

1. In disseminated intravascular coagulation (DIC), as a source of Factors V and VIII and fibrinogen.

2. In the treatment of mild to moderate Hemophilia A, as a source of Factor VIII.

3. In von Willebrand's disease, as a source of von Willebrand's factor.

Table 16–3. Replacement Therapy for Miscellaneous Hereditary Coagulation Disorders

Disorder	Hemostatic Level (% of Normal)	Therapeutic Material	Loading Dose	Maintenance Dose
Fibrinogen deficiency	10–25	Cryoprecipitate	4 bags/10 kg	1 bag/10 kg every other day
Prothrombin deficiency	20–40	Plasma (fresh frozen or cryoprecipitate-poor)	15 ml/kg	5–10 ml/kg daily
		Prothrombin complex	20 μ/kg	10 μ/kg daily
Factor V deficiency	15–25	Plasma (fresh frozen or cryoprecipitate-poor)	20 ml/kg	10 ml/kg every 12 hr
Factor VII deficiency	5–10	Plasma (fresh frozen or cryoprecipitate-poor)	10 ml/kg	Not required
		Prothrombin Complex	10 μ/kg	
Factor X deficiency	10–20	Plasma (fresh frozen or cryoprecipitate-poor)	15 ml/kg	10 ml/kg daily
		Prothrombin complex	15 μ/kg	10 μ/kg daily
Factor XI deficiency	10	Plasma (fresh frozen or cryoprecipitate-poor)	10 ml/kg	5 ml/kg daily
Factor XIII deficiency	2–3	Plasma (fresh frozen or cryoprecipitate-poor)	5 ml/kg every 2–3 wk	Not required

Reprinted from Guidelines to Transfusion Practices, Chap. 12 by D. Goldfinger and F. H. Britton. American Association of Blood Banks, 1980, p. 117.

4. In afibrinogenemia and hypofibrinogenemia, as a source of fibrinogen.

5. In the rare disorder of Factor XIII deficiency.

6. In the rare instance when it is necessary to provide the opsonization protein fibronectin.

Dose Calculation and Administration

The amount and frequency of cryoprecipitate administration depends upon the hemostatic level required, the metabolic half-life of the factor, and the initial distribution of the factor between the intravascular and extravascular spaces.

The hemostatic level of AHF required for minor trauma is 20 to 30 percent; for major trauma or surgery, it is 50 to 100 percent.

There are two methods by which the cryoprecipitate dose may be calculated: (1) by calculating the plasma volume, and (2) by using the formula that infusion of one unit of Factor VIII per kg raises the plasma level by 2 percent. An example of the first method follows: A child weighing 20 kg will have a plasma volume of 840 ml. To achieve a 100 percent Factor VIII level will require 840 U of AHF. Assuming that each bag of cryoprecipitate has 80 to 100 U, 8 to 10 bags will be required every 12 hours.

An example of the second method follows: A child weighing 10 kg will need 150 units of Factor VIII for the level to be raised by 30 percent over the existing level.

See Table 16–3 for the hemostatic levels, half-lives, and dosages of the various congenital factors.

Cryoprecipitate also contains ABO agglutinins; hence, it is preferable to use a group specific component. The small amount of red cell stroma present in the preparation has been known to cause Rh sensitization when transfused into Rh negative recipients. Therefore, Rh immunoglobulin prophylaxis must be considered.

ANTIHEMOPHILIC FACTOR (FACTOR VIII) CONCENTRATE

Antihemophilic factor (AHF) is prepared from batches of pooled plasma by various methods, including ethanol or ether fractionation, precipitation with polyethylene glycol, and filtration through agarose gel. AHF is available in packages of various sizes, from 200 to 300 U per vial to 800 to 1200 U per vial. Each vial's AHF activity is verified by the Bureau of Biologics. Most products have a half-life of 3 to 6 hours in the first phase, which consists of a rapid fall in the level of the factor as a result of the initial distribution between the extravascular and intravascular spaces. Biologic half-life in the second phase of intravascular disappearance is 12 hours. In vivo recovery is in the range of 90 percent.

Unlike cryoprecipitate, AHF concentrate has predictable potency and is easy to ship, store, and administer at home. These advantages have facilitated home infusion programs for hemophiliacs.

Because AHF is prepared from a large pool of donors, the risk for hepatitis is much greater than for plasma or cryoprecipitate. As a result, many of the transfused patients develop antibody to hepatitis B surface antigen (HbsAg). Most patients are asymptomatic; however, liver disease, ranging from mild elevation of transaminases to chronic hepatitis or cirrhosis, is not uncommon. Other complications include the development of AHF inhibitor.

AHF concentrates also contain anti-A and anti-B antibodies in a large enough concentration to cause hemolysis of the recipient's red cells when non–group-specific AHF concentrate is transfused in large amounts.

Several recent reports indicate that patients receiving AHF concentrates are at greater risk for developing acquired immune deficiency syndrome (AIDS). Reports also indicate that patients treated with AHF concentrates have reversal of their helper/suppressor T-cell ratio, as opposed to patients receiving cryoprecipitate. The causative agent is believed to be a retrovirus. Physicians should be aware of the risk.

AHF concentrate does not contain von Willebrand's factor and should not be used to treat von Willebrand's disease.

Indications

AHF concentrate is indicated in the following situations:

1. In patients with moderate to severe hemophilia A who require continuous home therapy.

2. For surgical intervention in hemophiliacs when it is impossible to achieve hemostatic levels with cryoprecipitate because of volume considerations.

3. In patients with hemophilia A when infection or bleeding changes the patient's AHF requirements.

Dose Calculations and Administration

AHF concentrate can be stored in a home refrigerator, reconstituted quickly, and administered with a syringe. See Table 16–3 for the hemostatic levels for other congenital Factor deficiencies.

As a result of repeated therapy, some children will develop Factor VIII inhibitors, the incidence of which is less than 4 percent in children younger than 10 years of age. Transfusion of Factor VIII in a child who already has the inhibitor will result in a rise of the titer. Minor bleeding in these children should be treated conservatively. Serious hemorrhage may be treated with large amounts of Factor VIII to overcome the inhibitor or may require other measures, such as bypassing the Factor VIII activity by activated Factor VIII products (Autoplex) or prothrombin complex concentrates, which are available commercially. A dose of 50 to 100 U of activated factor may be administered every 8 hours as needed for acute hemorrhage, provided that thrombogenicity is taken into consideration.

There are reports that plasmapheresis is also beneficial in reducing the titer of the inhibitor, thus making therapy more effective.

Occasionally, patients develop hemolytic anemia as a result of the infusion of anti-A and anti-B antibodies, which are present in the concentrates. Group-specific concentrates are available commercially and may be used in such circumstances, in addition to group O red cells as needed.

PROTHROMBIN COMPLEX CONCENTRATES

Prothrombin complex is a lyophilized concentrate manufactured from pooled plasma that contains Factors II, VII, IX, and X. Sensitive methodology for hepatitis testing has resulted in a decrease in the incidence of hepatitis. However, patients who receive prothrombin complex are still at higher risk for developing hepatitis than those who receive cryoprecipitate or plasma. Assayed vials for Factor IX activity have activity in the range of 500 U.

Indications

Prothrombin complex is used in the following ways:

1. To treat hemophilia B.
2. To bypass Factor VIII activity in hemophilia A with Factor VIII inhibitor.
3. To treat patients with liver disease who are actively bleeding before vitamin K therapy can be effective and if treatment with FFP is not correcting the coagulopathy.
4. To treat patients on oral anticoagulants.

Dose Calculation and Administration

See Table 16–3 for guidelines and calculations for administering prothrombin complex concentrates.

SERUM ALBUMIN AND PLASMA PROTEIN FRACTION

Serum albumin and plasma protein fraction (PPF) are purified products that are prepared from pooled plasma. These blood products are free of the risk for hepatitis because of the heat inactivation process (10 hr at 60°C).

Albumin preparation is available in 5 or 25 percent saline suspension in 50- to 250-ml vials. PPF also contains 5 percent albumin and contains small amounts of alpha and beta globulins. PPF has been known to contain bradykinin and other vasoactive substances known to cause hypotension. This complication is rare in albumin preparations.

Indications

Serum albumin and PPF are thought to be overused and abused. Appropriate indications are shock, extensive burns, adult respiratory distress syndrome (ARDS), and pump prime for cardiopulmonary bypass. Occasional use as supplemental therapy for hypoalbuminemia in acute liver failure, ascites, acute nephrosis, renal dialysis, and after surgery may also be justified when the serum albumin is less than 2.5 gm per dl.

Additional data are required for its use in hemolytic disease of newborns and in detoxification procedures as a binding protein. The use of serum albumin in hypoalbuminemia resulting from undernutrition, chronic cirrhosis, and chronic nephrosis is unjustified.

ADVERSE EFFECTS OF TRANSFUSION

Because each transfusion is in effect a transplant of homologous tissue, it is not surprising that adverse reactions occur. The incidence rate of reported transfusion reactions ranges from as low as 1 percent to 10 to 15 percent of transfused patients when disease transmission is included. Most reactions are harmless, with mild to moderate discomfort to the patient at the time, without any serious consequences.

Transfusion reactions can be caused by both cellular and noncellular elements. They can be immune-mediated or nonimmunologic, and immediate or delayed in relation to the transfusion event. See Table 16–4 for a suggested classification.

Acute Hemolytic Transfusion Reactions

Fortunately, this severe, potentially fatal reaction is rare. More than 85 percent of these reactions are due to human error and involve incorrect patient identification.

Unfortunately, there are no specific indications of serious hemolytic reaction, with the exception of hemoglobinemia and hemoglobinuria, which may not always be present. Fever, chills, back and chest pain, flushing, hypotension, dyspnea, and generalized oozing are some of the symptoms. Oozing from operative sites may be the only manifestation while the patient remains under anesthesia.

All reactions must be considered potentially hemolytic until proved otherwise. The exception is the presence of urticaria alone. In this case, the transfusion should be temporarily discontinued pending evaluation for hemolysis, which involves close communication between the transfusionist and the blood bank laboratory. Transfusion may be resumed if there is no evidence of hemolysis.

When attempting to find a suspected hemolytic transfusion reaction, stop the transfusion and follow these steps:

1. Keep the intravenous line open with normal saline solution.

2. Take vital signs, including temperature, blood pressure, and pulse.

3. Check for errors in identification of the unit and/or recipient. If an error is revealed, follow Step 6.

4. Collect an anticoagulated and clotted blood sample and a urine sample. (Catheterize if necessary.)

5. Spin the blood samples and urine sample and observe for hemolysis in the supernate (pink to red color indicates hemolysis).

6. If Step 3 or 5 reveals positive findings, dismantle the transfusion immediately and send the bag, the compatibility slip, and the reaction report to the blood bank.

7. Institute immediate steps to prevent shock, acute renal failure, and DIC.

8. If Steps 3 and 5 have negative results and if hemolysis is still suspected, follow Step 6, with additional tests for haptoglobin, BUN/creatinine, 6 hours post-transfusion; total and direct bilirubin; and Hb/Hct.

Severity of the reaction is directly proportional to the volume of incompatible red cells transfused. Renal failure and DIC occur commonly if more than 200 ml of red cells are transfused. After it has been confirmed that acute hemolysis has occurred, immediate steps must be taken to prevent these complications. See Chapters 38 and 50 for management of these complications.

Delayed Hemolytic Reactions

In contrast to acute hemolytic reactions, delayed hemolytic reactions are difficult to prevent in spite of sensitive laboratory techniques in pre-transfusion testing. This reaction is usually a result of an anamnestic response by the recipient to the antigens for which the recipient was previously sensitized. The antibody is usually of such concentration that it cannot be detected. Typically, it occurs 5 to 10 days after

Table 16–4. Classification of Adverse Effects of Transfusion

	Immunologic	Nonimmunologic
Immediate	Acute hemolytic transfusion reaction Nonhemolytic febrile reaction Urticarial (allergic) reaction Anaphylactic Noncardiogenic pulmonary edema	Circulatory overload Anticoagulant and storage effects Mechanical (nonimmune) hemolysis of transfused blood Bacterial contamination (rare) Air embolism (rare)
Delayed	Delayed hemolytic transfusion reaction Allosensitization Post-transfusion purpura Graft-vs.-host disease	Disease transmission Iron overload

the transfusion of an apparently compatible unit, at the peak of the antibody production. Hemolysis is usually extravascular, but intravascular hemolysis is known to occur with some antibodies, such as Kidd blood group antibodies.

Common symptoms include a fall in hemoglobin level, fever, headache, reticulocytosis, spherocytosis, and jaundice. When acute intravascular hemolysis occurs, renal failure and DIC are expected to occur. Recognition is important, because further transfusion of incompatible blood causes the condition to become worse.

Diagnosis depends upon laboratory demonstration of antibody in the serum or on red cells. Rarely, it may be necessary to show that the donor cells are being destroyed in the absence of detectable antibody.

Management involves supportive therapy and, if necessary, transfusion with compatible red cells selected to be negative for the antigens concerned.

Nonhemolytic Febrile Reactions

Fever and chills developing at the end of transfusion or within the next 4 hours are the common symptoms of nonhemolytic febrile reactions. Fever may persist for up to 8 to 10 hours.

These reactions are more common in multitransfused patients and account for 1 to 2 percent of all transfusion reactions. Etiology is commonly believed to be due to leukocyte antibodies of the recipient reacting with the leukocytes of the donor. It is not necessary or feasible to demonstrate these antibodies.

Treatment of the symptoms with antipyretics is all that is necessary after it has been confirmed that no hemolysis has occurred.

Prevention of future occurrences involves use of leukocyte-poor red cells and/or microaggregate filters. In the event of severe repeated reactions with leukocyte-poor red cells, it may be necessary to administer frozen deglycerolized red cells.

Allergic or Urticarial Reactions

These reactions are among the most common reactions, the incidence of which is 1 to 3 percent. They are believed to be caused by the soluble antigens in the plasma of the donor.

Symptoms include urticarial rash at the transfusion site, or the rash may cover the entire body surface.

Usually, slowing of the transfusion and administration of antihistamine will clear up the reaction. Future recurrences can be prevented by premedication with antihistamine.

Anaphylactic Reactions

Anaphylactic reactions are a rare complication of transfusion. They are most often seen in IgA-deficient patients with anti-IgA antibody as a result of previous sensitization.

Signs and symptoms include shock, respiratory distress, and airway obstruction. Management includes prompt discontinuation of the transfusion and treatment of anaphylaxis. See Chapter 11.

If IgA deficiency and antibody to IgA is confirmed by the laboratory, all future transfusions must be composed of frozen deglycerolized red cells, because even small amounts of plasma may cause a reaction. Components containing plasma must be derived from IgA-deficient donors.

Post-transfusion Purpura

This unusual complication manifests approximately 1 week after the transfusion, with thrombocytopenia and purpura. The etiology of post-transfusion purpura is thought to be allosensitization of platelet-specific antigen Pl^{A1} in a Pl^{A1}-negative patient. Because the incidence of Pl^{A1}-negative individuals is very low, this reaction is rare. The recipient forms the antibody and destroys the transfused platelets. The circulating immune complexes then attack and destroy the patient's own Pl^{A1}-negative platelets. This innocent bystander phenomenon is thought to be self-limiting.

Pulmonary Reactions

There are two types of pulmonary reactions: noncardiogenic pulmonary edema (NCPE) and pulmonary insufficiency following massive blood transfusion.

NCPE is characterized by the sudden onset of respiratory insufficiency, with diffuse bilateral pulmonary infiltrates associated with transfusion of whole blood or plasma-containing components. The etiology is believed to be leukocyte antigen–antibody reaction, with microembolization in the pulmonary vasculature. The antibody is usually thought to be in the plasma of the donor reacting with the patient's leukocytes. However, cases in which the reverse has occurred have also been described.

Leukocyte-poor blood should be used if it is known that the patient has the antibody. In cases in which the donor has the antibody, no special precautions are necessary because the donor is unlikely to come in contact with the same recipient.

The etiology of pulmonary insufficiency following massive blood transfusions is unclear. Several possibilities, including microaggregate emboli from stored blood, transfusion of 2,3-DPG–depleted red cells, and changes in osmotic gradient in pulmonary vasculature have been studied. No definitive causal relationship has yet been established. Insufficient pulmonary perfusion appears to be a common denominator in these patients and may be the common pathway.

Graft-Versus-Host Disease

The etiology of this condition is the engraftment of the donor lymphocytes in the recipient and rejection of the host tissue in an immunodeficient patient. Components that contain lymphocytes are platelets, granulocytes, red cell concentrates, and whole blood.

Signs and symptoms include fever, skin rash, diarrhea, infections, bone marrow depression, and abnormal results of liver function tests. Occasionally, circulating lymphocytes of the donor can be seen in the recipient. This complication can be fatal in severe, combined immunodeficient patients and in bone marrow transplant candidates. In a milder form, however, it may not be uncommon in children receiving high doses of chemotherapy.

Prevention of graft-versus-host disease is accomplished by irradiation of all lymphocyte-containing components.

Circulatory Overload

Circulatory overload may become a major concern in pediatric patients because of the smaller volume of blood in relation to the volumes of most components to be transfused.

Signs and symptoms include acute respiratory distress, hypertension, headache, and fever. Cardiac decompensation and pulmonary edema may result, although they are uncommon in children because of the excellent cardiac reserve in these patients. When overtransfusion is unrecognized, it may result in sudden death.

Careful monitoring and removal of excess plasma from the components will prevent circulatory overload. Management of incipient pulmonary edema consists of stopping or slowing the transfusion and administering diuretic.

Anticoagulant and Storage Lesions

Citrate toxicity, hypocalcemia, hyperkalemia, hypothermia, and initial acidosis with later alkalosis are some of the effects of anticoagulant and storage lesions.

Most of these reactions correct themselves without any intervention being necessary but they may require corrective action in exchange and massive transfusions.

Disease Transmission

At one time, hepatitis was the most common disease transmitted by transfusion. Sensitive techniques involving radioimmunoassay testing of donor units for HBsAg have reduced its incidence significantly. However, the incidence of non-A, non-B hepatitis still remains high. Some medical centers have begun to screen donor units for elevated levels of ALT (alanine amino transferase) as an indication of this disease. This procedure is expected to reduce the incidence of non-A, non-B hepatitis by one third.

Other infections transmitted by transfusion are cytomegalovirus (CMV), Epstein–Barr virus, malaria, syphilis, babesiosis, toxoplasmosis, salmonella, and AIDS. Transfusion-associated CMV infection occurs in immunocompromised individuals, especially in bone marrow transplant candidates and newborn infants. The prevalence of a CMV carrier state in donors is 3 percent, as measured by virus isolation from urine. A rise in anti-CMV antibody is sometimes seen in transfusion recipients who do not have post-transfusion hepatitis; however, such seroconversion is significantly higher in patients who have hepatitis.

Allosensitization

Transfusion recipients form antibodies to many constituents of transfused blood. The importance of these antibodies has been discussed in this chapter.

Iron Overload

Each unit of red cell concentrate contributes 225 mg of elemental iron to the body. Therefore, in long-term transfusion therapy, iron overload will result in hemosiderosis and its accompanying complications.

When preferentially harvested neocytes are available, iron overload may be reduced.

SUMMARY

Advances in the field of component transfusion therapy have made transfusion therapy practical, safe, and effective. Appropriate and timely component transfusions can save lives. Although transfusions are generally well tolerated, there are many attendant risks and they must be considered before transfusion is undertaken. The goal should be to treat the patient rather than be concerned with abnormal laboratory values.

SUGGESTED READING

Barnes, A., and Nelson, I.F.: Safe Transfusion. A technical workshop. Washington, D.C., American Association of Blood Banks, 1981.

Bove, J.R., Oberman, H.A., Holland, P.V., et al.: Report of the ad hoc committee on ALT testing. Transfusion 22:4, 1982.

Goldfinger, D.: Acute hemolytic transfusion reaction—a fresh look at pathogenesis and considerations regarding therapy. Transfusion 17:85, 1977.

Ingram, G.I.C., Brozovie, M., and Slater, N.G.P: Bleeding Disorders: Investigation and Management, 2nd ed. Oxford, Blackwell Scientific Publications, 1982.

Judd, J., and Barnes, A.: Clinical and Serologic Aspects of Transfusion Reaction. Washington, D.C., American Association of Blood Banks, 1982.

Luban, N.L.C., Kellehre, J.F., and Reaman, G.H.: Investigation of immune status in children and adolescents with hemophilia. Blood 60(Suppl): 216A, 1982.

Lusher, J.M., and Barnhart, M.I.: Acquired Bleeding Disorders in Children, Abnormalities of Hemostasis. Masson Monographs in Pediatric Hematology/Oncology 3, 1981.

McCullogh, J. (guest editor): Symposium on Blood Transfusion: Practice and Science, Clin. Hum. Pathol. Philadelphia, W.B. Saunders Company, Vol. 14, No 3, March 1983.

Mentor, J.E., Aster, R.H., Casper, J.J., et al.: T-lymphocyte subpopulation in patients with classic hemophilia treated with cryoprecipitate and lyophilized concentrate. N. Engl. J. Med. 308:83, 1983.

Myhre, B.A. (guest editor): Symposium on Blood Banking and Hemotherapy. Clin. Lab. Med. W.B. Saunders Company, Vol 2, No. 1, March 1982.

Rosen, R.C., Huestis, D.W., and Corrogen, J.J.: Acute leukemia and granulocyte transfusion of cells obtained from normal donors. J. Pediatr. 93:268, 1978.

Sherwood, C., and Cohen, A.: Transfusion Therapy: The Fetus, Infant, and Child. New York, Masson Publishing USA Inc., 1980.

Silver, H. (ed.): Blood, Blood Components, and Derivatives in Transfusion Therapy. A Technical Workshop. Washington, D.C., American Association of Blood Banks, 1980.

Umlas, J., and Silvergleid, A.J.: Transfusion for the Patient with Selected Clinical Problems. A Technical Workshop. Washington, D.C., American Association of Blood Banks, 1982.

Wolf, C.F.W., and Canale, V.C.: Fatal pulmonary hypersensitivity reaction to HLA incompatible blood transfusion. Report of a case and review of the literature. Transfusion 16:135, 1976.

Yeager, A.S., and Prober, G.C.: Prevention of transfusion—acquired cytomegalovirus infections in newborn infants. J. Pediatr. 98:281, 1981.

17

Infection Control

KEITH KRASINSKI, M.D.

Infection control was introduced in 1843 by Semmelweis when he showed that proper handwashing could reduce maternal mortality due to infection. Since that time, significant advances have been made in technique and antimicrobial chemotherapy has evolved. Shifts in the spectrum of nosocomial pathogens from gram-positive to gram-negative organisms and, more recently, multiple antibiotic resistant organisms have kept pace with the introduction of antimicrobial agents. The role of viral agents in nosocomial infections is difficult to assess because viral diagnostic measures are generally unavailable; however, it is likely to be much more significant than is apparent in published reports. Nosocomial infections in children are responsible for approximately 9 percent of all hospital-acquired infections. Patients in pediatric intensive care units (ICU) are particularly prone to develop infections. This predisposition exists because many pediatric patients are admitted for care of acute infectious diseases, may be compromised hosts by virtue of young age or disease, are frequently being treated with broad-spectrum antibiotics that tend to select for the development of resistant organisms, and are treated and monitored by many invasive devices such as intravenous lines, arterial lines, endotracheal tubes, and urinary catheters. Additional risk factors include crowding of patients, inadequate staffing, and intermixing of medical with surgical patients and of neonates with older patients. Even when these factors are strictly controlled, the very nature of care required for critically ill children frequently demands rapid crisis intervention, which may confound even the most well-designed infection control program.

GENERAL CONSIDERATIONS

In order to prevent or contain outbreaks of infections, hospitals must provide a clean physical environment in which crowding is avoided

and aseptic technique is advocated. However, the most important factor for infection control is the behavior of hospital personnel. Hospital infection control programs must promote a concerned consciousness about prevention of infection and encourage high standards of hygiene among staff members. Strict adherence to isolation policies also helps prevent transmission of infection. Effective infection control programs combine a system of surveillance to identify problems with an education program to reinforce prevention practices. Surveillance mechanisms should include review of culture results by the physician to identify low levels of endemic infections. Because the community is the substrate for hospital admissions, weekly review of outpatient visits for communicable diseases helps predict potential ICU problems. Similarly, weekly review of Employee Health Service visits may reveal potential exposures of patients to communicable diseases.

Frequent review of antibiotic usage provides information about the selective pressure exerted in a given area of the hospital and helps predict the patterns of antimicrobial resistance of pathogens. Knowledge of the antibiotics used in a specific patient also helps predict organisms that are likely to be the cause of intercurrent illness.

Physical Plant

The care of individual patients in ICUs requires sufficient room for adjunctive equipment such as ventilators, cardiac monitors, and cooling blankets. Minimally, 120 sq ft should be provided per patient, with 7 ft between each bed.

The importance of airborne transmission of infection varies with the type of patients being considered and is most important for patients with extensive burns and immunocompromised hosts. Current standards for ambient air ventilation specify a minimum of six air exchanges per hour for high-risk hospital areas. The American Hospital Association recommends at least 12 volumes of air exchange for areas where newborns receive care. Intensive care areas should be maintained at negative pressures with respect to the general hospital in order to prevent the escape of air. Potentially contaminated air should be exhausted directly to the outside. Similarly, areas set aside for isolation should also be maintained at negative pressures, with circulated air being vented directly to the outside. The door to each isolation room should remain closed and should have an adjacent anteroom in which personnel wash and gown. Many hospitals that do not have specific isolation areas are required to provide care for patients who have highly contagious diseases. In this setting, a private room separate from the ICU must be used.

The most important mechanism of transmission of infection seems to be direct contact of the hands of staff members with patients. Handwashing between patient contacts is the single most important method of infection control and is of critical importance in high-risk areas. Sinks should be provided in all patient areas, as well as at all entrances to the ICU. Hands should be lathered and vigorously rubbed together for a minimum of 15 seconds under a stream of warm water. Antiseptic soaps are recommended for use before any invasive procedure. Soaps without antiseptics may be used for routine handwashing. Hand-controlled faucets should be closed with a paper towel. Foot- or knee-controlled faucets are preferable. Another method for encouraging hand disinfection is to provide aerosol cans of antiseptic foam at each patient's bedside. Gloves are an effective barrier for the prevention of infection in many cases and should be mandatory for persons handling equipment such as endotracheal tubes and foley catheters, which invade sterile spaces. However, some organisms such as respiratory syncytial virus (RSV) survive better on gloves than on hands. Furthermore, gloves are expensive and frequently considered an impediment to patient care. The donning of gloves may be impractical in urgent situations such as cardiopulmonary resuscitation.

Indirect contact transmission of infection by fomes is also a potential ICU problem. Each patient should be provided with individual equipment such as stethoscopes, blood pressure cuffs, and ventilator tubing in order to prevent cross-contamination. Vascular pressure transducers should be cleaned and disinfected or sterilized between uses. All disposable components of such apparatus should be discarded and replaced. Incubators should also be dismantled, cleaned, and disinfected or sterilized.

Personnel

Prevention of nosocomial infection should be a major concern of all hospital personnel. One aspect of infection prevention is the state of health of individual staff members. Potential participants in health care delivery should undergo pre-employment medical evaluation to assess susceptibility to common communicable diseases. Immunization history should also be determined. Staff members working in pediatric areas should be immune by virtue of having had the disease or being immunized to measles, mumps, rubella, diphtheria, pertussis, tetanus, and polio. Staff members who are susceptible to such diseases should be immunized. Pertussis immunization is not recommended for adults although nonimmunized adults are a potential source for dissemination of the infection. Postexposure chemoprophylaxis may be useful for preventing the dissemination of pertussis. The presence and activity of tuberculosis and hepatitis B should be assessed. The new vaccine for hepatitis B will be very useful for the prevention of this infection in high-risk groups.

Intercurrent illnesses such as skin infections, flu, sore throat, diarrhea, and hepatitis are infection hazards. Common cold symptoms in staff members also increase the risk of infection to patients. Personnel who develop intercurrent illness require special attention. Depending upon the diagnosis and the duties of the staff member involved, it may be necessary to exclude the person from service until the danger of transmission has passed, to restrict his or her activity, or to impose extra precautionary measures to decrease the risk to patients and other staff members.

Postexposure prophylaxis and/or therapy for communicable diseases should be individualized according to the health status of the individual, the infecting agent, and the nature of the exposure. Infectious disease and infection control practitioners should be consulted by employee health services when problems arise.

Isolation

Infection control in pediatric ICUs poses some unusual problems, because patients may be admitted to these units for care of their acute infectious diseases. In addition, patients who are especially susceptible to such common childhood diseases as varicella may be cared for in the same environment as patients who are incubating the disease. Patients should be screened by their medical history for exposure and by physical examination for signs of communicable diseases before they are admitted to the ICU. Hospital policy should be liberal with regard to institution of isolation so that the supervisory nursing staff and physicians are able to establish isolation technique for suspected contagious diseases.

Isolation procedures for some types of infection are adaptable to the ICU. Wound and skin precautions, as well as secretion and excretion precautions, can be accomplished in a ward setting. Children who have no bowel control require private rooms for stool precautions. Respiratory isolation and strict isolation can not be accomplished effectively in a ward setting; individual rooms are required. Recommendations for specific diseases that require isolation and the procedures to be used for each are available in *CDC Guideline for Isolation Precautions in Hospitals.* After a particular type of isolation has been selected, all precepts must be followed. Isolation technique requires the cooperation of all contacts of the isolated patient. Laxity on the part of physicians, nurses, housekeeping, family members, or any other contacts may defeat the careful efforts of others.

In ICUs in which neonates are cared for with older infants and children or medical and surgical patients are intermixed, it may be desirable to obtain surveillance cultures to anticipate organisms that may become pathogens and to follow patterns of antibiotic resistance. Under these circumstances, it is advisable to cohort patients who are colonized with organisms that may cause potential problems. When cultures of patients' secretions or excretions reveal Pseudomonas or methicillin-resistant *Staphylococcus aureus,* isolation of the colonized patient may prevent spread of the organism to other patients who are at risk.

NOSOCOMIAL INFECTIONS

The following material is based on data collected during 1979 from acute care hospitals that participate in the national nosocomial infection survey (NNIS). The annual incidences of pediatric and nursery services are 1.6 and 1.2 nosocomial infections per 100 discharges, respectively. Approximately 9 percent of all hospital-acquired infections occurred on pediatric and nursery services. Children younger than 1 month had the greatest risk of developing infection. The body sites that are the most commonly infected are listed in Table 17–1. Infections with secondary bacteremia occurred in 11 percent of hospital-acquired infections of children, which is double the rate found in adults.

The most common pathogens isolated from infants and children with nosocomial infections are

> *Staphylococcus aureus*
> Klebsiella tribe
> > Klebsiella
> > Enterobacter
> > Serratia
> *Escherichia coli*
> Pseudomonas species
> Candida species
> Enterococcus
> Group B streptococcus
> Bacteroides species

Several cautions should be applied to the interpretation of these data. First, a substantial portion (12 percent) of the clinically apparent infections were not cultured. Second, infections resulting from viral agents tend to go unreported; for those that are reported, specific data on viral pathogens are not usually available because of the paucity of readily available viral diagnostic methods. Thirdly, neonatal infections that may be transmitted from mothers antepartum or intrapartum are classified by NNIS definitions as nosocomial infections. Finally, virtually any organism can be responsible for nosocomial infections.

Table 17–1. Nosocomial Infection Rates*

Site	Pediatrics	Nursery
Cutaneous	28.3	45.4
Lower respiratory	21.6	11.7
Urinary tract	21.4	6.2
Primary bacteremia	17.8	12.3
Surgical wound	17.0	4.5
Upper respiratory	13.2	1.6
Gastrointestinal	5.4	3.0
Cardiovascular	5.4	3.0
Central nervous system	3.2	3.1
Intra-abdominal	1.7	1.5
Burn wound	0.6	0.1
Gynecologic	0.1	0.1
Other sites	19.3	26.6
Secondary bacteremia	11.1	7.9

*Rate per 10,000 discharges

Intravenous Cannula–Associated Infections

Infections associated with the use of IVs include purulent thrombophlebitis and cellulitis. Both of these infections may be associated with secondary bacteremia with its attendant hazards. Factors influencing a patient's risk of acquiring IV-associated infections include the patient's innate susceptibility (state of immunosuppression), the type of cannula used (plastic catheters have a greater propensity for causing infection than steel needles), the method of insertion (the cutdown technique is a greater risk than percutaneous insertion), the duration of use (the risk of infection increases after 48 to 72 hours), the fluid being infused (hyperalimentation fluid is associated with infections resulting from Candida species), and the vascular channel being used (central venous lines have comparatively high infection rates). Cannula infections are usually characterized by warm erythematous skin overlying an indurated tender vein. Control measures for the prevention of IV-related infections include

1. Using metal needles when clinically feasible. Plastic cannulas should be reserved for clinical settings in which a secure vascular access is necessary or for cannulating central vessels.

2. Careful handwashing before IV insertion. Sterile gloves should be worn for cutdowns and for cannulation of central vessels.

3. Scrubbing the IV site with antiseptic solution (tincture of iodine, 1 to 2 percent; chlorhexidine; iodophore; or 70 percent alcohol) prior to venipuncture.

4. Stabilizing the cannula at the insertion site and applying and dating a sterile dressing. Many authorities recommend the use of a topical antibiotic or an antiseptic ointment at the IV site; however, this recommendation should not be considered standard practice.

5. Evaluating the IV site daily by inspection and palpation.

6. Completely changing the IV administration sets every 24 to 48 hours. Between changes, the IV system should be kept closed as much as possible. All medications and other entries into the system should be made through injection ports after they have been wiped with alcohol or another disinfectant.

All intravascular lines should be removed when they are no longer medically necessary or when they are strongly suspected of causing sepsis. Catheter tips may be culture positive in the absence of clinical signs of infection. The semiquantitative culture method of Maki will aid in interpreting a positive culture result.

Contamination of intravascular infusate is a rare cause of IV-associated infections. However, when infection of infusate occurs, it is generally epidemic in nature. Control measures for contaminated infusate are found mainly outside the ICU and depend upon adequate manufacturing safeguards and careful compounding in hospital pharmacies. ICU staff can minimize contamination by promptly using compounded parenteral solutions. Procedures that prevent in-use contamination include inspecting fluid containers for cloudy fluid, as well as for intact seals, cracks, and leaks. IV teams that are specifically trained and dedicated to insertion and maintenance of IV lines can reduce the risk of infection.

Cutaneous Infections

Infants and children develop pustules or impetigo and tend to have greater skin breakdown at pressure points than adults. Prevention of superficial infection involves recognizing and removing reservoirs of infecting organisms by bathing the patient daily and interrupting person-to-person transmission. In the event that a cluster of skin infections occur (usually resulting from staphylococci), it may be necessary to review infection control procedures, institute wound and skin precautions, establish contaminated and clean cohorts, and consider personal and environmental surveillance.

Respiratory Infections

Upper respiratory infections (URI) are erroneously regarded as innocuous, and, usually, either inadequate control measures or none at all are introduced. URIs are a true threat to hospitalized children because of the frequency of endemic URIs in the younger age group. In infants, URIs may progress to croup, bronchiolitis, and pneumonia. Viral respiratory pathogens are especially hazardous for patients with cyanotic congenital heart disease. RSV, adenoviruses, influenza A, parainfluenza viruses, and others have been associated with hospital outbreaks. Contact spread is most commonly responsible for respiratory cross infection. Airborne spread is possible but less likely.

Lower respiratory infections occur most often in patients who are already critically ill. The usual manifestations of nosocomial pneumonia include fever, changes in volume and consistency of secretions, increasing respiratory distress, and increasing ventilator requirements. Supporting laboratory data include a new infiltrate on chest roentgenogram and leukocytosis.

Normal children have a variety of mechanisms that prevent pulmonary infection: glottic closure to prevent aspiration of foreign material, cough reflex to expel any material that may pass the glottis, mucociliary clearance, and the cellular responses of pulmonary phagocytes. Many insults resulting from disease or therapeutic intervention, such as endotracheal intubation, anesthesia, intoxication with depressants, seizure disorders, and local irritants act to subvert these host defense mechanisms.

Airborne spread of infection may be important for some viral agents, Coxsackie viruses, and possibly adenoviruses; however, person-to-person transmission is important in the transmission of other viruses such as RSV, which does not survive in droplets. Transmission by direct contacts is promoted by the need for frequent airway manipulation of ill patients, which increases the likelihood of transmission of pathogens from the hands of staff members. Prolonged hospitalization, intubation, tracheostomy, and respiratory therapy in general are all strong forces that alter oropharyngeal flora. Contamination of nebulizers and ventilator surfaces, both internal and external, may serve as environmental sources of organisms.

Control measures for the prevention of infections associated with respiratory equipment include

1. Filling fluid reservoirs immediately prior to use. Reservoirs should be completely emptied prior to refilling while in use.

2. Draining the condensation in the tubing to the exterior. Retrograde flow into the patient or retrograde flow that may contaminate the reservoir should not be allowed.

3. Changing the nebulizer every 24 hours. Equipment that has been used should be replaced with disinfected or sterilized equipment.

4. Avoiding use of humidifiers that create droplets.

5. Cleaning reservoirs and oxygen outlets daily. Reservoirs should be rinsed and dried before being reused on the same patient.

6. Replacing all tubing between patient usage.

7. Changing all breathing circuits between patients and every 24 to 48 hours on the same patient.

Nebulizers aerosolize droplets of water for delivery to the alveoli and result in increased risk of infection. Ventilation–humidification systems without nebulizers have not been associated with outbreaks of pneumonia. Fluids used in respiratory equipment should be sterile and should be dispensed aseptically. Unused fluid from open containers should be discarded after 24 hours. Disposable equipment should not be reused. Reusable equipment should be thoroughly cleaned and subsequently disinfected or sterilized. Internal surfaces of ventilators should be cleaned according to the manufacturer's instructions. Tracheostomy care and patient suctioning should be accomplished using sterile supplies, aseptic technique, and a "no touch" approach to the patient. (After the tracheostomy wound has healed, a "no touch" technique is no longer necessary).

Urinary Tract Infections

Urinary tract infections (UTI) are usually preventable by adherence to strict indications for urinary tract instrumentation, stringent aseptic technique, and careful maintenance of closed urinary drainage systems. Pathogens responsible for infection (Enterobacteriaceae, enterococci, Pseudomonas species, staphylococci, and yeasts), either from a patient's indigenous flora or from hospital flora transmitted to patients, gain access to the urinary tract by 1) inadequate preparations of the periurethral area or skin, 2) contamination of catheters as a result of poor technique, 3) contamination of catheters when disconnecting the drainage tube, 4) retrograde flow of urine from bag and tube to patient, 5) occasional bowel perforation during suprapubic aspiration, and 6) secondary invasion of the kidney in bacteremic patients. Urethral and bladder mucosal erosions secondary to catheter trauma create an easy portal of entry into the systemic circulation for organisms. Many attempts have been made to prevent UTIs by giving prophylactic antibiotics or impregnating catheters with antibiotics. Only closed drainage systems and continuous catheter irrigation have proved to be effective. Closed drainage is considered superior to continuous irrigation. Criteria for effective maintenance of closed drainage systems include

1. Ensuring that the catheter junction and drainage tube remain closed.

2. Draining urine bags at 8-hour intervals, without contaminating the waste spigot.

3. Ensuring that bags are never raised to a position in which backflow of urine may occur.

4. Avoiding obstructions to urine flow in the tubing.

5. Keeping the urine bag off the floor.

Gastrointestinal Infections

Diarrhea and vomiting are the most common manifestations of gastrointestinal infections and occur frequently in pediatric patients. Water and food-borne outbreaks of illness occur, but the most common method of transmission is contact via the fecal–oral route. Pathogens associated with nosocomial pediatric gastrointestinal infections are listed in Table 17–2. The use of antibiotics may be associated with selection, perpetuation, and dissemination of bacterial pathogens and have been implicated in the pathophysiology of staphylococcal enterocolitis and pseudomembranous colitis. Neonatal necrotizing enterocolitis has also been associated with both viral and bacterial agents.

All patients with diarrhea should immediately be managed with stool precautions and should undergo appropriate diagnostic testing to establish the etiology of the symptom.

Surgical Infections

Surgical wound infections are an important source of morbidity and mortality. The most important factor influencing the rate of wound infection is the type of surgery. Procedures without transection of a viscus or mucosal surface or surgery in which no inflammation is encountered are much less likely to become infected than those operations in which a viscus is transected or gross contamination of a wound occurs. Other important factors chiefly under the influence of the surgeon include the length of the procedure and surgical technique. Rough treatment of tissue, residual foreign material, inadequate débridement, and incomplete closure of dead spaces are associated with increased risk of infection. Many of these factors are within the control of the surgeon. Most surgical infections are caused by the patient's own flora and are introduced at the time of surgery.

Most wound infections occur between 3 and 7 days postoperatively. Administration of antibiotics may delay the appearance of infection or alter the character of the infecting organisms. On newborn and pediatric services, Enterobacteriaceae, *Staphylococcus aureus,* and Pseudomonas species account for most infections. Streptococci groups A and B, Bacteroides species, Clostridia species, and many other organisms are occasionally isolated. Prophylactic administration of antimicrobial agents has reduced the infectious complications of specific surgical procedures; however, no controlled clinical trials have been performed for many of the procedures for which antibiotics are routinely prescribed. The decision to use antibiotic prophylaxis must take into account the risks of adverse drug reactions and the emergence of drug-resistant organisms.

If possible, surgical procedures should be carried out in specifically designed operating rooms. Because the morbidity of children, particularly neonates, is reduced by the presence of personnel who are trained to care for them and because transportation of critically ill infants to cold operating rooms are factors that increase morbidity and mortality, surgical procedures are occasionally performed in ICUs. Relatively major surgical procedures such as placement of a peritoneal catheter and ligation of a patent ductus arteriosis may be performed in ICUs. In these situations, sterile technique must be implemented with extreme care. A large area of the ICU that has no cross traffic should be set aside and equipped with all implements necessary to complete the operative procedures without contaminating either the patient or the environment.

Table 17–2. Agents Associated with Nosocomial Gastroenteritis

Bacterial
  Salmonella
  Shigella
  Escherichia coli
  Yersinia enterocolitica
  Staphylococcus aureus
  Clostridium difficile
Viral
  Hepatitis A
  Hepatitis B
  Enteroviruses
  Rheovirus-like agents
  Adenovirus
Parasitic
  Entamoeba histolytica

SUGGESTED READING

Bennett, J.V., and Brachman, P.S. (eds.): Hospital Infections, Boston, Little, Brown and Co., 1979.

Centers for Disease Control: Guidelines for the prevention and control of nosocomial pneumonia. Infect. Control 3:327, 1982.

Centers for Disease Control: National Nosocomial Infections Study Report, Annual Summary 1979. March, 1982.

Garner, S.J. and Simmons, B.P.: Guideline for isolation precautions in hospitals. Infect. Control 4 (Suppl):245, 1983.

Infection Control in the Hospital, Chicago, American Hospital Association, 1970.

TWO

SYSTEM–SPECIFIC PROBLEMS
Cardiocirculatory

Dysrhythmias in Children

DELORES DANILOWICZ, M.D.

Dysrhythmias in the pediatric age group were initially a minor problem, with a few infants presenting with paroxysmal supraventricular tachycardia and some children who had carditis presenting with atrial and/or ventricular ectopic beats. However, in the past few years, partly resulting from an increase in and partly resulting from better monitoring techniques, more children are being seen and treated for dysrhythmias. Many of these children are being seen secondary to surgical repair of underlying organic heart disease, either congenital or acquired. Some of these postoperative patients have introduced syndromes, such as the sick sinus, an almost exclusively adult problem, into the pediatric population.

Although many dysrhythmias do not present as an emergency situation, there are a few that do, including supraventricular tachycardia (paroxysmal atrial or junctional tachycardia, atrial flutter, and rarely, atrial fibrillation), ventricular tachycardia (often preceded by multifocal ventricular premature beats or as part of a cardiac arrest), and severe bradycardia (sinus or heart block). These dysrhythmias require rapid treatment or even immediate electrical cardioversion.

ETIOLOGY AND PHYSIOLOGY

To briefly review the conduction system, normal activation starts at the sinus node, which has the highest rate of automaticity. In descending order of automaticity are the atrial fibers, atrioventricular (AV) node, the bundle of His, and the ventricular Purkinje system. All portions of the cardiac conduction system, as well as the myocardial fibers, can act as pacemakers if the fibers above them fail or if block occurs. If irritation occurs at any level, tachycardia can result. Changes in threshold, length of refractory period, and chronotropy can be caused by systemic disease, electrolyte abnormality, drug ingestion, trauma, and so on. There are many causes of dysrhythmias, including

Organic heart disease, congenital or acquired
Myocarditis: infective or toxic
Cardiomyopathy
Hyperthyroidism
Pheochromocytoma
Accessory pathways
Post–open-heart surgery
Head trauma, increased intracranial pressure (ICP)

Trauma to chest or heart

Tumors: primary cardiac or metastatic

Infections

Invasive procedures: lines, cardiac catheter-ization, general anesthesia

Hypo- or hyperthermia

Drugs (digoxin, diuretics, tricyclic antide-pressants, stimulants)

Metabolic abnormalities (acidosis, hypoxia)

Electrolyte abnormalities (high or low po-tassium)

Familial conduction defects (QT prolonga-tion)

Anorexia nervosa

Emotional distress

Shock

Congestive heart failure (CHF)

Myocardial ischemia

Collagen diseases

Idiopathic

In addition to dysrhythmias that occur as direct effects on the conduction system or myo-cardial fibers are those produced if the blood supply to the nodes is damaged by disease or operation. The sinus node receives its blood supply from the right coronary artery in 55 percent of the population and from the left circumflex in 45 percent of the population. The AV node receives its blood supply mainly (90 percent) from the right coronary artery. In ad-dition to the normal conduction pathways, there can also be accessory pathways, which are often seen in infants younger than 6 months of age. However, these accessory pathways probably play no role in cardiac conduction. The accessory fibers may by-pass the AV node, originating in either the right or left atrium. Their importance lies in the fact that these pathways may precipitate a supraventricular tachycardia. Some accessory pathways make their presence known by changes on the scal-ar electrocardiogram (e.g., Wolff-Parkinson-White syndrome with a short P-R interval, delta wave, and prolonged QRS interval), but others may be found only by extensive and sophisticated electrophysiologic studies.

In normal older children and adults, the heart rate varies from 60 to 100 beats per minute. In newborn infants and younger children, the sinus rate is higher. Sinus arrhythmia is rare in newborns but becomes more common as the heart rate slows with age. Wandering pace-maker may also occur as a normal variant, with a change in the P-wave axis seen in the same lead. It may occur totally at an atrial rate (sinus node to coronary sinus area) or as atrial/junc-tional foci in individuals who have slower heart rates (e.g., athletes).

TYPES OF DYSRHYTHMIAS

Many of the following rhythm disturbances do not require emergency treatment; those that often *do* require emergency treatment are *des-ignated by an asterisk* and are discussed in more detail in the next section.

Sinus Tachycardia

With this condition, the heart rate is above normal for one's age but the P-wave axis is normal, with 1:1 conduction. Mild variation in rate may be seen or brought out by vagal maneuvers. It is usually a result of some un-derlying cause, often not cardiac (e.g., fever, hyperthyroidism), and treatment of the under-lying cause is the treatment of choice. Car-dioversion is obviously contraindicated, and specific cardiac drugs are rarely necessary. The exception might be the use of propranolol in a thyroid storm (See Chapter 34, Hyperthyroid-ism).

Sinus Bradycardia

The heart rate in sinus bradycardia is below normal for one's age but, again, the P-wave axis is normal, with 1:1 conduction. This is a normal occurrence in athletes and can result with any increase in vagal tone. Damage to the sinus node, increased intracranial pressure, and hypothermia are other causes. Drugs (propran-olol, digitalis) and electrolyte changes (in-creased potassium) may also be implicated. Again, treatment is ideally directed at the un-derlying cause. However, if the patient is symptomatic, the use of atropine is usually ef-fective. Pacing or stimulant drugs to the myo-cardium are rarely indicated.

Block

First Degree: A prolonged P-R interval is present with first-degree block, but with 1:1 conduction. No cardiac treatment is needed.

Second Degree: Variable block can be seen in both Mobitz type I or II, but the ventricular rate rarely is so slow as to require pacing or treatment. Again, atropine may be quite effec-tive.

Third Degree: There is no relation between the atrial P waves and the QRS complexes. The block may be high with a narrow QRS interval (junctional rate of 40 to 60 beats/minute) or low with a widened QRS interval (ventricular rate of under 40 beats/minute). Although the patient may be asymptomatic at rest, congestive failure and/or Adams-Stokes attacks often occur. Unless the cause of the block is thought to be reversible (recent myocardial infarction, elevated potassium, digoxin toxicity), a permanent pacemaker is the ultimate treatment.

Sick Sinus Syndrome

This condition has a variation in heart rate from sinus arrest/sinus bradycardia to tachycardias (with or without block). Symptoms may occur from either the bradycardia or the tachycardia, and it is often difficult to determine the choice of medical treatment. Treatment may need to be as radical as surgical ablation of the AV node, with placement of a permanent pacemaker. This is a rare condition in the pediatric age group and, when seen, it is often after Mustard repair for transposition of the great vessels or after repair of complex anomalous venous return.

*Supraventricular Tachycardias

Paroxysmal Atrial/Junctional Tachycardias

This is the most common dysrhythmia in children, with occurrence of 1 per 25,000. Approximately 5 percent of these cases have underlying heart disease. The heart rate is usually over 200 beats per minute, absolutely regular, and may break to normal sinus rhythm with an increase in vagal tone. Although supraventricular tachycardias often have narrow QRS complexes, aberrancy can occur with the QRS widened, suggesting a ventricular tachycardia. However, ventricular tachycardia is usually not as fast and shows some degree of irregularity.

Atrial Flutter

Atrial flutter is not as common in the pediatric age group but has been described, even in utero. The heart rate is often above 250 beats per minute if 1:1 conduction occurs; however, block is a common occurrence. Identification of the typical saw-tooth P waves (no isoelectric period between the P waves) can often be effected by increasing the degree of block by increasing vagal tone.

Atrial Fibrillation

This is the least common supraventricular tachycardia seen in children and has an atrial rate of over 300 beats per minute (random atrial baseline). Variable block occurs, but often, drugs are needed to slow the ventricular response rate.

*Ventricular Tachycardia

With ventricular tachycardia, the QRS complexes are always widened and the rate is rarely over 150 beats per minute. Mild variation in rate is seen, and it does not respond in any way to vagal maneuvers. Ventricular tachycardia may be triggered by a variety of etiologies resulting in myocardial irritability; multifocal or malignant ventricular premature contractions may precede the tachycardia and deterioration to ventricular fibrillation often occurs.

Premature Ectopic Depolarizations

Premature beats that are supraventricular are rarely dangerous in and of themselves. They may, however, lead to paroxysmal atrial tachycardia, especially if accessory pathways are present. With premature ventricular beats, one must distinguish between the benign and malignant groups (Table 18–1). In the case of malignant ventricular ectopic beats, treatment is indicated and may prevent the occurrence of ventricular tachycardia and sudden death. In the pediatric age group, this condition is being seen more often after complex open-heart surgery.

TREATMENT

Table 18–2 lists drugs, effects, dose ranges, toxicity, and the dysrhythmias most responsive

Table 18–1. Evaluation of Premature Ventricular Contractions

Benign	Malignant
No underlying heart disease	Heart disease
Fixed–coupling interval	Variable–coupling interval (parasystole)
Unifocal	Multifocal
Decreased or suppressed by exercise	Increased by exercise
Normal resting Q-T interval	Prolonged Q-T interval
No R-on-T phenomenon	R-on-T phenomenon

Table 18–2. Drugs Used in Dysrhythmias

Drug	Best Used For	EKG Changes	Cardiac Changes	Toxicity	Dose
Digoxin*	SVT, CHF	↑P-R ↓Q-T	↑BP ↑CO	Ectopics, SVT, VT, block / Vomiting / Vision disturbances	Varies with age / 0.02–0.04 mg/kg TDD IV / Increase 10–15% for p.o. / 0.001–0.0015 mg/kg/day-MDD
Quinidine†	VPC, VT APC, NPC, NT	↑QRS ↑Q-T	↓BP, CO ↑LVed	Asystole; neurologic and GI side effects. / Thrombocytopenia	15–60 mg/kg/day p.o.
Procainamide (Pronestyl)	same as quinidine	same as quinidine	same as quinidine	Asystole / Neurologic and GI side effects / Lupus-like syndrome	15–50 mg/kg/day p.o. / 3–6 mg/kg IV over 5 min.
Lidocaine (Xylocaine)	VT, VPC Dig. Tox. rhythms	↑QRS	↓BP, CO	Block, asystole, deafness, seizures, coma / Respiratory failure	1 mg/kg IV over 5 min.
Diphenyl hydantoin (Dilantin)	VT, VPC Dig. Tox. rhythms	↑QRS	↓BP ±→CO	Asystole / Gingival changes / Neurologic and GI side effects	2–5 mg/kg/day p.o. / 2–5 mg/kg IV over 5 min.
Propranolol (Inderal)	SVT Dig. Tox. rhythms	↓Q-T	↓BP, CO ↑LVed	Sinus arrest, asystole / Bronchospasm / Hypoglycemia	0.2–4 mg/kg/day p.o. / 10–20 ug/kg IV over 10 min.
Verapamil	SVT, esp. re-entry Dig. Tox. rhythms	↑P-R	↓BP, CO ↑LVed	Block / Variable CHF	40–80 mg/kg/day p.o. / 75–150 ug/kg IV over 5 min. (maximum 250)
Methoxamine (Vasoxyl)	SVT, esp. PAT	—	↑SVR, BP	Hypertension / Nausea, headache	0.1 mg/kg IV-titrate to BP
Edraphonium (Tensilon)	SVT, esp. PAT, AFl	—	minimal	Asystole	0.1 mg/kg IV given quickly as push; repeat in 2 min. if not effective
Atropine	SB, NB 2°HB	↓Q-T	minimal	Tachycardias / Bronchospasm	0.01 mg/kg s.c. IV child max. 0.4 mg adult max. 1.0 mg
Isoproterenol (Isuprel)	CHB or SB not responsive to atropine	↓Q-T ↓P-R	↑CO ↑PBF	VPC, SVT, VT, VF	5–10 mg/dose sublingual q 6–8 hr / 0.05–0.1 ug/kg/min-titrate to HR and ectopics

*Digoxin levels can decrease when quinidine or verapamil is added to the drug regimen.
†Hypersensitivity to quinidine can occur; a homeostatic dose should be given first, preferably in an office or hospital setting.
(AFl: atrial flutter; APC: atrial premature contraction; BP: blood pressure; CHB: complete heart block; CHF: congestive heart failure; CO: cardiac output; Dig. Tox.: digoxin toxicity; GI: gastrointestinal; HR: heart rate; IV: intravenous; LVed: left ventricular end diastolic pressure; max: maximum; MDD: maintenance digoxin dose; NB: nodal bradycardia; NPC: nodal premature contraction; NT: nodal tachycardia; PAT: paroxysmal atrial tachycardia; PBF: pulmonary blood flow; p.o.: by mouth; SB: sinus bradycardia; s.c.: subcutaneously; SVR: systemic vascular resistance; SVT: supraventricular tachycardia; 2°HB: second degree heart block; TDD: total digitalizing dose; VF: ventricular fibrillation; VPC: ventricular premature contraction; VT: ventricular tachycardia)

to each drug. In general, tachycardias can be treated by increasing the block at the AV node (digoxin) or by decreasing the irritability of the abnormal focus (propranolol, procainamide, or quinidine). Both types of drugs may be effective in interrupting accessory pathway conduction.

If the patient with tachycardia is very symptomatic or in critical condition, electrical cardioversion may be the initial treatment of choice. If electrical cardioversion is effective in restoring a more normal rhythm, there will be more time for evaluating and treating the patient. In the pediatric patient, a maximum of 2 to 3 watt-seconds per kg should be used, starting with 1 watt-second per kg, when possible. Higher doses are not more effective and may damage the chest wall and the myocardium. A loading dose of a negative inotropic drug (e.g., lidocaine or Inderal) is given just before the cardioversion. If the tachycardia recurs, additional drug management is required. If there is any chance that the tachycardia is a result of digoxin toxicity, the use of diphenylhydantoin as the loading agent is indicated. One must remember that cardioversion of a patient with digoxin toxicity may result in ventricular tachycardia or fibrillation. If fibrillation occurs, the cardioversion mode must be switched to defibrillate or the machine will not deliver a shock, having no complex from which to trigger. On the other hand, one does not wish to defibrillate a supraventricular tachycardia, because the shock may occur on the T wave and cause ventricular tachycardia or fibrillation. With supraventricular tachycardias, the cardioversion mode is used so the machine can deliver the shock on the QRS complex. Intravenous sedation is used as needed before the shock. If electrical cardioversion is not effective, it is important to check parameters that might be responsible such as hypoxia, acidosis, or abnormal electrolytes. Restoration to as near a normal condition as possible will make cardioversion more likely.

If the patient with a tachycardia is relatively stable, cardioversion can be posponed and further evaluation of the patient can be made. Identification of P waves from the standard electrocardiogram is often impossible. Special leads, especially an esophageal electrode hooked up to the C channel of the electrocardiogram machine, can be used to record P wave activity and to note its relationship to the QRS complexes. Saw-tooth flutter waves would diagnose atrial flutter; abnormal P wave axis would suggest an atrial or junctional focus for the tachycardia; random activity at over 300 beats per minute would confirm atrial fibrillation. The relationship of the P wave to the QRS response would establish whether 1:1 conduction exists or would reveal the presence of block. Increasing vagal tone can be a helpful diagnostic maneuver. Carotid massage, diving reflex, Tensilon, or methoxamine may be used. If paroxysmal atrial/junctional tachycardia is present, a break to normal sinus rhythm may occur (and may be therapeutic if it persists). The increase in block will allow one to see sawtooth flutter waves, whereas atrial fibrillation often shows no response or a minimal slowing during the vagal maneuver. After one has been convinced that a supraventricular tachycardia is present, treatment can be instituted. Intravenous propranolol or verapamil is often effective in breaking the tachycardia, and either of these drugs can then be used orally for chronic treatment. Although digoxin has been implicated in causing paroxysmal atrial tachycardia/ventricular tachycardia in adult patients with some forms of accessory pathways, this has not been an impressive feature in children.

Many pediatric cardiologists still use digoxin as the drug of choice in supraventricular tachycardias. The increase in block at the AV node usually reduces the ventricular rate and may allow cardioversion to normal sinus rhythm. In other cases, the additional use of procainamide or quinidine may be needed to effect cardioversion. If multiple drug therapy (with established therapeutic blood levels) is unsuccessful in restoring normal sinus rhythm, electrical cardioversion should be considered. If, however, it is believed that the tachycardia is a result of an acute process, cardioversion may be postponed to a later time if the patient can tolerate the dysrhythmia. Chronic cardiac conditions with long-standing dysrhythmias will rarely remain in normal sinus rhythm, even if they convert initially. Repeated recurrences of supraventricular tachycardias with symptoms may necessitate electrophysiologic studies to localize the irritable focus or the abnormal pathway. Multiple drug studies can be performed to assess effects. In some selective instances, surgical ablation of accessory pathways will be successful in preventing recurrences. If a patient with atrial flutter is already in some degree of block, one must be careful not to initially use medications that might slow the abnormal focus but allow a 1:1 conduction, thereby increasing the ventricular rate. In this instance, the patient would probably do better if he were initially treated with digoxin to maintain or increase the block. Only after therapeutic levels of digoxin are present should additional medications be used.

If the rhythm is determined to be ventricular tachycardia, it is more likely that the patient will be symptomatic, although some infants may do well for days. Electrical cardioversion is usually the treatment of choice and is performed following administration of lidocaine. If lidocaine converts the dysrhythmia to normal sinus rhythm, the drug can continue to be used as a titrated drip to control any ectopic beats or any further runs of ventricular tachycardia. If digoxin toxicity is suspected, dilantin should also be used. Chronic treatment will depend upon the response of the patient and the underlying cause for the tachycardia. Dilantin and propranolol are more effective agents for control of premature ventricular contractions in the pediatric age group than in adults and are often used first. If these are not effective, procainamide or quinidine is given. Additional, newer antidysrhythmic drugs are being used successfully in adults and will eventually be used in pediatric patients.

If bradycardia occurs and the patient becomes symptomatic, raising the heart rate with a drug that has the least number of side effects is the treatment of choice. Whenever the QRS is narrow or P-wave conduction can be identified, atropine is the drug of choice. In some instances, a widened QRS complex may occur, although the focus of origin is supraventricular (aberrancy). In this circumstance, a trial of atropine is worthwhile. A true slow ventricular rate, however, will not respond. If the rate is ventricular, direct stimulation with drugs such as Isuprel or epinephrine is suggested. The catheter used for infusion of these drugs should not be used for any other intravenous solution, because inadvertent flushing could deliver a fatal bolus of the drug. If the condition causing the bradycardia or block is presumed to be reversible, the placement of a temporary demand pacemaker offers a safer alternative to the prolonged intravenous infusion of potentially lethal drugs. A permanent pacemaker may later be needed if conduction does not return. In the case of block and/or recurrent ventricular irritability as a result of digoxin toxicity, a possible treatment, when all else fails, is the use of digoxin-specific antibodies.

CASE PRESENTATION 1

A 2-year-old boy is seen in the emergency room with a heart rate of 60 beats per minute. The mother states that she has never been told that he had heart disease and that the child has not been ill recently. This afternoon, while the child was walking with her, he fell to the ground and lost consciousness for a few seconds. There was no seizure activity and no postictal state. He has appeared normal since, but the mother carried him to the emergency room.

Examination

Examination reveals a normal 2-year-old white boy in no distress: heart rate (HR) = 52 beats/min, irregular; respiratory rate (RR) = 20 breaths/min, BP = 98/60 mm Hg. An electrocardiogram strip shows complete heart block with narrow QRS complexes and occasional premature ventricular contractions.

Assessment

Loss of consciousness associated with heart rate that is slow for his age.

Consider

Complete congenital heart block, which has manifested itself for the first time at this age with an Adams-Stokes attack. This can occur as an isolated finding (mother with lupus) or with associated heart disease (corrected transposition of the great vessels).

Complete heart block (acquired).
Seizure activity.
Breath-holding.
Hyperventilation.

Results of physical examination are normal except for slow irregular heart rate.

The history given by the mother is also not contributory; one must get more detailed information about the child's activity earlier that day and the immediate period preceding his loss of consciousness.

Electrocardiogram shows complete heart block with narrow QRS complexes and intermittent ventricular premature contractions (VPCs). Atrial rate is normal at 110 beats/per minute. Ventricular rate is 58/minute. Ectopic beats have widened QRS, with inverted T wave, and all have the same configuration in lead II. There is one ectopic for every two narrow QRS complexes. The coupling interval from the narrow QRS complex to the ectopic is not the same.

Consider

Complete heart block.
—narrow QRS complexes, so block is high with junctional rate.
—VPCs appear unifocal by configuration but do not have a fixed coupling interval, raising the possibility of parasystole (see Table 18–2).

Causes for complete heart block
1. Congenital with or without heart disease
2. Status/post open heart surgery
3. Coronary artery disease (Kawasaki's in children)
4. Myocarditis, myopathy—infectious, toxic
5. Hyperkalemia
6. Drug ingestion—digoxin, tricyclic antidepressants
7. Cardiac tumors—primary or metastatic
8. Collagen diseases
9. Trauma—head, heart

Causes for VPCs
1. Myocardial ischemia (CHF, coronary artery disease, myopathy)
2. Drugs
3. Electrolyte abnormalities (hypokalemia)
4. Mitral valve prolapse; status/post open heart surgery
5. Active myocarditis—(ARF) acute rheumatic fever, viral; (RHD) rheumatic heart disease
6. Accessory pathways
7. Tumors: primary cardiac or metastatic
8. Cardiac trauma
9. Hyperthyroidism
10. Pheochromocytoma
11. Hypoxia, acidosis
12. Pulmonary disease; cor pulmonale
13. Escape beats with complete heart block (not really ectopic)

Work-up
BUN, electrolytes, urinalysis; ESR (erythrocyte sedimentation rate)—all normal

Full EKG: within normal limits except for the rhythm described

Chest x-ray: cardiothoracic ratio (CTR) = 52%; normal lungs

Echo: Mild dilatation of left atrium and ventricle; otherwise normal except for heart block and ectopics

In ICU with IV in place; NPO; on monitor

At bedside: Emergency pacemaker tray.
Notify cardiology.
Lidocaine bolus (1 mg/kg) and lidocaine drip

While work-up is progressing, the patient's grandmother appears at the hospital and states that she had just gone to take her digitoxin tablet and found most of them gone from the container in her pocketbook. The boy had been with her from 9:00 to 11:00 A.M. that day. Since that time, he had lunch with his mother and lost consciousness at 1:00 P.M. It is now 3:00 P.M.

Consider

Diagnosis most likely is digitalis toxicity.

Send blood for digoxin level.

Give dilantin, 3–5 mg/kg as a slow IV push.

Maintain normal IV replacement solution and follow electrolytes.

Continue careful monitoring.

If any distress, check arterial blood gas.

Emesis and stomach lavage are not indicated because of the time lapse and meal in between.

Digoxin level comes back at 6 ng %, and during this time, the ectopic beats are occurring more frequently, now bigeminal, with overall heart rate about the same and BP still normal. In addition, on one EKG strip, two types of VPCs are seen.

Consider

Dialysis does not work for digoxin toxicity.

Continue dilantin; give lidocaine as IV drip to titrate against the VPCs; monitor BP carefully.

Cardioversion setup near at hand and functional.

Monitor serum K+ carefully.

Call nearest center and arrange to have digoxin-specific antibodies sent as soon as possible.

Remember that digitoxin preparations take much longer to clear (longer half-life) than digoxin.

Child remains stable on IV lidocaine with less VPCs; next digoxin level (2 hr after first) is 8 ng %; potassium, which was 4.2 and 4.0, is now 6.1. Digoxin-specific antibodies have arrived.

Consider

Use of digoxin-specific antibodies. Get informed consent from parents and test child for hypersensitivity.

As the previous step is being carried out, the child's HR slows to 38 beats/min with all complexes now wide. BP is 70/40, and the child becomes very anxious, passes out.

Consider

Give digoxin-specific antibodies. If BP and respiration are not maintained, start CPR. Notify cardiology for pacemaker if an elective pacemaker was not placed earlier.

Following the use of digoxin-specific antibodies, the potassium decreased to 4.0 and the digoxin level fell to 4 within the next few hours. This was accompanied by a return to sinus rhythm, with a HR of 90 beats/min.

Consider

Continued monitoring and treatment as needed until levels of digoxin are under toxic range. This may take a week or longer.

CASE PRESENTATION 2

A 4-month-old girl was brought to the pediatrician's office by her mother because of lethargy and poor feeding for 2 days. There has been no recent illness and the baby has no acute infection. She has not vomited and does not have diarrhea, and the mother has never been told of any cardiac problem. Early growth and development have been normal, and the pediatrician had never heard a murmur.

Examination

Examination reveals a tic-tac rhythm of the heart, too fast to count but over 220 beats per minute. RR = 50 breaths/min, with moderate retractions. The child's color is pale, and her extremities are cold. Pulses are barely palpable and BP is not obtainable by cuff. The liver is down 3 cm below the right costal margin, and diffuse rales are present over both lung fields. No edema is seen. An electrocardiogram strip shows a regular tachycardia of 280/minute with narrow QRS complexes. P waves cannot be seen.

Rapid heart rate with evidence of CHF and near shock.

Consider

Rapid heart rate is most likely the cause of the failure/shock.

Rate of over 200 beats/min makes ventricular tachycardia less likely.

Supraventricular tachycardias (SVT) include paroxysmal atrial tachycardia (PAT), atrial flutter, atrial fibrillation, and sinus tachycardia.

Admit child to ICU; place on monitor, with IV in place.

Results of physical examination are no different on unit than in the pediatrician's office. The child is tachycardic, dyspneic, pale and cool, cyanotic. BP by doppler is 50/30 mm Hg.

No further positive history is obtained from the mother or the pediatrician.

Electrocardiogram shows a regular tachycardia of 280/min with narrow QRS complexes. No P waves can be identified on the routine EKG. The remainder of the EKG appears normal for age.

Consider

Arterial blood gases (ABG). (SVT) supraventricular tachycardia present, most likely PAT.

Be sure that cardioversion machine is near and functional.

BUN; electrolytes, CBC.

Consider use of special esophageal electrode and/or the use of vagal maneuvers.

Bloods are drawn; chest x-ray is taken and reveals venous congestion of the lungs, cardiothoracic ratio (CTR) of 60%, generalized cardiomegaly. Echocardiogram is done but is not particularly helpful at a HR of 280; structures all appear to be present, with normal continuity. Esophageal lead cannot be found; cardiologist thinks the baby is too ill to wait around for this. Carotid massage is then done, no change occurs. A cold towel is placed over the baby's face; no response is noted. At this time, the ABG is phoned in. Results show a pH of 7.20, PCO_2 of 40, and PO_2 of 40.

Consider

Cardioversion after giving at least 1 mg/kg of bicarbonate; face mask oxygen.

IV dose of Tensilon can be given while cardioverter is being set up; also IV dose of Inderal or verapamil may be tried.

IV dose of Tensilon is given, and the baby's heart rate suddenly drops to 150 beats/minute. With this, the baby's BP is now reading 90/64 mm Hg. Cardioversion is postponed, and the oxygen is continued. Another ABG is sent. The results show a pH of 7.32, PCO_2 of 38, and PO_2 of 220.

Differential for PAT

1. Underlying heart disease
2. Infection: systemic, myocarditis
3. Electrolyte abnormalities (low potassium)
4. Metabolic abnormalities (hypoxia, acidosis)
5. Drugs: cardiac (through mother if breast-fed; stimulants, tofranil, elavil, digoxin)
6. Accessory pathways
7. Pheochromocytoma
8. Cardiac tumors
9. Trauma to chest, heart

While the differential is being considered and decisions are being made about the work-up and treatment, a repeat echocardiogram is done, with the child at a HR of 150. This is entirely normal for age with no evidence of underlying heart disease. Contractility is good. The baby is more alert and responsive; RR is down to 30 with minimal retractions, and the lungs are clear. BUN, electrolytes, CBC, and urinalysis are all normal. A repeat EKG shows flattened to slightly inverted T waves in leads avF, V4–6. Otherwise, it is normal for age. As a repeat chest x-ray is being taken, the nurse notifies you that the heart rate is back to 280 beats/minute. Another dose of Tensilon is given, with immediate break to 150.

Consider

Must use additional medication to keep the baby in normal sinus rhythm (NSR).

No obvious evidence from EKG or the changes in rhythm of accessory pathways.

Echo has ruled out heart disease.

EKG changes may reflect some residual ischemia due to the PAT; should be repeated after the child has been in NSR for several hours.

Draw bloods for thyroid screen.

Send urines for pheochromocytoma screen.

Mother denies use of any drugs. The baby is exclusively breast-fed.

The cardiologist elects to place the baby on digoxin, and this medication is given; 1/2 total digitalizing dose (TDD) stat and 1/4 q 6 hours intramuscularly. During this time, the baby goes in and out of tachycardia many times but converts back before Tensilon is given. By 12 hours after admission, there are only very short runs of PAT, lasting 6 to 8 beats, with most of the time spent in NSR. She is then placed on maintenance digoxin, p.o., observed in the ICU for another day with minimal dysrhythmias. She is then discharged to the ward, and two 24-hour Holter tapes are done. These show a rare short run of PAT occurring 2 to 3 times per day. During one of the breaks from PAT to NSR, three complexes with a short P-R interval are seen. All blood and urine tests are negative. Repeat EKG is normal. Repeat chest x-ray is normal.

Consider

Discharge on maintenance digoxin, with rise in dose to keep up with weight gain over at least the next 9 to 12 months.

Possibility of accessory pathway has been raised; if present, recurrent PAT may be a problem in the future and may not be able to be controlled with digoxin alone.

Careful follow-up should be maintained, with any prolonged tachycardia being seen in the emergency room.

If no recurrence in 1 year, consider stopping the digoxin and repeating two or three Holter tapes.

Child was followed for 1 year with no documented recurrences and with nothing on repeated EKGs suggestive of accessory pathways. Digoxin is stopped; Holter monitor reveals no dysrhythmias. The mother is advised that everything appears well and that recurrence is unlikely but still may occur.

SUGGESTED READING

Biller, J.A., and Yeager, A.M. (eds.): Harriet Lane Handbook, 9th ed. Chicago, Year Book Medical Publishers, Inc. 1981, pp. 111–198.

Doherty, J.E., Staub, K.D., Murphy, M.L., et al.: Digoxin–quinidine interaction. Am. J. Cardiol. 45:1196, 1980.

Dreifus, L.S., Haiat, R., Watanabe, Y., et al.: Ventricular fibrillation, a possible mechanism of sudden death in patients with Wolff-Parkinson-White syndrome. Circulation 43:520, 1971.

Hoffman, B.F., Rosen, M.R., and Wit, A.L.: Electrophysiology and pharmacology of cardiac arrhythmias. III.

The causes and treatment of cardiac arrhythmias. Part B. Am. Heart J. 89:253, 1975.

Hurwitz, R.: Cardiac arrhythmias in infants and children. *In* Current Problems in Pediatrics. Chicago, Year Book Medical Publishers, Inc., 1973.

James, T.N.: Cardiac conduction system: fetal and postnatal development. Am. J. Cardiol. 25:213, 1970.

Moller, J.H., Davachi, F., and Anderson, R.C.: Atrial flutter in infancy. J. Pediatr. 75:643, 1969.

Nadas, A.S., and Fyler, D.C.: Pediatric Cardiology: Arrhythmias, 3rd ed. Philadelphia, W.B. Saunders Company, 1972.

Roberts, N.K., and Gelband, H.: Cardiac Arrhythmias in the Neonatal Infant and Child. Norwalk, Conn, Appleton-Century-Crofts, 1977.

Rocchini, A.P., Chun, P.O., and Dick, M.: Ventricular tachycardia in children. Am. J. Cardiol. 47:1091, 1981.

Sapire, D.W., O'Riordan, A.C., and Black, I.F.S.: Safety and efficacy of short- and long-term verapamil therapy in children with tachycardia. Am. J. Cardiol. 48:1091, 1981.

Simche, A., and Bonham-Carter, R.E.: Paroxysmal atrial tachycardia in infants and children. Lancet 1:832, 1971.

Sloss, L.J., Greenwood, R.D., LaCorte, M.A., and Nadas, A.S.: Arrhythmias following Mustard's operation for transposition of the great arteries. Pediatr. Res. 9:271, 1975.

Talbot, S., and Dreifus, L.S.: Characteristics of ventricular extrasystoles and their prognostic importance: a reappraisal of their method of classification. Chest 67:665, 1975.

Wellens, H.J.J., and Durrer, D.: Effect of digitalis on atrioventricular conduction and circus movement tachycardias in patients with Wolff-Parkinson-White syndrome. Circulation 47:1229, 1973.

Zipes, D.P., and Troup, P.: New anti-arrhythmic agents. Am. J. Cardiol. 41:1005, 1978.

Zucker, A.R., Lacina, S.J., DasGupta, D.S., et al.: Fab fragments of digoxin-specific antibodies used to reverse ventricular fibrillation induced by digoxin ingestion in a child. Pediatrics 70:468, 1982.

Congestive Heart Failure

DELORES DANILOWICZ, M.D.

CONTRACTILITY OF THE HEART

The heart is a muscular organ that is responsible for pumping blood to the lungs and to the body at a rate commensurate with the body's metabolic demands. When this action cannot be sustained, signs and symptoms of congestive heart failure (CHF) occur.

Contractility of the heart is ultimately dependent upon sarcomere length and recruitment. Under electron microscopic examination, the sarcomere can be identified. This unit of the myocardial muscle makes up about 50 percent of the cardiac cell mass. Sarcomeres are 1.6 to 2.2μ in length and contain actin and myosin, the contractile proteins responsible for force generation. The sarcomere makes up the myofibril, which in turn forms the myocardial fiber. From sarcomere to the entire heart, a length/tension response can be shown (Starling's law). Optimal tension can be developed when the sarcomere is between 2 and 2.2μ in length. When the sarcomere is less than 2μ, there is a double overlap of the actin and myosin, with less force generation, possibly caused by a decrease in cross-links or a decrease in calcium binding. When a sarcomere exceeds 2.2μ in length, the number of cross-links decreases, as does the force generation. At 3.65μ, there are no cross-links remaining, and all force generation stops.

Starling's law of the heart applies to the most microscopic unit studied as well as to the myocardial fiber and to the heart as a whole. The number of sarcomeres recruited and their length determine the ultimate level of contractility. The position on the Starling curve at which a response occurs can be influenced by many underlying states, for example, sympathetic/parasympathetic tone, thyroid function, calcium ion, and drugs. However, the maximal response at any level of inotropy will depend upon sarcomere length. As the length is increased to 2.2μ, the force generated increases.

In the intact heart, this results in an increasing cardiac output as the pre-load volume is increased; this is accomplished with small changes in the left ventricular end–diastolic pressure until a level of approximately 12 mm Hg is reached. At this pressure level, sarcomere length has reached 2.2μ. After the sarcomere exceeds 2.2μ in length, the force generated decreases, and the left ventricular end–diastolic pressure of the intact heart will rise inordinately for the small amount of increase in pre-load. At this point, CHF may be seen, and the myocardial response is on the flat or descending limb of the Starling curve. Restoring function may be accomplished by decreasing pre-load, thus allowing sarcomere length to move back to between 2 and 2.2μ, which is optimal for force generation. Reducing afterload and providing positive inotropic stimulation may also allow some sarcomeres that are still in the 2 to 2.2μ length to increase their contractility. These principles become the rationale for treatment of CHF. The length of the sarcomere will determine contractile response, whereas the number of sarcomeres at any given length will serve as a functional reserve.

SIGNS AND SYMPTOMS

CHF may be right-sided, left-sided, or both; it may be high output or low output; and it may be chronic or acute. It will be manifested in different ways and will be due to various etiologies, including pressure and volume overloads as well as myocardial cell damage.

Although CHF may start as right- or left-sided, it will eventually involve both circulations. Left heart failure will be seen with a rise in left ventricular end–diastolic pressure and a decrease in forward flow. The increase in left ventricular end–diastolic pressure will be transmitted backward, with a resultant rise in left atrial pressure, pulmonary venous hypertension, rales, pulmonary arterial hypertension, and a rise in right ventricular systolic and then end–diastolic pressure, with secondary right heart failure. Initial or secondary right ventricular failure will be seen with an elevated right ventricular end–diastolic pressure, which will cause an increase in right atrial pressure and impede venous filling, with resultant increase in jugular venous pressure, hepatomegaly, edema, and ascites. As the right heart fails, forward flow through the lungs and into the left heart will decrease, leading to systemic hypotension and shock.

If a lesion progresses slowly, the heart will have a chance to adapt. Thus, there may be fewer symptoms for the amount of disease than if the same lesion occurred acutely, for example, mitral or aortic regurgitation following a myocardial infarction or bacterial endocarditis. A sudden increase in volume in a nondilated structure will cause a massive rise in pressure, with acute pulmonary edema if the failure is left-sided and a rapid shocklike state if it is right-sided. However, if accommodation and dilatation occur in response to a volume load over a period of time, the pressure rise is not rapid, and the patient will have fewer signs and symptoms in spite of a similar or even greater degree of disease. The same is true for acute pressure loads, such as in a patient with a pulmonary embolus in whom shock rapidly occurs, whereas a pulmonic stenosis with a much higher right ventricular systolic pressure will be well tolerated, having occurred over years of time with secondary hypertrophy.

High output failure is often seen in volume overload and hypermetabolic states. Pulses remain strong with good peripheral circulation, and contractility of the heart may actually be increased for a period of time before secondary impairment occurs. Examples of this are seen in patients with anemia, AV fistulae, hyperthyroidism, and patent ductus arteriosus. Treatment is best directed at removing the underlying cause, although reducing pre-load may be helpful for a period of time. If contractility is increased, use of a positive inotropic drug would not be helpful.

Low-output failure is seen in patients with damage to the myocardium (myocardial infarct, myocarditis) and in obstructive disease (pulmonary or systemic hypertension, valve stenoses.) It will also eventually replace the high-output failure of severe volume overload, leading to the typical situation involving vasoconstriction and poor pulses. When damage occurs to myocardial fibers, the myocardial fibers are replaced by noncontractile tissue, thus lowering the number of sarcomeres available for contractility. In addition, other cells that were not killed may be functioning poorly as a result of ischemia. Treatment should be directed toward lowering the workload of the heart, as well as increasing the contractility of the living cells. When systemic or pulmonary hypertension is the reason for the failure, lowering the resistance (afterload) is the treatment of choice, with secondary benefits from decreasing preload. If contractility has become impaired, an inotropic agent may also be helpful. If the resistance is due to valve stenosis, operative repair or replacement may be necessary, because often, medical assistance is not helpful over a long period of time.

When cardiac failure occurs, several secondary mechanisms are called upon to maintain cardiac output. Epinephrine and norepinephrine are secreted by the adrenals and cause an increase in heart rate and contractility. Vasoconstriction occurs, with redistribution of blood flow to the more vital organs. With prolonged failure, depletion of epinephrine and norepinephrine occurs and compensatory mechanisms fail. A patient in compensated failure, even when on treatment, remains at high risk, because additional insults such as fever, infection, or dysrhythmias may lead to rapid decompensation.

Symptoms of left-sided CHF include exertional dyspnea, orthopnea, paroxysmal dyspnea, dyspnea at rest, and acute pulmonary edema; all are caused by increasing degrees of pulmonary congestion. Fatigue and exercise intolerance are also seen. In infants, this is manifested as poor feeding, increased sweating, tachypnea, poor weight gain, and repeated respiratory infections. Because the infant's pulmonary bed is far more reactive than that of older children and adults, pulmonary hypertension and secondary right heart failure often occur quickly, with early hepatomegaly. However, because right atrial pressure in infants is normally 0 to 2 mm Hg, rarely is edema seen in a very young baby until the child is almost moribund from the failure, since the level at which tissue edema is seen is about 10 to 15 mm Hg. In right heart failure alone, pulmonary congestion is not seen. As systemic venous congestion occurs, hepatomegaly, edema, and ascites may occur. Fatigue and nausea are common. If the failure occurs rapidly, stretching of the liver capsule often results in abdominal pain. As the failure progresses, dyspnea and even orthopnea may occur as a result of anasarca, **ascites**, and hydrothorax.

Cardiac examination will also change as failure occurs. The first and second heart sounds may become muffled; as pulmonary hypertension develops, pulmonic closure will be louder than aortic closure. A diastolic gallop, S3 and/or S4 will be heard as compliance of the ventricles decreases. Murmurs of AV valve insufficiency (tricuspid or mitral regurgitation) can be heard as ventricular dilatation causes dilatation of the AV ring. The murmur of the underlying heart disease, however, may decrease as a result of low cardiac output. Pulse pressure may be narrow, with pulsus alternans and pulsus paradoxus occurring as the failure becomes more severe.

Laboratory evaluations of the patient in failure depend upon the chronicity and severity of CHF. Electrolyte changes and liver abnormalities are rarely seen in the early part of failure. A prolonged circulation time will be present in patients with congestion and low-output failure. The electrocardiogram will not diagnose congestive failure but is useful in assessing the underlying cause. It will also allow identification of any dysrhythmias or ischemic changes. Because of cardiac dilatation, the chest x-ray film will show cardiomegaly, right, left, or both. In left heart failure, there is pulmonary congestion, which manifests as a prominent venous pattern, then progresses to a redistribution of blood flow (apical more than basal) and eventually is revealed as overt pulmonary edema and pleural effusion. In right heart failure, although hydrothorax can occur in the very severe forms, pulmonary congestion is not seen. Echocardiography is very useful in evaluating cardiac function (ejection fraction) and in identifying anatomic abnormalities that may be responsible for the failure. Doppler flows, as well as shunts, can be used to evaluate stenosis and regurgitation. Pericardial effusion can be recognized early and followed easily. Thallium scans are useful for evaluating resting and exercise ejection fractions, especially after the failure has been treated, as well as providing information about regional ventricular contractility and coronary blood flow distribution.

TREATMENT

There are specific causes of CHF that require other than the usual means of treatment. For example, idiopathic hypertrophic subaortic stenosis with severe obstruction is best treated by decreasing contractility, and the patient in thyroid storm would have a good response to propranolol. On the other hand, a beta blocker would be expected to worsen the condition of most patients with CHF. Tachycardias and complete heart block can lead to failure, even if there is no underlying heart disease. Cardioversion, pharmacologically or electrically, is the treatment of choice for the tachycardias; placement of a pacemaker is best for heart block.

In general, CHF is treated by attempting to modify three parameters: contractility, pre-load, and afterload. A variety of drugs is available for this modification (Tables 19–1 through 19–3). Digitalis and other inotropic drugs such as amrinone, dopamine, and dobutamine can be used to increase contractility. Decreasing afterload is accomplished by decreasing the patient's activity, by having him lose weight, if applicable, and by using vasodilator drugs. Decreasing pre-load is accomplished by limiting sodium and fluid intake and by using diuretics. Mechanical removal of fluid (thoracentesis, paracentesis, dialysis, or phlebotomy) may be required at times. When all else fails, assisted circulation (balloon pumps, ventricular assist devices, cardiac transplant) is possible at some centers.

When possible, the best method of treatment of CHF is to remove the instigating or precipitating cause. This often means surgical intervention to relieve a stenosis, close a shunt, and so on. In high-output failure, treatment of the underlying cause is often the only effective means of treatment, especially if cardiac contractility is increased. Pre-load modification may be helpful for a period of time; however, closing the ductus, exchange transfusing the anemic patient, closing the AV fistula, or treating the hyperthyroidism is a better choice of treatment.

If hypertension is the major reason for the failure, vasodilators will be the most effective treatment, with secondary help obtained by reducing pre-load and perhaps by increasing contractility. Because drugs given to decrease pulmonary vascular resistance may also lower systemic vascular resistance, blood pressure must be monitored closely. It is often necessary to treat pulmonary hypertension in neonates, and drugs such as tolazoline or nitroprusside may also lower the systemic blood pressure to such an extent that volume infusion or use of dopamine/dobutamine may be necessary. When possible, the best pulmonary vasodilator is oxygen; it has few side effects when used acutely. Isoproterenol will also vasodilate the pulmonary bed without causing a drop in systemic blood pressure, but the patient must be watched for excessive tachycardia or any dysrhythmias. Prostacyclin has also been used re-

Table 19–1. Inotropic Drugs for Congestive Heart Failure

Drug	Dose	Side Effects
Digoxin	Digitalizing dose, p.o.	Dysrhythmias
	Prematures: 0.02–0.03 mg/kg	Heart block
	Full terms: 0.025–0.035 mg/kg	Nausea, vomiting
	1–24 months: 0.035–0.06 mg/kg	Vision changes
	2–5 years: 0.03–0.04 mg/kg	
	5–10 years: 0.02–0.035 mg/kg	
	older than 10 years: 0.01–0.15 mg/kg	
	Use 80% of the above dose when giving intramuscularly (IM) or IV	
	Use 20–30% of total digitalizing dose as maintenance, divided q 12 hr, p.o.	
Amrinone	No established pediatric dosage	Thrombocytopenia, reversible
	Experimental drug	Others to be evaluated
	Adult dose: 1.6–4 mg/kg, p.o.	
	40 μgm/kg/min, IV	
Isoproterenol (Isuprel)	0.05–0.1 μgm/kg/min, as IV drip	Tachycardia Dysrhythmias
Dopamine	5–10 μgm/kg/min, as IV drip	Increases renal blood flow Tachycardia, dysrhythmias Vasoconstriction, vomiting
Dobutamine	2–10 μgm/kg/min, as IV drip	Tachycardia, dysrhythmias
Epinephrine	0.1–1 μgm/kg/min of 1:50,000 solution, as IV drip	Tachycardia, dysrhythmias

cently, but with marked variability in response in neonates. Many drugs used to decrease systemic vascular resistance have unacceptable side effects, for example, propranolol will increase CHF and cannot be used in asthmatics; beta blockers and diuretics raise the level of serum cholesterol and low-density lipoproteins. Recently, the alpha-antagonist, prazosin, has been used with good results and, to date, with fewer side effects.

When CHF is due to cell damage and loss, inotropic help to the remaining cells may be useful, but reducing the workload by lowering the afterload is often a better solution. A variety of vasodilators (hydralazine, nitroprusside, nitrates, captopril) can be used while monitoring blood pressure. In adults with coronary artery disease, these drugs can relieve angina and improve exercise tolerance. If cell loss is excessive, assisted circulation and cardiac transplant may be necessary.

It is important to recognize that modification of one modality may lead to a secondary change in another. An increase in contractility often results in diuresis, as renal flow improves. This lowering of pre-load can allow a decrease in cardiac dilatation, thus influencing sarcomere length and making force generation more efficient.

When more than one drug is used, the possibility of drug interaction must be considered. Both quinidine and verapamil will cause an increase in digoxin levels in a patient who is already on digoxin, because of the competition for renal excretion; the level of digoxin may rise to toxic levels.

Table 19–2. Diuretic Drugs for Congestive Heart Failure

Drug	Dose	Side Effects
Furosemide (Lasix)	1 mg/kg, IV 2 mg/kg, p.o.	Ototoxicity; keeps ductus open in prematures Depletes volume and potassium Increases glucose and bilirubin Increases lipids, uric acid, and calcium
Ethacrynic Acid (Edecrin)	1 mg/kg, IV 2 mg/kg, p.o.	Volume and potassium depletion
Chlorthiazide (Diuril)	20–25 mg/kg/day, p.o. given o.d. or q 12 hr	Increases bilirubin and glucose Increases lipids and uric acid Increases calcium Can deplete potassium on chronic basis
Spironolactone (Aldactone)	1.5–3.5 mg/kg/day p.o. q 6–8 hr	Gynecomastia Can elevate potassium levels

Table 19–3. Vasodilator Drugs for Congestive Heart Failure

Drug	Dose	Side Effects
Pulmonary		
Oxygen	High flow by face mask or closed hood	Neonate: retrolental fibroplasia (chronic) bronchopulmonary dysplasia
Isoproterenol (Isuprel)	0.05–1.0 μgm/kg/min, as IV drip	Tachycardias, dysrhythmias
Tolazoline (priscoline)	1 mg/kg, as IV bolus, preferably into the lungs directly	Systemic hypotension
Prostacyclin	Experimental drug; no established pediatric dosage	Nausea, vomiting Flushing, headache
	Adult dose: 2–12 μgm/kg/min, IV	Systemic hypotension
Systemic		
Captopril (Capoten)	No established dosage for pediatrics	Nausea, vomiting
	Adult dose: 25–100 mg/day, p.o.	Systemic hypotension, renal toxicity
Prazosin (Minipres)	No established dosage for pediatrics	Marked systemic hypotension
	Adult dose: 1 mg h.s. to start and increase slowly to 6–15 mg/day, p.o.	Fluid retention
Propranolol (Inderal)	0.01–0.25 mg/kg/dose, IV 0.5–3 mg/kg/day, p.o. q 6 hr	Bronchospasm; hypoglycemia Nausea, vomiting, slow heart rate Systemic hypotension; CHF
Systemic and Pulmonary		
Nitroprusside (Nipride)	1 μgm/kg/min—titrate to BP, IV	CNS seizures; cyanide toxicity Systemic hypotension
Hydralazine (Apresoline)	0.75–7.5 mg/kg/day, p.o. q 6 hr 0.15 mg/kg/dose q 4 hr, IM or IV	Lupus-like syndrome Drug fever, nausea, vomiting
Nitrates	No established dosage for pediatrics Adult dose: 10–100 μgm/min, IV 0.3–0.6 mg q 2 hr, S.L. 2.5–6.5 mg q 6 hr, p.o.	Headaches, flushing Postural hypotension, dizziness

MEDICATIONS

Digitalis

Digitalis is used to increase contractility and to slow heart rate. Because the tachycardia of CHF is a method of increasing cardiac output, the heart rate must not be slowed to a dangerous level, which can occur with digitalis toxicity. It is best to use one preparation of digitalis (e.g., digoxin) so concentrations are readily known and easily remembered in calculating dosages. Orders for digoxin should always be written in both milligrams and milliliters so that errors are minimal. Digitalis must be used selectively, depending upon the clinical circumstances. If a child is in severe failure with vasoconstriction, intravenous digoxin should be used at 80 percent of the calculated oral digitalizing dose, because neither oral nor intramuscular medication will be absorbed well. Premature infants and patients with depressed renal function must be given lower loading doses and less frequent maintenance doses. In patients with myocarditis, a loading dose of digoxin may be contraindicated, because increased myocardial irritability may lead to premature ventricular beats, ventricular tachycardia, or ventricular fibrillation. Often, it is better to put these patients on a low maintenance dose and allow the digoxin level to rise slowly to a therapeutic level. This may also be true in patients with CHF after a myocardial infarct, as in Kawasaki's disease. Obviously, premature atrial and ventricular beats can be secondary to the failure and, if so, may disappear with the use of digoxin. If toxicity does result, the drug should be stopped, and dilantin can be used to decrease the irritability of the myocardium. The occurrence of life-threatening dysrhythmias may require the use of Fab digoxin–specific antibodies.

In routine pediatric use, digoxin is calculated on a per kilogram basis, depending upon age. Half the calculated dose is usually given stat, with quarter doses given as needed every 4 to 8 hours until clinical improvement or early toxicity occurs. Digoxin levels can be helpful, although higher levels are often needed in children. The drug can be continued past the 2 ng percent level if no toxicity is observed and if clinical improvement has not yet resulted. A lower dose range is used in premature infants, because renal immaturity leads to a longer half-life of digoxin in this group. The highest dose level is used in children from 1 month to 2 years of age. By preadolescence, an adult range is used, with the upper limits for a total digitalizing dose being between 1 and 2 mg per day, regardless of weight. Maintenance dose is usually 25 to 30 percent of the digitalizing dose, given orally every 12 hours.

Amrinone

In the past several years, an inotropic drug, amrinone, has been tested in some patients with chronic CHF who have responded poorly to the drugs that are normally given for CHF. Amrinone has a positive inotropic response that is an additive to digoxin, without incurring any significant dysrhythmias. The drug is available as both an intravenous and an oral preparation, and the only reported side reaction is thrombocytopenia, which resolved when the drug was stopped. The inotropic response is thought to be due to increased uptake of calcium by the red blood cells. Peak action is within an hour and is sustained up to 7 hours in some patients. Because the drug is still under investigation, no set regimen has been formulated for its use.

Other Inotropic Drugs

If digoxin alone is not helpful, there are many additional drugs that can be used, all as titrated drips requiring careful monitoring. Epinephrine, norepinephrine, isoproterenol, dopamine, and dobutamine can be used acutely to increase and maintain cardiac output. In some instances, a central venous line, a Swan–Ganz catheter, and an arterial line should be available to monitor the response to these medications.

In the newborn period, a variety of abnormalities can depress myocardial contractility. These abnormalities, including hypoglycemia, hypoxia, hypocalcemia, and acidosis, should be ruled out because the treatment is specific.

Diuretics

Drugs often used in pediatrics to reduce the pre-load include chlorothiazide (Diuril), furosemide (Lasix), ethacrynic acid (Edecrin) and spironolactone (Aldactone). Given intravenously at 1 mg per kg, Lasix and Edecrin will produce a rapid diuresis, starting within 15 minutes of when the dose is given. Excessive loss of potassium can result with use of both of these drugs, and supplementation is needed when either drug is used chronically. Diuril has less of a potassium-depleting effect, because the diuresis is not as massive. Aldactone is a potassium-sparing diuretic, occasionally leading to an elevation in potassium levels. Decreasing sodium and fluid intake is helpful acutely but is rarely used as a chronic method of treatment in the pediatric age group.

Vasodilators

Vasodilators have been used in pediatrics for reduction of pulmonary vasoconstriction, but only recently have they been used to lower systemic vascular resistance as a method of treating chronic CHF. They have been useful in children after myocarditis and in those with myopathies in whom surgical intervention is not possible.

Drugs effective in treating increased pulmonary vascular resistance include oxygen, isoproterenol, prostacyclin, nitroprusside, hydralazine, and tolazoline. Unfortunately, none of these drugs have been shown to have a consistent lowering response in older patients with primary or secondary pulmonary arterial hypertension, although a study with prostacyclin is currently being done. The best effects of these drugs have been found in the neonatal period and in the postoperative period in younger children when pulmonary vascular resistance is due to muscular vasoconstriction, not intimal thickening. When pulmonary vasoconstriction is treated, the systemic blood pressure must be watched closely because it may drop. This may be a result of incomplete activation of the drug by passage through the lungs or, in neonates, to residual right-to-left shunting at the atrial or ductal levels.

Drugs that have been used to reduce systemic vascular resistance include nitroprusside, hydralazine, nitrates, captopril, prazosin, and propranolol. There are limitations with some of these drugs, because nitroprusside can be used only intravenously, and propranolol cannot be used in asthmatics or in patients with significantly decreased myocardial contractility. Hydralazine can cause a lupus-like syndrome, whereas captopril may cause renal damage. Nitrates can be used as intravenous, sublingual, oral, or cutaneous preparations, but they have been used infrequently in children. Most of these medications have been used effectively in adults, especially in patients with coronary artery disease. More recently, they have been used with reasonable results in children, but the doses of many of these drugs become a trial-and-error situation in small children or infants. When the standard means of controlling CHF have not been successful, the use of afterload reducers should be attempted. At the present time, initiation of this therapy is probably best carried out in the hospital under careful observation until a dosage response and regimen are established.

CASE PRESENTATION 1

A 4-month-old white boy is admitted to the pediatric intensive care unit after being seen in the pediatrician's office. The mother had noted poor feeding for about 1 month and had found the child in bed "soaked in sweat" several times during the past week. This morning, he was febrile to 102°F and brought to the office. When seen, the temperature was 104°F, HR = 180 beats/min, RR = 72 breaths/min, and BP could not be obtained by a regular cuff. The baby was pale, irritable, and immediately admitted to the ICU.

Examination

Physical examination shows a HR = 180 beats/min; RR = 62/min; BP = 80 mm Hg, systolic; T = 104°F; and Wt = 8 lb.

This small, pale, and irritable 4-month-old white boy has moderate intercostal and subcostal retractions. His color is dusky, but there is no edema or clubbing. Pulses are present but are weak in all extremities; there is marked vasoconstriction. The liver is 3 cm below the right costal margin (RCM). The lungs are clear anteriorly but have rales posteriorly at both bases, more so on the left than on the right. HEENT (head, ears, eyes, nose, and throat) are normal; fontanelle is full but not bulging. The PMI (point of maximal impulse) is in the 6th LIS, AAL with a right ventricular impulse present at the LLSB. The first sound is normal; the second sound is single and loud. A diastolic gallop is present at the apex. A grade 2/6 systolic murmur is present along the LSB with minimal radiation. No diastolic murmur is heard.

The child is obviously in CHF with poor pulses, tachycardia, tachypnea, gallop, and a nonspecific murmur. No obvious source of the fever has been found.

Consider

Start IV with low maintenance fluids; put NPO; on monitor.

Give acetaminophen for fever; oxygen for duskiness and distress.

Get further history from mother.

History

The child was the product of a normal, full-term spontanous delivery, first child, BW-6 lb, 10 oz. Neonatal course was normal; no murmur was mentioned. He was seen at 6 weeks for his first well baby check-up; his weight was 7 lb, 14 oz, and there was no distress. A 3/6 holosystolic murmur was heard at the LLSB. The mother missed her next appointment and did not phone in for another until the present time. Family history is negative.

Test Results

Laboratory Data

ABG (air) pH = 7.32, P_{O_2} = 50 mm Hg, P_{CO_2} = 32 mm Hg.

BUN, 22 mg/dl; K, 4 mEq/L; C1, 102 mEq/L; Na, 138 mEq/L; creatinine, 0.6 mg/dl.

Urinalysis normal, SG 1.012.

Hgb, 9.2 gm/dl; hmt, 27%; RBC microcytic, hypochromic.

WBC 16,000, with 42% polys, 26% bands, 28% lymphs, 0.5% reticulocytes, platelets 300,000.

LP negative.

Blood cultures pending.

EKG

HR = 180 beats/min, sinus tachycardia

Tall R waves with small S in V3R, V1, and upright T waves.

Tall and deep R/S complexes V2–4.

Tall R waves with small S wave in V5–6; T waves flat.

Broad P wave in II; deep negative P in V1.

Chest X–ray

Cardiothoracic ratio = 68%, generalized enlargement.

Increased pulmonary vascularity with effusion in the fissure; streaking and air bronchogram in the parenchyma on the left.

Echo

Dilated left atrium and left ventricle; dilated right ventricle.

Left atrium/aortic (LA/Ao) ratio = 1.5

Left ventricular ejection fraction (LVEF) = 55%

On sector, large dropout in ventricular septum, high.

Possible dropout in midatrial septum.

Problem List

Anemic, probably iron deficient, dilutional?

Desaturation probably secondary to failure ± LLL pneumonia and/or atelectasis.

High WBC with shift to left, CHF?, infection?.

BUN elevated, but creatinine normal.

EKG: LAH, BVH, ischemic T-wave changes.

Chest x-ray: Increased flow, large heart with effusion and possible LLL pneumonia.

History suggestive of VSD; echo confirms this.

Heart dilated with decreased EF. Atrial dropout may be ASD or stretched foramen.

Lack of typical murmur now due to low cardiac output and pulmonary hypertension.

Treatment

Lasix or edecrin, 1 mg/kg IV stat; then p.r.n. depending upon weight and clinical course. Maintenance fluids.

Start digoxin at 0.04–0.05 mg/kg as digitalizing dose and give half stat IV; give remaining quarters q 4–6 hr IV depending upon child's clinical response and lack of toxicity (rhythm strip before each dose for P-R interval, block, ectopics).

Continue antibiotics IV until blood culture results are obtained.

Oxygen and acetaminophen p.r.n.

Keep NPO while there is respiratory distress.

Consider transfusion with packed cells.

24 hours later

Blood cultures are negative. ABG is normal on room air. Wt = 7 lb, 4 oz. T = 99.8°F; HR = 140 beats/min; RR = 38 breaths/min, with fewer retractions; BP = 108/68 mm Hg. The patient is still pale but not dusky; pulses are good. Repeat hgb = 10.2 gm/dl; hmt = 30%. Liver is 2 cm below RCM, and there is now a 4/6 holosystolic murmur heard along the LLSB, with widespread precordial radiation. Diastolic sound is still present.

Treatment

Maintenance digoxin started at 30% of digitalizing dose; given q 12 hr, IV or IM; when switch made to p.o., increase dose by 20%, check digoxin level.

Give packed cell transfusion at 5 ml/kg, slowly.

Start on clear fluids, and if no distress, start formula with added iron.

24 hours later

Blood cultures are still negative. Murmur is the same in systole and 2/6 mid-diastolic murmur is present at the apex. HR = 120 beats/min; RR = 24 breaths/min; BP = 100/66 mm Hg; T = 98.8°F; Wt = 7 lb, 5 oz.

Hgb = 12 gm/dl, gm and hmt = 35%. Repeat EKG is the same, with slower HR and T waves upright in V4–6. Repeat chest x-ray showed CTR of 65%, with increased vascularity, LLL density, and no pleural effusion. EF on echocardiogram is now 66% with LA and LV still dilated; RV is normal. Baby is feeding well, on maintenance digoxin p.o. Antibiotics switched to IM; IV is discontinued; and baby is transferred to ward.

Follow-up

The baby continued to do well on the ward. The digoxin level came back at 1.8 ng%. Antibiotics were continued for 10 days and then stopped, with no return of fever or distress.

He was sent home on maintenance digoxin, and iron was added to his diet. Reticulocyte count was 4% at discharge.

When seen by his pediatrician 2 weeks later, the baby's weight was 8 lb, 3 oz, and his vital signs were normal. The VSD murmurs were the same.

Final Assessment

Because the child has responded well to medical management, he will be followed clinically, with plans to do a catheterization in 1–3 months. If the pulmonary artery pressures are normal, the child will be followed clinically, with elective closure of the VSD at between 3 and 5 years of age if it remains a significant shunt (repeat catheterization will be done before surgery). If the pulmonary artery pressures are elevated, the catheterization will be repeated when the baby is 12–18 months of age. If the pulmonary artery pressure is still high, early closure of the defect will be done.

In spite of the history of failure, the defect can still go on to spontaneous closure. In this baby, the failure was probably precipitated by pneumonia and was possibly made worse by the anemia.

CASE PRESENTATION 2

A 4-year-old white girl is seen in her pediatrician's office with a history of fatigue for 1 week, demanding to be carried for the past day. Her appetite has been poor, and she has had a cough for the last 3 nights. This child and several other members of the family had "colds" about 10–14 days ago. All are well now, and the child is not febrile. The child's past history is benign, and the family history is negative. There is one older sibling, a 10-year-old brother.

Examination

Physical examination shows a HR = 120 beats/min; RR = 20 breaths/min; BP = 90/60 mm Hg; T = 98.8°F; Wt = 40 lb.

This well-developed (w/d), well-nourished (w/n) "washed-out" looking 4-year-old white girl is somewhat irritable and fussy. HEENT are normal. Color is good with no edema or clubbing. The lungs are clear. The liver edge is at the RCM and is not tender. Pulses are palpable, equal, and normal. Heart sounds are muffled with a gallop heard at the apex. There is no murmur. The PMI cannot be felt, but cardiac dullness extends to the AAL.

The child is sent for a chest x-ray, and the CTR is 75%; what lung can be seen appears normal. She is then admitted to the ward and placed on bedrest while the work-up is started.

The question of an enlarged heart versus a pericardial effusion is presented by both the examination and the chest x-ray. The history of a previous respiratory infection raises the possibility of a viral myocarditis/pericarditis. A regular diet can be continued with daily weighings. If needed, a cardiac monitor can be placed.

Test Results

Laboratory Data

WBC 4500, with 20% polys, 60% lymphs, 15% monos, 3% bands, 2% eos. Hgb, 12.2 gm/dl; hmt, 36%. Some atypical lymphs; reticulocytes and platelets, normal.

BUN, electrolytes, liver chemistries, all normal. Urine, normal. Mono spot and strep titers, negative. ESR, 15 mm/hr; CPK, normal; MB, not done. Viral studies, sent.

EKG

Low voltage in limb leads and precordial leads; no axis deviation. S-T segments, normal. T waves inverted in V4–6, II, III, avF. P waves, normal. Rare unifocal VPC.

Echo

Large LV with EF 42%. Mild to moderate pericardial effusion but no tamponade. LA, aorta, RV, all normal in size. No anatomic abnormalities seen.

Assessment Treatment

Lasix or edecrin, 2 mg/kg p.o. stat.

Start digoxin at 0.01 mg/kg/day in q 12-hr doses to avoid loading dose, which may cause dysrhythmia in myocarditis. Check digoxin level in 3–4 days. Bedrest on monitor; daily weighing.

Regular diet with maintenance fluids; no salt on tray.

3 days later

Digoxin level is 1.5 ng %, with no dysrhythmias noted. EKG shows a normal P-R interval, T waves are now flat in V4–6, no longer inverted, and HR is down to 80 beats/min. Voltage in precordial leads is better. Weight is down to 38.5 lb. There is still no murmur, but the gallop persists. Echocardiogram is repeated and shows no residual pericardial fluid, but the LV is still dilated, and the EF is 45%. The heart size on chest x-ray is not appreciably changed.

Comment.

Child is discharged after 7 days and sent home on maintenance digoxin, 2 mg/kg/day p.o., o.d. every other day of Lasix with 1 mEq/L K+/kg/day on the days Lasix is given. Activity is to be restricted.

4 weeks later

Child is seen in the office with normal vital signs. No murmur is heard, but gallop is still present. Viral studies are not helpful. LV EF on echo was 50%, and the CTR on x-ray was 70%. The child was started on prednisone, 2 mg/kg/day p.o., t.i.d. The remainder of the medications were left the same, and the parents were advised to watch for fluid retention. Restricted activity is to be continued.

2 weeks later

Two weeks after prednisone was started, the child developed a fever to 102°F and complained of an earache. When seen in the pediatrician's office, her HR was 150 beats/min; RR was 28 breaths/min; and BP was 80/50 mm Hg. Her T was 102.8°F, and her eyes were puffy. There was no edema elsewhere, and her color was good. She was readmitted to the hospital, started on antibiotics for the otitis, and the prednisone was decreased to 1 mg/kg/day. The child's weight on admission was 41 lb.

Laboratory Data.

WBC 12,000, with shift to left; ESR, 40 mm/hr.

BUN, electrolytes, normal. Beta hemolytic streptococcus is grown from the throat culture but strep titers, negative.

Blood cultures × 3, negative.

Digoxin level is 1.4 ng%.

EKG.

T waves still flat in V4–6; voltage increased over last EKG but not in limits for LVH. Sinus tachycardia, with NAD. P waves borderline for LAH.

Chest x-ray.

CTR 70%; no parenchymal disease. Pulmonary venous pattern increased, but no fluid in fissure.

Echo.

No pericardial effusion; LV dilated, with EF 38%.

Treatment

Lasix, 1 mg/kg given IM stat; p.o. dose of lasix is increased to o.d., with K+ supplement also increased to daily dose.

Bedrest on monitor, with no salt diet.

24 hours later

Weight is down to 39 lb, and puffiness is gone. HR = 110 beats/min; RR = 18 breaths/min; T = 99°F. Cardiac examination is the same with no murmur, persistent gallop. Chest x-ray shows the same heart size but a decrease in the congestion.

The child is observed for 5 days. She stays afebrile and does not reaccumulate fluid. She is discharged on antibiotics to be continued for another 5 days, maintenance digoxin, daily Lasix, and K+ supplements, 1 mg/kg/day of prednisone to be tapered over the next month.

3 months later

The steroids were tapered and cut without any problem. No change occurred in the clinical picture, and the child was referred for cardiac biopsy because of persistent cardiomegaly and poor exercise tolerance. The procedure was well tolerated but showed nonspecific fibrosis.

Over the next 3 months, poor exercise tolerance continued, and a 2/6 systolic murmur at the apex was heard for the first time. At this point, an echocardiogram was repeated and showed a dilated LV with EF of 52%. Doppler ultrasound confirmed the presence of mitral regurgitation. The EKG now shows left atrial and left ventricular hypertrophy; T waves are still flat in the left precordial leads. At this time, hydralazine was added to her medications. Her blood pressure remained stable, and her exercise tolerance improved. She was subsequently able to attend a half-day session in kindergarten without symptoms; her physical activity was restricted.

Final Assessment

The child now has chronic myocarditis, with poor EF. It is unlikely that much further improvement will occur. If she can live through adolescence, a cardiac transplant may be feasible. Amrinone might be attempted if increasing failure occurs before that time.

SUGGESTED READING

Berman, W., Jr., Yabek, S.M., Dillon, T., et al.: Effects of digoxin in infants with a congested circulatory state due to a ventricular septal defect. N. Engl. J. Med. 308:363, 1983.

Braunwald, E.: Pathophysiology of heart failure. *In* Heart Disease: A Textbook of Cardiovascular Medicine. Philadelphia, W.B. Saunders Company, 1980, pp. 453–471.

Braunwald, E.: Clinical manifestations of heart failure. *In* Heart Disease: A Textbook of Cardiovascular Medicine. Philadelphia, W.B. Saunders Company, 1980, pp. 493–508.

Braunwald, E., Sonnenblick, E.H., and Ross, J., Jr.: Contraction of the normal heart. *In* Braunwald, E. (ed.): Heart Disease: A Textbook of Cardiovascular Medicine. Philadelphia, W.B. Saunders Company, 1980, pp. 426–448.

Goetzman, B.W., Sunshine, P., Johnson, J.D., et al.: Neonatal hypoxia and pulmonary vasospasm: response to tolazoline. J. Pediatr. 89:617, 1976.

Klein, H.O., Lang, R., Weiss, E., et al.: The influence of verapamil on serum digoxin concentration. Circulation 65:998, 1982.

Lang, D., and Von Bernuth, G.: Serum concentration and serum half-life of digoxin in premature and mature newborns. Pediatrics 59:902, 1977.

Leahey, E.B., Jr., Bigger, J.T., Jr., Butler V.P., Jr., et al.: Quinidine–digoxin interaction: time course and pharmacokinetics. Am. J. Cardiol. 48:1141, 1981.

LeJemtel, T.H., Keung, E., Ribner, H.S., et al.: Sustained beneficial effects of oral amrinone on cardiac and renal function in patients with severe congestive heart failure. Am. J. Cardiol. 45:123, 1980.

Okun, R.: Effectiveness of prazosin as initial antihypertensive therapy. Am. J. Cardiol. 51:644, 1983.

Rogers, M.C., Willerson, J.T., Goldblatt, A., Smith, T.W.: Serum digoxin concentrations in the human fetus, neonate, and infant. N. Engl. J. Med. 287:1010, 1972.

Rubin, L.J., Groves, B.M., Reeves, J.T., et al.: Prostacyclin-induced acute pulmonary vasodilation in primary pulmonary hypertension. Circulation 66:334, 1982.

Smith, T.W., and Braunwald, E.: The management of heart failure. In Braunwald, E. (ed.): Heart Disease: A Textbook of Cardiovascular Medicine. Philadelphia, W.B. Saunders Company, 1980, pp. 509–570.

Smith, T.W., Butler, V.P., Jr., Haber, E., et al.: Treatment of life-threatening digitalis intoxication with digoxin-specific Fab antibody fragments. N. Engl. J. Med. 307:1357, 1982.

Stemple, D.R., Kleiman, J.H., and Harrison, D.C.: Combined nitroprusside–dopamine therapy in severe chronic congestive heart failure. Am. J. Cardiol. 42:267, 1978.

Nursing Process for Patient Care:
Congestive Heart Failure

Congestive heart failure (CHF) occurs when the heart is unable to adequately pump blood to the lungs and to the body in response to metabolic demands. Failure may be right-sided, left-sided or both. It usually begins as right- or left-sided but progresses to involve both sides.

CARDIOVASCULAR

Assess, Monitor and Document

Rate
Rhythm
Quality
Heart sounds
Perfusion: color, skin condition

Blood pressure
Temperature
Activity tolerance
Response to pharmacologic management:
  drugs (inotropic, diuretic, vasodilator)

Anticipate

Alteration in cardiovascular status
  Left heart failure: dyspnea, fatigue, exercise
    intolerance, pulmonary edema
  Right heart failure: distended neck veins,
    hepatomegaly, edema (uncommon), as-
    cites (rare)

Systemic hypotension
Shock
Dysrhythmias
Cardiac arrest

RESPIRATORY

The pulmonary status is directly and rapidly affected by a change in cardiac function. As the heart fails in its ability to pump efficiently, pulmonary congestion increases. The signs and symptoms occur as a consequence.

Assess, Monitor, and Document

Respiratory rate
Dyspnea: exertional, paroxysmal, orthopnea
Breath sounds
Color

Arterial blood gases
Fatigue
Exercise intolerance: poor feeding, increased
  sweating

Anticipate

Pulmonary edema: tachypnea, rales, rhonchi,
  increased secretions

Respiratory failure
Respiratory arrest

FLUID AND ELECTROLYTE BALANCE

The fluid and electrolyte status of the child becomes significant as pulmonary congestion and systemic venous congestion occur. One of the basic tenets in the management of CHF is to reduce pre-load. This is accomplished by limiting sodium and fluid intake and by using diuretics.

Assess, Monitor, and Document

Weight
Urine output
Urine specific gravity
Fluid intake: accurate administration of parenteral fluids (use infusion pump if available) and oral fluids, maintenance of fluid limit
Response to pharmacologic management
Serum electrolytes

Anticipate

Fluid overload: weight gain
Pulmonary edema: tachypnea, rales, rhonchi, increased secretions
Serum electrolyte abnormalities: decreased potassium, dysrhythmias

RESPONSE OF CHILD

The age and developmental level of the child, along with the degree of respiratory distress, will significantly influence the child's response and will determine the child's ability to understand the illness, the need for hospitalization, and the therapeutic modalities, for example, mist tent and face mask. The ability of the child to comply with the therapeutic regimen is also a product of his or her developmental level.

The degree of respiratory distress contributes to the child's emotional response. Nursing interventions that deal with the child's response and that facilitate coping must be developed and implemented.

Assess, Monitor, and Document

Developmental level: verbal, psychosocial, cognitive, fears
Behavioral response: anxious, fearful, calm, compliant
Response to nursing intervention

Anticipate

Emotional distress
Inability to cope

RESPONSE OF FAMILY

The nurse must be aware of the many factors that influence the behavioral response of parents. After assessment of the response, nursing strategies to facilitate coping and to prepare for discharge can be developed and implemented.

Assess, Monitor, and Document

Behavioral response of parents: anxiety, fear, disappointment
Level of knowledge of disease and condition of child
Expected outcome
Ability to cope
Learning needs related to discharge: signs and symptoms of distress, medication administration, diet
Response to nursing interventions

Anticipate

Family crisis
Inability to cope
Learning needs related to discharge planning
Referral: social service

MIND SET

Assess

Cardiovascular status
Respiratory status

Fluid and electrolyte balance
Response of child and family

Anticipate

Alteration in cardiac function
    Left heart failure: increased pulmonary
      congestion
    Right heart failure
    Shock
    Dysrhythmias
    Cardiac arrest

Alteration in respiratory status
    Respiratory failure
    Respiratory arrest
    Fluid overload
    Electrolyte abnormalities
Emotional distress of child
Family crisis

20

Hypertension

DANIEL A. NOTTERMAN, M.D.

Hypertension denotes an elevation of the systolic or diastolic blood pressure. Normal blood pressure in children increases with age; therefore, the diagnosis of hypertension rests upon comparison of the patient's blood pressure with age-related norms (Fig. 20–1). A child is hypertensive when either the systolic or diastolic blood pressure is greater than the 95th percentile for age.

Hypertension occurs as a primary disease (essential hypertension) or as a process that is secondary to a well-defined pathophysiologic disturbance such as renal artery stenosis. Alternately, hypertension may be an acute complication of severe, often multisystem, illness. This is the usual presentation in the setting of a pediatric intensive care unit (ICU). Thus, elevations of blood pressure are common in children with serious intracranial disturbances and in those with multiple trauma who must undergo prolonged skeletal traction. Severe hypertension occurs in most children who have undergone repair of aortic coarctation and frequently complicates other cardiovascular procedures. Diseases of the kidney such as poststreptococcal glomerulonephritis, obstructive nephropathy, and renal vein thrombosis may be associated with extreme elevations of blood pressure. *Essential* hypertension that is severe enough to warrant admission to an ICU is rare in the pediatric age group. Most hypertensive emergencies, therefore, are secondary to a recognizable underlying disorder. Processes that may be associated with hypertension are listed in Table 20–1.

Hypertension that complicates critical illness is usually acute; thus, it is limited in duration and can be expected to abate with resolution of the underlying illness. For this reason, efforts at controlling blood pressure are directed toward preventing acute, rather than chronic, sequelae.

Whatever the underlying illness, hypertension per se may induce serious target organ injury. The goal of therapy is to prevent this secondary injury. The areas that are principally affected are the central nervous system, the kidneys, and the heart. The secondary injury may inhibit recovery from the underlying illness and may directly threaten life. For this reason, extreme or symptomatic elevations in blood pressure must be treated aggressively. Conversely, because hypertension in the critically ill child is usually limited in duration, modest elevations in blood pressure are best treated expectantly.

EVALUATION

Diagnostic

Evaluation of the hypertensive child must begin with accurate measurement of the blood pressure. The cuff should be appropriate for the size of the child: bladder width two thirds of the arm upper length; the bladder should encircle the arm. The child should be supine and as relaxed as the clinical situation permits. An agitated, screaming child will have an elevated blood pressure, and occasionally it will be necessary to offer sedation and analgesia before meaningful measurements can be made. Unless the elevation is extreme or the child is symptomatic, the blood pressure should be taken three times over a 1-hour period, and the results should be averaged before the diagnosis of hypertension is made. Evaluation should include a meticulous physical examination, with special emphasis on neurologic function (level of consciousness, focal deficits, reflexes) and the condition of the retina. Disturbances in neurologic function that are secondary to hypertension are ominous and mandate immediate therapy, as does the presence of advanced grades of hypertensive retinopathy (Table 20–2).

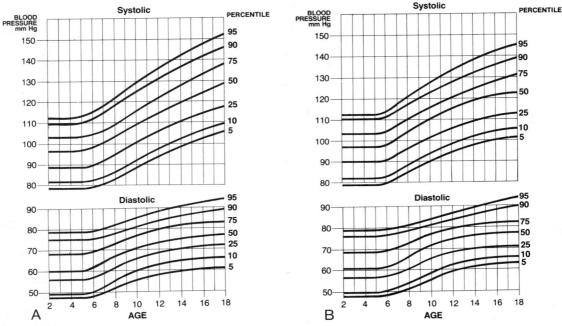

Figure 20–1. *A*, Percentiles of blood pressure measurement in boys (right arm, seated). *B*, Percentiles of blood pressure measurement in girls (right arm, seated). (From Standards for Children's Blood Pressure. Pediatrics [Suppl.] 59:803, 1977. Used by permission.)

Initial laboratory studies should include: 1) serum electrolytes, calcium, BUN, and creatinine; 2) urinalysis; 3) chest x-ray; 4) EKG; and 5) CBC. Abnormalities suggested by the history and physical examination or those detected by the initial laboratory investigation should be clarified by appropriate studies. If the results of initial evaluation are negative and if a specific, treatable cause of hypertension is not suggested by the history or physical examination, further diagnostic studies are not indicated and serve only to disrupt essential care. The major exception to this advice concerns the child in whom the only sign of disease is acute severe hypertension. Such individuals may harbor a serious process such as pheochromocytoma or renal artery stenosis. They should undergo an aggressive diagnostic evaluation, perhaps including intravenous urography and renal angiography.

Therapeutic

The intensity of antihypertensive therapy should be modulated by the magnitude of the elevation and the presence of target organ dysfunction. The initial physical and laboratory evaluations serve to stratify patients into the following categories (Table 20–3).

Malignant Hypertension. The presence of hypertensive encephalopathy, grade IV retinopathy, or severe end-organ dysfunction denotes malignant hypertension. Patients who fall into this category require *emergent therapy.*

Hypertensive encephalopathy may manifest by headache, emesis, diminished mentation, visual disturbances, or seizures. Although the pathophysiology of this disturbance is not clear, it probably results from impaired cerebral autoregulation and consequent cerebral hyperfusion and edema.

Hypertension may trigger dysfunction in other organs systems: *renal*—azotemia, hematuria, proteinuria; *cardiac*—heart failure, myocardial ischemia, left ventricular hypertrophy; and *hematopoetic*—microangiopathic hemolytic anemia. Extreme disturbances in these target organs place the patient in the category of malignant hypertension.

Accelerated Hypertension. Patients with hypertensive retinopathy grade III, moderately severe target organ dysfunction, or severe elevation of blood pressure (e.g., greater than 160/110) have accelerated hypertension. This category also includes patients who are at unusual risk from hypertension, for example the child with pre-existing left ventricular dysfunction. Patients with accelerated hypertension require *urgent* therapy.

Table 20–1. Diseases Associated With Acute Hypertension

Renal
  Post-streptococcal glomerulonephritis
  Hemolytic uremic syndrome
  Renal vein thrombosis
  Arteritis
  Henoch–Schönlein purpura
  Acute or chronic renal failure
  Excessive fluid administration
  Renal artery stenosis
Neurologic
  Intracranial hypertension of any cause (cerebral edema, tumor)
  Intracranial hemorrhage
  Spinal cord injury
  Post-craniotomy (brain stem or posterior fossa manipulation)
  Guillain-Barré syndrome
Orthopedic
  Skeletal traction
Endocrinologic
  Congenital adrenal hyperplasia
  Cushing's syndrome
  Hyperplaosteronism
  Exogenous corticosteroid administration
  Pheochromocytoma/Neuroblastoma
  Hypercalcemia
Cardiovascular
  Coarctation of the aorta
  Post-PDA (patent ductus arteriosus) repair
  Post-coarctation repair
  Essential hypertension
Drugs
  Pressor infusions
  Intoxications
  Antihypertensive medication withdrawal
  Corticosteroids

Simple Acute Hypertension. Hypertension that is not associated with target organ dysfunction is termed simple acute hypertension. Patients with this condition may or may not require therapy depending upon the intensity and duration of hypertension, as well as associated medical or surgical conditions.

THERAPY

Emergent Therapy

Patients with malignant hypertension require immediate control of blood pressure. The goal is not to normalize blood pressure but to reduce it to a level that relieves acute symptoms. Usually it is not necessary to acutely reduce the diastolic pressure below 90 mm Hg. Two agents, nitroprusside and diazoxide, are available for this purpose (see Tables 20–4 and 20–5).

Nitroprusside. The agent of choice for malignant hypertension is sodium nitroprusside. This drug causes a prompt (within seconds) increase in venous capacitance and a decrease in arterial resistance. There is a moderate increase in heart rate. In patients with normal myocardial function, the cardiac output is unchanged or slightly reduced. Patients in heart failure may experience a beneficial increase in cardiac output.

The half-life of nitroprusside is quite short. The fall in blood pressure is almost immediate, and blood pressure rises promptly when the infusion is reduced or terminated. These characteristics allow the physician to titrate the patient's blood pressure to the desired range.

Side effects are uncommon. Nausea, diaphoresis, palpitations, and chest pain are related to a too rapid reduction in blood pressure and are ameliorated by reducing the rate of infusion. Hypotension may occur but is quickly (within minutes) reversed upon stopping the medication. Nitroprusside is metabolized to cyanide and thiocyanate, and cyanide intoxication may occur. Accumulation of cyanide is unusual during short-term therapy; if the agent is required for more than 72 hours when there is hepatic dysfunction, it is prudent to determine the blood cyanide level on a daily basis. Poor renal function may cause accumulation of thiocyanate and subsequent toxicity. Patients with reduced glomerular filtration rate (GFR) should have daily thiocyanate levels performed, and

Table 20–2. Hypertensive Retinopathy

	A/V Ratio	Hemorrhage	Exudate	Papilledema
Normal	3/4	0	0	0
Grade I	1/2	0	0	0
Grade II	1/3	0	0	0
Grade III	1/4	+	+	0
Grade IV	Fine cord	+	+	+

Modified from Thorn, G.W. ed.: Principles of Internal Medicine. New York, McGraw-Hill, Inc. 1977.

Table 20–3. Diagnostic Categories for Acute Hypertension

Malignant Hypertension
Hypertension with
Encephalopathy *or*
Grade IV retinopathy *or*
Severe end-organ damage (i.e., acute CHF, azotemia, intravascular hemolysis) *or*
Pronounced risk of progression (i.e., post-aortic coarctation repair)
Accelerated Hypertension
Hypertension with
Grade III retinopathy *or*
End-organ damage *or*
Marked acute elevation of BP (i.e., 160/110) *or*
Increased risk from hypertension (i.e., leaking aneurysm, after intracranial surgery)
Simple Acute Hypertension
Hypertension with none of the previous factors

---

the infusion should be stopped if levels exceed 10 mcg per dl.

Dosage and Administration. The infusion is compounded by adding the contents of one vial (50 mg) to the desired amount of 5 percent dextrose, D5W, (usually 250 ml). The solution is photosensitive and must be protected from light by wrapping the IV bottle in an opaque material such as foil. Diluted nitroprusside has a faint brownish tint; if highly colored, the solution should be discarded. The mixture is stable for 24 hours after preparation. Nitroprusside should be administered by a separate IV catheter; it should not be piggybacked into other solutions.

The starting dosage is 0.5 mcg per kg per minute. The dosage should be increased at 10-minute intervals until the desired blood pressure is reached. The average therapeutic dosage is 3 μg per kg per minute; it is not advisable to exceed 10 μg per kg per minute.

As soon as a stable, safe blood pressure is achieved, the patient should be started on other antihypertensive medication (usually hydralazine or methyldopa) so that the nitroprusside can be gradually tapered and discontinued.

Nitroprusside is exceptionally potent; therefore, it must be administered only in a critical care area that is capable of providing continuous (1:1) nursing and physician surveillance. Blood pressure should be monitored continuously by means of an indwelling arterial catheter. In cases that are complicated by myocardial dysfunction, it is prudent to monitor the central venous pressure (CVP) or, if possible, the mean capillary wedge pressure (MCWP) and cardiac output by means of a pulmonary artery catheter.

Diazoxide. This drug is an alternative to nitroprusside for control of malignant hypertension or severe accelerated hypertension. Diazoxide is chemically related to the thiazide diuretics. It causes direct dilatation of arterioles but has little effect upon venous capacitance vessels. It does not affect autonomic function, and cardiovascular reflexes are not disturbed. When injected intravenously, there is a prompt (1 to 5 minutes) reduction in systolic and diastolic blood pressure and a concomitant rise in pulse and cardiac output. In the absence of fixed arterial stenosis, regional blood flow is preserved. The drug is extensively protein bound, and its pharmacologic effect depends upon the concentration of free or unbound drug. For this reason, rapid (30 seconds), bolus injection is said to be necessary for maximal effect. The half life of diazoxide is 28 hours, and the duration of action is 2 to 12 hours.

Serious adverse effects include hypotension and coronary or cerebral ischemia. The effect upon hemodynamics is such as to increase sheer forces upon the aortic wall. Thus, diazoxide is contraindicated in the presence of dissecting aortic aneurysm or after recent vascular surgery.

Diazoxide causes salt and water retention, and a diuretic may become necessary after 24 hours of therapy. Other effects include hyperglycemia (very common); hyperuricemia; gastrointestinal disturbances; and, rarely, hypersensitivity reaction. Extravasation of the drug produces severe pain.

Dosage and Administration. In the past, the entire dosage (adult: 300 mg; child: 5 mg per kg was administered as a single bolus. This practice was irrational and dangerous. Currently, repetitive smaller dosages are favored. An initial IV bolus of 1 to 2 mg per kg (maximum 75 to 150 mg) is administered. Blood pressure is monitored continuously. The same dosage is repeated every 5 to 15 minutes until a satisfactory blood pressure is achieved. After the blood pressure has been lowered to a safe level, repeated injections of diazoxide are given as needed every 4 to 24 hours. Alternative oral or parenteral therapy (usually with methyldopa) should be started as soon as it is practical. Diazoxide may potentiate the action of other antihypertensives; thus, the initial dosage of these agents should be reduced by one half.

Therapy with diazoxide should not be continued for more than 2 or 3 days. The dosage of the drug should be reduced in the presence of uremia or other conditions known to affect protein binding.

The potential for serious hypotension mandates that diazoxide be used only in the setting of a critical care unit by physicians familiar with its use. In my judgment, nitroprusside, is the agent of choice for treatment of malignant hypertension.

Urgent Therapy

Patients with **accelerated hypertension** require urgent control of blood pressure. This means that the diastolic blood pressure should be reduced to 90 mm Hg within 4 to 6 hours. Two agents, hydralazine and methyldopa, are valuable for this purpose (Tables 20–4 and 20–5).

Hydralazine. This agent lowers blood pressure by causing arteriolar dilatation. The systemic vascular resistance decreases, and heart rate and cardiac output may be increased.

When administered by vein, the antihypertensive effect begins within 15 to 30 minutes and persists for 3 to 4 hours. As with other agents that cause arteriolar dilatation, hydralazine promotes salt and water accumulation. The other significant side effect is reflex tachycardia. This increase in heart rate may augment the cardiac output so much that the hypotensive effect of hydralazine is blunted. The reflex may be offset by concomitant treatment with a beta-adrenergic blocking agent such as propranolol. However, oral propranolol acts too slowly to be of value in acute hypertension, and IV propranolol is too hazardous to be recommended for routine use. Thus, in the context

Table 20–4. Drugs for Hypertensive Emergencies

Drug	Dosage	Onset	Peak	Side Effects
Vasodilators				
Hydralazine	0.2–0.8 mg/kg/dose q 4–6 hr (maximum 3.2 mg/kg/ 24 hr) PO/IM/IV	IV, 15–30 min	IV/IM/PO 3–4 hr	Tachycardia, fluid retention, GI disturbance, headache, myocardial ischemia, lupus-like syndrome
Nitroprusside	IV infusion, 0.5–10 mcg/ kg/min titrated to response, average dosage = 3 mcg/kg/min	Immediate	—	Hypotension, tachycardia, fluid retention, nausea, headache, palpitation, chest pain, cyanide or thiocyanate intoxication
Diazoxide	IV bolus, 1–2 mg/kg (maximum 75–150 mg), repeat q 5–15 min until BP is controlled	1–5 min	—	Hypotension regional ischemia, fluid retention, hyperglycemia, hyperuricemia, hypersensitivity
Sympatholytics				
Methyldopa	5–10 mg/kg/dose (maximum 500 mg) q 4–6 hr IV/PO	IV, 1–2 hr	3–4 hr	Sedation, nasal stuffiness, Coombs' + hemolytic anemia, liver dysfunction, paradoxic hypertension (IV)
Reserpine	0.02–0.07 mg/kg/dose IM/PO (maximum first dose 0.5 mg)	2–4 hr (IM)	4–8 hr (IM) (weeks, PO)	Sedation, depression, nightmares, abdominal cramps, peptic ulcer
Propranolol	PO, 0.5–2 mg/kg/day q 6–12 hr IV, 0.1 mg/kg/dose (maximum 1.0 mg) (use extreme caution)	IV, Immediate PO, 4–6 hr	—	Bronchospasm, heart block, asystole, CHF, hypoglycemia
Diuretics				
Chlorothiazide	PO, 10–20 mg/kg/day q 12–24 hr	1 hr	—	Azotemia, hypokalemia, hyperglycemia, hyperuricemia, hypercalcemia, blood dyscrasia, hypersensitivity (rash, photosensitivity), pancreatitis
Furosemide	IV/PO, 1 mg/kg/dose q 6–12 hr	IV, 1–2 min PO, 1 hr	2 hr (IV) 6 hr (PO)	Hypokalemia, hyperglycemia, hyperuricemia, blood dyscrasia, dermatologic reactions, ototoxicity, dehydration, interstitial nephritis

Table 20–5. Treatment of Acute Hypertension

Malignant Hypertension
  Sodium nitroprusside (drug of choice)
  Diazoxide
  Use diuretic only if there is evidence of fluid retention
Accelerated Hypertension
  Methyldopa or hydralazine
  If response is inadequate, use both concurrently
  If response to combination therapy is inadequate, use
    nitroprusside or reserpine
  Add diuretic after 48 hr
Simple Acute Hypertension
  Treat if persistent
  Begin therapy with diuretic
  Subsequent management as for chronic hypertension

of *acute* hypertension, marked tachycardia should prompt consideration of an antihypertensive agent other than hydralazine.

Other side effects of hydralazine include headache, which can be minimized by gradual increases in dosage, gastrointestinal disturbances, rash, and blood dyscrasias. A lupus-like syndrome (fever; arthralgia; positive antinuclear antibody) has been noted and is dose related.

The initial IV dosage is 0.2 mg per kg given over a 1-minute period. This amount can be repeated hourly to a maximum of 0.8 mg per kg over a 6-hour period if the initial response is unsatisfactory. The total amount required to achieve control is then administered every 6 hours as a single dose.

If therapy with hydralazine is continued for more than 48 hours, a diuretic should be added (usually thiazide) to offset fluid accumulation. After satisfactory control of blood pressure has been achieved and when the child's overall condition permits, the drug can be given orally. The dosage is the same as that effective by vein and is administered in three or four divided doses.

Methyldopa. This is a centrally acting agent that decreases sympathetic tone and peripheral vascular resistance. Heart rate and cardiac output may be reduced, but renal blood flow is maintained. IV administration produces a fall in blood pressure that begins within 1 to 2 hours and persists for 4 to 6 hours. After oral administration of the drug, blood pressure begins to fall in 4 hours, reaches a nadir in 6 to 8 hours, and returns to baseline in 12 to 24 hours. With repetitive doses, a maximal effect is recorded in 3 to 5 days.

A major side effect is sedation, which occurs soon after therapy is initiated and may be desirable in critically ill children. Other effects include dryness of the mouth, nasal congestion, and a positive result of a Coombs' test. The latter occurs in about 20 percent of patients who receive the drug. Unless there is evidence of hemolysis, a positive reaction from a Coombs' test is not an indication to discontinue the drug. Paradoxical hypertension has been noted after IV administration of methyldopa. Treatment of this unusual response includes cessation of the methyldopa infusion and initiation of a different agent, usually hydralazine. Other adverse effects include drug-induced hepatitis, drug fever (often pronounced), blood dyscrasias, and myocarditis. Impotence and orthostatic hypotension occur, but not frequently; neither is relevant in critically ill children.

Therapy for accelerated hypertension should begin with a slow IV infusion of 5 to 10 mg per kg. If the blood pressure is not at a satisfactory level within 2 hours, the dose can be repeated. Subsequent doses should be given every 6 hours, with a maximum daily dosage of 40 mg per kg (2 gm).

After the blood pressure has been lowered to an acceptable level and the patient is otherwise stable, the medication can be switched to the oral form in the same daily dosage. Methyldopa promotes retention of salt and water. If therapy continues for more than 48 hours, diuretic therapy should be added, generally with a thiazide.

Occasionally, methyldopa or hydralazine given alone is insufficient to cause adequate reduction in blood pressure. In this circumstance, the drugs should be used concurrently, given alternately every 3 hours.

Rarely, even combination therapy with methyldopa and hydralazine is ineffective in lowering blood pressure. In this circumstance, sodium nitroprusside will provide immediate reduction of blood pressure and will do so in a safe, controlled manner. If this agent is chosen, both hydralazine and methyldopa should be continued. After a period of stabilization on the nitroprusside, the infusion should be tapered and discontinued. After the blood pressure has been controlled on nitroprusside, it will usually remain at an acceptable level during subsequent therapy with methyldopa and hydralazine.

Reserpine is an alternative to sodium nitroprusside in cases of accelerated hypertension that do not respond to methyldopa and hydralazine.

Reserpine. This drug is a rauwolfia alkaloid that causes depletion of catecholamine stores. This produces a reduction in peripheral vascular resistance, slowing of the heart rate, and a decrease in cardiac output. Side effects that are dose related and relatively common include sedation and psychic depression. Reserpine augments gastrointestinal tone and stomach acid secretion. For these reasons, the drug should not be given to patients with a history of depression or peptic ulcer disease. Other adverse effects include nasal congestion, nightmares, and water retention. The dosage is 0.02 to 0.07 mg per kg per dose (maximum of 0.5 mg). For acute hypertension, the drug is given by intramuscular (IM) injection (*never* IV). The onset is 2 to 4 hours, the maximal effect is 4 to 6 hours, and the duration of action is 10 to 12 hours. It is best to begin with a dosage of 0.02 mg per kg (maximum 0.5 mg); if the blood pressure is not appreciably lower in 3 to 4 hours, a dose of 0.04 to 0.07 mg per kg (maximum 1 mg) can be given. As soon as possible, reserpine should be discontinued in favor of agents with fewer adverse effects.

Therapy of Simple Acute Hypertension

Treatment of children with no evidence of target organ damage must be individualized. Many children with mild to moderate acute elevations of blood pressure do not require therapy. Often, adequate sedation and analgesia will produce satisfactory reduction in blood pressure. If this is not the case and the elevation is moderately severe or persistent, specific therapy may be indicated (Table 20–5). Methyldopa or hydralazine, in the dosages outlined previously, will usually prove effective. Although IV administration usually results in more rapid reduction in blood pressure, most patients in this category are satisfactorily controlled on oral therapy. If treatment is continued for more than a few days, a diuretic (usually a thiazide) should be added. If hypertension persists beyond the acute illness, the patient should be classified as having chronic hypertension. A complete diagnostic evaluation is indicated. Details about the evaluation procedure can be found in several reviews of the subject.

CASE PRESENTATION

Malignant Hypertension

A 10-year-old boy underwent surgery for repair of aortic coarctation. Preoperatively, the blood pressure in his upper extremity was 120/85, and in his lower extremity, the blood pressure was 65/40. He weighed 32 kg. There were no complicating conditions. The patient tolerated the procedure well and was extubated 8 hours after leaving the operating room. Upon admission to the pediatric ICU, his blood pressure was 135/90 by radial arterial catheter. The results of laboratory tests, including CBC, SMA–6, and urinalysis were all normal. Within 4 hours of admission to the unit, however, the patient complained of severe frontal headache and began to retch. BP was 170/115 mm Hg, pulse was 120 beats/min, and T was 100°F. The neck was supple, but examination of the fundi revealed arteriolar narrowing. Results of the general physical examination were not contributory. Neurologic examination disclosed a disoriented child. There were no focal motor deficits. Deep tendon reflexes were symmetrically increased, and a Babinski sign was present on the right. Arterial blood gas results were normal. Except for 2+ hematuria, other laboratory tests were unchanged.

The diagnosis was malignant hypertension with hypertensive encephalopathy. This finding was based upon the severity of blood pressure elevation and the neurologic findings of headache, emesis, and hyperreflexia. The etiology of the hypertension was ascribed to excision of the coarctation.

A second IV catheter was inserted, and the patient was placed in a reverse Trendelenburg position. The arterial blood pressure was continuously monitored by the child's physician, who remained at the bedside. Sodium nitroprusside was started at an initial dosage of 16 mcg per minute (0.5 mcg per kg per min). The dosage was increased by 0.5 mcg per kg per minute at 10-minute intervals until the blood pressure fell to 140/90. A dosage of 96 mcg per minute (3 mcg per kg per min) was required to achieve this response. Over the next 60 minutes, the blood pressure remained stable, although small adjustments in the rate of infusion were necessary. The child's neurologic symptoms abated. After 12 hours of therapy with nitroprusside, the patient was placed on methyldopa, 10 mg per kg IV every 6 hours. With this regimen, it was not possible to substantially reduce the dosage of nitroprusside. Hydralazine was added, at a dosage of 0.8 mg per kg every 6 hours, alternating with the methyldopa. Subsequently, it was possible to taper and discontinue the nitroprusside over a 24-hour period. At this time, the blood pressure was 140/85. After an additional 24 hours, the antihypertensive medications were changed to the oral route. Six months after surgery, the patient is hemodynamically normal and does not require antihypertensive medication. His blood pressure is 120/75.

SUGGESTED READING

Balfe, J.W., and Rance, C.P.: Recognition and management of hypertensive crises in childhood. Pediatr. Clin. North Am. 25:159, 1978.

Gilman, A.G., Goodman, L., and Gilman, A.: The Pharmacological Basis of Therapeutics. New York, Macmillan Publishing Co., Inc., 1980.

Palmer, R.J., and Lasseter, K.C.: Sodium nitroprusside. N. Engl. J. Med. 292:294, 1975.

Reisman, L., and Selden, R.: Management of systemic hypertension in children. Pediatr. Ann. 11:604, 1982.

The Medical Letter: Drugs for hypertension. 23:45, May 15, 1981.

Recommendations of the Task Force on Blood Pressure Control in Children. Pediatrics 59:797, 1977.

Nursing Process for Patient Care:

Hypertension

The usual presentation of hypertension in the pediatric critical care unit is in response to some severe illness. It can be anticipated in children with neurologic, neurosurgical, and cardiovascular problems. Hypertension can also occur as a result of renal pathophysiology.

The mind set that emerges focuses on the significance of the elevation of the blood pressure as it relates to other organs.

BLOOD PRESSURE

Assess, Monitor, and Document

Blood pressure
 Serial measurement
 Appropriate cuff size (bladder width 2/3 the upper arm length; bladder length encompasses the arm circumference)

Appropriate procedure: child supine, relaxed (as possible)
Response to pharmacologic intervention

Anticipate

Blood pressure elevation
 Malignant hypertension: encephalopathy, severe end-organ dysfunction
 Accelerated hypertension: Blood pressure

> 160/110 and moderately severe organ dysfunction
Simple acute hypertension: no target organ involvement

NEUROLOGIC

Neurologic dysfunction occurs with significant elevation of blood pressure. The pathophysiology of the disturbance is not clear. It is thought to occur as a result of impaired cerebral autoregulation and consequent cerebral hyperperfusion and edema. Disturbances in neurologic function are ominous and mandate immediate therapy.

Access, Monitor, and Document

Headache
Vomiting
Level of consciousness

Pupillary activity
Reflexes
Focal deficits

Anticipate

Hypertensive encephalopathy: altered level of consciousness, seizures

CARDIOVASCULAR

Assess, Monitor, and Document

Rate
Rhythm

Perfusion
Breath sounds

Anticipate

Heart failure
Dysrhythmias

RENAL

Assess, Monitor, and Document

Urine output: specific gravity, protein, glucose, blood
Serum electrolytes, BUN, creatinine, osmolality

Urine electrolytes and osmolality
Fluid intake
Weight

Anticipate

Azotemia
Hematuria
Proteinuria

RESPONSE OF CHILD AND FAMILY

Hypertension in the pediatric intensive care unit (ICU) usually occurs as a result of an underlying problem; it is not generally a primary medical problem. Consequently, nursing activities that were previously implemented to deal with the emotional aspects of this illness and hospitalization must be altered so that hypertension can be treated.

Assess, Monitor, and Document

Behavioral responses: anxiety, fear, anger, disappointment
Ability to cope with secondary diagnosis

Strategies used to facilitate coping: provide information, listen, support

Anticipate

Emotional distress

MIND SET

Assess

Blood pressure: serial measurement, appropriate procedure, response to pharmacologic intervention
Neurologic status

Cardiovascular status
Renal status
Response of child and family

Anticipate

Blood pressure elevation
Hypertensive encephalopathy
  headache
  altered level of consciousness
  seizures
Alteration in renal function
  azotemia
  hematuria
  proteinuria
Alteration in cardiovascular status
  Heart failure
Alteration in child's and family's response to
  diagnosis of hypertension as a complication
  of the underlying problem

Common Complications in Infants with Cyanotic Congenital Heart Disease

MONIKA RUTKOWSKI, M.D.

Cyanosis secondary to congenital heart disease is due to intracardiac right-to-left shunting. Admixture of desaturated blood with saturated blood results in an arterial oxygen saturation under 90 percent. Cyanotic heart disease can be divided into two groups of anatomic defects that cause either diminished pulmonary blood flow (group I) or increased pulmonary blood flow (group II). The most common defects in group I are tetralogy of Fallot, pulmonary atresia with intact ventricular septum, and tricuspid atresia, whereas transposition of the great arteries, total anomalous venous return, and truncus arteriosus most frequently represent the defects in group II. Tables 21–1 and 21–2 list the different defects, with their respective findings on noninvasive examination.

Many of these infants may rapidly deteriorate at the time that the ductus arteriosus or patent foramen ovale closes and may then require early intervention to improve their systemic hypoxemia. It is, therefore, common practice to establish a definitive diagnosis with a cardiac catheterization during the neonatal period, even if the cyanotic infant appears stable.

The most frequently performed procedures for the cyanotic defects are listed in Tables 21–3 and 21–4. Most of these are surgical interventions, so-called palliative procedures, with the important exception of balloon septostomy for transposition of the great arteries. The most recently introduced administration of prostaglandin E has improved the outcome of the group I lesions by ensuring the patency of the ductus arteriosus until a shunt can be established.

After he is beyond the neonatal age, the infant with cyanotic heart disease is still at risk of developing complications, some of which are direct sequelae of a particular cardiac lesion; some are common to all cyanotic defects. Typical for the infant with tetralogy of Fallot is the cyanotic spell. One of the underlying mechanisms is a spasm of the right ventricular infundibular area, decreasing the pulmonary flow even further and increasing the right-to-left shunting at the ventricular level. The patient becomes severely hypoxic and, depending upon the length of the spell, acidotic. Cyanotic spells are usually first seen at the age of 3 to 5 months. Most first spells are not fatal but are a reflection of severe infundibular hypertrophy and an indication for surgical intervention. The acute treatment for the cyanotic spell aims at alleviating the infundibular spasm, establishing a normal respiratory pattern, and increasing the pulmonary blood flow (Table 21–5). After the spell is reversed and the condition is stabilized, a complete repair or a shunt procedure, depending upon the severity of the pulmonary artery hypoplasia, is undertaken. If a shunt is selected in the hope of increasing the growth of the pulmonary arteries with the increased flow, the patient must be carefully followed for shunt obstruction. Slowly increasing cyanosis and a diminishing amplitude of the shunt murmur will indicate shunt occlusion. A repeat surgical procedure, usually repair, can be scheduled electively. Repair of tetralogy of Fallot removes the right ventricular outflow obstruction and closes the ventricular septal defect (VSD). In general, the procedure will result in an acyanotic patient with a good exercise tolerance.

Table 21–1. Cyanotic Congenital Cardiac Defects with Decreased Pulmonary Blood Flow

Cardiac Lesion	Physical Examination	EKG	X-ray	Echocardiogram
Tetralogy of Fallot	Systolic ejection murmur	RVH		Overriding aorta, VSD
Pulmonary atresia with intact septum	No significant murmur	RAH ?RVH		Atretic PV
Tricuspid atresia	Murmur of VSD or PDA	LDEA; RAH; LVH		Atretic TV, minute RV

Key: RVH = right ventricular hypertrophy, VSD = ventricular septal defect, RAH = right atrial hypertrophy, PV = pulmonic valve, PDA = patent ductus arteriosus, LDEA = left axis deviation, LVH = left ventricular hypertrophy, TV = tricuspid valve, RV = right ventricle.

A hemodynamically very different problem is encountered in patients with transposition of the great arteries. Fibrosis or an inadequate balloon septostomy may lead to a decrease or complete closure of the atrial communication. Life, however, is dependent upon the exchange of blood between the pulmonary and systemic circuit across the atrial defect in the simple transposition. With a diminishing exchange, the infant will become increasingly cyanotic, irritable, unable to feed, and dyspneic. If these signs are not recognized, the infant will become acidotic and will eventually succumb. Balloon atrial septostomy is rarely successful at this age. Surgical atrial septectomy (Blalock–Hanlon procedure) or preferably a complete repair (Senning or Mustard procedure) should be performed. The complete repair creates a new systemic venous atrium, with its drainage across the mitral valve into the left ventricle and a pulmonary venous atrium draining, via a tricuspid valve, into the right ventricle, in essence a switch of the venous return to the heart. One commonly encounters atrial dysrhythmias in the postoperative period, and very rarely, a sick sinus syndrome with brady- and tachydysrhythmias. Most of these dysrhythmias can be controlled medically; rarely is a pacemaker needed.

All defects in group II are characterized by a markedly increased pulmonary blood flow. The volume overload often leads to congestive heart failure (CHF), with its onset usually at the end of the neonatal period. Digitalization and appropriate diuretic therapy are indicated (Table 21–6).

Common to all cyanotic congenital heart disease is the cerebral vascular accident (CVA), occurring in infants younger than 2 years of age. The infant may be well but then suddenly develops convulsions and hemiplegia. The etiology of the CVA is not entirely clear but is thought to be secondary to anoxia, cerebral thrombosis, or embolism. Occasionally, a relationship to hot weather or diarrhea with dehydration is found. Conservative therapy with oxygen, cautious hydration, and surgical procedures to improve the systemic desaturation are indicated. It is of utmost importance to rule out the presence of a brain abscess, which, al-

Table 21–2. Cyanotic Congenital Cardiac Defects with Increased Pulmonary Blood Flow

Cardiac Lesion	Physical Examination	EKG	X-ray	Echocardiogram
Transposition of great arteries	No significant murmurs	RVH		Transposed arteries
Total anomalous pulmonary venous drainage	No significant murmurs	RAH, RVH		Abnormal structures posterior to La
Truncus arteriosus	Systolic click Single S_2	RVH or LVH		Overriding aorta VSD

Key: RVH = right ventricular hypertrophy, RAH = right atrial hypertrophy, LVH = left ventricular hypertrophy, La = left atrium, S_2 = second heart sound, VSD = ventricular septal defect

though an unusual occurrence in those younger than the age of 2 years, would require very active intervention.

The following case reports underline the clinical aspects and management of some of the more common complications of infants with cyanotic heart disease.

Table 21–3. Palliative Procedures for Cyanotic Defects

Defect	Procedure
Tetralogy of Fallot	Blalock–Taussig shunt (subclavian artery to pulmonary artery) Central shunt (Gore-Tex graft between aorta and pulmonary artery)
Pulmonary atresia	Shunt procedures as above plus valvulotomy
Tricuspid atresia	Shunt procedures as above Glenn procedure after age 4 months (anastomosis of superior venae cava to right pulmonary artery)
Transposition of great arteries	Atrial balloon septostomy Blalock–Hanlon procedure (surgical atrial septectomy)
Truncus arteriosus	Banding of pulmonary artery

CASE HISTORY 1

Tetralogy of Fallot (TOF)

H.E. is the product of a normal spontaneous delivery and gestation with a birth weight of 3.2 kg. Circumoral cyanosis and a grade 2/6 holosystolic

Table 21–4. "Complete Repair" for Cyanotic Defects

Defect	Procedure
Tetralogy of Fallot	Closure of VSD, resection of infundibular hypertrophy, reconstruction of pulmonary valve and pulmonary arteries
Pulmonary atresia	Insertion of valved conduit into right ventricle
Tricuspid atresia	Fontan procedure (connection of right atrial appendage to left pulmonary artery)
Transposition of great arteries	Senning or Mustard procedure (switching of venous return to the heart and creation of new atria)
Truncus arteriosus	Closure of ventricular septal defect, insertion of valved conduit into right ventricle
Total anomalous pulmonary venous return	Anastomosis between pulmonary venous channel and left atrium

Table 21–5. Management of the Cyanotic Spell

Measures	Effect
Oxygen by mask	Increase of the free dissolved plasma oxygen
Knee–chest position	Increase of systemic resistance and venous return
Morphine sulfate (0.2 mg/ kg, SC)	Central sedation of respiratory center
Propranolol (0.15–0.25 mg/kg, IV)	Relaxation of infundibular spasm
Sodium bicarbonate (1 mEq/kg, IV)	Correction of acidosis

Table 21–6. Treatment for Group II Defects

Digitalization
Total digitalizing dose (TDD) for infants younger than 2 yr
50–60 μg/kg, po
50 μg/kg, IV
TDD is divided into 1/2, 1/4, and 1/4 and is given in 6 to 8-hour intervals
Maintenance—10 μg/kg/day, divided into two doses, po
Diuretic Therapy
Furosemide 0.5–1 mg/kg/dose, IV
2–4 mg/kg/dose, po

murmur along the left sternal border are noted in the first hour of life. An arterial blood gas shows the arterial PO_2 to be 42 mm Hg and 45 mm Hg in 0.8 FIO_2 The EKG is normal for age, the chest x-ray film shows a "boot-shaped" heart with decreased pulmonary blood flow, and the echocardiogram is pathognomonic for TOF. The cardiac catheterization demonstrates severe infundibular hypertrophy and obstruction, a small pulmonic valve annulus and pulmonary artery branches, a large ventricular septal defect, and an overriding aorta. The infant is comfortable and able to feed fairly well in spite of the cyanosis. During the following 4 months, the infant's general condition remains stable with a slow, steady weight gain. Mild cyanosis at rest and moderately severe cyanosis with crying persist. The hematocrit at 4 months of age is 48 percent.

At age 5 months, the infant suddenly became irritable, hyperpneic, with a severe increase in the cyanosis, and then limp and unconscious when picked up from his crib in the morning. The episode lasted about 5 minutes. By the time the parents reached the hospital, the infant was in his usual state of health, alert and playful. Three hours later, following a bowel movement, a similar episode occurred. At that time, the examination revealed a severely cyanotic, hypotonic, comatose infant, in whom no heart murmur could be detected. There was no seizure activity.

A cyanotic spell was diagnosed. The infant was immediately put into knee–chest position, and an oxygen mask was held over the face. One mg of morphine sulfate (0.2 mg/kg; 4.8 kg) was given subcutaneously. An intravenous line was established, and 1 mg of propranolol (0.2 mg/kg) was given intravenously. An arterial blood gas revealed a PO_2 of 33 mm Hg and a pH of 7.21. Five mEq of bicarbonate was given intravenously. Within 2 minutes of the propranolol injection, a systolic murmur became audible at the upper left sternal border, indicating a reopening of the infundibular area. The infant's color improved, and the respiratory rate was decreased to normal levels. The infant was arousable

but sleepy. A repeat arterial blood gas showed a pH of 7.33 and a PO_2 of 42 mm Hg. One hour later, the infant was fully awake, playful, and without neurologic defects. A repeat catheterization done the following day showed that the infundibular obstruction had become much more severe. The main pulmonary artery and the pulmonary artery branches were still very small, as was the pulmonic annulus. It was therefore decided to perform a Blalock–Taussig shunt rather than complete repair at this stage.

CASE HISTORY 2

Transposition of the Great Arteries (TGA)

D.A. is the product of an uncomplicated pregnancy and delivery with a birth weight of 4 kg. At 2 hours of age, he is noted to be tachypneic and cyanotic. Lungs are clear, and there is no heart murmur. The EKG shows the normal right ventricular preponderance for a newborn, and the chest x-ray reveals an increase in heart size, with a narrow mediastinum and increased pulmonary vascularity. The echocardiogram shows a TGA, a patent foramen ovale, and an intact ventricular septum. An arterial gas in room air shows a Pa_{O_2} of 26 mm Hg, a PCO_2 of 22 mm Hg, and a pH of 7.30. The patient is taken to the catheterization laboratory where the diagnosis of TGA is confirmed, and a balloon atrial septostomy is performed. Immediately following the procedure, the Pa_{O_2} is 40 mm Hg. The infant's general condition is improved, with fair feeding capability. Digitalization brings the respiratory rate down to an average of 50 breaths per minute.

Over the next 8 weeks, the infant becomes increasingly cyanotic, with a rising hematocrit, 55 percent, and poor intake. The weight gain has leveled off. A repeat echocardiogram at age 9 weeks suggests complete closure of the atrial septal defect. The infant is irritable, tachypneic, and very blue. The arterial Pa_{O_2} is 26 mm Hg, the PCO_2 is 21 mm Hg, and the pH is 7.34. By the time the infant reached the ward, he appeared grey and cyanotic, and had poor reflexes and a respiratory rate of 110 breaths per minute. An arterial blood gas revealed a pH of 7.18 and a PO_2 of 21 mm Hg. An IV line was established and 5 mEq of bicarbonate were given. The FIO_2 was increased to 1.0. An infusion of prostaglandin E (0.1

μg/kg/min) was begun, with the scant hope of reopening the ductus arteriosus. Five mg of furosemide (1 mg/kg) were given IV. The infant was typed and crossmatched, and the cardiovascular surgeon was notified. A repeat blood gas showed a pH of 7.28, a PO_2 of 22 mm Hg, and a PCO_2 of 55 mm Hg. There were bilateral rales, with increasing retractions and fatigue of the infant. An elective intubation was undertaken. The infant's condition stabilized over the next 3 hours, with a borderline pH and scant urinary output of 15 ml. At that time, the infant was taken to the operating room for a Senning procedure.

In summary, acute problems in infants with cyanotic heart disease, that is, anoxic spells, shunt obstruction, or closure of an atrial septal defect frequently occur and must be recognized as such and treated as emergencies.

SUGGESTED READING

Engle, M.A.: Pediatric Cardiovascular Disease. *In* Brest, A.N. (ed.): Cardiovascular Clinics. Philadelphia, F.A. Davis Co., 1981, pp. 323–336, 337–342, 343–352, 353–364.

Gersony, W.M.: A practical approach to the neonate with cyanosis. Res. Staff Phys. Dec., 59, 1976.

Moss, A.J., Adams, F.H., and Emmanouilides, G.C.: Heart Disease in Infants, Children, and Adolescents, 2nd ed. Baltimore, Williams & Wilkins, Chapters 17–19 and 27, 1977.

Roberts, W.C., Mason, D.T., Engle, M.A., and Cohn, L.H.: Cardiology 1981. Yorke Medical Books, pp. 262, 269–276, 277–279, 284–285, 1981.

Common Complications in Infants with Cyanotic Congenital Heart Disease

Cyanotic congenital heart disease involves lesions in which a right-to-left shunt occurs. The admixture of saturated blood with desaturated blood results in cyanosis. These lesions are further divided anatomically into two groups. In the first group are those defects that cause a decrease in pulmonary blood flow; in the second group are those defects that cause an increase in pulmonary blood flow. The nurse must know the hemodynamics involved in the basic defect to be able to determine assessment parameters.

Common complications are associated with cyanotic congenital heart disease and may be the result of a particular lesion or common to all cyanotic defects. Nursing management must include anticipation of these complications.

CARDIOPULMONARY

Assess, Monitor, and Document

Rate
Rhythm
Perfusion: presence and quality of peripheral
    pulses
Blood pressure
Respiratory rate
Respiratory pattern

Work of breathing
Breath sounds
Color
Level of consciousness
Response to medical and pharmacologic
    management

Anticipate

Cyanotic spell (tetralogy of Fallot, TOF)
Hyperpnea
    Increased cyanosis
    Altered level of consciousness: lethargy,
        syncope
Deterioration in status secondary to closure
    of atrial communication (Transposition of
    the Great Arteries, TGA) or palliative shunt
    occlusion

    Increased cyanosis, dyspnea, irritable, dif-
        ficult to feed.
Congestive heart failure (truncus arteriosus,
    Transposition of the Great Arteries)
    Difficult to feed, poor weight gain, irritable,
        tachypnea, diaphoresis

NEUROLOGIC

All children with cyanotic congenital heart disease are at risk for neurologic sequelae secondary to thrombotic or embolic phenomenon and brain abscess.

Assess, Monitor, and Document

Level of consciousness: restless, irritable,
    lethargic, unresponsive
Pupillary activity
Reflexes

Motor responses
Blood pressure
Pulse
Respiratory rate and pattern

Anticipate

Cerebral vascular accident or brain abscess
    Altered level of consciousness
    Altered motor responses: paresis, plegia

Seizures
Coma

169

RESPONSE OF CHILD

The response of the child with a congenital cyanotic cardiac defect to the hospitalization experience is dependent upon many factors, including his or her age and developmental level. The nurse must know normal growth and development patterns in order to anticipate potential problems related to the child's fears, fantasies, and perception of events. The child's physical condition is also important. How the child feels influences his or her response. A warm, sensitive approach will enhance the implementation of a plan of care.

Assess, Monitor, and Document

Developmental level: verbal, and psychosocial, cognitive, fears
Behavioral response: anxious, fearful, withdrawn, passive, aggressive
Response to nursing interventions

Anticipate

Emotional distress
Disruption of normal growth and development

RESPONSE OF FAMILY

The responsibility of parenting a child with a congenital cyanotic cardiac defect is great. Hospitalization related to complications of defects can conjure all types of feelings, which can influence parental reactions. The nurse must be sensitive to the parents' needs for obtaining accurate information, reassurance, and emotional support. A plan of care that meets the needs of the family and that facilitates coping should be developed and implemented. The parents may have a need for further information related to the underlying problem and concerning home management. All needs should be assessed and incorporated into the plan of care.

Assess, Monitor, and Document

Behavioral response of parents: anxiety, fear, guilt
Level of knowledge of disease and condition of child
Expected outcome
Ability to cope
Learning needs related to discharge: signs and symptoms of complications, medication administration
Response to nursing interventions

MIND SET

Assess

Cardiopulmonary status
Neurologic status
Response of child and family

Anticipate

Alteration in cardiac status
  Cyanotic spell (Group 1, TOF)
  Worsening hypoxemia secondary to closure of atrial communication (Group II, TGA) or palliative shunt occlusion
  Congestive heart failure (Group II)
Alteration in neurologic function
  Cerebral vascular accident
  Brain abscess
Emotional trauma
Family crisis

Postoperative Care of Infants and Children After Open-Heart Surgery

MICHAEL A. LaCORTE, M.D.
ROBERT A. BOXER, M.D.

Many advances in the surgical management of congenital heart disease have been made in the last three decades. The development of cardiopulmonary bypass in the 1950's has enabled surgeons to correct defects within the heart. The introduction of deep hypothermia and circulatory arrest has allowed surgical correction of both simple and complex defects in the smallest infants. The intraoperative success of such surgery is the result of the expertise of pediatric cardiovascular surgeons and the development of new techniques to protect the myocardium during surgery. Critical to the perioperative survival of these patients is the delivery of expert postoperative care. Prompt recognition and treatment of problems in the immediate postoperative period are the responsibility of both the physicians (including pediatric cardiologist, pediatric house officer, and surgeon) and the nursing staff. All personnel involved in postoperative care must be familiar with monitoring techniques and equipment and must understand the principles of postoperative care in these patients.

CARDIOVASCULAR MONITORING

All patients undergoing cardiac surgery should have monitoring of the following parameters to ensure optimal care in the perioperative period.

Electrocardiogram

Heart rate and rhythm are monitored constantly via leads applied to the chest or extremities. Full 12-lead electrocardiagrams are obtained before surgery, immediately after surgery, and every 24 hours for 3 days postoperatively.

Respiratory Rate

Respiratory rate is monitored when the patient is receiving ventilator support and after extubation.

Body Temperature

Rectal temperature may be monitored continuously via rectal probe or hourly for the first 12 hours and every 4 hours thereafter if the clinical condition is stable.

Blood Pressure

Systemic arterial blood pressure (systolic, diastolic, and mean arterial pressure) should be monitored by an indwelling catheter inserted via cutdown in an artery or percutaneously, usually the radial or femoral artery. Cuff blood pressure may not be accurate in the immediate postoperative period because of systemic vasoconstriction.

Left Heart Filling Pressure

Left atrial pressure is continuously monitored by a catheter inserted into the left atrium at the time of surgery. The distal end of this catheter is externalized through a small incision in the chest wall and is attached to a continuous heparin infusion. In older patients, left heart filling pressure may alternatively be measured by a Swan–Ganz catheter advanced to the pulmonary artery wedge position. Extreme care must be taken not to allow air or particulate matter to enter this line in order to prevent systemic embolization.

Right Heart Filling Pressure

In certain conditions, right atrial pressure will be monitored continuously. This may be accomplished by an indwelling line placed in the right atrium at the time of surgery or by a central venous line advanced to the right atrium.

Pulmonary Artery Pressure

Pulmonary artery pressure (systolic, diastolic, and mean) is often monitored via inserting a pressure line at the time of surgery into the pulmonary artery or by advancing a flow-directed, balloon-tipped catheter into the pulmonary artery. Measurement of pulmonary artery pressure is most useful in patients with preoperative pulmonary hypertension or patients undergoing repair of tetralogy of Fallot.

Care of Pressure Lines

All pressure lines are maintained by a slow constant infusion (3 ml or less per hour) of heparinized saline. At our institution, a solution of normal saline with 100 units of heparin per 500 ml is used. With all indwelling pressure lines, care should be taken to withdraw samples from a portal as close to the patient as possible. In order to compensate for any dilution of the blood by the constant infusion of saline, an appropriate amount, usually 3 to 5 ml must be withdrawn from the lines before obtaining any blood samples for analysis. Careful measurements of amounts of blood drawn through the pressure lines should be made, and these amounts should be replaced with equal volumes of colloid. After the sample is withdrawn from the pressure line, the line should be flushed immediately to maintain patency.

Cardiac Output

Cardiac output may be monitored in the postoperative period by the thermodilution technique. This is accomplished by placement of a thermistor probe in the pulmonary artery at the time of surgery or by the use of a multilumen thermodilution catheter inserted intravenously by cutdown or the percutaneous technique in the internal or external jugular vein immediately prior to surgery. Cardiac output is determined by rapid injection of a known volume of cold solution (5 percent dextrose in water, D5W, or saline) into the right atrium. Cardiac output is determined by a bedside computer attached to the thermistor catheter.

Urinary Output

Urinary output is monitored continuously by a Foley catheter inserted in the bladder at the time of the operative procedure. Whenever there is a drop in the urine output, the possibility of a catheter obstruction should be ruled out before more serious reasons, such as low cardiac output or renal failure, are considered.

Chest and Mediastinal Drainage

Plastic mediastinal and pericardial chest tubes are routinely used postoperatively to collect and measure fluid drainage from the pericardial and pleural spaces. These tubes are connected to underwater drainage systems under negative pressure. In order to maintain patency and prevent clot formation in the tubes, they should be stripped frequently. Fluid output from these tubes should be recorded and replaced with appropriate volumes of colloid. The choice of replacement fluid will depend upon the patient's hematocrit and status of the clotting mechanism. These tubes are removed when there is minimal drainage, usually after a minimum of 24 hours postoperatively. The intracardiac catheters should be removed prior to discontinuing the chest tubes. Care should be taken to prevent pneumothorax at the time of removal of tubes inserted into the pleural spaces.

Pacing Wires

Temporary epicardial ventricular pacing wires are routinely inserted into the ventricular myocardium at the termination of the operative procedure. Occasionally, atrial wires may also be put in at the time of surgery to perform atrial pacing or sequential atrial/ventricular pacing or to record atrial electrograms. The distal end of the pacing wire is externalized through a small incision in the chest wall. These distal ends should be wrapped in nonconducting material to prevent contact with electrical equipment. A temporary pacemaker should be readily available in case there is a need for pacing. The pacemaker wires may be removed 24 hours or more after surgery by gentle traction on the wires at the skin surface. Because these wires are extremely thin and not put into the cavity of the ventricle, their removal is not associated with cardiac tamponade.

Ventilatory Support

Preferably, all patients are intubated by the nasotracheal route and connected to a ventilator for a variable period postoperatively. The duration of intubation and ventilatory support depend upon the patient's preoperative condition, complexity of the operation, duration of cardiopulmonary bypass, and hemodynamic state, postoperatively. Weaning from the respirator and extubation depend upon the results of arterial blood gas studies, state of consciousness, and the hemodynamic state. It is imperative that the endotracheal tube be suctioned hourly or more frequently depending upon the amount of secretions. If there is an abrupt deterioration of the ventilatory status, obstruction of the endotracheal tube must immediately be ruled out.

Laboratory Studies

Postoperative blood studies should include arterial blood gases, mixed venous blood gas (if there is a pulmonary line in place), complete blood count, platelet count, clotting studies (prothrombin time, activated partial thromboplastin time, fibrinogen), serum sodium, potassium, chloride, BUN, creatinine, and calcium. These studies should be repeated at frequent intervals postoperatively depending upon the hemodynamic state of the patient. A chest x-ray should be obtained immediately postoperatively and after chest tube removal. Additional chest x-rays may be needed if pneumothorax, pleural effusion, cardiac tamponade, or change in location of the endotracheal tube, are suspected.

GENERAL CONSIDERATIONS

Before the patient arrives in the pediatric intensive care unit (ICU) after open-heart surgery, monitoring equipment should be ready and pressure transducers should be prepared. Upon arrival to the pediatric ICU, the infant or child is prepared for postoperative monitoring. Pressure lines are connected to the transducer, and the electrocardiogram and pressures are displayed on the ICU multichannel monitor. The Foley catheter, nasogastric tube, and chest tube are drained appropriately. The patient must be adequately restrained. A proper ambient temperature is provided; in small infants, a radiant warmer is often needed to ensure adequate body temperature control. After these initial procedures are accomplished, blood gases, electrolytes, and clotting studies are drawn. Attention is then directed toward specific organ systems and their management after open-heart surgery.

MANAGEMENT OF THE CARDIOVASCULAR SYSTEM

Problem Recognition

The greatest concern in the immediate postoperative period is the maintenance of adequate cardiac output. The infant or child with a satisfactory cardiac output will have warm extremities with good peripheral pulses and good capillary refill. Blood pressures measured with an intra-arterial catheter will be normal (infants younger than 1 year of age: systolic pressure is greater than 80 mm Hg; children older than 1 year of age: systolic pressure greater than 90 mm Hg) and urine output will be at least 1 to 2 ml per kg per hour. In addition, arterial blood gas determination shows no evidence of metabolic acidosis (absence of negative base excess), and mixed venous PO_2 (a measure of tissue extraction of oxygen and an indirect measure of cardiac output) is over 30 mm Hg. The presence of cool extremities with poor peripheral pulses, oliguria, hypotension, or metabolic acidosis should make one suspicious of the presence of low cardiac output. The presence of an indwelling thermodilution catheter to measure cardiac output serially at the bedside is of great aid in the recognition of a low cardiac output state and is used routinely in many centers. A cardiac index of less than 2.5 L per minute per m^2 or a steady downhill trend in the cardiac output measurement is indication for prompt intervention.

Etiology and Therapy

Low cardiac output in the immediate postoperative period may result from hypovolemia, myocardial dysfunction, elevated peripheral vascular resistance, cardiac tamponade, and dysrhythmias.

Hypovolemia

One of the most frequent causes of low cardiac output in the immediate postoperative period is hypovolemia, which may be secondary to increased losses (i.e., postoperative bleeding) or inadequate volume administration after cardiopulmonary bypass. The placement of intracardiac catheters in the right and left atrium during surgery is important in the recognition of hypovolemia after surgery. In general, one should maintain filling pressures of 5 to 10 mm Hg. Clearly, if there is an adequate cardiac output, with filling pressures below 5 mm Hg, additional volume replacement is not needed. However, when there is a low cardiac output, low filling pressures indicate that primary therapy should be directed toward increasing diastolic volume (pre-load) and augmenting stroke volume via the Starling mechanism. Volume replacement with packed red blood cells (if the patient's hematocrit is less than 35) or fresh frozen plasma or albumin (hematocrit greater than or equal to 35) can be given in the amount of 5 to 10 ml per kg either as a rapid bolus over a 5- to 10-minute period or more gradually (30 to 60 minutes), depending upon the clinical situation. In general, crystalloid should be restricted to two-thirds maintenance in the first 24 hours and should not be used to augment intravascular volume.

Myocardial Dysfunction

In the patient with evidence of low cardiac output in whom filling pressures (especially left atrial pressure) are elevated (greater than 12 to 15 mm Hg), primary myocardial dysfunction is likely. Myocardial dysfunction may be a result of prolonged ischemic time, preoperative myocardial injury, or poor hemodynamic repair. Our philosophy is that therapy to increase cardiac contractility should be started as soon as myocardial dysfunction is suspected. Urinary output of less than 1 ml per kg per hour or borderline hypotension in the presence of left atrial pressure greater than 10 mm Hg indicates that a positive inotropic agent should be initiated. We believe that increasing left atrial pressure to levels of 15 mm Hg or greater with volume replacement and distention of the left ventricle is not the preferred method of management in this situation. Dobutamine, a powerful synthetic inotrope with little chronotropic action and no peripheral vascular effect, is the drug we prefer to institute at doses beginning at 10 mcg per kg per minute; it may be increased up to 30 to 40 mcg per kg per minute. Dopamine, another positive powerful inotropic agent, selectively causes renal vascular dilatation in doses up to 5 mcg per kg per minute. However, in larger doses, dopamine causes peripheral alpha-receptor stimulation and is more dysrhythmogenic than dobutamine. Isuprel, a powerful beta-agonist, can be used to increase cardiac output, but its vasodilating effect may result in a decrease in blood pressure. We use Isuprel (0.1 to 0.5 mcg/kg/min) to increase heart rate in patients with junctional or sinus bradycardia and as an adjunct to dobutamine or dopamine therapy to augment cardiac output.

It is of great importance in patients with decreased myocardial contractility to maintain serum calcium levels above 9.0 mg per dl. This is accomplished by giving calcium gluconate in doses of 100 mg per kg or calcium chloride in doses of 10 mg per kg every 4 to 6 hours.

Of great concern in the patient with myocardial dysfunction is the maintenance of an adequate urine output. The combination of borderline low cardiac output and hemoglobinuria after cardiopulmonary bypass may result in renal failure. In addition to increasing cardiac output with positive inotropic agents, diuretics should be used to increase urine output to at least 2 ml per kg per hour to possibly prevent renal failure by maintaining a forced diuresis. Furosemide, 1 to 2 mg per kg per dose, can be given as frequently as every 3 to 4 hours. The combination of mannitol, 0.5 gm per kg, and furosemide, 1 mg per kg, is a very effective means of maintaining satisfactory urine output in cases of borderline cardiac output.

Finally, patients with depressed myocardial function should be digitalized in the immediate postoperative period. Patients previously on digoxin should be restarted on this medication at maintenance levels. Patients who have never received digitalis should be digitalized via the IV route at total digitalizing doses (TDD) of 30 mcg per kg for patients younger than 2 years of age and 20 to 25 mcg per kg for patients older than 2 years of age. The TDD is given in 3 equally divided doses at 8-hour intervals. The maintenance digoxin dose is begun 12 hours after the last third of the TDD. If there is compromised renal function, electrolyte imbalance, or bradydysrhythmias (such as second- or third-degree heart block), digitalis administration should be postponed. It should be understood that digoxin is not a substitute for the powerful positive inotropic agents mentioned previously, but it will be effective 48 to 72 hours after surgery when the patient is weaned from inotropic support. When patients are weaned from inotropic support, doses should be decreased very gradually over a minimum 24-hour period, with monitoring of filling pressures and clinical parameters of cardiac function.

Elevated Peripheral Vascular Resistance

Until now, the discussion of cardiac output manipulation postoperatively has centered around adjustments of pre-load and contractility. There are patients, however, with low cardiac output who have an inordinately high peripheral vascular resistance postoperatively. These patients have manifestations of low cardiac output with normal-to-increased blood pressure and benefit from afterload reduction with nitroprusside, 1 to 8 mcg per kg per minute. Afterload reduction therapy is particularly useful in patients in whom afterload was markedly reduced preoperatively (i.e., mitral insufficiency). In most patients, afterload reduction is used in conjunction with a positive inotropic agent. It is important to carefully monitor blood pressure and provide adequate filling pressures during administration of afterload-reducing agents.

Cardiac Tamponade

An important and potentially lethal cause of low cardiac output is cardiac tamponade. In patients with evidence of low cardiac output and elevated right- and left-sided filling pressures, tamponade must be considered. An increasing mediastinal shadow on x-ray examination may be helpful in diagnosis; pulsus paradoxus may be present but is often a late finding in this setting. In patients with increased postoperative bleeding and decreased cardiac output associated with a sudden decline in chest tube drainage, one may be dealing with clotting of the chest tube and impending cardiac tamponade. The danger of tamponade is always present in patients with excessive bleeding. Reoperation for hemorrhage should be performed if blood loss is greater than 10% of blood volume per hour and if it does not consistently decrease each hour after clotting studies have normalized.

Dysrhythmias

Another major cause of decreased cardiac output postoperatively is cardiac dysrhythmias. Bradydysrhythmias include sinus bradycardia, junctional rhythm, and second- and third-degree heart block. Tachycardias include supraventricular tachycardia, atrial fibrillation, atrial flutter, and ventricular tachycardia. In all cases of dysrhythmias, electrolyte disturbances, especially hypokalemia and hypocalcemia and acid-base imbalances, should be corrected. In patients with either sinus bradycardia or slow junctional rhythm in which the bradycardia may be compromising cardiac output, Isuprel therapy may be used, but pacing may be necessary to adequately increase the heart rate. In cases of second-degree heart block, Isuprel may increase AV conduction, resulting in one-to-one conduction. Complete heart block is usually treated with pacing unless there is an adequate ventricular response with normal cardiac output. Supraventricular tachycardia is often not well tolerated postoperatively. Cardioversion (1 watt/sec/kg) followed by digitalization or digitalization alone will usually control the dysrhythmia. Digitalis is also used to control atrial fibrillation and atrial flutter. The use of quinidine, Inderal, and Pronestyl is avoided, if possible, in the immediate postoperative period in the management of supraventricular tachydysrhythmias because of their negative inotropic effect. Ventricular premature beats should be controlled with lidocaine therapy or rapid pacing. In cases of ventricular tachycardia, lidocaine, pacing, or cardioversion are used.

MANAGEMENT OF THE RESPIRATORY SYSTEM

After open-heart surgery, almost all infants and children return to the pediatric ICU intubated nasotracheally and on a ventilator. The type of ventilator used varies from center to center, but usually the volume ventilator is preferred. The initial tidal volume is generally placed at 10 ml per kg, with an additional volume added for dead space. We usually set the initial rate at 20 breaths per minute in infants and 15 breaths per minute in children older than 2 years of age. The FI_{O_2} is usually placed at 100 percent initially and positive end–expiratory pressure is placed at 5 cm of water. Arterial blood gases are obtained at least once every hour in the first 12- to 24-hour period postoperatively, and adjustments are made in the ventilator settings based upon the blood gas determination. In general, the FI_{O_2} is lowered by 5 percent decrements, keeping arterial PO_2 approximately 100 mm Hg in patients without residual right-to-left shunting. The respiratory rate, intermittent mandatory ventilation, IMV, is decreased by 2 breaths per minute decrements, keeping the PCO_2 less than or equal to 45 mm Hg.

The decision to extubate a patient is based upon a number of factors. The patient must be hemodynamically stable, with satisfactory filling pressure and adequate blood pressure, and on no, or minimal, doses of pressor agents. The patient should be alert, breathing comfortably, able to clear secretions, and able to maintain good blood gases on minimal ventilator settings (rate less than or equal to 5; FI_{O_2} less than or equal to 0.4). A short trial of continuous positive airway pressure (CPAP) may be tried prior to extubation. Just prior to extubation, the stomach should be emptied, the patient should be ambu bagged with oxygen, and the endotracheal tube should be suctioned.

Inadequate Ventilation

Problem Recognition

Often, the first clue to inadequate ventilation is restlessness and agitation. Cyanosis may be present. Auscultation of the chest reveals decreased breath sounds. Arterial blood gases reveal respiratory acidosis (increased PCO_2), hypoxemia, and at times, a metabolic acidosis.

Etiology and Therapy

Inadequate ventilation may be a result of many causes. Obstruction of the endotracheal tube is a common problem, especially in small infants, and is suggested by difficulty in passing the catheter during routine suctioning and by an increase in peak airway pressure needed to deliver the required tidal volume. If airway obstruction is secondary to a plugged endotracheal tube, tubes should be changed as expeditiously as possible. Poor endotracheal tube position, another cause of inadequate ventila-

tion, is suggested by poor air entry on one side (usually the left side), and is confirmed by a chest x-ray. A chest x-ray film may also reveal parenchymal disease such as atelectasis and interstitial or pulmonary edema, problems that may cause inadequate ventilation. Adjustment of ventilator settings is usually the solution to these problems. Problems within the pleural cavity (pneumothorax, pleural effusion) may also make ventilation difficult. After the chest tube is inserted to decompress the pneumothorax or drain the effusion, adequate ventilation can be re-established.

Often, an alert infant or child may fight the respirator, making adequate ventilation difficult. If the decision is made to keep the child intubated, sedation with morphine (0.1 mg/kg) and/or Valium (0.1 mg/kg) IV is indicated. We have also had success with a combination of morphine and droperidol.

Right–To–Left Shunting

Problem Recognition

Right-to-left shunting is recognized by persistent hypoxemia in the presence of high inspiratory oxygen. In some patients, the PO_2 will not approach 100, even with administration of 100 percent oxygen.

Etiology and Therapy

Right-to-left shunting may be intrapulmonary or intracardiac. In most patients, after open-heart repair, right-to-left shunting is transient. Contrast echo-cardiogram, with injection into central venous or right atrial catheters, will reveal right-to-left atrial or ventricular shunting secondary to a persistent patent foramen ovale or transient patch leak. This phenomenon is most commonly seen in patients with depressed right ventricular function or significant residual right ventricular overflow obstruction. Continued ventilatory support and maintenance of cardiac output will usually result in a gradual disappearance of the shunt.

MANAGEMENT OF THE RENAL SYSTEM

As discussed earlier, the urine output postoperatively is an important guide to the status of the circulatory system. In the first 3 to 4 hours after surgery, there is usually a large diuresis resulting from the osmotic load of glucose and mannitol administered during cardiopulmonary bypass. After this initial diuresis, urine output usually decreases to levels of 1 to 2 ml per kg per hour when there is satisfactory cardiac output. Oliguria (urine output less than 1 ml/kg/hour) usually reflects an inadequate cardiac output or impending renal failure. In cases of low cardiac output, the decreased urine output is accompanied by sodium retention and decreased urinary sodium. Therapy to increase cardiac output will result in increase in urinary output. If cardiac output remains inadequate for several hours or if periods of significant hypotension occur, especially in the presence of hemoglobinuria, oliguria will progress (possibly to anuria) and become a manifestation (along with increased creatinine and sodium wasting) of renal failure. How effective are diuretics such as Lasix and mannitol in the prevention of renal failure? In many situations, renal failure cannot be prevented if cardiac output is not improved. However, we believe that occasionally in situations with borderline cardiac output in patients who have had long operative procedures with significant hemoglobinuria, forced diuresis with a combination of Lasix and mannitol may prevent acute tubular necrosis. If acute tubular necrosis does occur, a renal failure regimen, including fluid restriction, therapy for hyperkalemia, and, in some instances, dialysis, is instituted (see Chapter 15, Acute Peritoneal Dialysis).

MANAGEMENT OF THE HEMATOLOGIC SYSTEM

The major hematologic problems postoperatively concern excessive bleeding, which may be of several etiologies. Excessive bleeding from the chest tubes and/or wound sites may be due to poor hemostasis at suture lines in the heart surface, in the mediastinum, at the sternal closure, or in the layers of skin closure. This prolonged bleeding may be due to medical causes such as 1) inadequate reversal of heparin, which is given during cardiopulmonary bypass; 2) platelet dysfunction, quantitative and/or qualitative; 3) dilutional coagulopathy; and 4) increased fibrinolysis.

If the aforementioned causes of prolonged bleeding are ruled out and there is excessive ongoing blood loss through the chest and mediastinal tubes, inadequate surgical control of hemostasis must be assumed.

The sites of excessive hemorrhage could potentially involve any tissue plane incised during the operative procedure, such as the sternal edges, the atriotomy site, the aortotomy site, the site of a ventriculotomy, or sites of entry of pressure lines into the heart.

In evaluating postoperative bleeding, it is essential to obtain a prothrombin time (PT), activated partial thromboplastin time (APTT), thrombin time (TT), and fibrinogen and platelet counts. Treatment for bleeding will depend upon abnormalities of the aforementioned tests. If heparin excess is suspected (very prolonged APTT, PT relatively unaffected), protamine sulfate should be administered IV in a slow drip because it may cause hypotension. Dilutional coagulopathy (moderately prolonged PT and APTT) can be corrected with fresh frozen plasma. Thrombocytopenia may be corrected by administering platelet concentrate at a dose of 1 U per 5 kg. Occasionally, consultation with a pediatric hematologist may be necessary to select the mechanism for prolonged postoperative bleeding.

If the laboratory evaluation of the clotting system proves to be normal and the bleeding is ongoing and excessive, surgical re-exploration of the chest should be done to locate the sources of bleeding and to prevent the life-threatening sequelae of cardiac tamponade.

SPECIAL CONSIDERATIONS

The Chronically Ill Child

Most infants and children recover quickly after open-heart surgery. After 48 to 72 hours, most patients have been extubated and intracardiac lines and chest tubes have been removed, oral intake has been started, and most patients are transferred out of the ICU. However, occasionally, a patient will require prolonged intubation and/or ventilatory support and remain in the ICU for an indefinite period of time. Many problems arise in these patients, and a complete discussion of them is beyond the scope of this chapter. Two major considerations in these patients should be mentioned: risk of infection, and need for nutrition. In patients in whom intracardiac catheters and endotracheal tubes are left in place for a prolonged period, infection is a major risk. Although all patients receive prophylactic systemic antibiotics for 1 to 3 days after surgery (cephalosporins are currently used), in chronically ill patients, specific organisms must be sought and treated aggressively. Attention must also be paid to each patient's nutritional status. Adequate caloric intake must be provided if recovery is to occur. Total parenteral nutrition or nasogastric (or nasojejunal) feedings should be used 5 to 7 days after surgery if oral alimentation cannot be initiated.

SUGGESTED READING

Applebaum, A., Blackstone, E.H., Kouchoukos, N.T., and Kirklin, J.W.: Effect of afterload reduction on cardiac output in infants after intracardiac surgery. Circulation 51, 52 (Suppl II):11–151, 1975.

Argarwala, B.N.: Postoperative management of open heart surgery in infants and children. Hosp. Pract. 17: 40C-40R, 1982.

Downes, J.J., Nicodemus, H.F., Pierce, W.S., and Waldhausen, J.A.: Acute respiratory failure in infants following cardiovascular surgery. J. Thorac. Cardiovasc. Surg. 59:21, 1970.

Feeley, T.W., and Hedley-Whyte, J.: Weaning from controlled ventilation and supplemental oxygen. N. Engl. J. Med. 292:903, 1975.

Kouchoukos, N.T., Shephard, L.C., and Kirklin, J.W.: Effect of alteration in arterial pressure on cardiac performance early after open intracardiac operations. J. Thorac. Cardiovasc. Surg. 64:563, 1972.

Lister, G.: Perioperative care of infants and children in thoracic and cardiovascular surgery. In Glenn, W., Barre, A., Geha, A., et al. (eds.): Thoracic and Cardiovascular Surgery. 4th ed. Norwalk, Conn., Appleton-Century-Crofts, 1983, pp. 626–639.

Mills, L.J., Newfield, E.A., Mast, C.P., and Carew, J.: Cardiothoracic surgery. In Levin, D., Morriss, F., and Moore, G. (eds.): A Practical Guide to Pediatric Intensive Care. St. Louis, The CV Mosby Co., 1979, pp. 224–237.

Parr, G.V.S., Blackstone, E.H., and Kirklin, J.W.: Cardiac performance and mortality early after intracardiac surgery in infants and young children. Circulation 51:867, 1975.

Sade, R.M., Cosgrave, D.M., and Casteneda, A.R.: Infant and Child Care in Heart Surgery. Chicago, Year Book Medical Publishers, Inc., 1977.

RESPIRATORY

Adult Respiratory Distress Syndrome

ELAINE ZOBERMAN, M.D.
SOL S. ZIMMERMAN, M.D.

Adult respiratory distress syndrome (ARDS), or shock lung, is the clinical condition resulting from acute damage to the pulmonary capillary endothelium and alveolus. This damage may result from a variety of direct or indirect pulmonary insults (Table 23–1), but most often is secondary to hypoperfusion, hypoxia, or sepsis. Despite progress in understanding its pathogenesis and advances in therapy, ARDS carries a 40 to 60 percent mortality rate.

PATHOLOGY

ARDS evolves in a sequence of pathologic stages characterized by initial injury to the pulmonary capillary endothelium, subsequent interstitial edema and microatelectasis, and final alveolar damage with edema and possible hyaline membrane formation.

All the antecedent events (shock, trauma, sepsis, near-drowning) associated with ARDS have in common the ability to destroy capillary endothelial integrity. The damaged endothelial cells swell and lose their intercellular adherence, allowing fluid to leak from the capillary into the interstitium. Endotoxin and vasoactive substances such as histamine, serotonin, and bradykinin have been postulated as having a direct role in altering capillary permeability. Complement activation and neutrophil release of proteases and superoxide radicals are additional proposed mechanisms of endothelial cell injury.

As increasing amounts of fluid, protein, and even red blood cells leak into the interstitial space, lung compliance decreases and microatelectasis occurs. Oxygen diffusing capacity decreases, and clinical symptoms may first become evident.

Alveolar cell damage ensues, and fluid passes from the interstitial space into the alveolus. Direct injury to type II pneumocytes and the presence of proteinaceous fluid in the alveolus result in loss of surfactant by inactivation and inhibition of synthesis. Progressive atelectasis and pulmonary edema further impair ventilation and gas exchange.

With time, the intra-alveolar fluid and protein may go on to the hyaline membrane formation that initially likened the disease to neonatal respiratory distress syndrome (RDS). An overreactive reparative response to the lung injury may result in interstitial and alveolar fibrosis in a disordered manner.

In summary, the underlying pathology consists of increased interstitial and alveolar fluid, progressive atelectasis, and reduced lung compliance and functional residual capacity (FRC). Profound hypoxemia is the consequence of increased intrapulmonary shunting.

CLINICAL PRESENTATION

The clinical manifestations of ARDS evolve in stages that parallel the described pathologic changes (Table 23–2). There is an initial serious insult associated with hypoperfusion and tissue hypoxia, which results from shock states (hypovolemic, septic, or cardiogenic), reflex vasoconstriction (head trauma), or asphyxia

179

Table 23–1. Causes of ARDS

Shock
  Hypovolemic
  Septic
  Cardiogenic
Tissue Injury
  Trauma (lung, brain, bone)
  Burns
Sepsis
Aspiration
  Gastric contents
Near Drowning
Toxins
  Drug overdose (heroin, methadone, barbiturates, salicylates)
  Inhalants (oxygen, hydrocarbons)
Microthrombi
  Disseminated intravascular coagulation
  Post-cardiopulmonary bypass
  Multiple transfusions
Fat Emboli
Uremia
Increased Intracranial Pressure

(near-drowning, strangulation). Following appropriate resuscitative measures, the physical examination is generally unremarkable, with the lung fields clear upon auscultation. The chest x-ray is usually interpreted as negative, and arterial blood gases demonstrate normal or mildly decreased oxygen tensions and low normal carbon dioxide tension.

Over the subsequent 48 to 72 hours, a period that corresponds to the progressive accumulation of interstitial fluid, tachypnea disproportionate to the degree of fever, anxiety, or discomfort becomes evident. This is generally the first clinical sign, and although increased respiratory rate can be a nonspecific finding, in this setting it indicates the onset of severe respiratory distress. Physical examination reveals tachypnea but no other signs of respiratory difficulty, and auscultation of the chest may disclose only sparse rales. Chest x-ray examination results may still be normal or pertinent for small, patchy infiltrates ascribed to atelectasis or pulmonary vascular congestion. Arterial blood gases are consistent with the clinical picture of hyperventilation, demonstrating a significant hypocarbia; there is a mild to moderate degree of hypoxemia.

At the end of this relatively "subclinical" period, severe respiratory distress becomes apparent. Although the respiratory difficulty appears to have an acute, explosive onset, careful monitoring of vital signs, chest radiographs, and arterial blood gases would have clearly forecast the sequence of events. Physical examination now reveals labored respirations with flaring of the alae nasi and intercostal retractions. Diffuse rales are audible upon auscultation. On chest x-ray examination, the previously noted infiltrates coalesce and a pul-

Table 23–2. Clinical Stages of ARDS and Pathologic Correlates

Stage	Pathology	Clinical Manifestations and Laboratory Data

Immediate stage postrecovery from initial insult	Disruption of endothelial cell integrity with leak of fluid and protein into interstitial space	Physical examination and chest x-ray negative unless initial insult was pulmonary
		Arterial blood gas:
		  Normal–mildly decreased PO_2
		  Low normal PCO_2

Intermediate progressive but "subclinical" stage	Progressive accumulation of interstitial fluid
	Microatelectasis
	Decreased lung compliance
	Decreased functional residual capacity
		Tachypnea disproportionate to fever, anxiety, and discomfort
		Auscultation may reveal sparse rales
		Chest x-ray may be normal or pertinent for patchy infiltrates representative of atelectasis or pulmonary vascular congestion
		Arterial blood gas:
		  Mild–moderate hypoxia
		  Hypocarbia

Final stage of overt respiratory distress	Alveolar cell damage and passage of fluid from interstitial space into the alveolus
	Pulmonary edema
	Loss of surfactant
	Hyaline membrane formation
		Nasal flaring and intercostal retractions
		Diffuse rales on auscultation
		Chest x-ray: pulmonary edema and progression of infiltrates to "white-out"
		Arterial blood gas:
		  Moderate–severe hypoxia
		  Hypocarbia → normocarbia

monary edema pattern is present. The films may progress to a complete "white-out." Metabolic acidoses, hypocarbia, and marked hypoxemia are evident on arterial blood gas analysis. The pulmonary shunt may be in excess of 30 to 40 percent. As the disease progresses, the shunt fraction may increase and the CO_2 tension returns to normal or becomes elevated. Marked hypercarbia is considered a poor prognostic sign.

TREATMENT

Therapy for ARDS is directed at supporting the patient and ensuring adequate oxygenation by treating pulmonary edema, reopening atelectatic areas, and returning functional residual capacity to normal. Recognition of both the patient population at risk and the time course of the syndrome, and therapeutic intervention before clinical decompensation becomes obvious are the most effective ways to reduce morbidity and mortality.

Arterial oxygen tension should be maintained at greater than 60 mm Hg and hemoglobin should be kept above 10 to 12 gm per dl to maximize oxygen content. If conventional criteria for mechanical ventilation are used (F_{IO2} greater than 0.5 to maintain Pa_{O2} greater than 60 mm Hg, Pa_{CO2} greater than 60 mm Hg, or intrapulmonary shunt greater than 15 percent), intervention will be reserved until the last stage, when the syndrome is far advanced. Intubation and institution of positive airway pressure therapy when the hyperventilation and mild hypoxia characteristic of the "subclinical" phase become evident may be optimal management.

Ventilation is best achieved with a volume-cycled mechanical ventilator set to deliver relatively high tidal volumes of 10 to 15 ml per kg with a low flow rate (less than 20 L per min) and a prolonged inspiratory plateau (greater than 0.8 sec). The slow rise in inspiratory pressure that results improves gas distribution and reduces the risk of barotrauma. The addition of positive end–expiratory pressure (PEEP), however, is the mainstay of therapy, expanding atelectatic alveoli and thereby increasing FRC and improving oxygenation. The presence of PEEP permits the use of a lower F_{IO2} and reduces the risk of oxygen toxicity. PEEP is introduced at a pressure of 5 cm of H_2O and increased in increments of 3 to 5 cm H_2O to levels of 20 cm H_2O or above, as needed. Optimal PEEP for a given patient is that which maximizes lung compliance and systemic arterial oxygen transport.

The disadvantages of high PEEP are an increased risk of barotrauma and, more importantly, hemodynamic compromise secondary to increased intrathoracic pressure. Venous return to the heart may be reduced and right and left ventricular compliance may be altered, with the net effect being decreased cardiac output and oxygen delivery. Therapeutic intervention to maintain cardiac output may require volume expansion to increase pre-load, administration of dopamine or dobutamine for inotropic action, or infusion of nitroprusside for afterload reduction. In cases requiring PEEP greater than 15 cm H_2O, a pulmonary artery (PA) catheter (Swan–Ganz catheter) should be placed for monitoring of pulmonary artery and pulmonary capillary wedge pressures and cardiac output. The noncardiogenic pulmonary edema of ARDS is characterized by pulmonary artery hypertension, with low to normal capillary wedge pressure. Because of its associated complications, use of the pulmonary artery catheter should be limited to 48 to 72 hours. The incidence of pulmonary artery rupture, thrombocytopenia, and infection increase dramatically with duration of catheterization.

Other therapeutic modalities include bronchodilators if bronchospasm is evident, fluid management of pulmonary edema, early recognition and antibiotic treatment of infectious processes, and possible use of steroids. Fluid restriction and diuretic therapy, guided by data from CVP or PA catheters, are directed at decreasing pulmonary edema while maintaining adequate tissue perfusion and urine output. High-dose steroids (greater than 30 mg/kg/dose of methylprednisolone) have been advocated in the treatment of ARDS because of their ability to stabilize membranes and interfere with neutrophil production of superoxide, but there is no evidence to firmly support their efficacy. The possible role of steroids in preventing the evolution of ARDS, if administered immediately following the primary insult, must also be further evaluated.

Systems other than respiratory may be involved as a consequence of the initial injury or secondary to progression of the syndrome, requiring close monitoring of renal, hepatic, neurologic, and hematologic functions. Early recognition of potential organ failure and aggressive treatment are necessary to prevent these complications from contributing to the high mortality rate.

CASE PRESENTATION

A 3 ½-year-old girl, 2 years post medulloblastoma resection, was admitted to the hospital for re-evaluation of her tumor status. A recurrence deemed inoperable was noted several months prior to this admission, and *cis*-platinum therapy was instituted. Chemotherapy was discontinued when deterioration of renal function became evident.

On Day 2, she was sedated with chloral hydrate and sent for a CAT scan. Immediately after intravenous administration of contrast material, she became dusky and diaphoretic. Blood pressure was determined to be 30 per palp. Epinephrine was given subcutaneously, colloid was infused for volume expansion, and oxygen was administered by face mask. A second dose of epinephrine and an additional "push" of colloid were required before vital signs were restored to normal. Because of an episode of emesis during the resuscitation, a chest x-ray was obtained. The lung fields were clear upon auscultation. She was admitted to the ICU for observation and transferred back to the ward the following day after an uneventful course.

On Day 4, tachypnea to 45 breaths per minute was noted; the remaining vital signs were BP = 100/60 mm Hg, HR = 120 beats/min, and T = 99° F. Results of physical examination were pertinent only for her chronic neurologic findings, and a repeat chest x-ray was negative. An arterial blood gas revealed: pH = 7.42, PO_2 = 82 mm Hg, and P_{CO_2} = 30 mm Hg. The tachypnea was attributed to separation anxiety, and no therapy was ordered.

Nasal flaring and subcostal retractions became apparent that night. Vital signs were: BP = 100/65 mm Hg, HR = 150 beats/min, RR = 50 beats/min, and T = 100° F. Basilar rales were audible bilaterally, and chest x-ray examination revealed patchy infiltrates in both lung fields. Arterial blood gas in room air revealed: pH = 7.35, PO_2 = 49 mm Hg, and PCO_2 = 35 mm Hg. With 40 percent oxygen delivered by face mask, the arterial blood gas revealed: pH = 7.36, PO_2 = 78 mm Hg, and PCO_2 = 33 mm Hg. Other laboratory results included: WBC = 6,900, with 64 segmented neutrophils, 18 bands, 10 lymphocytes, and 8 monocytes; platelets 272,000, hematocrit 30 percent; sodium 141 mEq per L; potassium 4.4 mEq per L; chloride 101 mEq per L; CO_2 19 mEq per L; BUN 34 mg per dl; and creatinine 1.4 mg per dl.

She was transferred back to the ICU, and over the next 8 hours, her pulmonary status deteriorated. Rales were audible over both entire lung fields, findings of chest x-ray films progressed to generalized opacification bilaterally, and hypoxemia was increasingly refractory to high FI_{O_2} delivered by nasal prongs. She was intubated, and arterial and central venous catheters were placed. Initial CVP determination was 5 to 6 cm H_2O. An echocardiogram demonstrated normal contractility.

Problem List

Intake and Output

The patient was placed on a mild fluid restriction of D5W/ 1/2 NS + 10 mEq KCl/500 ml at two-thirds maintenance rate. Furosemide was given as needed to maintain CVP less than or equal to 5 cm H_2O and a urine output of greater than 1 ml/kg/hr. Serum electrolytes were determined q 6 hr and KCl supplementation was administered when indicated.

Respiratory

She was placed on a volume ventilator set to deliver a tidal volume of 15 ml/kg; an F_{IO_2} of 0.45, an IMV of 20, and a PEEP of 10 cm H_2O. The initial peak inspiratory pressure was 30 cm H_2O. The arterial blood gas corresponding to these settings was: pH = 7.45, PO_2 = 62 mm Hg, and PCO_2 = 41 mm Hg.

Peak inspiratory pressures rose to 50 cm H_2O, and oxygen tensions fell as the lung compliance decreased. PEEP was increased to 15 cm H_2O, and FI_{O_2} was increased to 1.0, but oxygenation remained inadequate. Pancuronium and morphine were administered, and a Swan–Ganz catheter was placed. PEEP was then increased to 18 to 20 cm H_2O. Cardiac index, pulmonary capillary wedge pressure, systemic arterial pressure, and urine output remained within the normal ranges. Her calculated pulmonary shunt was in excess of 60 percent. Carbon dioxide tensions progressively rose, despite changes in IMV and expiratory time. On the morning of Day 7, she developed a large pneumomediastinum but no pneumothorax.

Infectious Disease

Shortly after transfer to the ICU, she became febrile to 102° F. Cultures of blood, tracheal aspirate, and urine were obtained. Broad spectrum antibiotic coverage was begun, with aminoglycoside dose corrected for renal function. Blood and urine cultures ultimately were negative, whereas the initial tracheal aspirate grew *Streptococcus viridans*.

Hematologic

She required several transfusions of irradiated packed red blood cells to maintain a hemoglobin greater than 12 gm per dl. Her platelet count progressively dropped, declining to less than 20,000 by Day 7, despite multiple platelet transfusions. Prolongation of prothrombin and partial thromboplastin times, reduced fibrinogen, and elevated fibrin split products were all consistent with disseminated intravascular coagulation. Vitamin K and fresh frozen plasma were given, but the coagulopathy was not reversed. Petechiae were present on the thorax, pulmonary secretions were blood tinged, microscopic hematuria was evident, and stools were guaiac positive.

Cardiac

Myocardial function remained adequate, and pressors were not required. The Swan–Ganz catheter was removed on Day 7, when thrombocytopenia became more severe.

Neurologic

On Day 7, generalized tonic-clonic seizures were noted and she was placed on phenobarbital. Her clinical status did not permit CAT scan evaluation of a possible intracranial hemorrhage.

Nutrition

Nasojejunal feedings were instituted on Day 5 but were discontinued when the presence of blood in the stool was detected on Day 7.

Outcome

Throughout the course of Day 7, her pulmonary and neurologic status deteriorated. Severe hypoxemia and metabolic acidosis were refractory to all therapeutic efforts, and the child expired late in the day.

SUGGESTED READING

Holbrook, P.R., Taylor, G., Pollack, M.M., and Fields, A.I.: Adult respiratory distress syndrome in children. Pediatr. Clin. North Am. 27:677, 1980.

Lyrene, R.K., and Truog, W.E.: Adult respiratory distress syndrome in a pediatric intensive care unit: predisposing conditions, clinical course, and outcome. Pediatrics 67:790, 1981.

Moss, G.: Shock lung: a disorder of the central nervous system? Hosp. Pract. 77:86, 1974.

Petty, T.L., and Ashbaugh, D.G.: The adult respiratory distress syndrome: clinical features, factors influencing prognosis, and principles of management. Chest 60:233, 1971.

Pfenninger, J., Gerber, A., Tschappeler, H., and Zimmerman, A.: Adult respiratory distress syndrome in children. J. Pediatr. 101:352, 1982.

Sladen, M.: Methylprednisolone: pharmacologic doses in shock lung syndrome. J. Thorac. Cardiovasc. Surg. 71:800, 1976.

Suter, P.M., Fairley, H.B., and Isenberg, M.D.: Optimum end–expiratory airway pressure in patients with acute pulmonary failure. N. Engl. J. Med. 292:284, 1975.

Nursing Process for Patient Care:

Adult Respiratory Distress Syndrome

The key elements in the nursing management of patients with adult respiratory distress syndrome (ARDS) are recognition of the events that lead to this condition and anticipation of the progression of the syndrome through its three characteristic stages. In addition, it is important to recognize the effect of the primary and/or subsequent insults on organ systems other than respiratory.

RESPIRATORY

Assess, Monitor, and Document

Respiratory rate
Work of breathing
  Retractions
  Nasal flaring
Breath sounds

Secretions: amount, description
Level of consciousness
Color
Arterial blood gases

Anticipate

Subtle signs of respiratory distress
  Tachypnea disproportionate to fever, anxiety, and discomfort
  Sparse rales
  Arterial blood gases: mild to moderate hypoxia, hypocarbia

Progression to fulminant respiratory distress
  Nasal flaring
  Intercostal retractions
  Diffuse rales
  Arterial blood gases: moderate to severe hypoxia, hypocarbia to normocarbia
  Respiratory failure

POST-INTUBATION

Assess, Monitor, and Document

Patency of tube
Position of tube
Breath sounds
Secretions: amount, description
Response to chest physical therapy and pulmonary hygiene

Ventilator settings: tidal volume, flow rate, inspiratory pressure, FI_{O_2}, IMV (intermittent mandatory ventilation), PEEP (positive end–expiratory pressure)

Anticipate

Self-extubation
Hemodynamic compromise: decreased cardiac output

Pneumothorax

CARDIOVASCULAR

Both the underlying respiratory pathology and the ventilatory therapy required for its treatment can result in decreased cardiac output.

Assess, Monitor, and Document

Rate
Rhythm
Blood pressure: arterial, central venous, pulmonary artery, capillary wedge

Perfusion: peripheral pulses, color, skin condition, capillary filling

Anticipate

Alteration in cardiovascular status
Decreased cardiac output: increased cardiac rate, decreased arterial blood pressure
Decreased peripheral perfusion: weak pulses, cool skin, mottled, dusky skin, poor capillary refill
Dysrhythmias
Cardiac arrest

FLUID AND ELECTROLYTE BALANCE

The fluid and electrolyte balance of the child is always an important parameter. The underlying respiratory pathology necessitates the manipulation of fluid balance as a therapeutic modality.

Assess, Monitor, and Document

Weight
Urine output (hourly, including specific gravity)
Urine electrolytes
Fluid intake: accurate administration of parenteral fluids (use infusion pump if available)
Serum electrolytes

Anticipate

Alteration in fluid and electrolyte status
Response to pharmacologic management:
diuretics (if appropriate)

NEUROLOGIC

Assess, Monitor, and Document

Level of consciousness: lethargy, stupor
Pupillary activity
Reflexes
Motor responses

Anticipate

Altered level of consciousness
Seizures

INFECTIOUS PROCESS

The multiplicity of invasive equipment and procedures in addition to the general condition of the child and the location in the pediatric ICU should generate concern regarding the potential for infection.

Assess, Monitor, and Document

Temperature
Secretions: amount, description (consistency, color, odor)
Insertion sites of catheters: description (color, warmth, edema)
Urine: description (color, odor)

Anticipate

Presence of infectious process
Fever
Positive cultures of blood, wounds, secretions, urine

HEMATOLOGIC

An adequate hemoglobin is essential to oxygen transport. Disseminated intravascular coagulation (DIC) may be the consequence of the initiating insult or may be present during the course of ARDS.

Assess, Monitor, and Document

Signs of bleeding
  Intravenous or arterial catheter insertion sites
  Venipuncture site
  Petechiae
  Gastrointestinal: nasogastric, rectal

Laboratory
  Hemoglobin
  Platelets
  Prothrombin Time (PT), Partial Thromboplastin Time (PTT)
  Fibrinogen
  Fibrin split products

Anticipate

Altered hematologic status
  Anemia
  DIC: bleeding, decreased platelets, prolonged PT and/or PTT, decreased fibrinogen, increased fibrin split products

RENAL

Assess, Monitor, and Document

Urine output: amount (hourly), description, specific gravity, dipstick for blood and protein
Urine electrolytes and osmolality

Serum electrolytes, BUN, creatinine, osmolality
Status of hydration: weight, blood pressure

Anticipate

Alteration in renal function
  Acute renal failure: acute tubular necrosis (decreased urine output, weight gain, increased blood pressure)

RESPONSE OF CHILD

The response of the child will be determined by such factors as age, developmental level, and physical condition. Because ARDS usually occurs in response to another problem, the existing care plan must be modified to support the child emotionally through this crisis.

Assess, Monitor, and Document

Developmental level: verbal, motor, psychosocial, cognitive

Behavioral response: fearful, anxious, tearful
Response to nursing interventions

Anticipate

Emotional distress
Inability to cope

RESPONSE OF FAMILY

Because ARDS occurs as a consequence of a primary insult and is not the presenting complaint, nursing interventions that have been previously implemented will be continued and modified so that ARDS can be treated. The severity of the respiratory problems and of the child's general condition render this situation a crisis for the family.

Assess, Monitor, and Document

Behavioral response of parents: anxious, fearful, verbal, angry, disappointed
Level of understanding of child's condition

Expected outcome
Response to nursing interventions

Anticipate

Inability to cope
Family crisis

MIND SET

Assess

Respiratory status
Cardiovascular status
Fluid and electrolyte balance
Neurologic status

Infectious disease status
Hematologic status
Renal function
Response of child and family

Anticipate

Alteration in respiratory status
  Subtle signs of respiratory distress: tachypnea
  Progression to fulminant respiratory distress: pulmonary edema, respiratory failure, intubation, mechanical ventilation
Alteration in cardiovascular status
  Decreased cardiac output

Alteration in fluid and electrolyte balance
Alteration in neurologic status
Infectious process
Alteration in hematologic function
Alteration in renal function
Emotional trauma
Family crisis

Status Asthmaticus

HARRIS E. BURSTIN, M.D.
DANIEL A. NOTTERMAN, M.D.

Status asthmaticus denotes a condition of severe acute asthma that is refractory to a therapeutic regimen of sympathomimetic medication. Such a regimen may involve the conventional subcutaneous administration of epinephrine or the inhalation of beta-agonists. Implicit in the diagnosis is the physician's concern about the patient's unstable ventilatory status and the possibility of abrupt deterioration into acute respiratory failure. Management of such a patient must be instituted quickly and conducted in a setting that permits continuous medical and nursing supervision.

PATHOPHYSIOLOGY

The underlying derangement in asthma is constriction of small- and medium-sized airways, which results from bronchospasm, mucosal edema, and hypersecretion of mucus. Because the intrapulmonary airways are narrower during expiration than inspiration, obstruction to air flow is relatively greater during expiration. Air-trapping ensues, and the functional residual capacity of the lung volume increases. Consequently, a more negative intrapleural pressure is needed to effect the same tidal volume and the work of breathing increases. Because airway narrowing is not uniform in extent and because some alveoli are atelectatic, ventilation is uneven and ventilation/perfusion ($\dot{V}/\dot{Q}$) mismatching occurs.

Early in an acute episode, hypoxemia predominates as a consequence of $\dot{V}/\dot{Q}$ mismatching. Hyperventilation results in initial hypocarbia and further contributes to the increased work of breathing. After a variable amount of time, the patient becomes exhausted. Normocarbia and then hypercarbia supervene, and the patient enters the terminal phase of illness, acute respiratory failure.

These perturbations in respiratory function induce important derangements in cardiovascular and metabolic function. The child with status asthmaticus takes fluid poorly, if at all. Insensible water loss is augmented by tachypnea and fever, if present. Emesis occurs in most patients, often as a result of therapy. Higher than normal energy consumption, resulting from the increased work of breathing, coupled with dehydration, promotes accumulation of lactic acid. Hypocarbia, present initially, limits conservation of bicarbonate ion by the kidney. Consequently, most severely affected patients have some degree of metabolic acidosis.

As noted previously, an early consequence of airway obstruction is abnormally negative intrapleural pressure, which interferes with resorption of interstitial lung fluid. Fluid accumulates in the pulmonary interstitium and, ultimately, in the alveoli. In extreme cases, pulmonary edema may result.

X-RAY EXAMINATION

The need for x-ray evaluation is dictated by the results of the physical examination and clinical condition. Routine chest x-rays should be discouraged. In the absence of physical findings such as rales, decreased breath sounds, or increased tympany, x-ray films most often do not add significant information. An x-ray examination is indicated with impending respiratory failure or following intubation. Unless discretion is used, a young patient with chronic asthma will receive large doses of radiation over the course of time.

THERAPEUTIC MODALITIES
Oxygen

The importance of arterial blood gas samplings cannot be overstated in the management of severe status asthmaticus. As previously discussed, most patients in status asthmaticus are hypoxemic, even in the absence of severe distress. Underestimation of arterial desaturation is frequent, even with experienced examiners. Oxygen should be the first therapeutic modality in any severe asthma attack. Giving cardiotonic medications such as epinephrine in the presence of a hypoxic myocardium can induce serious dysrhythmias. Oxygen should not be withheld pending receipt of the arterial blood gas analysis.

Antibiotics

There is no place for the uncritical use of antibiotics in status asthmaticus. Bacterial infections, including pneumonia, rarely cause exacerbations of asthma. There have been many studies attempting to evaluate the role of infections in asthmatics. The consensus is that viral infections play a major role but bacterial infections do not.

Fluids

The administration of fluids is another area in which clinical discretion is needed. As a consequence of the previously discussed predisposition for pulmonary edema in asthmatics, the rate and composition of fluid administration should be based on the usual clinical and laboratory indices of hydration. Volumes greater than maintenance should not be used unless the patient is dehydrated.

Simply stated, with regard to x-rays, antibiotics, and fluids, asthmatics should be treated in the same way as other patients. Clinical judgment is crucial.

Sedation

Agitation is a response to hypoxemia and dyspnea and should be treated by specific measures to correct these disturbances. Sedation of any kind is *contraindicated.* Sedation is one of the most common factors implicated in in-hospital mortality from asthma.

Theophylline

Theophylline is the mainstay of therapy for acute severe asthma. A methylxanthine, it inhibits the intracellular enzyme phosphodiesterase, thereby increasing the levels of cyclic AMP (adenosine 3'5'-cyclic monophosphate). Increased cyclic AMP, in turn, promotes relaxation of bronchial smooth muscle, thereby causing bronchodilatation. This leads to decreased airway resistance and improved ventilation. Hypoxemia and hypercarbia lessen, and the work of breathing decreases.

There is significant variability in the rate of theophylline elimination in patients. In general, younger patients eliminate theophylline more rapidly than older patients. This age-related difference in elimination rate requires corresponding adjustments in dosages. Although Table 24–1 lists age-appropriate average dosages of theophylline, it is important to recognize that large, unpredictable differences in theophylline elimination exist. Therefore, the table provides only a rational *starting* dosage for patients. Subsequent adjustments in dosage depend upon clinical response and blood theophylline levels.

The elimination rate of theophylline is rapid in children ($t_{1/2}$ = 3 to 4 hr). In order to avoid undesirable fluctuations in theophylline level, the drug should be administered by continuous infusion. This continuous infusion should be preceded by a loading dose to quickly achieve therapeutic theophylline levels.

Table 24–1. Theophylline Dosage for Pediatric Patients

Group	Loading Dosage	Maintenance Dose (By Ideal Body Weight)
Children 1–9 yr	5 mg/kg (6)*	1.0 mg/kg/hr (1.2)*
Children 9–16 yr	5 mg/kg (6)	0.85 mg/kg/hr (1.0)
Young adults 16 yr and older	5 mg/kg (6)	0.6 mg/kg/hr (0.7)
Patients with CHF, liver disease	5 mg/kg (6)	0.4 mg/kg/hr (0.5)

*Equivalent aminophylline dosage indicated in parentheses

Administration

If the patient has been receiving a theophylline-containing product, a serum theophylline level is drawn. Patients who have not received theophylline for 6 to 8 hours receive a full loading dose of 5 mg per kg (aminophylline, 6 mg/kg). Patients who have received a short-acting preparation within the past 4 hours or a long-acting preparation within 8 hours should receive a reduced loading dose of 2.5 mg per kg (aminophylline, 3.0 mg/kg).

If the pre-loading theophylline level is immediately available, the correct loading dose can be calculated exactly: for each 1 mg per kg of theophylline administered as a loading dose, the serum theophylline level will increase by about 2 mcg per ml. Thus, if the patient's preloading level is 8 mcg per ml and if a concentration of 15 mcg per ml is desired, the patient should receive 3.5 mg per kg.

The loading dose is diluted in 50 ml of the patient's intravenous fluid and administered over 20 minutes by infusion pump. Too rapid infusion of the loading dose is dangerous, because it can precipitate cardiac dysrhythmias and seizures.

At the conclusion of the loading dose, a theophylline level is drawn and a continuous infusion is started. The infusate is compounded by adding 500 mg of aminophylline to 500 ml of the patient's standard IV fluid. This solution contains aminophylline at a concentration of 1 mg per ml. The dosage, and thus the rate of infusion, is selected by reference to Table 24–1. Aminophylline contains 80 percent theophylline by weight. Thus, the dose of aminophylline is 20 percent greater than the dose of theophylline. It is important to recognize that the mg per kg dosage of aminophylline is referenced to the *lean* body weight (LBW). For obese individuals, the LBW is assumed to be the 50th percentile weight for the patient's measured height.

Adjustments in the rate of infusion are guided by the serum theophylline level and by the clinical response. The therapeutic serum concentration of theophylline is 10 to 20 mcg per ml. Above 20 mcg per ml, pronounced tachycardia, palpitations, headache, and gastrointestinal disturbances are noted. More serious toxic manifestations usually occur at concentrations greater than 30 mcg per ml, but occasionally, they may precede the minor effects just noted. These serious toxic effects include cardiac dysrhythmias and generalized convulsions. *Any* evidence of toxicity, including emesis or marked tachycardia, should prompt a serum theophylline level and a reduction in the rate of infusion.

Monitoring Therapy

Continuous monitoring of the electrocardiogram is important during infusion of theophylline. Blood pressure should be obtained every hour initially, and arterial blood gases should be obtained as dictated by the clinical status. Theophylline levels should be drawn at the conclusion of the loading dose and after 6, 12, and 24 hours of continuous infusion. For seriously ill patients, it is appropriate to strive for a serum theophylline level of 15 to 20 mcg per ml.

Changing to Oral Therapy

When the patient is able to breathe without distress and to accept oral feeding, the theophylline infusion should be stopped. Patients who are to receive a long-acting preparation should receive their first oral dose at the time that the infusion is terminated. Patients who are to receive a short-acting preparation should receive their first dose 4 hours after the infusion is stopped. The total daily oral dosage is the same as the total daily IV dosage. Thus, a child who required 1 mg per kg per hour of theophylline by infusion to achieve a serum level of 15 mcg per ml should receive the same dosage (24 mg/kg/day) of an oral preparation.

Beta-Agonists

Beta-agonists have become useful adjuncts to theophylline therapy. Though no pure beta-2 sympathomimetic drug exists, the newer agents have increased selectivity for beta-2 activity on bronchial muscles and decreased beta-1 effects on the heart compared with a nonselective beta-agonist such as isoproterenol. There are essentially four preparations in clinical use (see Table 24–2).

Metaproterenol is probably the most widely used beta-2 agonist. It is available as an oral liquid, tablet, inhalant solution, and metered dose inhaler. When compared with isoproterenol as an inhalant, metaproterenol has fewer cardiotoxic effects and a longer duration of action (up to 4 to 6 hours).

Isoetharine is available only for inhalation use and has no advantages over metaproterenol.

Table 24-2. Beta-Agonists in Theophylline Therapy

Beta-Agonist	Brand Name	Rate of Administration	Dosage	Frequency of Administration
Metaproterenol	Alupent	MDI*	1–2 puffs	every 4–6 hr
	Metaprel	Inhalant solution	0.1–0.5 ml in 2.5 ml NS†	every 4–6 hr
		Syrup, 10 mg/5 ml	↓ 27 kg = 10 mg	every 6–8 hr
		Tablets, 10 mg/20 kg	↑ 27 kg = 20 mg	every 6–8 hr
Terbutaline	Brethine	Injectable	0.01 mg/kg	every 20–30 min
			max = 0.25 mg SC‡	
		Scored 5-mg tablets	2.5–5 mg	every 8 hr
Isoetharine	Bronkosol	MDI	0.5 ml in 2.5 ml NS	every 4–6 hr
		Inhalant solution		
Albuterol (salbutamol)	Proventil	MDI	1–2 puffs	every 4–6 hr
	Ventolin	Scored 2-mg tablets	? dosage in children	

*MDI = metered dose inhaler
†NS = normal saline
‡SC = subcutaneous

Terbutaline, as an oral preparation, is as effective as metaproterenol but has a longer duration of action. However, it has a high incidence of causing tremors and is not available in a liquid form. Injectable terbutaline has limited, if any, benefits over epinephrine. An inhalant solution is available in Europe.

Albuterol (salbutamol) has recently become available in the United States. It is as versatile as metaproterenol and has been used extensively in Europe and Canada. It may soon replace metaproterenol as the most widely used beta-2 agonist in the United States.

In our institution, a beta-2 agonist is routinely used in conjunction with aminophylline therapy for the treatment of status asthmaticus. When there is no contraindication, the patient is placed on an oral preparation. Children 6 to 9 years of age (under 27 kg) are placed on 10 mg of metaproterenol every 6 hours. Children 9 to 12 years of age (over 27 kg) or older are placed on 20 mg every 6 hours. Though metaproterenol has not been studied extensively in children younger than 6 years of age, we have had excellent results with daily dosages of 2 mg per kg divided every 6 hours. Terbutaline may be used in patients older than 12 years of age at a dosage of 2.5 to 5 mg every 8 hours.

Patients in respiratory distress have difficulty using metered dose inhalant pumps. An inhalant solution of metaproterenol can be delivered by a nebulizer through a mouthpiece or face mask and is well tolerated. The nebulized solution is administered every 4 hours along with IV aminophylline therapy. In the patient who is taking oral aminophylline and metaproterenol and is "breaking through" therapy, nebulized metaproterenol may be given every 4 hours on a p.r.n. basis.

We usually give 0.3 to 0.5 ml of metaproterenol in 2.5 ml of normal saline (NS) in older children and 0.1 to 0.3 ml in 2.5 ml of NS in younger children. Dosage should be lowered when given directly via an endotracheal tube.

Steroids

Corticosteroids are known to be effective in the therapy of chronic asthma. Their role in acute asthma is less well defined, and the use of these agents in this condition is controversial. There is evidence that corticosteroids reduce the duration of hypoxemia in children with status asthmaticus, and that they are synergistic with agents operating at the β-adrenergic receptor. They have not been shown to reduce the duration of an acute episode or, when used intermittently, to favorably affect the overall course of the disease. There is no evidence that corticosteroids, when used intermittently for short periods of time, promote or cause a condition of "steroid dependence."

We do not use corticosteroids for all patients with acute severe asthma. Rather, their use is limited to the following circumstances:

1. Pa_{O_2} less than 65 mm Hg after oxygen administration and the loading dose of aminophylline.

2. Pa_{CO_2} greater than 35 mm Hg in the presence of hypoxemia or marked tachypnea.

3. No improvement after 8 to 12 hours of conventional therapy.

4. Patients receiving or recently receiving chronic steroid therapy.

The dosage is 2 mg per kg per day of methylprednisolone. If the duration of therapy is less than 5 days, no taper is necessary. For longer acute courses, it is wiser to taper the drug over 3 to 4 days.

RESPIRATORY FAILURE

Respiratory failure in an asthmatic is defined as refractory hypoxemia (PaO_2 < 60 mm Hg, FiO_2 0.5) or hypercarbia ($PaCO_2$ > 40 mm Hg). Occasionally, an asthmatic, even though treated with aminophylline, metaproterenol, and methylprednisolone, will progress to respiratory failure or present to the emergency room in respiratory failure.

Classically, patients in respiratory failure are managed by mechanical ventilation via an endotracheal tube. Neuromuscular blockade is usually a necessary adjunct. This therapy, even in the most experienced hands, is accompanied by the dangers of subcutaneous emphysema and pneumothorax as well as the risks of intubation (see Chapter 2).

Continuous isoproterenol intravenously is cited as a safer alternative to the management of respiratory failure in children with status asthmaticus. Aminophylline is continued intravenously while a second intravenous line is started for isoproterenol. A drip is begun at 0.1 mcg per kg per minute and is increased by 0.1 mcg per kg per minute every 10 to 15 minutes until the desired response is effected or the heart rate reaches 200 beats per minute. Most asthmatics do not respond until their heart rate is above 180 beats per minute. Constant cardiac monitoring is necessary, and the drip is decreased at the first sign of dysrhythmia. Two IV's must always be maintained, because interruption of this isoproterenol drip causes rebound bronchospasm.

After stabilization, the drip is tapered at a rate calculated to end the infusion in 24 to 36 hours. A dose of subcutaneous terbutaline or inhaled metaproterenol is helpful just prior to when the isoproterenol drip is discontinued. If isoproterenol and aminophylline are not successful in preventing respiratory failure, mechanical ventilation is begun as previously outlined.

CASE PRESENTATION

A 10-year-old boy presents to the pediatric emergency service in severe respiratory distress.

The patient has a 5-year history of chronic asthma and is on theophylline and metaproterenol chronically. Over the past few days, the patient has had rhinitis, cough, and a low-grade temperature. He took his last dose of theophylline 3 hours before presentation and has vomited twice since then.

Examination

The patient is in obvious respiratory distress. Although he is alert and walked into the treatment room, he is retracting and is air hungry. Pertinent findings on physical examination were nasal congestion, supra- and subcostal retractions, and diffuse high-pitched wheezing, with marked prolongation of both inspiration and expiration. He weighs 35 kg.

Problem List

Respiratory

The patient is in severe distress and upon arrival to the treatment area *oxygen* at an FiO_2, 0.35 is administered.

Epinephrine, 1:1000 0.3 ml, is given SC stat, and an arterial blood gas (ABG) is obtained with the following report: pH = 7.30, PO_2 = 54 mm Hg, and PCO_2 = 55 mm Hg.

Because of minimal response to epinephrine and the ABG demonstrating hypoxia and hypercarbia, the patient is admitted and epinephrine is not repeated.

An IV is started, and the patient is given 6 mg/kg or 210 mg of aminophylline over 20 minutes. A repeat ABG 15 minutes later shows the following results: pH = 7.34, PO_2 = 59 mm Hg, and PCO_2 = 47 mm Hg.

The FiO_2 delivered is increased to 0.5. Methylprednisolone, 1 mg/kg or 35 mg, is given IV stat. After the aminophylline has been administered, an aminophylline drip consisting of 500 mg in 500 ml of fluid is started at 1 mg/kg/hr or 35 ml/hr.

Metaproterenol inhalant solution, 0.3 ml in 2.5 ml of NS, is given via nebulizer, and an ABG is performed. The results are pH = 7.39, PO_2 = 66 mm Hg, and PCO_2 = 42 mm Hg.

The patient appears more comfortable and is transferred to the pediatric ICU for further management.

Cardiac

A cardiac monitor is placed on the patient at the time of epinephrine injection. The HR is 110–130 beats/min, with a normal sinus rhythm. Before each medication is given, pulse and BP are obtained. Both are stable.

Intake and Output (I&O)

The patient clinically appears hydrated, with moist mucous membranes and good skin turgor. A urine specimen is obtained, with a specific gravity of 1.014. Electrolytes are sent for evaluation.

D5 1/3 NS, with 10 mEq/KCl/500 mg, is started after the patient voids at 75 ml/hr (maintenance) and the aminophylline bolus has been given.

The aminophylline drip is set to run at 35 ml/h and contains D5 1/3 NS and 500 mg aminophylline/500 ml of fluid. Forty ml/hr. of D5 1/3 NS and 10 KCl/500 mg is provided in addition.

Hematologic

A CBC was sent to the lab. Hand-spun hematocrit is 44.

Infectious

The patient appears to have a URI (upper respiratory infection). Coryza, cough, and low-grade temperature support the diagnosis. There is no evidence to suggest bacterial infection.

Final Assessment

The patient arrives at the pediatric ICU in stable condition. He is still quite dyspneic, with RR = 47 breaths/min, HR = 110 beats/min, and BP = 107/70 mm Hg.

Respiratory

An ABG on arrival at the pediatric ICU reveals pH = 7.31, P_{O_2} = 69 mm Hg, and P_{CO_2} = 51 mm Hg.

There is marked diminution in audible breath sounds, especially on the right side. A stat chest x-ray film reveals hyperinflated lungs with no pneumothorax.

A percutaneous arterial line is placed in the right radial artery. IV methylprednisolone at 2 mg/kg/day divided every 6 hours is ordered.

Because of signs of progressive respiratory failure and hypercarbia, the patient is placed on an isoproterenol drip.

A second peripheral IV is placed, and an isoproterenol drip is begun at a rate of 0.1 mcg/kg/min.

The repeat ABG showed a P_{CO_2} of 54 mm Hg. The isoproterenol drip was raised by 0.1 mcg/kg/min every 20 minutes. At 0.5 mcg/kg/min, the patient began to become less dyspneic.

An ABG revealed pH = 7.40, P_{O_2} = 87 mm Hg, and P_{CO_2} = 38 mm Hg. On auscultation, the chest now showed good air entry bilaterally, with diffuse wheezes.

Cardiac

On 0.5 mcg/kg/min, the HR rose into the 180 to 190 beats/min range. EKG monitoring revealed sinus tachycardia. There was no evidence of dysrhythmia.

Over the next 24 hours, the patient was weaned off isoproterenol and transferred to the pediatric floor in stable condition. Metaproterenol, 10 mg every 6 hours, was begun by mouth.

The next morning, IV aminophylline and methylprednisolone were stopped, and the patient was placed on 250 mg of slow release theophylline and 10 mg of metaproterenol every 8 hours.

He was discharged the next morning.

SUGGESTED READING

Estelle F., Simons R., Pierson, W.E., and Bierman, M.D., Respiratory failure in childhood status asthmaticus. *Am. J. Dis. Child.*, 131:1097, 1977.

Leffert, F.: The management of acute severe asthma. *J. Pediatr.*, 96:1, 1980.

Parry, W.H., Martorano, F., and Cutton E.K.: Management of lifethreatening asthma with intravenous isoproterinol infusions. *Am. J. Dis. Child.*, 130:39, 1976.

Weingerber, M., Hendeles, L., and Abrens, R.: Clinical pharmacology of drugs used for asthma. Pediatr. Clin. North Am., 28:217, 1981.

Nursing Process for Patient Care

Status Asthmaticus

Hospital admission of a child with the diagnosis of status asthmaticus is a true emergency. Constant assessment and anticipation in terms of the child's ventilatory status is crucial to a positive outcome. The major system involved is the respiratory system, with the constriction of the small and medium airways being the underlying pathophysiologic process. Obstruction of airflow results in the appearance of characteristic signs and symptoms.

RESPIRATORY

Assess, Monitor, and Document

Respiratory rate
Pattern
Work of breathing: retractions, nasal flaring
Breath sounds: wheeze, rales, rhonchi
Color
Heart rate

Level of consciousness
Arterial blood gases
Response to medications: oxygen, epinephrine, metaproterenol inhalant, aminophylline, isoproterenol

Anticipate

Alteration in respiratory status
  Rate
  Pattern: prolongation of expiratory phase
  Work of breathing
  Breath sounds
  Color

Level of consciousness: restless, irritable, lethargic
Alteration in arterial blood gases
  Acidosis
  Hypoxia
  Hypercarbia

CARDIOVASCULAR

Alterations in respiratory function have a significant impact upon cardiovascular function. The child in status asthmaticus is usually hypoxic and acidotic. The myocardium is sensitive to these problems.

Assess, Monitor and Document

Rate
Rhythm
Quality
Perfusion

Blood pressure
Response to pharmacologic management: aminophylline, metaproterenol inhalant, isoproterenol

Anticipate

Dysrhythmias

FLUID AND ELECTROLYTE BALANCE

The child in status asthmaticus is usually dehydrated. However, with the predisposition for pulmonary edema, the administration of fluids must be carefully managed. The volume and composition are based upon the usual clinical and laboratory indices of hydration.

Assess, Monitor, and Document

Weight
State of hydration
Urine output
Urine specific gravity

Fluid intake: accurate administration of parenteral fluids (use infusion pump if available)
Laboratory data: serum electrolytes

Anticipate

Alteration in fluid and electrolyte balance
Pulmonary edema

RESPONSE OF CHILD

Assess, Monitor, and Document

Developmental level: verbal, cognitive, motor, psychosocial, normal fears
Behavioral response: anxious, fearful, angry, compliant

Response to nursing interventions

Anticipate

Emotional distress

RESPONSE OF FAMILY

Assess, Monitor, and Document

Behavioral response: anxious, angry, verbal
Level of understanding of the child's condition

Expected outcome
Response to nursing interventions

Anticipate

Family crisis

MIND SET

Assess

Respiratory status
Cardiovascular status

Fluid and electrolyte balance
Emotional response of child and family

Anticipate

Acute respiratory failure
Dysrhythmias
Pulmonary edema

Emotional distress
Family crisis

Bronchiolitis

HARRIS E. BURSTIN, M.D.

Bronchiolitis is a lower respiratory tract infection characterized by inflammatory obstruction of the terminal airways. Affected children are usually younger than 1 year of age, with the incidence of disease markedly decreased after age 18 months. The etiology is viral, with respiratory syncytial virus (RSV) the most common cause; parainfluenza and adenoviruses play a lesser role. Though there is minimal associated mortality, there can be significant morbidity, especially in the young infant.

Increased airway resistance, increased work of breathing, distal air-trapping, and atelectasis are consequences of bronchiolar obstruction caused by edema and accumulation of mucus and cellular debris. Alveolar hypoventilation results in hypoxia, but hypercarbia generally does not occur because the infant compensates by increasing his minute volume and is thereby able to hyperventilate those alveoli that are relatively less obstructed. If the infant becomes fatigued and is unable to maintain an increased minute volume or if a greater number of alveoli become affected by progressive airway obstruction, respiratory failure supervenes.

The typical clinical presentation is that of a tachypneic infant, with flaring of the alae nasi and suprasternal, intercostal, and subcostal retractions. The chest appears hyperinflated. Auscultation reveals diffuse wheezes and rales. A decrease in breath sounds is an ominous sign and occurs when airway obstruction is almost complete.

Most infants with bronchiolitis have only mild respiratory distress and do not require hospitalization. Close observation by the parents and regular communication with the pediatrician are sufficient precautions. Criteria for admission to a hospital include significant tachypnea (greater than 60 breaths per minute) in a small infant and/or respiratory distress requiring oxygen therapy or further respiratory support. A bronchiolitic who appears fatigued or cyanotic or has respiratory acidosis and hy-

percarbia evident on arterial blood gas (ABG) should be admitted to the intensive care unit (ICU). The infants in this group tend to be younger than 4 or 5 months of age and may require intubation and mechanical ventilation (see Chapter 3). Neuromuscular blockade may be a necessary adjunct to respiratory therapy.

Oxygen is the mainstay of therapy for bronchiolitis. Most bronchiolitics admitted to a hospital are hypoxic with PO_2 values between 50 and 60 mm Hg. ABGs, therefore, are crucial both on admission and later, as indicated to guide oxygen therapy. Although at present the most common form of oxygen administration is in a tent, it is less than an optimal delivery system in view of "leaks" and fluctuations in FI_{O_2} resulting from opening of the tent to gain access to the patient. With smaller infants, a plastic head box system of delivery should be used.

Mist has traditionally been used, but with no good scientific basis. Recent studies have shown that it is not effective, because it does not reach the lower airways and may be detrimental by inducing bronchospasm. Mist is probably not indicated, and humidified oxygen alone is sufficient.

The risk of aspiration in infants who have marked tachypnea and significant respiratory distress precludes oral feedings, making intravenous fluids essential. Fluid accumulates in the lung as a consequence of the great negative intrathoracic pressure generated during inspiration and the hyperdynamic circulatory state present in patients with severe bronchiolitis. Determination of IV infusion rates, therefore, should be based upon the patient's state of hydration. Overhydration should be avoided, because it can adversely affect the respiratory status.

A chest x-ray should be obtained upon admission. It will classically demonstrate hyperinflation of the lungs, an increased anteroposterior chest diameter, flattening of the diaphragms, and increased interstitial markings. Antibiotics (e.g., ampicillin) are indicated only if an infiltrate is seen.

The use of bronchodilators in bronchiolitics is controversial. Controlled studies have generally shown no beneficial effect in infants younger than the age of 12 to 18 months. A trial of subcutaneous epinephrine or a nebulized beta-agonist may be warranted, depending upon the patient's clinical status. If there is improvement, IV aminophylline may be started, with the infant's special aminophylline pharmokinetics kept in mind. Serum theophylline levels should be followed frequently.

It has been postulated that the small infant's bronchial muscles are immature and thus unresponsive to bronchodilators. A more plausible explanation is that the principal pathologic mechanism of bronchiolitis is the inflammation and edema resulting in obstruction rather than bronchospasm.

The use of corticosteroids is another area of controversy. Controlled studies show them to be ineffective, though many clinicians may still opt to use them in a very sick bronchiolitic because of the inflammatory nature of the disease and the lack of toxicity in short-term steroid usage.

Isolation techniques are extremely important when dealing with RSV, especially in an intensive care unit (ICU). A nosocomially acquired RSV infection in a debilitated ICU patient can have devastating consequences. Respiratory isolation techniques should be strictly followed.

CASE PRESENTATION

A 6-month-old girl is brought to the pediatric emergency service by her parents for an increased respiratory rate and a whistling sound in her chest. Physical examination reveals an uncomfortable-appearing infant in respiratory distress with:
Substernal and supraclavicular retractions noted
Vital Signs: T = 102.7°F; HR = 160 beats/min; RR = 70 breaths/min; Wt = 7.2 kg
HEENT: nasal congestion
Neck: supple; Cor: RR, with no murmurs noted
Chest: diffuse rhonchi and wheezing
Abdomen: soft; Neuro: intact
An arterial blood gas, CBC, and electrolytes are obtained. The patient is started on oxygen, and a portable chest x-ray is obtained. The patient is then transferred to the pediatric floor.

Problem List

Respiratory

The results of ABG are pH = 7.34, P_{CO_2} = 33 mm Hg, and P_{O_2} = 62 mm Hg. The baby was placed in a tent with 35 percent humidified O_2. The chest x-ray film is read as hyperinflation with a possible patchy infiltrate in the right middle lobe.

Intake and Output (I & O)

The baby is made NPO and placed on IV D5W 1/5 NS with 10 mEq of KCL per 500 ml, added after she voids at maintenance rate. The specific gravity is 1.030, and the electrolytes are normal. The fluids are raised to 1 1/4 maintenance.

Infectious

The baby is placed in respiratory isolation. The CBC reveals:

WBC = 9,500 (50 segs, 10 bands, 35 lymph, 5 monos)
Platelets = 250,000; Hct = 36%
After the chest x-ray film has been read, a blood culture is obtained and the patient is started on ampicillin, 100 mg/kg/day divided every 6 hours.

In spite of O_2 therapy, the patient's respiratory rate is still in the 70's, with continued retractions. The repeat ABG reveals: pH = 7.31, P_{CO_2} = 40 mm Hg, and P_{O_2} = 74 mm Hg. Because of the increased P_{CO_2} and continued respiratory distress, the patient is moved to the pediatric ICU for closer observation.

A dose of nebulized metaproterenol is given, with no symptomatic relief, and the P_{CO_2} continues to hover around 40 mm Hg, in spite of tachypnea. By 8 hours post-admission, the patient has not improved; there are increasing signs of respiratory distress and there is a rise in P_{CO_2} to 61 mm Hg. The patient is electively intubated, and assisted mechanical ventilation is begun with improvement in her blood gases. Methylprednisolone is begun at 2 mg/kg/day, divided every 6 hours intravenously.

The baby is able to be extubated 2 days later and is sent to the ward the following day in good condition.

SUGGESTED READING

Brooks, L.S., and Cropp, G.J.A.: Theophylline therapy in bronchiolitis. Am. J. Dis. Child 135:934, 1981.
Stalcup, S.A., and Mellins, R.B.: Mechanical forces producing pulmonary edema in acute asthma. N. Engl. J. Med. 297:592, 1977.
Whol, M.E., and Chernick, V.: State of the art bronchiolitis. Am. Rev. Respir. Dis. 118:759, 1978.
Workshop on Bronchiolitis. Pediatr. Res. 11(3): March 1977, Part 2.

Nursing Process for Patient Care:

Bronchiolitis

The child admitted to the unit with a diagnosis of bronchiolitis presents with some degree of respiratory distress. The focus of attention in terms of assessment, monitoring, and anticipation is clearly respiratory. The young age of the child and the severity of the illness can have a profound effect on the child and the parents. Attention to the emotional effects of this illness and hospitalization is important in providing comprehensive care to the child and family.

RESPIRATORY

Assess, Monitor, and Document

Respiratory rate
Pattern
Work of breathing: retractions, nasal flaring
Breath sounds: rhonchi, wheezes
Color

Heart rate
Level of consciousness
Response to medications: oxygen, nebulized metaproterenol, aminophylline

Post–Intubation

Endotracheal tube
   Patency: suction as needed

Position: breath sounds, equal chest excursion

Anticipate

Acute respiratory failure
   Altered level of consciousness
   Restlessness
   Agitation
   Decreased respiratory rate
   Decreased or absent breath sounds

Cyanosis
Arterial blood gases: hypoxemia, hypercarbia, acidosis
Airway obstruction: plugged endotracheal tube

CARDIOVASCULAR

Assess, Monitor, and Document

Heart rate
Rhythm
Quality

Perfusion
Blood pressure

Anticipate

Tachycardia
Dysrrhythmias

FLUID AND ELECTROLYTE BALANCE

Fluid balance is a key issue in infants with severe bronchiolitis. Fluid accumulates in the lung as a consequence of the negative intrathoracic pressure generated during inspiration and the hyperdynamic circulatory state. Overhydration must be prevented. Careful assessment and monitoring of the child's fluid status is important.

Assess, Monitor and Document

Fluid intake: accurate administration of parenteral fluids (use infusion pump if available)
Weight

Urine output
Urine specific gravity
Laboratory data: serum electrolytes

Anticipate

Fluid overload: weight gain
Pulmonary edema

INFECTION

Assess, Monitor, and Document

Temperature
WBC
Appropriate cultures
Isolation techniques

Anticipate

Fever
Secondary infection

RESPONSE OF CHILD

Assess, Monitor, and Document

Developmental level: cognitive, psychosocial, normal fears
Behavioral response: anxious, tearful, angry, compliant
Response to nursing interventions

Anticipate

Emotional distress

RESPONSE OF FAMILY

Assess, Monitor, and Document

Behavioral response: anxious, angry, verbal
Level of understanding of the child's condition

Expected outcome
Response to nursing interventions

Anticipate

Family crisis

MIND SET

Assess

Respiratory status
Cardiovascular status
Fluid and electrolyte balance

Presence of infection
Response of child and family

Anticipate

Acute respiratory failure
Aspiration
Decreased cardiac output

Infection
Emotional distress
Family crisis

Bronchopulmonary Dysplasia

MICHAEL GRAFF, M.D.

Advances in the care of sick neonates over the past 20 years have resulted in a lower mortality rate. Improved survival among low birth weight infants has led to the emergence of bronchopulmonary dysplasia (BPD), a chronic respiratory disease affecting the lung parenchyma and airways. The incidence of BPD is difficult to ascertain. Those at highest risk for BPD are the smallest and most ill of the premature infants. In these neonates, the incidence may be 15 to 20 percent. However, any newborn with lung disease may develop BPD; some centers report a 5 percent incidence in their ventilated newborns, independent of birth weight.

BPD was first described in 1963. The initial description divided the disease into four radiographic stages, each serving as a prognostic indicator of progression of the disease (Table 26–1). These subdivisions are imprecise, with a large amount of overlap between the different stages.

PATHOGENESIS

Although 20 years have passed since BPD was first described, the pathogenesis remains elusive. Although numerous etiologies have been suggested, a few warrant more detailed examination.

Barotrauma

Barotrauma caused by positive pressure ventilation has been proposed as playing a major role in the pathogenesis of BPD. Neonates who received intermittent positive pressure ventilation (IPPV) have been shown to have a significant increase in airway resistance (Raw) at 7 months of age when compared with infants managed with continuous positive airway pressure (CPAP) or oxyhood alone. An etiologic role for barotrauma is also suggested by the

absence of BPD in infants treated with negative pressure ventilators. It must be noted, however, that no controlled study has been performed comparing positive and negative pressure ventilation and that the smallest and sickest neonates always require positive pressure ventilation. Although it appears that barotrauma plays a role, the pathogenesis of BPD cannot be exclusively explained by the use of IPPV, because the disease has occurred in newborns treated without positive pressure ventilation.

Oxygen Toxicity

Oxygen has been shown to be toxic to lung tissue. Newborn animals kept in an environment of greater than 95 percent oxygen for 24 hours have a pulmonary disorder similar clinically and histologically to BPD. Premature infants are thought to be particularly susceptible to elevated oxygen concentrations. This increased susceptibility may result from their lack of superoxide dismutase or their low vitamin E levels, both of which act to protect the lung from the oxidative damage caused by free oxygen radicals. Although oxygen appears to play a role in the pathogenesis of BPD, no direct relationship between duration of exposure to oxygen and the frequency of developing BPD has been shown.

Patent Ductus Arteriosus

The fact that some newborns who are ventilated with positive pressure and who receive oxygen do not develop BPD suggests that other factors may be necessary in conjunction with these primary causes. The persistence of the patent ductus arteriosus (PDA) has been implicated as such a factor. As many as 80 percent of newborns who subsequently develop BPD have a significant ductus arteriosus. The ductus may contribute to the development of BPD by

Table 26–1. Bronchopulmonary Dysplasia–Staging

Stage I: Period of Acute Respiratory Distress Syndrome (1–3 days of age)
  Radiographic findings: "classic" radiographic findings of RDS
    Increased opacity
    Reticular granular pattern
    Presence of air-bronchograms
  Pathology
    Hyaline membranes
    Hyperemia
    Atelectasis

Stage II: Period of Regeneration (4–10 days of age)
  Radiographic findings
    Nearly complete opacification
    Obscured cardiac silhouette
  Pathology
    Necrosis with repair of alveolar epithelia
    Persistence of hyaline membrane
    Emphysematous coalescence of alveoli
    Delicate focal thickening of capillary basement membranes

Stage III: Period of Transition (10–20 days of age)
  Radiographic findings
    Radiolucent bullae distributed throughout both lungs
    Areas of irregular densities alternating with hyperaeration
  Pathology
    Widespread bronchial and bronchiolar mucosal metaplasia
    Alveolar coalescence with groups forming areas of emphysema
    Thickening and widening of basement membrane

Stage IV: Period of Chronic Disease (1 month of age)
  Radiographic findings
    Enlargement of radiolucent bullae
    Decreased number of areas of radiodensity
    Cardiomegaly
  Pathology
    Focal areas of emphysema
    Hypertrophy of peribronchiolar smooth muscle
    Perimucosal fibrosis and widespread metaplasia
    Generalized basement membrane thickening

---

causing an increase in pulmonary blood flow and a secondary decrease in pulmonary compliance. The decrease in pulmonary compliance may then lead to increased respiratory support, including higher peak pressures and $F_{I_{O_2}}$. Because the recent trend is for earlier ductal ligation, the role of the ductus in the development of BPD may soon be modified.

In summary, a single entity is probably not the cause of BPD. The pathogenesis appears to originate from an interplay of several events that act on a very immature lung and disrupt its extrauterine adaptation.

CLINICAL AND RADIOGRAPHIC CORRELATION

According to the classification system devised by Northway, BPD can be divided into four stages. The best way to understand the classification is to correlate the stages of BPD with concurrent radiographic findings. It must

be emphasized, however, that not all patients with BPD progress through each stage and not all are necessarily oxygen dependent.

Stage I: Acute Respiratory Distress (2–3 days)

Stage I is indistinguishable clinically and radiographically from hyaline membrane disease (HMD). The patients present with tachypnea, grunting, retractions, and cyanosis. The radiographic findings show a ground glass appearance with air bronchograms.

Stage II: Recovery Phase (4–10 days after onset)

Stage II can be subdivided into two groups according to the clinical outcome. Stage IIA is composed of those infants who progressively improve. Initially, they are oxygen dependent, but their oxygen demands decrease as their respiratory condition improves. Radiographically, Stage IIA is indistinguishable from Stage I, with progressive clearing and complete resolution. Stage IIB is composed of those infants who fail to improve clinically and eventually become oxygen dependent. Radiographically, Stage IIB is characterized by either interstitial emphysema or increasing opacification. Air-trapping is frequent during this phase, and the incidence of spontaneous pneumothorax is increased.

Stage III: Transitional Stage

Stage III includes those infants who have passed through Stage II and continue to require oxygen and occasionally ventilatory support. Radiographically, Stage III is characterized by cystic areas alternating with those of increased consolidation.

Stage IV: Chronic Phase

Stage IV represents the chronic phase of BPD. Infants in this stage generally are respirator dependent and have some evidence of right-sided heart failure and pulmonary hypertension. Infants in Stage IV may slowly progress to an improved status, but frequently show a stepwise progression during the course of their improvement, with frequent periods of regression. The survival rate for this stage has been reported to be approximately 50 percent, with some of the surviving infants demonstrating oxygen dependency for as long as 2 years. Radiographically, Stage IV is characterized by areas of atelectasis interspersed with cystic areas of hyperaeration. It is important to note that the radiographs, even in those infants successfully weaned from oxygen, may continue to reveal increased areas of hyperaeration interspersed with fibrosis.

MANAGEMENT

Management of patients at risk for BPD must be twofold: it must alleviate the potential causes of BPD, and it must treat the disturbed physiology without causing further damage.

Stages I and II are treated in the same manner as HMD. Ventilator settings and oxygen content should be the minimal needed to provide adequate oxygenation and gas exchange. Attempts should be made to ventilate with the lowest pressures and frequencies possible, thereby minimizing barotrauma. If the radiograph reveals a progression to Stage IIB, an increased effort must be made to wean the patient from the ventilator. Arterial blood gases should be monitored, and the oxygen concentration should be regulated to maintain partial oxygen pressures (P_{O_2}) of 50 to 60 mm Hg. Nutritional support should be provided as soon as possible.

As the disease progresses to the more chronic stages (III and IV) and oxygen dependence becomes established, the patient should be continued on settings that provide the minimal ventilatory support to maintain an adequate P_{O_2}. During the chronic stages of BPD, arterial blood gases become more difficult to obtain. Falls of 20 mm Hg or greater in Pa_{O_2} have been noted to occur during these procedures. Transcutaneous oxygen monitors and earlobe oximeters can be useful in this context by providing daily trends of oxygenation and by minimizing the number of blood gases needed.

Patients with BPD often display evidence of fluid retention and require intermittent diuretic therapy. Furosemide (Lasix) has been shown to be useful at a dose of 1 mg per kg per dose whenever a diuretic is clinically indicated. For those infants who display chronic right heart failure, a chronic regimen of diuretic therapy is needed; oral Lasix given every 6 hours has been used. The use of chronic diuretic therapy is not without risks, and the patients should be monitored for hyponatremia, calcium wasting and urolithiasis. Recently, theophylline has been advocated for use in patients with Stage IV (chronic) BPD. The mode of action of theophylline in these patients is not known, but the beneficial effect may be secondary to its acting as a mild diuretic, its bronchodilator activity, or its ability to improve minute ventilation by increasing CO_2 sensitivity.

As with any chronic illness, nutrition plays a vital role. It is imperative to provide optimal nutrition to these patients as soon as possible. Because these infants are often unable to tolerate enough calories enterally to sustain growth, supplemental parenteral alimentation should be used until good growth is seen.

Patients that require chronic respiratory care are prone to respiratory infections. Frequently, patients with BPD are operating at maximal respiratory capacity and any increase in demand, such as is induced by a lower respiratory tract infection, may cause respiratory failure. It is difficult, however, to diagnose respiratory infections in these infants. Temperature instability, tachypnea, and rales are features of the underlying disease process. The radiographic diagnosis is also difficult, because features commonly associated with pneumonia are masked by the underlying chronic pulmonary changes. It is important that clinicians maintain a high index of suspicion regarding even minimal deterioration in their respiratory status. Empiric antibiotic therapy plays an important adjunctive role in managing periodic episodes of respiratory decompensation.

Nursing care plays a major role in the management of BPD. Suctioning and chest physiotherapy are necessary in all stages. General supportive care is crucial to achieve a successful outcome and must include infant stimulation. Although parents are encouraged to visit as often as possible, nurses and other hospital personnel play the important role of surrogate parents, providing the infants with the tactile, visual, and auditory stimulation needed for optimal growth.

Some institutions advocate the use of home care for their chronic patients. Parents should be taught how to provide suctioning and chest physiotherapy as well as to recognize subtle changes in clinical status. It is advisable to have the parents stay with the child for several days in the controlled environment of the hospital to ease the transition to home care and to monitor the parents' abilities to cope with the increased needs of an ill child.

Those children who are sent home, on or off oxygen, continue to require intensive follow-up. Children with BPD have been noticed to have an increased incidence of respiratory failure. Occasionally, a common URI can progress rapidly to pneumonia with concomitant respiratory failure. Parents should be warned to remain alert for signs of infection and respiratory distress, and they should be encouraged to seek aid early in the disease process.

PREVENTION

Prevention of BPD is not yet possible. Although ventilators and oxygen play a role in the development of BPD, no alternative mode of therapy currently exists for the treatment of severe respiratory illness in newborns.

Ventilator care has been improved in recent years. The recent development of mean airway pressure (MAP) monitors may provide a way to decrease peak airway pressure without sacrificing oxygenation. Extracorporeal membrane oxygenation (ECMO) has been used experimentally for the care of sick newborns and may provide a tool in the future for oxygenating the smallest and sickest infants without causing pulmonary damage.

Vitamin E has been suggested as a means of preventing BPD. Infants who are at risk for BPD are generally preterm and relatively deficient in vitamin E. The use of vitamin E during the acute phase of respiratory distress syndrome (RDS) has been advocated and preliminary reports reveal some decrease in the incidence of BPD in those groups treated with vitamin E. Vitamin E therapy may be a way of minimizing the effect that oxygen plays in the pathogenesis of BPD.

CASE PRESENTATION

Presentation

A 6-month-old boy arrived in the pediatric emergency room with a chief complaint of increasing respiratory distress. A nursing triage revealed a small infant with acute respiratory distress, nasal flaring, grunting, and intercostal retractions. Vital signs were: HR = 160 beats/min, RR = 65 breaths/min, BP = 95/65 mm Hg, and a rectal temperature of 101.8°F.

History

A history, provided by the mother, was pertinent to the infant's being a product of a 28-week gestation and acutely ill at birth. He had been maintained on a ventilator with high levels of oxygen for several weeks of life and continued to require oxygen therapy until 5 months of age. Two weeks before this emergency room visit, he was discharged from the hospital.

Examination

Physical examination revealed a 3.5 kg male with bilateral wheezing, scattered coarse rhonchi, and basilar rales. A I to II/VI systolic ejection murmur was noticed at the lower left sternal border and a 2- to 3- cm liver edge was palpable below the right costal margin. The other results of the physical examination were noncontributory.

Emergency chest x-rays were ordered and a request was sent for the patient's old hospital records. The chest x-ray was remarkable for areas of consolidation alternating with cystic areas of hyperlucency and with a large area of consolidation at the right base. A worsening of the infant's respiratory status was noted, and a re-examination revealed an increase in the amount of wheezing and slight perioral cyanosis. Emergency blood work and cultures were obtained, and the patient was placed in an oxyhood and transferred to the pediatric ICU.

In the pediatric ICU, it was noted that the patient had symptoms of acute respiratory distress. Vital signs were: RR = 75 breaths/min, HR = 165 beats/min, BP = 100/65 mm Hg. Physical examination revealed an acutely ill, agitated infant with tachypnea, nasal flaring, and intercostal and subcostal pleural retractions. He had bilateral wheezing, with rales noted in the right base of the chest.

Problem List

Intake and Output (I & O)

A history taken from the mother was pertinent to the fact that the child's intake had been poor for the 12 hours prior to admission. The patient was bagged for a urine analysis and stat electrolytes were drawn. An IV line was placed, and fluids were administered at maintenance requirements. An adequate diuresis was noted, but because of worsening of his respiratory status, a 1 mg/kg dose of furosemide was given. Fluids were subsequently restricted to two-thirds maintenance, with close monitoring of his hydration status. All electrolytes remained in the normal range.

Respiratory

Comparisons of the patient's previous x-rays and the one obtained on the day of admission revealed a similar pattern of hyperlucency alternating with areas of consolidation but without the right lower lobe infiltrate.

The patient arrived in the pediatric ICU in a oxyhood in 40 percent oxygen. An arterial blood gas obtained in 40 percent oxygen had a pH of 7.56, PO_2 of 40 mm Hg, and a PCO_2 of 45 mm Hg. The oxygen concentration was increased to 65 percent.

The patient's clinical condition continued to deteriorate. Arterial blood gases revealed persistent hypoxemia, and a physical examination showed an increased amount of wheezing and the presence of basilar rales. A stat dose of furosemide was given and was followed by a large diuresis and slight clinical improvement. IV theophylline and nasal CPAP were begun, and over the next 12 hours, clinical improvement was noted.

Infectious

The chest x-ray film was evaluated as a right lower lobe pneumonia superimposed on a chronic lung condition consistent with BPD. A blood culture, throat culture, and CBC were obtained and appropriate antibiotics were begun.

Cardiac

A cardiologist was consulted to evaluate the heart murmur and the possibility of congestive heart failure (CHF). A cardiac ultrasound demonstrated right ventricular hypertrophy and pulmonary hypertension. The recommendation was that digitalis not be used and that intermittent diuretic therapy be used as needed.

The patient's clinical condition improved over the subsequent 3 days, oxygen therapy was stopped and feedings were begun.

Hospital Course

When the child had been weaned to room air, the nurses noted that feedings and crying episodes were accompanied by perioral cyanosis. An earlobe oximeter was placed to record trends in his oxygen saturation for the subsequent 8 hours. Oxygen saturation was noted to be 90 to 95% while the patient was resting, decreasing to 50% when he was agitated or fed. It was decided to provide oxygen to the patient during feedings or whenever excessive exertion was noted.

Reports from the bacteriology laboratory revealed a gram-positive organism in the blood cultures, later identified as pneumococcus. The same organism was noted in the throat culture and was sensitive to penicillin. A repeat blood culture was taken, and antibiotics were changed to penicillin G. A 10-day course of IV penicillin was completed.

Continued improvement was noticed until Day 14 of hospitalization, when he was noticed to be more irritable, tachypneic, and tachycardic.

A physical examination revealed the presence of basilar rales and fine expiratory wheezing. A stat injection of intramuscular furosemide was given. It was followed by a large diuresis and clinical improvement.

Intermittent bouts of mild respiratory distress continued to occur over the following days, but each episode was followed by spontaneous improvement. During hospitalization, the theophylline was discontinued; the patient was discharged after 3 weeks of hospitalization.

Follow-up was continued in an outpatient clinic specializing in the care of premature infants. At 1 year of age, because of a subsequent episode of respiratory distress and wheezing, theophylline therapy was begun and maintained.

SUGGESTED READING

Ehrenkranz, R.A., Bonta, B.W., Ablow, R.C., et al.: Amelioration of bronchopulmonary dysplasia after vitamin E administration. N. Engl. J. Med. 299:564, 1978.

Markestad, T., and Fitzhardinge, P.M.: Growth and development in children recovering from bronchpulmonary dysplasia. J. Pediatr. 98:597, 1981.

Northway, W.H., Rosan, R.C., and Porter, D.Y.: Pulmonary disease following respirator therapy of hyaline membrane disease. N. Engl. J. Med. 276:357, 1967.

Taghizadeh, A., and Reynolds, E.O.R.: Pathogenesis of bronchopulmonary dysplasia following hyaline membrane disease. Am. J. Pathol. 82:241, 1976.

Workshop on Bronchopulmonary Dysplasia. J. Pediatr. 95:815, 1979.

Nursing Process for Patient Care:
Bronchopulmonary Dysplasia

Bronchopulmonary dysplasia (BPD) is a chronic respiratory disease that is a sequela primarily of respiratory distress syndrome (RDS) in premature infants. Oxygen and barotrauma caused by positive pressure ventilation have been implicated as etiologic factors in the development of BPD. The persistence of a patent ductus arteriosus may be a contributing factor.

Some children with BPD have residual respiratory failure that requires suctioning, chest physiotherapy, and oxygen administration at home. Others have a lesser degree of respiratory insufficiency but decompensate in the presence of infection.

RESPIRATORY

Assess, Monitor, and Document

Respiratory rate
Pattern
Work of breathing: retractions (substernal, suprasternal, intercostal, midclavicular), nasal flaring
Breath sounds
Color

Skin condition
Restlessness
Agitation
Level of consciousness: activity
Arterial blood gases
Response to medications

Post–Intubation

* Patency of tube: equal chest excursion, breath sounds present in all areas, suction catheter passes easily
Response to pulmonary toilet

Ventilator settings: oxygen concentration, flow rate, inspiratory pressure, IMV
Response to ventilatory management

Anticipate

Acute respiratory failure
  Restlessness
  Hypoxia: cyanosis
  Hypercarbia
  Increased work of breathing

Fatigue
Obstruction of tube
Displacement of tube
Accidental extubation

FLUID AND ELECTROLYTE BALANCE

Assess, Monitor, and Document

Weight
Urine output
Urine specific gravity
Fluid intake: accurate administration of parenteral fluids (use infusion pump if available)

Serum electrolytes
Urine electrolytes
Response to medications: furosemide, theophylline

Anticipate

Fluid overload

RESPONSE OF CHILD

Assess, Monitor, and Document

Developmental level: fears, response to separation; psychosocial, motor, and verbal skills
Response to nursing interventions

Anticipate

Emotional distress
Disruption of normal growth and development

RESPONSE OF FAMILY

Assess, Monitor, and Document

Behavioral response: anxiety, fear, disappointment, despair
Level of knowledge of BPD and child's condition and expected outcome
Ability to cope
Ability to relate to child and foster normal growth and development

Learning needs related to discharge
    Assessment of child's respiratory status
    Signs of respiratory distress
    Utilization of special equipment
    Special techniques: pulmonary toilet
Nursing strategies used to facilitate coping and to prepare for discharge

Anticipate

Family crisis
Inability to cope

Learning needs related to discharge and home management

MIND SET

Assess

Respiratory status
Cardiovascular status

Fluid and electrolyte balance
Response of child and family

Anticipate

Alteration in respiratory status
    Acute respiratory failure
    Respiratory infection
Alteration in cardiovascular status
    Congestive heart failure (CHF)

Alteration in fluid and electrolyte balance
    Fluid overload
Emotional distress
Family crisis

Croup and Epiglottitis

ALAN G. KULBERG, M.D.

Obstruction of the upper airway secondary to bacterial epiglottitis or viral laryngotracheitis may develop rapidly and pose a threat to life. The intensive care unit (ICU) shares the responsibilities of establishment and, more so, preservation of a patent airway in these situations.

ANATOMY AND PATHOPHYSIOLOGY OF THE UPPER AIRWAY

Knowledge of the anatomy and pathophysiology of the upper airway is crucial to understanding the symptoms of the various disorders that can produce obstruction of the airway. The upper airway has extrathoracic and intrathoracic components. The supraglottis (area above the vocal cords) and the glottis (the vocal cords) are purely extrathoracic (Fig. 27–1), whereas the infraglottis (area below the cords, including the trachea) has both extrathoracic and intrathoracic parts. On inspiration in children, the walls of the extrathoracic airway tend to collapse toward the lumen because of the softness and flexibility of these tissues. At the same time, the intrathoracic airway tends to expand with thoracic expansion. The opposite holds true during expiration, with the caliber of the intrathoracic trachea decreasing and that of the extrathoracic airway increasing. When there is intact innervation by the recurrent laryngeal nerves, the vocal cords will remain in the abducted position during both phases of respiration, providing a constant space for airflow.

The relatively small cross-sectional area of the upper airway in pediatric patients is the critical factor predisposing to airway obstruction by superimposed inflammatory processes. The pressure required to produce a given flow through a tube, and similarly the resistance to flow in the tube, varies directly with the length of the tube and inversely with the fourth power of the radius, as described by the following relationship:

$$\Delta P \; \alpha \; \frac{l \, V}{r^4}$$

where

ΔP = pressure gradient

l = length of tube

V = airflow

r = radius of tube

The radius of the tube assumes the greatest importance in determining resistance to flow. If the length of the tube is increased fourfold, the pressure must be increased fourfold to maintain constant flow, but if the radius of the tube is halved, the pressure must be increased sixteenfold to maintain constant flow.

Clinically, the patient must significantly increase airway pressure to overcome the resistance produced by the presence of a stenotic lesion. To do so requires the use of the accessory muscles of respiration in the neck, thoracic cage, and abdomen; that is, the patient will exhibit retractions. Given the same absolute decrease in the radius of the airway of both an infant and an older child, the infant will experience greater resistance to flow, because the infant's airway is intrinsically smaller and a greater proportion of the lumen is compromised. One mm of mucosal edema will reduce the glottic airway in the newborn infant to almost one third the normal size. Obviously, the older child will tolerate the same encroachment better.

Stridor, the noisy inspiratory "crow" or expiratory "bark," is the most significant indicator of upper airway obstruction. In general,

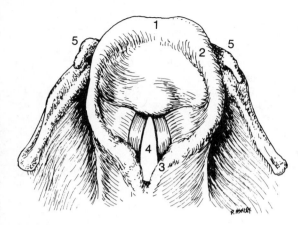

Figure 27–1. Glottis and supraglottis (posterosuperior view; 1 = epiglottis, 2 = aryepiglottic fold (right), 3 = arytenoid cartilage (right), 4 = vocal cords, 5 = hyoid bone)

the higher the level of obstruction, the more prominent is the inspiratory sound; the lower the obstruction, the more noticeable is the expiratory effort, with wheezing present at times. With obstruction in the middle region of the upper airway, the patient may show signs in both phases of respiration. Involvement of the vocal cords with an inflammatory process produces hoarseness.

VIRAL LARYNGOTRACHEITIS (CROUP)

Viral laryngotracheitis, or laryngotracheobronchitis, commonly referred to as *croup,* is a disease usually caused by the parainfluenza or influenza virus. It is characterized by an inflammatory process that produces edema and fibrinous exudate mainly in the glottic and subglottic regions. Children younger than the age of 3 years are most often affected. The major clinical signs of crowing stridor on inspiration, a cough that sounds like the bark of a seal, and hoarseness are signs that typically develop after a febrile upper respiratory illness of about 1- to 3-day duration. The pattern of illness ranges from an acute and fulminant course producing obstruction in less than a day to a more subacute progression over several days. In the latter situation, the danger is not only from obstruction but also from hypoventilation, because the child fatigues as a result of the increased work of breathing. Although emotional agitation will cause an exaggeration of the stridor, hypoxemia should be ruled out as a sole or contributing factor before ascribing the agitation to emotion. A more accurate assessment of the severity of the disease can be obtained when the child is in a calmer state. Hypercarbia should be regarded as an ominous feature, signifying either fatigue-induced hypoventilation or severe airway obstruction.

Acute pulmonary edema (APE) has been described in association with the croup syndrome caused by adenovirus. For therapy of APE, see the discussion of treatment of pulmonary edema in the section on epiglottitis.

Therapy

Patients with relatively mild viral laryngotracheitis do well with simple supportive therapy. Almost universally recognized as a therapeutic adjunct, nebulized mist often provides some relief of obstruction by improving local airway hydration and facilitating the expectoration of secretions.

The intensive care patient, however, usually qualifies for more advanced forms of therapy. Racemic epinephrine, a 1:1 mixture of the L (active) and D (inactive) isomers of epinephrine, is an effective therapeutic modality for croup. It is safest when delivered by face mask. The solution to be delivered is prepared by mixing 0.2 to 0.5 ml of the 2.25 percent racemic epinephrine with 2.5 ml of normal saline (NS). A single inhaled dose of racemic epinephrine produces an effect that peaks in 10 to 30 minutes and has an overall duration of 1 to 2 hours. A rational plan for administration consists of a dose every 1 to 2 hours as clinically indicated. More frequent administration should be discouraged. The ICU is the safest place to deliver this therapy, because some patients may experience a rebound phenomenon, becoming more obstructed after a dosing interval than at the onset of therapy. Close observation is essential.

Pharmacologic doses of corticosteroids (dexamethasone, hydrocortisone, or methylprednisolone) may be a helpful adjunct when the child requires more than inhalation therapy. Although their efficacy has not been proved conclusively, corticosteroids are commonly used in cases of severe upper airway obstruction. Given the abundance of favorable experience reported and the lack of any documented danger in its use, steroid therapy may be helpful in avoiding intubation in very ill children.

The definitive form of therapy, placement of an artificial airway, should be reserved for severely ill children in whom medical management is unsuccessful, yet there should be no delay whenever clinical indications are evident. These indications include steady deterioration of arterial blood gases and exhaustion of the patient. Intubation and tracheostomy, although potentially lifesaving, have long been feared as methods of therapy for viral laryngotracheitis because of the risk of developing subglottic stenosis as a consequence of trauma to an inflamed airway. In the hands of a skilled anesthesiologist, however, nasotracheal intubation can provide a reliable patent airway, with minimum complications. Firmly taping the tube to the nose will prevent movement and reduce trauma to the wall of the airway. The tube should be 1 mm smaller in diameter than would otherwise be selected for the child to prevent scarring secondary to ischemia from pressure applied to airway mucosa.

Sedation is contraindicated unless the patient has an artificial airway in place.

Infants and children who have recurrent, severe stridor, with or without a febrile upper respiratory infection, should be evaluated for the presence of a congenital obstructive lesion (web, stenosis). Such patients should be referred for otolaryngologic evaluation.

EPIGLOTTITIS

The term *epiglottitis* describes a cellulitis of the supraglottic airway, caused almost exclusively in childhood by *Hemophilus influenzae* type B. The disease process involves not only the epiglottis but also the other soft tissues above the glottis, including the aryepiglottic folds. Involvement of these folds contributes more to the actual obstruction than the epiglottis itself. The disease can strike at any age, although the mean age of those affected is 3 to 4 years. It affects both sexes almost equally and does not have a seasonal predilection.

The fulminant nature of epiglottitis qualifies it as a true emergency; establishment of a reliable airway is the first priority.

The clinical picture is usually that of an acutely ill child with onset of symptoms within the previous 12 to 24 hours. The child is febrile and often chooses to sit up and lean forward with the tongue partially extruded, emitting a low-pitched flutter on inspiration and a strangled, garbled noise on exhalation. Because of throat pain and swelling partially obstructing the esophageal inlet, the child may drool saliva.

Infections that have been noted in association with epiglottitis are acute otitis media and pneumonitis, sometimes with a pleural effusion. Fortunately, meningitis due to *Hemophilus influenzae* type B is a rare concomitant, and the patient should receive a lumbar puncture only if the clinical condition warrants it.

The diagnosis of epiglottitis can be confirmed by a lateral x-ray of the neck. Positive findings include effacement of the vallecula, swelling of the epiglottis and aryepiglottic folds, and distention of the hypopharynx. At times, reversal of the normal cervical lordotic curve is evident, reflecting the child's position of comfort.

Therapy

The role of the ICU in cases of children with epiglottitis is airway maintenance, which begins when the child returns from the operating room, where an artificial airway has been established (Table 27–1). A well-coordinated protocol combining the efforts of the pediatrician, otolaryngologist, anesthesiologist, and radiologist, all understanding the swift progression of the disease, is the best way to avoid needless mortality from epiglottitis.

Although tracheostomy was long considered the airway of choice, increased experience has made nasotracheal intubation a routine procedure in many large institutions. The type of airway used is the choice of the person performing the procedure. When performed by competent personnel, endotracheal intubation and tracheostomy have similar mortality rates.

Upon the patient's arrival at the ICU with the artificial airway in place, the lungs are auscultated to ensure that there is equal air entry. An anteroposterior chest film is obtained to confirm that the tip of the endotracheal tube is midway between the vocal cords and the carina. The tube can be marked with an indelible pen on tape where it emerges from the mouth or nose, so that its proper position in the airway can be restored if it accidentally moves. Furthermore, the chest film may reveal acute pulmonary edema, which has been described in patients with epiglottitis following intubation and is presumably a result of the rapid transudation of fluid from the pulmonary capillary bed into the alveoli as central venous return suddenly increases following relief of the airway obstruction.

Post-intubation pulmonary edema can be treated by increasing the continuous positive airway pressure (CPAP) from the 2 cm H_2O

Table 27–1. Role of the Intensive Care Unit in a Multidisciplinary Protocol for Epiglottitis

Emergency Service
Diagnosis is made clinically and/or radiographically.
Child is kept calm, in a comfortable sitting position, with nebulized O_2, if tolerated.
Anesthesiology and otolaryngology consultants are assembled in the emergency service, with airway equipment.
Child is transported, with consultants, to the operating room.

Operating Room
Child is anesthetized with halothane and O_2, and an IV cannula is inserted.
The airway is visualized, and an artificial airway is established.
  The airway is securely taped in place.
Blood specimens are drawn, and IV antibiotic therapy is begun.

Intensive Care Unit
Self-extubation is prevented by sedating child and splinting both elbows with armboards.
After at least 36–48 hours of appropriate antibiotic therapy, the airway is revisualized, preferably in the operating room, and if found to be satisfactorily improved, extubation (or decannulation) is performed. This step can be performed in the ICU, provided that all necessary personnel and equipment for artificial airway reinsertion, in case that is necessary, are present.
Child is observed in the ICU for 24 hours for development of post-airway edema.
When child can take oral antibiotics, therapy is switched to oral for a total of 7–10 days.

pressure used to maintain functional residual volume in the intubated patient to 4 to 8 cm H_2O pressure. For the refractory patient, mechanical ventilation and diuretics (furosemide, 1 mg/kg/dose IV) may be useful therapeutic modalities.

The patient should have continuous cardiac monitoring during the initial critical period as well as during the entire ICU course. Frequent arterial blood gas (ABG) measurements may be needed for patients with pulmonary complications; this may require placement of an indwelling arterial catheter.

The nursing staff is responsible for meticulous care of the endotracheal tube or tracheostomy cannula. Suctioning should be performed when necessary and should be preceded by positive pressure ventilation with 100 percent oxygen delivered by bag apparatus. Normal saline (1 to 2 ml) may be instilled into the airway to facilitate removal of accumulated secretions.

General guidelines for admitting patients to the ICU follow:
1. Every child with epiglottitis
2. Viral laryngotracheobronchitis with:
 Hypoxemia, Pa_{O_2} < 70 mm Hg.
 Hypercarbia, or progressively rising Pa_{CO_2}.
 Moderate to severe retractions at "rest."
 Unresponsiveness to plain nebulized mist, when child might require racemic epinephrine.
3. The infant with known or suspected congenital airway stenotic lesion who develops an upper respiratory infection.

In the ICU every effort should be made to prevent the intubated child from self-extubating. The methods used are based upon individual preference as well as the nurse/patient ratio. If the choice is sedation, it should be given on a round-the-clock basis. Combinations of morphine sulfate, 0.1 mg per kg IV or IM (intramuscular) q 3 to 4 hours, with diazepam, 0.2 mg per kg IV q 4 hours, hydroxyzine, 1 mg per kg q 6 hours IM, or chloral hydrate, 15 to 25 mg per kg q 6 hours, are effective in producing sedation without respiratory depression. The endotracheal tube is attached to a T piece with humidified gas. If the choice is to allow the child to remain awake, a nasotracheal tube should be used and cut flush with the nostril, with no connector piece attached for the child to potentially grab. Heavy-duty sutures are placed through the end of the tube and knotted, and the long suture ends are taped securely to the cheek and nose (see Fig. 27–1). With either method, the child's elbows should be splinted with armboards as extra ensurance against self-extubation. In the event of premature extubation, there may be enough airway lumen caused by the space-occupying effect of the tube to allow a "grace period" for reintubation, either in the ICU or in the operating room. If assisted ventilation is required immediately and an anesthesiologist is not present, positive pressure bag–mask ventilation may be a satisfactory substitute in the interim. A tracheostomy tray should be available at the bedside at all times.

Final extubation is usually possible after 2 to 3 days, although some patients may require the tube for 5 days or more. It may be done in the ICU or in the operating room, provided that the proper equipment and personnel are on hand for reintubation, if necessary. Any sedation should be withheld for 6 to 8 hours prior to the planned extubation. When the patient is ready to have the tube removed, thiopental, 3 to 4 mg per kg IV push is given and the patient is laryngoscoped. If the supraglottic edema has subsided adequately, the tube can be removed. A chest x-ray is then obtained to determine the presence of any residual atelectasis.

Post-extubation stridor can be treated with nebulized racemic epinephrine. In the cases in which initial intubations are thought to be traumatic and problems are anticipated following extubation, systemic corticosteroids may be helpful if started 24 hours prior to extubation. If the extubated patient shows increasing stridor unresponsive to medical management, reintubation should be performed with the smallest possible tube and the procedure should be attempted again in 48 to 72 hours.

Antibiotics

After blood cultures have been drawn (after airway insertion), chloramphenicol, 100 mg per day IV, divided q 6 hours, is begun. Chloramphenicol is used because of the ubiquity of β-lactamase-producing *H. influenzae*. If the organism is recovered and found to be sensitive to ampicillin, the chloramphenicol can be discontinued. The dose of ampicillin is 200 to 300 mg per kg per day IV, divided q 6 hours. After the airway has been removed and the child is able to drink, the medication can be continued orally at home for a total of 7 to 10 days.

CASE PRESENTATION

B.L., an 11-month-old male, presented to the emergency service in respiratory distress. The current illness began 3 days prior to admission with rhinorrhea and a cough productive of clear sputum. Fluid intake was below normal. Fever during this period ranged from 37.8° to 38.5°C. Beginning approximately 12 hours prior to admission, the patient developed a barking cough with increased inspiratory effort.

At 4 months of age, the patient reportedly had an episode of "croup" that responded well to vaporizer therapy at home.

Examination

Physical examination revealed an anxious ill-appearing child, with pale, diaphoretic skin. Vital signs revealed: T = 38°C, BP = 90/50 mm Hg, pulse = 144/min, and RR = 30 breaths/min. The child showed moderately severe respiratory difficulty, with marked suprasternal, substernal, and intercostal retractions. There was a loud, high-pitched crowing sound on inspiration; a deep, paroxysmal, barking cough; and a hoarse cry. The remainder of the examination was pertinent for rhinorrhea and decreased air entry, with transmitted adventitious upper airway sounds on lung auscultation.

Test Results

Laboratory values on admission included a CBC, with a WBC count of 14,100/cu mm, 45 polys, 8 bands, 47 lymphs. Hemoglobin was 13.2 gm/dl, and hematocrit was 40 percent. Platelet count was estimated as adequate. Urinalysis revealed dark yellow urine with a specific gravity of 1.032, a pH of 5, and dip-positive for 1 + ketones. Microscopic examination revealed 0–2 WBC, 0–1 RBC/hpf. ABG on room air revealed: pH = 7.41, P_{CO_2} = 30 mm Hg, P_{O_2} = 60 mm Hg.

A lateral neck x-ray film showed a normal-sized epiglottis, with barely visible aryepiglottic folds. An anteroposterior film of the chest was read as normal.

Problem List

Respiratory

The child is obviously dyspneic, with signs compatible with upper respiratory obstruction due to viral laryngotracheitis (stridor, retractions, hoarseness, URI prodrome) and negative evidence for epiglottitis (no drooling, nonmuffled voice, normal lateral neck film). Although the ABG indicates adequate alveolar ventilation (P_{CO_2} = 30 mm Hg), the child is hypoxemic secondary to ventilation/perfusion mismatch. The patient should be given supplemental humidified oxygen.

Intake and Output (I & O)

Because of his respiratory distress, the child was unable to drink his normal quota of fluids. The increased respiratory rate also increased his insensible water loss in the form of water vapor. The hematocrit of 40 percent is slightly higher than normal for this age group and is consistent with hemoconcentration resulting from dehydration. The elevated urine specific gravity supports this conclusion. The child should be given enough IV fluids to establish a urine output of about 1 ml/kg/hr. The humidified oxygen will now decrease the insensible pulmonary water loss.

Neurologic

When there is mild hypoxemia, anxiety can probably be attributed to an emotional cause. The frightening feeling of breathing against an obstructed airway combined with unfamiliar people (personnel) and separation anxiety common to an 11-month-old are all contributory causes. The child should be made as comfortable as possible and should not be separated from his parents.

B.L. appeared to improve following the administration of 30 percent O_2 by mask; the severity of the retractions decreased slightly while he was allowed to sit on his parent's lap. He was admitted to the general ward. One hour later, the retractions worsened and he appeared slightly cyanotic around the mouth and nose. ABG results showed pH = 7.28, P_{CO_2} = 39 mm Hg, and P_{O_2} = 50 mm Hg.

The child was transferred to the ICU. The inspired oxygen concentration was increased to 45 percent. Racemic epinephrine in a 1:8 dilution with normal saline (NS) was given by hand-held nebulizer. After 10 minutes the child's color improved markedly and his state of agitation lessened. The racemic epinephrine therapy had to be repeated in 45 minutes and again 2 hours later, but each time there was a good clinical response. Only three more doses had to be given over the next 12 hours.

Eighteen hours after admission to the ICU, the child was only mildly stridorous and had good ABG while inhaling 28 percent oxygen.

His clinical course gradually improved and he was sent home 46 hours after admission.

A similar episode occurred 1 month later. Because of the recurrent nature of his upper airway disease, bronchoscopy was performed after clinical improvement, revealing a circumferential congenital sublgottic stenosis 2.5 cm below the level of the vocal cords.

SUGGESTED READING

Cantrell, R.W., Bell, R.A., and Morioka, W.T.: Acute epiglottitis: intubation versus tracheostomy. Laryngoscope 88:994, 1978.

Gross, C.W.: Medical management, nasotracheal intubation, and tracheotomy in the treatment of upper airway obstruction in children. Otolaryngol. Clin. North Am. 10:157, 166, 1977.

Hannallah, R., and Rosales, J.K.: Acute epiglottitis: current management and review. Can. Anaesth. Soc. J. 25:84, 1978.

Holinger, P.H., and Brown, W.T.: Congenital webs, cysts, laryngoceles, and other anomalies of the larynx. Ann. Otolaryngol. 76:744, 1967.

Shann, F.A., Phelan, P.D., Stocks, J.G., et al.: Prolonged nasotracheal intubation or tracheostomy in acute laryngotracheobronchitis and epiglottitis? Aust. Paediatr. J. 11:212, 1975.

Taussig, L.M., Castro, O., Beaudry P.H., et al.: Treatment of laryngotracheobronchitis (croup): use of intermittent positive-pressure breathing and racemic epinephrine. Am. J. Dis. Child 129:790, 1975.

Westley, C.R., Cotton, E.K., and Brooks, J.G.: Neubulized racemic epinephrine by IPPB for the treatment of croup: a double-blind study. Am. J. Dis. Child 132:484, 1978.

Croup and Epiglottitis

Viral laryngotracheobronchitis and bacterial epiglottitis set a stage for airway obstruction that can occur at any time. The prodrome may be several days for croup or several hours with epiglottitis. The presentation is usually dramatic, with the child in obvious distress. The mind set that emerges is almost entirely respiratory.

RESPIRATORY

Assess, Monitor, and Document

Respiratory rate
Heart rate
Work of breathing: nasal flaring, inspiratory stridor, retractions (substernal, suprasternal, intercostal)

Color
Level of consciousness: restlessness, lethargy, agitation
Arterial blood gases
Response to medications

Anticipate

Alteration in respiratory status
  Acute respiratory failure
  Sudden airway obstruction

Hypoxia, hypercarbia
Cardiac arrest

Post–Intubation

Patency of artificial airway: equal breath sounds, equal chest excursion, suction catheter passes easily, amount and consistency of secretions

Security of artificial airway: tube in place, child restrained appropriately
Response to pulmonary toilet
Response to medications

Anticipate

Obstruction of tube
Self-extubation
Post-intubation pulmonary edema

FLUID AND ELECTROLYTE BALANCE

Children in respiratory distress are usually dehydrated in relation to their inability to drink and to increased insensible water loss caused by their increased respiratory rate. Secretions are more difficult to manage in a dehydrated child. The presence of thick secretions in an already compromised airway can be dangerous.

Assess, Monitor, and Document

Weight
Fluid intake: accurate administration of parenteral fluids (use infusion pump if available)
Mucous membranes
Skin turgor
Tears
Thirst

Urine output
Urine specific gravity
Blood pressure
Pulse
Serum electrolytes
Hematocrit

Anticipate

Alteration in fluid and electrolyte status
  Dehydration
  Decreased urinary output

Increased urine specific gravity
Dry mucous membranes
Poor skin turgor

RESPONSE OF CHILD

Assess, Monitor, and Document

Developmental level: verbal, motor, psycho-social, cognitive
Degree of distress

Behavioral response: fearful, anxious, angry, compliant
Response to nursing interventions

Anticipate

Emotional distress

RESPONSE OF FAMILY

Assess, Monitor, and Document

Behavioral response: verbal, anxious, angry
Level of understanding of child's illness and condition

Expected outcome
Response to nursing interventions

Anticipate

Family crisis
Inability to cope

MIND SET

Assess

Respiratory status
Fluid and electrolyte status
Response of child and family

Anticipate

Alteration in respiratory status
  Acute respiratory failure
  Sudden airway obstruction
  Cardiorespiratory arrest

Pulmonary edema (post-intubation)
Emotional distress
Family crisis

28

Pulmonary Embolism

SOL S. ZIMMERMAN, M.D.

Pulmonary embolism is recognized as a leading cause of morbidity and mortality in the adult population, with approximately 500,000 cases and 50,000 fatalities occurring annually. With such a high incidence, the frequency of underdiagnosis is striking; over 50 percent of acute emboli diagnosed at autopsy were not diagnosed prior to death. Difficulty of diagnosis results from the lack of specific clinical and routine laboratory findings. In the pediatric population, in whom the incidence of pulmonary embolism is only a small fraction of that in the adult, only a very high index of suspicion will lead to early diagnosis and appropriate intervention.

ETIOLOGY

Pulmonary emboli are the consequence of venous thrombosis, primarily in the deep veins of the lower extremities. Less common sites include the pelvis, abdomen, and right atrium. Because venous thrombosis is the primary process and embolism is the complication, attention must be directed to those factors that contribute to thrombus formation: stasis, hypercoagulability, and altered vascular integrity.

Stasis is the primary predisposing factor in both children and adults. Patients at increased risk of thrombosis on this basis include those with spinal cord injury; prolonged states of unconsciousness; abdominal, pelvic, and lower extremity trauma; burns; and neuromuscular diseases (Guillain-Barré syndrome, Werdnig-Hoffmann disease). Patients with altered states of consciousness and those with sensory deficits (spinal cord trauma, spina bifida, Guillain-Barré syndrome) will be unable to perceive any discomfort arising from deep vein thrombosis and associated phlebitis. Even in the presence of intact sensation, however, venous thrombosis is frequently silent. Stasis may result not only from the bedridden status of the patient

but also from increased viscosity of blood. Polycythemia and hyperproteinemias, therefore, predispose to thrombus formation.

Hypercoagulable states, such as those associated with oral contraceptives and antithrombin III deficiency, contribute to a higher incidence of venous thrombi. Because there is widespread use of birth control pills among adolescent females, this age group is among those people considered at greater risk for deep vein thrombosis and pulmonary embolism.

Altered vascular integrity in pediatric patients is most often the consequence of an indwelling venous catheter causing local trauma to the vessel wall. Such catheters include those placed for hyperalimentation, determination of central venous pressure, and shunting of cerebrospinal fluid to the right atrium. When venous catheters are in place, the anatomic sites of deep venous thrombosis change from those described previously, because these catheters are generally not placed in the lower extremities. Hydrocephalic patients with ventriculoatrial shunts must be included in the group considered at higher risk for pulmonary embolism.

DIAGNOSIS OF DEEP VENOUS THROMBOSIS

Deep venous thrombosis most often occurs without significant complaint or obvious physical findings. An acute increase in the size of a lower extremity, sudden venous prominence, or focal tenderness over the inguinal vessels would simplify the diagnosis, but these signs occur infrequently. Currently, the diagnosis of venous thrombosis rests upon four possible modes of evaluation: Doppler ultrasound, plethysmography, labeled-fibrinogen scanning, and contrast venography.

The Doppler technique, using ultrasound, and plethysmography, using impedance, both measure venous obstruction by detecting a less than anticipated increase in venous flow following removal of an induced obstruction (blood pressure cuff). These procedures are most accurate for detection of thrombi in the venous system of the thigh, but false-negative results will occur whenever there is significant collateral circulation. The reliability of the Doppler method is highly dependent upon the experience of the operator; this factor must be considered when selecting technique or interpreting results. Both procedures can be accomplished at the patient's bedside.

Fibrinogen scanning techniques rely upon the incorporation of intravenously administered ^{125}I-labeled fibrinogen into a forming thrombus. A baseline scan is obtained immediately following the infusion, and a second scan is obtained following a 24-hour interval. This technique is useful primarily in the detection of deep venous thrombi in the lower thigh and calf. The presence of extensive vasculature in the upper thigh and pelvis creates a "background count," which entirely negates the use of this technique in those areas. The 24-hour interval necessary to accurately interpret the results of these scans is an additional drawback, because heparin therapy must be withheld so that it does not interfere with fibrinogen incorporation into a clot.

Contrast venography is the most accurate method of thrombus detection, because it "visualizes" the thrombus and its scope includes the entire deep venous network. Of all the procedures, however, it is the most invasive and includes the infusion of contrast material. As such, it has some associated morbidity.

PATHOPHYSIOLOGY

Pulmonary embolism results from loosening or fragmentation of the thrombus and migration through the vena cava, right atrium, and right ventricle to a branch of the pulmonary artery. Vascular flow distal to the embolism is interrupted, creating an area of dead space (ventilation but no perfusion). Infarction, however, occurs in fewer than 10 percent of the cases. Resulting hemodynamic effects such as pulmonary hypertension are dependent upon the extent of vascular obstruction and the degree of associated hypoxia. The pulmonary vascular bed is so extensive that in most people who do not have pre-existing cardiopulmonary disease pulmonary arterial pressures generally do not become significantly elevated. This is the case with most pediatric patients. In people who have pre-existing cardiopulmonary dis-

ease, most often adults, the resulting increase in pulmonary vascular resistance acutely increases the work of the right ventricle, possibly causing decompensation to the point of cor pulmonale.

The mechanical concept of the effects of embolism on the lung, however, is an oversimplification. The embolus contains platelets that degranulate, releasing chemical mediators such as histamine, prostaglandins, and serotonin. These substances produce both bronchoconstriction and pulmonary vasoconstriction. The bronchoconstriction primarily affects the most distal airways, because these airways are perfused by branches of the pulmonary artery. The proximal airways receive their blood flow from branches of the bronchial artery. Peripheral bronchoconstriction results in an acute diminution of lung volume. Over the course of the subsequent 24 to 36 hours, lack of adequate perfusion will reduce surfactant synthesis, contributing to additional atelectasis. The net effect upon the arterial blood gas is to decrease the Pa_{O_2}, although a few patients may maintain a Pa_{O_2} greater than 85 to 90 mm Hg. The Pa_{CO_2} is generally lower than normal as a consequence of the tachypnea present with embolism. Significant hypoxia is often present with relatively small pulmonary emboli where the local lack of perfusion seems inadequate to explain the profound reduction in arterial oxygen tension. Other areas of ventilation/perfusion ($\dot{V}/\dot{Q}$) mismatch, therefore, must occur as a consequence of the embolism but are less obvious.

DIAGNOSIS

There are no clinical findings pathognomonic of pulmonary embolism. The textbook triad of shortness of breath, pleuritic chest pain, and hemoptysis is present in only a minority of cases. Dyspnea is the most common symptom but may be of only brief duration. Chest pain of a pleuritic nature is a frequent, but not consistent, complaint. Tachypnea and tachycardia are almost uniformly present, but these findings are not specific for pulmonary embolism. Physical findings of wheezing and pleural friction rub rarely occur. Auscultation may reveal a loud P_2 (pulmonic second sound) in the presence of pulmonary hypertension. Fever is a frequent occurrence but, again, is nonspecific.

The chest x-ray film is often interpreted as "normal," but retrospective evaluation may reveal subtle findings such as slight elevation of a hemidiaphragm (secondary to decreased volume), widening of a pulmonary artery segment, or relative radiolucency of a lung field. A peripheral infiltrate may be evident especially in the presence of an infarct or atelectasis. Most often the chest x-ray film will be helpful by ruling out other causes of acute pulmonary disease such as pneumonia or pneumothorax.

The electrocardiogram generally reveals only nonspecific ST-segment and T-wave changes. An S_I–Q_{III} pattern rarely occurs. The classic description of right axis deviation, right ventricular strain pattern, and P pulmonale is infrequent, even in the adult population.

Arterial blood gas (ABG) determinations will generally reveal an acute hypoxemia, but a normal Pa_{O_2} does not exclude the possibility of embolism. The Pa_{CO_2} will usually be low, as in any circumstance where there is significant tachypnea. White blood count, erythrocyte sedimentation rate and fibrin split products may be elevated, but these findings are nonspecific. With the lack of specificity of the history, physical examination, chest x-ray, electrocardiogram, and other laboratory data, it is incumbent upon the physician to maintain a certain vigilance as to the possibility of embolism. Only with this awareness will the appropriate steps be taken to make the diagnosis.

The next step in the diagnosis is performing a perfusion lung scan. This entails the administration of isotopically labeled ^{99m}Tc macroaggregated albumin through an IV infusion. Gamma camera imaging is then utilized to show functional pulmonary blood flow. The typical scan consists of six views: anterior, posterior, both laterals, and both obliques. A scan revealing no perfusion defect rules out the diagnosis of clinically significant pulmonary embolism. A positive scan, however, does not confirm the diagnosis, because perfusion defects on scanning may result from other forms of pulmonary pathology, such as pneumonia. If the accuracy of diagnosis is to be increased, a ventilation scan using ^{133}Xe should be combined with the perfusion study. If pulmonary embolism exists, an area of abnormal perfusion will be normally ventilated. This is known as ventilation/perfusion ($\dot{V}/\dot{Q}$) mismatch. With most other forms of pulmonary pathology, abnormal perfusion is paired with abnormal ventilation and forms a $\dot{V}/\dot{Q}$ match.

If the diagnosis of pulmonary embolism is being seriously considered and the perfusion scan is suggestive but no ventilation scan is available or if the ventilation/perfusion scan is nondiagnostic, the most definitive study is the pulmonary angiogram. This procedure will allow direct visualization of any existing embolus by demonstrating intravascular filling defects and/or complete pulmonary arterial occlusion. The angiogram, however, is an invasive procedure that carries an associated morbidity and mortality. It should be considered in circumstances in which the diagnosis of pulmonary embolism is not certain and the risk of anticoagulant therapy for that particular patient is great.

TREATMENT

Management of patients with pulmonary embolisms is generally directed more toward prevention of further deep venous thrombosis than toward resolution of the existing embolus. IV heparin is administered in an initial dose of 100 U per kg, followed by a continuous infusion of 25 U per kg per hr. Efficacy of heparinization can be determined by following the partial thromboplastin time (PTT), which should be maintained in the range of 1.5 to 2 times the control value. This range, however, does not imply safety, and surveillance for bleeding complications must be included in the management plan.

An initial high dose bolus of heparin (15,000 to 20,000 U in adult patients) has been advocated to prevent further platelet aggregation and to minimize the effect of thrombin upon platelet degranulation. The result should be a decreased release of vasoactive substances from the embolus. The continuous infusion is begun two hours following the initial bolus. Such high-dose therapy has not been completely standardized in the treatment of adults, and experience with pediatric patients is minimal.

The continuous infusion of heparin is generally continued for 7 to 10 days. The duration of anticoagulant therapy beyond the acute period is controversial and must be evaluated for each patient. Consideration must be given to the acute and chronic condition and circumstances of the patient and the risk of long-term therapy. In the absence of persistent risk factors for deep venous thrombosis, the existing data suggest that anticoagulant therapy, in the form of oral coumarin, should be continued for at least 2 to 3 months.

Therapy specifically directed to the existing embolus involves the use of enzymes such as streptokinase and urokinase, which act by converting plasminogen to the fibrinolytic agent plasmin. In studies of adults, these agents have been shown to be equally efficacious. Pulmonary emboli resolve more rapidly in adults treated with these agents compared with those treated with heparin alone. However, administration of enzyme has not led to a demonstrable decrease in overall mortality from pulmonary embolus, and this therapy should probably be reserved for massive pulmonary embolus as an alternative to surgical embolectomy. Neither the enzyme nor surgical approach to treatment has had any widespread use in the pediatric population.

Other modalities of therapy are supportive in nature: oxygen for hypoxia, mechanical ventilation for respiratory failure, infusion of inotropic agents for hypotension, diuretics for congestive heart failure, and analgesics for pain.

The prophylactic administration of "minidose" heparin subcutaneously has been evaluated in adults deemed at high risk for pulmonary embolism and has been found to be efficacious. There has been little experience with such prophylactic protocols in the pediatric population. However, as pediatricians become more aware of the possibility of embolism in their patients, identification of "highrisk" groups may lead to the use of low-dose heparin prophylaxis.

CASE PRESENTATION

A 13-year-old male was brought to the emergency room with headache, confusion, and progressive lethargy for several hours' duration. Upon arrival he was noted to be unresponsive to all but painful stimuli. He was tachycardic to 170 beats/min, tachypneic to 48 breaths/min, and febrile to 108°F. and had minimally responsive pupils, decerebrate posturing, and positive Babinski signs bilaterally. Weight upon admission was 50 kg. An emergency craniostomy was performed, with insertion of a ventricular catheter. Grossly bloody cerebrospinal fluid was drained via the catheter. A CAT scan revealed a left parietal lobe intracerebral hemorrhage, with communication into the ventricle. Medical management subsequently included assisted ventilation, high-dose steroids, fluid restriction, diuretics, phenobarbital, Dilantin, aminocaproic acid (Amicar), fresh frozen plasma, and antibiotics.

Examination and Test Results

The patient remained ventilator dependent for 10 days. On Day 14, he acutely became tachypneic to 52 breaths/min and tachycardic to 140 beats/min. Blood pressure was 110/68 mm Hg. Temperature was 101.6°F. Diffuse rhonchi and decreased breath sounds at the bases were evident upon auscultation of the lungs. There were no rales, wheezes, or friction rubs. Cardiac examination revealed no murmurs, rubs, gallops, or change in intensity of the heart sounds. Examination of the extremities failed to show any evidence of phlebitis or deep venous

thrombosis. An ABG in room air revealed pH = 7.41, Pa_{O_2} = 37 mm Hg, and Pa_{CO_2} = 32 mm Hg. Increasing the Fi_{O_2} sequentially to 0.70 led only to a modest increase in Po_2 to 65 mm Hg. A chest x-ray film was interpreted as normal, with no infiltrates, atelectasis, pneumothorax, vascular congestion, or cardiomegaly present. An EKG demonstrated an S_I–Q_{III} pattern not previously present. An emergency perfusion scan revealed absent flow to the right upper lobe. This finding combined with the negative chest x-ray led to the diagnosis of pulmonary embolism.

Upon return to the ICU from the perfusion scan, the patient was noted to have very shallow respirations and to be pale in color. Blood pressure now was 80/40 mm Hg, and temperature was 104.8°F. Urine output had decreased to 12 ml over the preceding hour.

Problem List

Respiratory

Because of his shallow respirations and deteriorating condition, the patient was reintubated and placed on a mechanical ventilator with an IMV = 25 breaths/min, and an Fi_{O_2} = 1.00. Repeat ABG on these settings were: pH = 7.36, Pa_{O_2} = 95 mm Hg, and Pa_{CO_2} = 40 mm Hg.

Pulmonary embolus: heparin, 5,000 U (100 U/kg) was given as a bolus, followed by 1,250 U/h (25 U/kg/hr) continuous infusion. Coagulation profile to be obtained 4 hr following onset of therapy. Stool guaiacs, urinalyses, and arterial and venous puncture sites are to be observed for evidence of bleeding. Bloody secretions from the endotracheal tube may be the result of the embolus, anticoagulation, or local trauma from intubation and suctioning.

Cardiac

Hypotension: Volume expansion with normal saline (NS), 20 ml/kg, was administered with no increase in either BP or urine output. A dopamine infusion at 10 mcg/kg/min was begun with increase in BP to 115/58 mm Hg. A central venous catheter, already in place, did not fluctuate well, and readings were unreliable. This catheter was removed, because it did not contribute to the monitoring of the patient and could have an etiologic role in the pulmonary embolism. Because interpretation of central venous pressure can be difficult when there is a massive pulmonary embolus, the central venous line was not replaced. A Swan–Ganz catheter was placed so that cardiac output could be more appropriately followed.

Renal

In the presence of dopamine infusion, urine output rose to 1 ml/kg/hr. Serum electrolytes were: Na = 135 mEq/L, K = 5.1 mEq/L, Cl = 99 mEq/L, CO_2 = 21 mEq/L, BUN = 30 mg/100ml, and creatinine = 1.2 mg/100 ml. Both the BUN and creatinine were significantly elevated from laboratory determinations performed on the previous day

(BUN = 14, creatinine = 0.7), giving the impression of acute renal failure. Urine is sent to the laboratory for determination of sodium concentration, as an additional confirmation of renal failure. IV infusion rates are to be decreased in accordance with decreased urine output.

Hematologic

Hematocrit = 36 percent. White blood count = 22,500, with 20 segmented, 55 bands, 20 lymphs, and 5 monocytes. Platelet count = 223,000 cu mm. The coagulation profile obtained as the baseline was control for both prothrombin time (PT) and partial thromboplastin time (PTT). Repeat coagulation profile is to be obtained 4 hr following institution of heparin therapy.

Neurologic

There was no acute change noted in neurologic status. The use of anticoagulants in a patient with a recent intracranial hemorrhage warrants close monitoring. Repeat CAT scan will be necessary following onset of therapy. If there is a change in neurologic status, an intracranial pressure transducer may have to be used to assist in monitoring medical and/or surgical therapy for increased intracranial pressure.

Deep Vein Thrombosis

Because pulmonary embolism is the consequence of venous thrombosis, possible sources must be evaluated. A Doppler study of the lower extremities was interpreted as "normal."

Hyperpyrexia

Acetaminophen was administered with no defervescence. A hypothermia blanket was placed to reduce the elevated temperature. The etiology of the fever could be the embolus, but all appropriate cultures should be obtained to evaluate infectious causes. Antibiotic therapy was instituted.

SUGGESTED READING

Buck, J.R., Connors, R.H., Coon, W.W., et al.: Pulmonary embolism in children. J. Pediatr. Surg. 16(3):385, 1981.

Firror, H.V.: Pulmonary embolization complicating total intravenous alimentation. J. Pediatr. Surg. 7:81, 1972.

Jones, D.R.B., and MacIntyre, I.M.C.: Venous thromboembolism in infancy and childhood. Arch. Dis. Child. 50:153, 155, 1975.

Jones, R.H., and Sabiston, D.C.: Pulmonary embolism in childhood. Monogr. Surg. Sci. 3:35, 51, 1966.

Moser, K.M.: Diagnosis and management of pulmonary embolism. Hosp. Pract. 15:57, 1980.

Wolfe, W.G., and Sabiston, D.C.: Pathogenesis, incidence, and clinical significance of pulmonary embolism. *In* Pulmonary Embolism, Major Probl. Clin. Surg. 25:9, 1980.

Nursing Process for Patient Care:
Pulmonary Embolism

Pulmonary embolism, as a primary diagnosis, rarely appears in the pediatric population. When it does occur, it is a complication of another underlying problem. Because it is relatively rare, nurses do not ordinarily anticipate its occurrence. However, it should be anticipated and added to the mind set of spinal cord injury; multiple trauma, especially of the abdomen, pelvis and lower extremity; neuromuscular disorders; and prolonged states of unconsciousness. It should also be anticipated in those children with indwelling venous catheters for hyperalimentation, central venous pressure monitoring, and shunting of cerebrospinal fluid to the right atrium.

When pulmonary embolism occurs, it does so with devastating effects. Although the respiratory system is primarily affected, pulmonary embolism also has an effect on cardiovascular status. Further sequelae, in terms of acute renal failure, may also occur.

RESPIRATORY

Assess, Monitor, and Document

Respiratory rate
Dyspnea
Chest pain
Hemoptysis
Breath sounds: wheezing, pleural friction rub

Heart rate
Temperature
Color
Arterial blood gases

Anticipate

Alteration in respiratory status
Acute respiratory failure: altered level of consciousness, restlessness/agitation, lethargy, cyanosis, bradycardia

Post–Intubation

Patency of tube
Placement of tube: equal bilateral chest excursion, equal breath sounds
Response to pulmonary toilet

Anticipate

Obstruction of tube

CARDIOVASCULAR

Although pulmonary hypertension is rare, it can occur. It is usually dependent upon the extent of vascular obstruction and the degree of associated hypoxia. Nursing personnel must be aware of the consequences of pulmonary hypertension on the right ventricle.

Assess, Monitor, and Document

Heart rate
Blood pressure
Central venous pressure

Distended neck veins
Response to medications

Anticipate

Alteration in cardiac status
  Congestive heart failure: increased heart rate, decreased blood pressure, increased central venous pressure, distended neck veins, hepatomegaly, peripheral edema

HEMATOLOGIC

IV heparin therapy is administered in an attempt to prevent further deep vein thrombosis. Heparin is administered in an initial bolus, followed by a continuous infusion.

Assess, Monitor, and Document

Rate of flow hourly (use infusion pump)
Intake hourly
Signs of bleeding secondary to anticoagulant therapy: petechiae, bruises, oozing from puncture sites, hematuria, stools/guaiac, gastric aspirates, pulmonary secretions
Laboratory data: partial thromboplastin time (PTT)

Anticipate

Bleeding: overt, occult

RENAL

Declining urinary output and rising serum BUN and creatinine are clues to the fact that the kidneys may have suffered an insult.

Assess, Monitor, and Document

Weight
Urine output
Urine specific gravity
Blood pressure
Heart rate
Breath sounds
Serum electrolytes, BUN, creatinine, and osmolality
Urine electrolytes and osmolality

Anticipate

Alteration in renal status
  Acute renal failure: decreased urine output, increased urine specific gravity, hypertension, weight gain, breath sounds (rales, rhonchi)

DEEP VEIN THROMBOSIS

Assess, Monitor, and Document

Extremities for redness, edema (measure thighs and calves at least once each shift), pain, prominent veins

Anticipate

Pulmonary embolism
Continuation of embolic phenomenon

NEUROLOGIC

The underlying problem of this child was an intracranial hemorrhage with considerable neurologic deficits. The neurologic status of the child must be assessed and monitored.

Assess, Monitor, and Document

Level of consciousness
Response to painful stimuli
Pupillary response
Movement of extremities

Blood pressure
Heart rate
Respiratory rate

Anticipate

Alteration in neurologic status
   Increased intracranial pressure: altered level of consciousness, absence of re-flexes, increased blood pressure, decreased pulse, decreased respiration and altered pattern

RESPONSE OF CHILD AND FAMILY

Assess, Monitor, and Document

Behavioral response: anxious, angry, verbal
Level of understanding of child's condition, treatment, and prognosis

Expected outcome
Ability to cope

Anticipate

Family crisis
Inability to cope

MIND SET

Assess

Respiratory status
Cardiovascular status
Hematologic status
Renal status

Deep vein thrombosis
Neurologic status
Response of child and family

Anticipate

Alteration in respiratory status
   Acute respiratory failure
Alteration in cardiovascular status
   Decreased cardiac output
Alteration in hematologic status secondary to therapy

Bleeding
Alteration in renal status
   Acute renal failure
Continuation of embolic phenomenon
Emotional distress
Family crisis

29

Apnea in Infants and Children

HEDI L. LEISTNER, M.D.

Although apnea has long been reported as a significant cause of morbidity and mortality in premature infants, it has been recognized only recently as an important event in term newborns, infants, and older children. The evaluation of apnea can pose both diagnostic and treatment dilemmas. The etiology of apnea often remains elusive and unclassifiable. A lack of consensus on the scientific worth of some diagnostic procedures and treatment often makes management difficult. Yet, it is important to recognize and treat the causes, because the consequences of apnea can include neurologic sequelae, cor pulmonale, and sudden death. In this chapter, many of the physiologic factors that predispose children, especially infants, to apnea will be explored; a diagnostic approach to children presenting with apnea will be outlined; and some common clinical presentations of apnea will be discussed, with suggested therapeutic interventions.

NORMAL RESPIRATION

The regulation of respiration will be reviewed briefly to aid in understanding the factors that predispose children to apnea.

Dorsal and ventral groups of nerve cell bodies located in the pontomedullary tegmentum fire rhythmically. These phasic impulses descend down the bulbospinal tracts to the anterior horn cells of the phrenic and intercostal nerves to cause muscular contraction and respiratory effort. If the airways are patent and the lungs are sufficiently compliant, air will move into the lungs to provide gas exchange.

Ventilation depends upon the orderly sequence of muscular contraction. The upper airway will collapse if the muscles stabilizing the upper airway fail to contract (analogous to trying to drink through a wet paper straw). The negative pressure generated by the diaphragm during inspiration will be dissipated if the intercostal muscles fail to contract and stabilize the chest wall. Finally, the diaphragm must generate sufficient negative intrathoracic pressure to move air into the lungs.

The phasic impulses coming from the respiratory centers in the brain stem are very dependent upon afferent inputs from chemoreceptors (both peripheral and central) and airway and lung receptors, as well as influences from the cerebral and reticular activating systems. The importance of this afferent input and higher brain activity in controlling the rhythmicity of the respiratory centers was demonstrated by Sullivan and associates, who decreased the spontaneous respiratory rate in dogs to 1 per minute by modifying the afferent information reaching the respiratory centers in the pontomedullary area.

Normal sleep produces changes in muscular tone as well as in the control of ventilation. During rapid eye movement (REM) sleep, there is a depression of all skeletal muscle tone, including the upper airway and intercostal muscles. In contrast, the phasic inspiratory discharges of the upper airway and intercostal muscles are intact during non-REM sleep. A decrease in the ventilatory response to hypercarbia and hypoxia is also seen during REM sleep, and the arousal response to hypercarbia, hypoxia, and airway stimulation is depressed. Respiratory control during non-REM sleep is similar to that in the awake state, although there is a slightly lower level of ventilation at rest and during hypercarbia and hypoxia.

ABNORMAL RESPIRATORY PATTERNS

Normally, breathing is regular in people who are awake and at rest. Changes in the rhythm of breathing may occur in a variety of conditions, including central nervous system disease, congestive heart failure (CHF), and normal sleep. Apnea has been defined by various researchers as a respiratory pause lasting from 3 to 20 seconds, which emphasizes the arbitrary nature of the definition. Apneas during sleep may be present in healthy people and are especially common in young infants and older adults. The significance of even numerous apneic episodes in asymptomatic individuals is unknown. It has been proposed that more than 30 apneic episodes during a 7-hour nocturnal study are abnormal, but this definition is also arbitrary and not universally accepted, especially for children. The normative data for children, especially term infants, are limited.

Three types of apnea have been described: 1) *central apnea,* the absence of respiratory efforts and airflow; 2) *obstructive apnea,* the absence of airflow in spite of often extreme respiratory effort; and 3) *mixed apnea,* the absence of respiratory effort and airflow, followed by the resumption of respiratory effort without airflow. Some researchers have suggested that all three types of apnea may have the same significance, because all three types have been observed in the same patient. In addition to these apneas, another type of abnormal respiratory pattern is *hypopnea,* inadequate minute ventilation with oxygen desaturation. Hypopnea commonly results from partially obstructed breathing.

Bradycardia is seen in all three types of apnea and is the result of absent or ineffective respiratory effort and the resulting hypoxemia. Atropine and supplemental oxygen will attenuate the bradycardia seen during apnea, although oxygen administration will prolong the length of apnea. Bradycardia is not seen with hypopnea.

PATHOPHYSIOLOGY

Newborn and young infants are especially vulnerable to apneic episodes, because the afferent inputs from the chemoreceptors, lung and airway receptors, and central nervous system are immature. Maturational changes in the response to hypercarbia and hypoxia are seen in newborns. A mature response depends upon both gestational and postnatal age and may reflect changes in neurologic development as well as in pulmonary mechanics.

Apnea has been reported to occur in a variety of disease processes affecting infants, especially premature infants. These causes are summarized in Table 29–1. According to this table, several factors appear to be very important in the pathophysiology of apnea. The first factor

Table 29–1. Causes of Apnea in Infants

Systemic Processes
Sepsis
Hypothermia
Hypoglycemia, hyponatremia, hypocalcemia
Pulmonary Disease
Pneumonia
Respiratory distress syndrome
Cardiac Disease
Congestive heart failure (CHF)
Left-to-right shunt
Neurologic Disease
Seizures
Intracranial hemorrhage
Meningitis
Gastrointestinal Disease
Gastroesophageal reflux
Abnormal coordination of swallowing
Botulism
Normal Reflexes
Suctioning of nasopharynx and trachea
Stimulation of laryngeal chemoreceptors
Control of Ventilation
Depressed response to hypoxia
Depressed response to hypercarbia
Environmental Conditions
Ambient temperature changes
Posture
Head flexion

is the role of hypoxia and hypoxemia. When given hypoxic gas mixtures to breathe, the newborn is unable to sustain the normal hyperventilation and will hypoventilate and suffer apneas. This paradoxical and inappropriate response to hypoxia may be secondary to central nervous system depression caused by the hypoxemia.

This abnormal response to hypoxia is important, because infants are prone to hypoxemia. Airway closure and consequently a fall in PO_2 is frequently seen in infants because of several factors. The immature development of elastic fibers in the septae of the alveoli surrounding the conducting airways allow these airways to collapse. This tendency for airway collapse is aggravated by the frequently low lung volumes in infants. Low lung volumes result when infants are placed in a supine position, and a further fall in thoracic gas volumes is seen during REM sleep.

Infants depend upon the intercostal muscles to stabilize their very compliant rib cages. During REM sleep, there is a selective inhibition of all skeletal muscles, including the intercostals, which results in an unstable rib cage and a fall in lung volumes. Infants spend a large portion of their time sleeping, and much of this sleep time is in REM. Thus, low lung volumes and immature development of elastic fibers act in synergism to produce airway closure. Furthermore, infants are very susceptible to many disease states, such as pneumonia and congestive heart failure (CHF), that result in hypoxemia and are more likely to develop respiratory muscle fatigue because of the decreased number of type I high oxidative fatigue-resistant fibers. In premature infants, even the decrease in oxygen-carrying capacity caused by anemia (less than 10 gm per dl hemoglobin) may result in apnea.

Another mechanism that may produce apnea in infants is normal reflexes overriding respiratory drive. Stimulation of the nasopharynx or trachea during suctioning as well as other vagal stimuli such as defecation can produce apnea, especially in premature infants. Animal studies suggest that reflex apnea can occur by stimulation of the laryngeal chemoreceptors and pulmonary receptors. The apnea observed in infants during feeding and in infants with pulmonary edema and pneumonia may be related to these observations. Blowing cool air on the face of a young infant and temperature changes caused by the cycling of the isolette heater may produce apnea. The significance or even the existence of the diving reflex (apnea, bradycardia, and redistribution of the cardiac output with a water stimulus to the mouth or nose) in human infants remains speculative but is a proposed theory for a cause of sudden infant death syndrome (SIDS). In both animal and human infants, reflex apnea becomes less frequent with increasing postnatal age.

The role of defective control of ventilation as a result of immaturity or some other mechanism also must be considered. Abnormal responses to hypoxia and hypercarbia have been shown to occur in premature infants with apnea. An abnormal response to carbon dioxide has been seen in some infants who present with prolonged sleep apnea and require resuscitation and may also be secondary to immaturity or abnormal maturation. Defective control of ventilation, that is, a blunted response to hypoxia and hypercarbia, has been reported in family members and may produce apnea. Another type of abnormal control of ventilation is seen in infants with congenital central hypoventilation (often called Ondine's curse) who have apnea only when they are asleep.

Finally, unlike the obstructive apnea in adults, anatomic abnormalities of the upper airway are common in children with obstructive sleep apnea. The most frequent abnormality in the upper airway resulting in apnea in children is hypertrophy of the tonsils and/or adenoids.

Facial abnormalities such as micrognathia, macroglossia, and temporomandibular joint an-

kylosis are also important in the etiology of obstructive sleep apnea in children. Obstructive sleep apnea has also been described after velopharyngeal incompetence surgery and other cleft palate repairs. These anatomic abnormalities narrow the upper airway. Sleep-related changes in the patency of the upper airway, that is, decrease in the muscle tone in the genioglossus and oropharyngeal muscles, compromise the already narrowed upper airway, resulting in obstructive breathing.

DIAGNOSTIC APPROACH

History

Because apneic episodes are usually not observed by trained medical personnel, the physician is dependent upon the observations of the parents or caretaker, who may be emotionally upset. Therefore, obtaining a detailed history is essential in determining the condition of the child (Table 29–2). This history must include questions concerning the child's sleeping habits, including snoring, choking, mouth breathing, restlessness, unusual sleeping positions, and enuresis. A detailed, carefully obtained history often suggests the etiology of the apneic episodes. Key answers to be obtained include the state of consciousness and activity prior to, during, and after the apneic episode; changes in motor tone or color of the skin; the type and duration of the apnea; whether these apneas have occurred previously; and the type of resuscitation required, if any. Throughout the history taking, one must make a careful judgment as to the validity of the parents' or caregiver's observations.

Physical Examination

A thorough physical examination, including a careful neurologic and upper airway evalu-

Table 29–2. Key Factors in Evaluating a Child with Apnea

State of consciousness
Asleep, awake, postictal
Activity
Feeding, burping, crying, sleeping
Motor tone
Stiff, limp, normal
Color
Pallor, cyanosis, facial rubor
Type of apnea
Duration of apnea
Previous episodes
Type of resuscitation, if any

ation is essential. At times, findings of the physical examination will suggest the cause of the apnea such as sepsis, pneumonia, CHF, and so on. It is not uncommon, however, for the results of physical examination to be entirely normal, even on the initial presentation.

Laboratory Evaluation

Using the findings of the history and physical examination, a laboratory evaluation can usually focus on several possible etiologies. Routine screening tests should include a complete blood count, serum glucose and electrolytes, chest x-ray, arterial blood gas, electrocardiogram, and Holter monitor. If infection is suspected, blood, urine, and spinal fluid cultures should be obtained. In children with normal results of physical examination, one must rely upon the history alone to direct the laboratory evaluation.

COMMON CAUSES

Common conditions associated with apnea in children are gastroesophageal (GE) reflux, incoordinated feeding, seizures, and sleep-related apnea. These causes of apnea are discussed in detail in the sections that follow and are summarized in Table 29–3. These divisions are somewhat arbitrary; for example, GE reflux and seizures can occur during and may be aggravated by sleep.

Gastroesophageal (GE) Reflux

The incidence of GE reflux in infants is unknown, but it is probably common. Most infants spit up sometimes, and every parent knows the consequences of shaking a recently fed infant. It is possible that infants with GE reflux–induced apnea are more sensitive to stomach contents in the oropharynx and larynx, inducing a reflex similar to that observed in experimental animals. Aspiration of small quantities of the refluxed material may also play a role. GE reflux–induced apnea occurs in infants, especially young infants.

Description

The description of an infant with apnea caused by GE reflux may vary. The apneas seen in GE reflux may be central or obstructive; the infant may be described as having difficulty catching his or her breath. The infant may be asleep or awake. Cyanosis, pallor, or facial rubor may be present. The muscle tone may be increased or decreased. Gagging, choking, burping, or vomiting may be reported, although some infants demonstrate none of these signs. GE reflux apnea may occur either right after feeding or several hours later.

Evaluation

In addition to the screening tests previously listed, the laboratory evaluation of an infant suspected of having GE reflux–induced apnea should include a test for blood in the stool to check for esophagitis and several tests of esophageal function. A combination of cine-esophagram with barium, pH monitoring in the esophagus (the Tuttle test), and manometric measurements in the esophagus and cardioesophageal sphincter will provide a more reliable estimation of clinically significant reflux than any single test. Whether GE scintiscanning will be useful in detecting and quantitating GE reflux in infants remains to be seen; a negative test result does not completely exclude reflux with aspiration, because peristalsis may have emptied the radionuclide from the stomach prior to the reflux episode. The cine-esophagram with barium is the least reliable test for determining GE reflux. Monitoring the pH during sleep is important, because this is the time of increased risk for reflux. Reflux associated with dilatation of the esophagus and reflux associated with apnea and/or aspiration are considered significant. Simultaneous recording of heart rate, respiratory rate and pattern, and esophageal pH may be especially helpful in recognizing clinically significant reflux. Esophagoscopy may be necessary if esophagitis is suspected.

Treatment

Treatment of GE reflux–induced apnea consists of upright positioning and small frequent feedings of formula thickened with cereal. In preventing reflux, the upright prone position is superior to the upright supine position. Antacids are usually not necessary and must be used with caution to prevent milk–alkali syndrome. There may be a role for pharmacologic agents such as bethanechol in patients who continue to experience reflux and apnea in spite of feeding changes. Surgery to perform a fun-

Table 29–3. Clinical Features of Types of Apnea in Children

Feature	GE Reflux Apnea	Feeding Apnea	Seizures Apnea	Prolonged Sleep Apnea	Obstructive Sleep Apnea
Description	Usually infant Usually after feeding May be any time Apneic or dyspneic Facial rubor, pale, or cyanotic Coughing, gagging Limp or stiff	Usually infant During nipple feeding Apneic or dyspneic Usually cyanotic Gagging, choking Sometimes stridor Usually limp	Any age Asleep or awake Central or obstructive apnea Cyanotic or pale Stiff or normal tone Drooling, sucking, atypical cry Extraocular movements	Infant Asleep Usually central apnea Cyanotic or pale Usually limp	Any age Snoring during sleep Obstructive apnea Disturbed sleep pattern Cyanosis Enuresis
Physical Findings	Usually none	Premature infant Neurologically impaired if severe, failure to thrive	May be none ± Neurologic signs	Usually none	Failure to thrive Neurologic dysfunction Pulmonary and systemic hypertension Cor pulmonale
Evaluation	Stool guaiac Cine-esophagram pH monitoring with HR, RR* Manometric measurements ? GE scintiscanning	Barium swallow under fluoroscopy Record HR, RR during feeding	EEG awake and asleep ? Sepsis work-up	Sleep study of HR, RR, O$_2$ Cinefluoroscopy of upper airway during sleep Endoscopy	Sleep study of HR, RR, O$_2$ Cinefluoroscopy of upper airway during sleep Endoscopy
Therapy	Upright position Thickened, small frequent feedings ? Bethanechol Fundoplication	Change nipple, position, thicken formula NG or NJ feedings Gastrostomy	Anticonvulsant medication	? Home monitoring ? Theophylline	Nasopharyngeal airway Tonsillectomy and adenoidectomy Reconstructive surgery Tracheostomy

* HR = heart rate and EKG; RR = respiratory rate and pattern.

doplication may be necessary if medical therapy is unsuccessful or if the GE reflux is especially severe, causing failure to thrive or esophagitis.

Incoordinated Feeding

Incoordinated feeding may cause apnea. This type of apnea is usually seen in infants. Nipple feeding requires the complex coordination of breathing, sucking, and swallowing. The performance of this complex activity depends upon intact sensory, motor, and central nervous systems. Feeding-induced apnea occurs most frequently in premature infants and infants with neurologic problems; central nervous system immaturity or dysfunction, neuromuscular weakness and incoordination, and prominent laryngeal and vasovagal reflexes may play a role in feeding-induced apnea.

Description

Typically, an infant will become symptomatic while feeding and may be described as being apneic or having difficulty catching his or her breath. The infant may gag and choke and may be cyanotic or pale.

Evaluation

Diagnostic tests that may be useful include recording heart rate and respiration rate during an observed feeding and fluoroscopic examination of swallowing. Thick barium is easier to swallow; therefore, barium should be thickened to a consistency similar to that of formula. A cine-esophagram should also be performed to rule out concurrent significant GE reflux.

Treatment

Thickening the formula with cereal, changing the type of nipple or formula used, and changing the position of the infant during feeding are often successful in treating feeding-induced apnea. If medical therapy does not eliminate the apnea or if the nutrition of the infant is inadequate, a nasogastric (NG) or nasojejunal (NJ) tube should be used for feeding. If there is no improvement in the infant's ability to feed with a nipple, a feeding gastrostomy should be considered.

Seizures

Seizure-induced apnea can occur at any age. There may be no history of seizures, and tonoclonic movements are not necessarily present. In evaluating a child with apnea and seizures, there is always the question of whether the seizure caused the apnea or was secondary to a prolonged apnea and the resulting hypoxemia. Although it may sometimes be difficult to answer this question, usually one can infer from the clinical presentation and laboratory evaluation which came first. Possible mechanisms by which seizures cause apnea include central nervous system depression and upper airway obstruction.

Description

The clinical presentation of seizure-induced apnea can be variable. Apnea associated with seizure may be central, obstructive, or a combination of both. The child may be asleep or awake. The muscle tone may be increased or normal. Some children may demonstrate extraocular movements, drooling, sucking, or an abnormal cry, but these signs may be absent, especially in infants. The color of the skin may be cyanotic, pale, or normal.

Evaluation

An awake and sleeping electroencephalogram (EEG) may be helpful in determining whether the apnea is secondary to a seizure or vice versa. It is rarely necessary to sedate an infant for an EEG, because most infants will lie quietly and fall asleep after feeding; sedation may make the interpretation of the EEG more difficult. A normal EEG does not exclude a seizure disorder in young infants, because early in life, the EEG often remains normal. In addition to the routine screening tests, a sepsis work-up should be considered in younger infants.

Treatment

Therapy includes the use of anticonvulsant drugs. However, before prescribing anticonvulsants, other causes of apnea must be excluded, because these medications may cause respiratory depression in susceptible children.

Sleep-related Apnea

Irregularity in the respiratory pattern is common during sleep. In normal children, apneic episodes are commonly seen at onset of sleep and accompanying bursts of REM. These apneas are not pathological. Many term infants and almost all premature infants show a periodicity to their breathing during REM sleep. In contrast to the apnea of prematurity, apneas in periodic breathing are short (5 to 10 seconds) and are not associated with bradycardia. The incidence of periodic breathing decreases with increasing postconceptual age, and the phenomenon usually disappears after 52 weeks post conception. Disease processes such as upper respiratory infections, pneumonia, and CHF may produce clinically significant sleep apnea when superimposed upon sleep-related changes in the central nervous system, chemoreceptors, and pulmonary mechanics. The most common clinical presentations of apnea during sleep in children are obstructive sleep apnea and prolonged sleep apnea of infancy.

Obstructive Sleep Apnea

Obstructive sleep apnea (OSA) is being recognized with increasing frequency in children from infancy through adolescence. In contrast to adults with OSA in whom the etiology of apnea often remains obscure, most children with OSA have anatomic abnormalities, such as hypertrophy of tonsils and/or adenoids, micrognathia, dysmorphic facial development, chronic nasal obstruction, muscular hypotonia, and macroglossia. Sleep-related changes in the patency of the upper airway compromises the already narrowed upper airway, resulting in obstructed breathing during sleep. The most common anatomic abnormality of the upper airway in OSA in children is tonsillar and/or adenoidal hypertrophy. The increased incidence of OSA in children may be due to increased physician awareness of sleep apnea and the decline in the number of tonsillectomies and adenoidectomies performed in recent years. Other predisposing conditions to OSA in children include craniofacial abnormalities such as Crouzon's disease, micrognathia such as in Pierre Robin syndrome, and temporomandibular joint ankylosis, macroglossia, muscular hypotonia, chronic nasal obstruction from allergy, and deviated nasal septum.

Description

Loud snoring with recurrent periods of silence (the apnea) are almost always present in OSA. The parents will frequently describe periods of increasing chest wall movement without airflow. These apneas are terminated by a loud snort or choking and sometimes by arousal. Cyanosis is often present during these periods. Disturbed sleeping habits are frequent and include restlessness; frequent arousals, often with crying; and bizarre sleeping positions (e.g., sleeping in a chair with one's head on the bed). Children with OSA are frequently difficult to arouse and may be confused in the morning. In children older than 4 years of age, enuresis is also common. Children with OSA frequently suffer from failure to thrive and exhibit developmental delays and poor school performance. Obesity and daytime hypersomnolence are less common in children with OSA than in adults with OSA.

EVALUATION

Often the diagnosis of OSA can be confirmed simply by observing the sleep in a suspected case. Polysomnogram recording of heart rate, respiratory rate, and respiratory pattern (requiring monitoring of chest and abdominal movement and airflow at the mouth and nares) during sleep will quantitate and verify the clinical impression of OSA. Measurement of oxygen saturation by ear oximeter or determination of transcutaneous oxygen levels is also helpful in determining significant OSA and episodes of hypopnea caused by partially obstructed breathing. Cinefluoroscopic examination of the upper airway during sleep is very useful in determining the site of obstruction. Endoscopy during sleep and while awake is another method of confirming the site of obstruction. Because the signs of respiratory failure can be subtle, an arterial blood gas should be performed. An echocardiogram is a more sensitive test than a chest x-ray or an electrocardiogram (EKG) for detecting early cor pulmonale.

TREATMENT

In cases of severe OSA with respiratory failure and cor pulmonale (or biventricular failure), the initial intervention should be the establishment of a patent airway. A temporary nasopharyngeal tube or a tracheostomy should be performed before any diagnostic testing is carried out. Surgical removal of the hypertrophied tonsils and adenoids is clearly indicated in children with the sequelae of OSA. Whether these lymphoid tissues should be removed in children with OSA who have no signs of impairment is unknown. Usually both the tonsils and the adenoids need to be removed to completely alleviate the OSA. In children with craniofacial anomalies who are too young for the definitive correction, tonsillectomy and adenoidectomy will often improve airway patency. Tracheostomy will prevent upper airway obstruction, but this therapy is reserved for cases refractory to other modalities. Some patients with OSA also have central apneas. Often, these central apneas resolve with the resolution of OSA. If the central apneas persist, respiratory stimulants such as theophylline, progesterone, and almitrine should be considered.

Prolonged Sleep Apnea of Infancy

Prolonged sleep apnea can occur in any age group. Infants presenting with apnea associated with cyanosis or pallor and requiring some form of resuscitation are frequently called aborted SIDS or "near-miss" SIDS infants. Unfortunately, this designation assumes a relationship with SIDS that has not been proved and adds emotional connotations. In fact, a recent prospective study of 24-hour recordings in infants at home failed to document apnea in any of the infants who subsequently died of SIDS.

Proposed mechanisms for these apneic episodes include central nervous system immaturity or dysfunction, immature or abnormal chemoreceptors, reflex apnea, and airway obstruction.

Attempts at characterizing infants with prolonged apnea requiring resuscitation have produced conflicting results. The reported observations by some investigators of an abnormal response (increased and decreased) to carbon dioxide, increased levels of periodic breathing and apnea, and the occurrence of obstructive apnea in these so-called aborted SIDS infants have not been confirmed by others.

To date, on the basis of these conflicting findings, one cannot explain the apneic episode, predict which infants are likely to have additional episodes, or recommend a clearly indicated treatment plan for most infants.

This heterogeneity in results may be caused by several factors. First, infants with apnea originating from different causes may have been included in the group. The nature of the presentation requires reliance upon parental observations. Duration of study, daytime nap vs. nighttime monitoring, home vs. laboratory recordings, steady state vs. incremental increases in carbon dioxide, and method of measuring ventilation are only a few of the differences in methodology that may contribute to the diversity in results. There is also the problem of defining "normal" from a relatively small number of infants. Variability exists not only from infant to infant but also from study to study in the same infant. Finally, there is lack of agreement concerning the definition of such terms as *apnea* and *bradycardia*.

DESCRIPTION

The presentation of infants with prolonged sleep apnea may be variable. Cyanosis or pallor may be present, and muscle tone may be increased, decreased, or unchanged. There is no apparent relationship to feeding. Some form of resuscitation, ranging from shaking the infant to mouth-to-mouth resuscitation, was believed to be necessary by the person in the room with the infant.

EVALUATION

To exclude known causes of apnea, the screening tests listed in the section entitled "Laboratory Evaluation" should be performed. Recording heart rate, respiratory rate, and respiratory pattern during sleep may be helpful in diagnosing the different types of sleep apnea. Examination of the upper airway using cinefluoroscopy, bronchoscopy, and laryngoscopy should be considered in cases of obstructive apnea.

TREATMENT

The efficacy and safety of drug therapy for treatment of obstructive or central apnea in infants has not been established. Theophylline has been advocated in cases of prolonged central apnea, but care must be taken to exclude infants with GE reflux, because theophylline may aggravate the reflux. Although some researchers believe that home monitoring of heart rate and respiration rate is useful in all infants who present with prolonged apnea, the scientific merit of home monitoring for all these infants is questioned by other investigators.

The efficacy of home monitoring has yet to be proved. To date, there is no method of distinguishing between those infants who will have another apneic episode and those who will die. Tracheostomy or an oropharyngeal tube may be necessary in the rare case of an infant with obstructive apnea.

CASE PRESENTATION

L.R. is a 3½-month-old male infant who was brought to the emergency room because of an apneic episode. One-half hour after feeding, he was found to be not breathing. He was pale, stiff, and drooling and his eyes were rolled up. When seen 10 minutes prior to the episode, he was alseep. No crying or abnormal sounds were heard. His mother slapped him on the back, shook him, and then started mouth-to-mouth breathing. After several mouth-to-mouth breaths, he gasped and started to cry. His color returned about 1 minute after he started to cry. In the emergency room, his physical examination was negative. He was afebrile.

History

L.R.'s past medical history was significant for periodic regurgitation and vomiting, with burping, after feeding. His mother noted noisy breathing and mucus production for several days prior to his apneic episode. He was the full-term product of a pregnancy monitored by prenatal care for only the last month and complicated by moderate alcohol consumption by his mother.

Test Results

Laboratory evaluation revealed normal results of chest x-ray examination and arterial blood gas, CBC, glucose, and electrolyte studies. The infant was admitted to the intensive care unit (ICU) for observation.

Problem List

Neurologic

The description of the stiffening, eye rolling, and drooling suggested a seizure. Phenobarbital therapy was instituted, and awake and asleep EEGs were scheduled.

Cardiac

An EKG and a Holter monitor study were ordered to rule out any dysrhythmia as a possible etiology.

Gastrointestinal

Because of the history of periodic regurgitation and the proximity of this episode to a feeding, a cine-esophagram was ordered.

The awake and asleep EEGs, the EKG, and the Holter monitor study were all negative. The cine-esophagram revealed a dilated esophagus, with barium refluxing to the level of the carina.

Final Assessment

L.R. was treated with upright positioning and frequent small thickened feedings. Phenobarbital was discontinued. After an in-hospital observational period of 1 week, he was discharged. Two weeks later, he was brought to the emergency room, again with the complaint of apnea. His father had laid him flat after feeding him to change his diaper. No other episodes occurred. At 1 year of age, he had normal developmental milestones and a normal physical examination.

SUGGESTED READING

Berger, A.J., Mitchell, R.A., and Severinghaus, J.W.: Regulation of respiration. N. Engl. J. Med. 297:92–97, 138–143, 194–201, 1977.

Brouillette, R.T., Fernbach, S.K., and Hunt, C.E.: Obstructive sleep apnea in infants and children. J. Pediatr. 100:31, 1982.

Frank, Y., Kravath, R.E., Pollak, C.P., and Weitzman, E.D.: Obstructive sleep apnea and its therapy: clinical and polysomnographic manifestations. Pediatrics 71:737, 1983.

Gould, J.B., Lee, A.F.S., James, O., and Sander, L.: The sleep state characteristics of apnea during infancy. Pediatrics 59:182, 1977.

Guilleminault, C., Ariagno, R., Korobkin, R., et al.: Sleep parameters and respiratory variables in near-miss sudden infant death syndrome infants. Pediatrics 68:354, 1981.

Guilleminault, C., Eldridge, F.L., Simmons, F.B., and Dement, W.C.: Sleep apnea in eight children. Pediatrics 58:23, 1976.

Haddad, G.G., Leistner, H.L., Lai, T.L., and Mellins, R.B.: Ventilation and ventilatory pattern during sleep in aborted sudden infant death syndrome. Pediatr. Res. 15:879, 1981.

Kelly, D.H., and Shannon, D.C.: Periodic breathing in infants with near-miss sudden infant death syndrome. Pediatrics 63:355, 1979.

Phillipson, E.A.: Control of breathing during sleep. Am. Rev. Respir. Dis. 118:909, 1978.

Shannon, D.C., Kelly, D.H., and O'Connell, K.: Abnormal regulation of ventilation in infants at risk for sudden infant death syndrome. N. Engl. J. Med. 297:747, 1977.

Southall, D.P., Richards, J.M., de Swiet, M., et al.: Identification of infants destined to die unexpectedly during infancy: evaluation of predictive importance of prolonged apnea and disorders of cardiac rhythm or conduction: first report of a multicentered prospective study into the sudden infant death syndrome. Br. Med. J. 286:1092, 1983.

Sullivan, C.E., Kozar, L.F., Murphy, E., and Phillipson, E.A.: Primary role of respiratory afferents in sustaining breathing rhythm. J. Appl. Physiol. 45:11, 1978.

Nursing Process for Patient Care:

Apnea in Infants and Children

The infant or young child admitted to the ICU with a history of an apneic episode requires close observation. Continuous monitoring is important to determine the cause of apnea and to prevent serious neurologic sequelae.

APNEA

Assess, Monitor, and Document

Respiratory rate
Respiratory pattern
Heart rate
Circumstances preceding episode of apnea: alert, asleep, feeding, crying, seizure, position
Apneic event: duration, associated bradycardia, color, muscle tone

Termination of episode: spontaneous, stimulation, resuscitation
Condition of child following episode of apnea: level of consciousness, respiratory rate, respiratory pattern, heart rate, color

Anticipate

Central nervous system sequelae: dysfunction, seizures
Cor pulmonale

Respiratory arrest
Cardiac arrest

RESPONSE OF CHILD

Assess, Monitor, and Document

Development level: verbal, motor, cognitive, psychosocial, fears
Behavioral response: crying, fearful, withdrawn, passive
Response to nursing interventions

Anticipate

Emotional distress
Disruption in normal growth and development

RESPONSE OF FAMILY

An episode of apnea in a child can be devastating for the parents. Today, parents are very aware of sudden infant death syndrome (SIDS) and the consequences of oxygen deprivation on the central nervous system. Parents become involved in the crisis and their need for information, reassurance, and support is great while the physician attempts to determine the cause and treatment of apnea in their child. After the cause has been identified, parents must be prepared to manage the child at home. The child may now have special needs in terms of diet, position, medication, and home monitoring. Parents must also be prepared to perform basic life support.

Assess, Monitor, and Document

Behavioral response: verbal, anxious, fearful
Level of knowledge of apnea and child's condition
Expected outcome
Ability to cope

Learning needs related to discharge and home management: diet, medications, body positioning, apnea monitor, basic life support
Response to nursing interventions

Anticipate

Emotional distress
Family crisis

Inability to cope
Learning needs related to discharge planning

MIND SET

Assess

Respiratory rate
Respiratory pattern
Heart rate
Circumstances preceding episode of apnea

Apneic event: duration, bradycardia, color, termination (stimulation, resuscitation)
Condition of child after episode of apnea
Response of child and family

Anticipate

Central nervous system sequelae: dysfunction, seizures
Cor pulmonale

Respiratory arrest
Cardiac arrest

Near-Drowning

ALAN G. KULBERG, M.D.

Drowning, defined as death within 24 hours by suffocation due to submersion in water, is a leading cause of mortality in childhood. Near-drowning implies survival, for at least 24 hours, following asphyxia secondary to submersion in water. Near drowning is associated with significant morbidity in the form of central nervous system injury. This results largely from the pulmonary insult which produces hypoxemia, hypoperfusion and acidosis. In its most severe expression, near-drowning can produce multisystem failure stemming from a profound hypoxic insult. The main goal of treatment is cerebral salvage, with the major therapeutic effort directed at controlling the pathophysiologic processes that lead to cerebral edema.

ASSOCIATED FACTORS

A variety of medical and environmental factors may either predispose to or complicate the management of the nearly drowned individual. Alcohol abuse, exhaustion, seizure disorders, and suicidal intent may play a role. The child who hyperventilates prior to diving into the water places himself at risk; oxygen utilization may result in hypoxemia before Pa_{CO_2} reaches levels high enough to create an overwhelming stimulus to resume breathing, and the child "blacks out" under water. Another unfortunate situation is near-drowning as a result of child abuse or neglect. Suspicion of abuse or neglect may be based on a history that seems improbable given the child's developmental capabilities or when there is a discrepancy among reports of those providing the history. The physical examination may reveal evidence of other injuries that are suggestive of being inflicted, especially scald burns from bathtub water that is too hot. A parental history of psychiatric illness or drug abuse should arouse one's suspicion of abuse or neglect, although these features are often absent.

Hypothermia, a common complication of near-drowning in cold water, may have a beneficial impact on morbidity and mortality. Management considerations with respect to hypothermia are discussed in a later section of this chapter and in Chapter 13.

Last but perhaps most important is the possibility of cervical spine injury, which should not be overlooked in any patient, particularly the victim of a diving accident. Awareness of the potential for cervical injury should begin at the time of initial resuscitation and should continue when the patient arrives at the hospital. A cervical collar should be placed if there is suspicion of cervical spine injury, or if more urgent airway considerations supersede its use, at least appropriate care should be taken to prevent motion of the neck. In either case, cervical spine x-ray films should be obtained as soon as it is feasible.

PATHOPHYSIOLOGY

The actual sequence of events that develops in the drowning or near-drowning episode is difficult to confirm in any individual patient, but animal studies and observations of human cases have elucidated several stages. Initially, the victim attempts to struggle for freedom and, by gasping, may immediately inhale water leading toward respiratory and cardiac arrest or he may reflexively swallow large amounts of water, vomit, and aspirate gastric contents and/or water. In either event, hypoxia ensues, the victim becomes unconscious, and reflexes are lost, with gasping and further aspiration of fluid.

As a final event, water may passively enter and flood the lungs. In approximately 10 to 15 percent of patients, early laryngospasm may completely prevent aspiration. This is commonly referred to as *dry drowning,* in contrast to *wet drowning* with aspiration. Whether the episode is "wet" or "dry," the final hypoxic insult is the same.

Much has been written about the potential differences between near-drowning in salt water and in fresh water. Animal studies have suggested that hypertonic salt water in the lungs, by virtue of its oncotic and hydrostatic effects, would favor passage of fluid from the intravascular space into the alveoli, thereby flooding the lungs. In contrast, with fresh water, oncotic pressures would favor free fluid shifts *into* the intravascular space with volume overload, hemolysis, hyperkalemia, and hemoglobinuria being the predicted results. In humans, these fluid shifts probably occur to some degree, but the patient who survives long enough to be transported to the hospital has probably not aspirated enough water for them to be of major concern. There is a tendency toward a dilution of serum sodium in fresh water aspiration and hyperconcentration with salt water, but they are almost never life-threatening. Hypermagnesemia and mild to moderate rises in the hematocrit have been observed in submersion accidents in extremely hypertonic water, such as that in the Dead Sea. The long-held belief that dysrhythmias seen with fresh water aspiration are secondary to hyperkalemia has been disproved; these cardiac effects are most likely due to hypoxia. Similarly, the renal failure seen is predominantly on the basis of hypoxic tubular damage.

The pathophysiologic derangements seen in the lung in both salt water and fresh water near-drownings are relatively similar although the pathogenetic mechanisms may differ somewhat. Decreased pulmonary compliance and increased airway resistance, intrapulmonary shunting, dead space to tidal volume ratio, and ventilation/perfusion mismatch are present in each. Aspiration of salt water causes direct chemical injury to the alveolar capillary membrane, which, along with the oncotic effects of the water, permits passage of protein-rich fluid into the alveoli. In addition, seawater may contain algae, sand, bacteria, and pollutants that can exacerbate the inflammatory response in the lung or even cause structural obstruction of the airways. Fresh water aspiration, on the other hand, causes a washout of surfactant, the surface-active phospholipid that serves to decrease the surface tension at the gas–fluid interface of the alveoli, resulting in atelectasis and disruption of alveolar cells. With the alveolar lining disturbed, pulmonary edema may develop. Special situations that may pose a problem in terms of surfactant disruption include near-drownings in soapy bathtub water or in water, usually lakes, where motor boats have discharged gasoline (see Chapter 62).

CLINICAL CONSIDERATIONS

Clinical evaluation of the nearly drowned patient begins with assessment of the vital signs, including an initial check of airway patency, breath sounds, and blood pressure. Hypothermia may be so profound that accurate readings of body temperature can be made only with a rectal thermocouple probe. Abdominal distention may be indicative of a large volume of swallowed water or possibly occult trauma. When indicated, a thorough search for other signs of trauma should be made. The neurologic examination should be thorough, noting the mental status in terms of responsiveness to stimuli and the presence of focal deficits. The pupils should be tested for size and reactivity, and the fundi should be examined to detect signs of increased intracranial pressure, such as blurring of the optic disc margins and absence of venous pulsations.

While carrying out the clinical evaluation, one should keep an open mind to the possibility of an associated factor that may have an effect on the results of the examination. For instance, the condition of a patient, with small reactive pupils, found lying face up and unresponsive in a bathtub may be better explained by a drug overdose or a postictal state rather than by submersion injury.

RADIOLOGIC CONSIDERATION

A chest x-ray should be obtained routinely in any patient suspected of having a submersion injury, regardless of the mental status on admission. Perihilar or generalized pulmonary edema may be seen. Widespread atelectasis is consistent with loss of surfactant or with the presence of foreign matter in the airways. Dissociation of the clinical and radiologic findings may occur; a normal chest film may be seen early in patients with significant aspiration or in victims of "dry" drowning. Vigorous prehospital cardiopulmonary resuscitation may leave its scars, including fractured ribs, pneumothorax, or pneumomediastinum. As emphasized previously, a cervical spine series may be the only reliable way of ruling out the possibility of fracture or subluxation.

MONITORING AND MANAGEMENT

Hypothermia in patients who require full-scale cardiopulmonary resuscitation dictates that the resuscitative effort should be complete and sustained at least until the core temperature is rewarmed to 92° to 95°F. Survival with good neurologic outcome has been well documented with submersion for 40 minutes in cold water followed by more than 2 hours of resuscitation, during which time the rewarming process continued. Simply, a patient should not be declared dead if he or she is cold. The protective effects of hypothermia include a decrease in the cerebral oxygen requirement, coupled with a preferential shunting of cardiac output to the brain and heart. Also, because the hypothermic patient may be refractory to cardiostimulatory medications, care should be taken not to give many repeated doses of inotropic or chronotropic medications; their sudden mass action on the heart when the patient is warm may produce intractable dysrhythmias.

Arterial blood gases (ABG) should be monitored at least every hour until the patient is stable. When multiple samples are required, an indwelling peripheral arterial line should be placed. Hypoxemia should be treated with as high an F_{IO_2} as necessary to maintain an adequate Pa_{O_2}, although more moderate F_{IO_2} values may suffice if the patient is supplemented with some form of positive airway pressure, such as continuous positive airway pressure (CPAP). The alert, awake patient may tolerate CPAP by wearing a tight-fitting face mask. CPAP or positive end–expiratory pressure (PEEP) may be delivered via endotracheal tube for patients unable to normalize the Pa_{O_2} and Pa_{CO_2} by mask, for patients with significant depression in mental status, or for ease of suctioning. Intubation by the nasotracheal route is preferred when there is a cervical spine injury. Assisted ventilation should be achieved with a volume-controlled ventilator. Potential dangers of positive pressure ventilation include decreases in cerebral venous return and cardiac output. Decreased cerebral venous return increases intracranial pressure, complicating hypoxic cerebral edema.

Rational fluid management, which, on the one hand, should be parsimonious to help control cerebral edema, should be aggressive if the patient shows signs of poor peripheral perfusion. Clinically, peripheral capillary filling can be monitored as an index of cardiac output. When there is evidence of poor perfusion early in the patient's course of treatment, volume-expanding solutions should be infused at a rapid rate, even prior to obtaining specific hemodynamic parameters. This may be done even without precise knowledge of the etiology of the hypoperfusion, whether it is due to pump failure secondary to hypoxia and acidosis, sequestration of fluid in the lungs, hemorrhage secondary to trauma, or even cervical spine disruption. Determinations of central venous pressure (CVP) and ABG (to assess the presence of metabolic acidosis) generally suffice to guide fluid therapy. Occasionally, measurements of cardiac output and pulmonary capillary wedge pressure are necessary to determine the optimal balance between ventilator settings and fluid requirements; a Swan–Ganz catheter should be passed for these purposes (see Chapter 6). Metabolic acidosis should be treated aggressively with sodium bicarbonate. (A more complete discussion of the relationship of ventilator and hemodynamic management can be found in Chapter 3.)

The patient should be constantly monitored with an electrocardiogram (EKG); initially, at least, a 12-lead tracing should be obtained and repeated when necessary. Although dysrhythmias may respond to the standard medications (except in the presence of hypothermia), the common underlying causes, such as hypoxemia, acidosis, hypoperfusion, and occasionally electrolyte abnormalities, should be treated vigorously.

Hourly monitoring of urine output is crucial, because renal compromise is common after severe hypoxia. The urine should be tested periodically with a dipstick to screen for hemoglobin, red blood cells, and protein. Concomitant measurements of serum and urine osmolality can be useful in diagnosing the syndrome of inappropriate antidiuretic hormone secretion (SIADH), which may be secondary to either increased intracranial pressure or severe lung disease (see Chapter 31). Standard tests for renal function, blood urea nitrogen (BUN), and serum creatinine should also be carried out.

Other parameters that should be closely watched are serum electrolytes, hemoglobin and hematocrit, and white blood cell count and differential. Additional chest x-rays should be obtained if there is any significant clinical or laboratory change in pulmonary status or suspicion of pneumonitis.

The phenomenon of so-called "secondary" drowning refers to a deterioration in pulmonary function, with pulmonary edema and atelectasis, sometimes associated with hemodynamic changes, that occurs from 15 minutes to 72 hours after the submersion episode. It occurs more commonly after salt water aspiration and is thought to result from an intense chemical alveolitis and bronchiolitis.

Control of increased intracranial pressure resulting from hypoxic cerebral edema is one of the major therapeutic goals, because it has been shown that control of cerebral edema improves the neurologic outcome of survivors. Despite this, there is still a high morbidity and mortality rate in near-drowning victims who require cardiopulmonary resuscitation (CPR), have a pH of less than 7.00, or have fixed, dilated pupils at the time that they present to the emergency room. These are general rules, however; a few cases of survival with good neurologic function have been reported in patients who had such poor prognostic indices. If the patient is hypothermic, these factors may be completely invalid. For these reasons, *all* patients who are brought to the emergency room deserve a full resuscitative effort.

In patients who have one of these poor prognostic factors, some degree of cerebral edema is inevitable. Several measures, including hyperventilation, fluid restriction, osmotic diuretic therapy, steroid administration, therapeutic hypothermia to 92°F, and barbiturate therapy, are commonly used to control intracranial pressure. Intracranial pressure monitoring devices such as the intraventricular cannula or subarachnoid bolt are used to guide therapy (see Chapter 12). Unfortunately, there is no single parameter or set of parameters that is 100 percent predictive of a poor outcome, although coma for more than 2 days in the intensive care unit (ICU) and certain electroencephalogram EEG patterns reported by Janati and Erba have been proposed as useful considerations when deciding on the feasibility of aggressive life support.

Additional problems encountered in nearly drowned patients include disseminated intravascular coagulation, hyperthermia, and hyperrigidity. A protocol addressing, in particular, the latter two complications has been devised by Conn and colleagues.

CASE PRESENTATION

A 3-year-old male is found floating face down in cold water in the bathtub in his house. His father has no idea how long the child has been there. The emergency paramedics are called, and they arrive approximately 10 minutes later to find the child cyanotic and without spontaneous respirations and palpable pulse. They take him out of the water, wrap him in a blanket, and commence CPR, using a bag–mask apparatus with oxygen. On the way out of the house, one of the paramedics notices an open medication bottle and yellow tablets on the floor of the parents' room.

The child arrives in the emergency service 7 minutes later, with CPR continuing.

Examination reveals a slightly cyanotic child with dilated, sluggishly reacting pupils. Chest x-ray examination discloses diffuse coarse rhonchi in both lung fields. The abdomen is scaphoid. Neurologically, he is unresponsive, with generalized moderate extensor rigidity and no shivering.

Problem List

Respiratory

Near-drowning is a good possibility, with aspiration of fluid into the lungs. Despite artificial ventilation with oxygen, the child is clinically cyanotic. Endotracheal intubation should be performed to ensure adequacy of ventilation and a route for pulmonary suctioning. Other considerations that may account for the altered mental status are aspiration of gastric contents or the direct effects of a drug ingestion—these may possibly be related. After intubation, an ABG study should be obtained. Failure to achieve a satisfactory PO_2 on a volume-controlled ventilator might require the addition of PEEP to maintain alveolar expansion during expiration. A chest x-ray should be obtained to assess the baseline extent of the pulmonary injury and endotracheal tube positioning.

Fluids and Electrolytes

The most important issue here is clinically determining the adequacy of peripheral perfusion. Volume-expanding–type fluids (Ringer's lactate, normal saline, plasmanate) should be pushed if the blood pressure is low or if nail bed capillary perfusion is poor. Balancing the need to *provide* fluids are the reasons for *restricting* fluids, such as the potential for posthypoxic cerebral edema, the lung edema secondary to injury to the alveolar–capillary membrane, and the potential for inappropriate secretion of antidiuretic hormone. Placement of a CVP catheter may be required. Serum electrolyte determination should be done, with special regard for the serum sodium, potassium, and bicarbonate. Urine flow is monitored with an indwelling catheter, and a nasogastric tube is placed and connected to low suction to decompress the ileus that inevitably develops.

Hypothermia

On admission, the core temperature is 84°F (29°C). At this level, shivering is abolished and generalized rigidity is common. Rewarming may be accomplished passively by use of blankets and actively by use of heating blankets and radiant warmers. If the core temperature is successfully raised by 1 to 1.5°F per hour, more invasive techniques such as gastric warming, heated IV solutions, or warm enemas should not be necessary and may, in fact, be dangerous. A sedative drug ingestion could exacerbate hypothermia.

Neurologic

The extent of neurologic recovery is impossible to predict given this child's history and findings upon physical examination. The possibility of a drug ingestion and the hypothermia make it difficult to determine the precise etiology of the comatose state. Indeed, the Glasgow Coma Scale should *not* be applied in this situation, because it would tend to assign a false, poorer prognosis than the patient would receive if these complicating factors were not present. The development of severe cerebral edema is likely, considering the prolonged period of cardiorespiratory arrest. To monitor and treat the cerebral edema, an intracranial pressure monitoring device should be placed. Finally, the potential for head trauma complicating this child's condition must be considered and a computed tomography (CT) scan should be done to detect a neurosurgically treatable lesion.

SUGGESTED READING

Conn, A.W., Edmond, J.F., and Barker, G.A.: Cerebral resuscitation in near-drowning. Pediatr. Clin. North Am. 26:691, 1979.

Hoff, B.H.: Multisystem failure: a review with special reference to drowning. Crit. Care Med. 7:310, 1979.

Janati, A., and Erba, G.: Electroencephalographic correlates of near-drowning encephalopathy in children. Electroencephalogr. Clin. Neurophysiol. 53:182, 1982.

Levin, D.L.: Near-drowning. Crit. Care Med. 8:590, 1980.

Nursing Process for Patient Care:

Near–Drowning

Submersion in water results in pulmonary injury that can cause central nervous system damage resulting from hypoxia and acidosis. Other organ systems may also be affected by the hypoxic insult.

RESPIRATORY

In most cases, water is either inhaled or swallowed, vomited, and aspirated into the lungs. The pathophysiologic changes that occur are relatively similar in both salt water and fresh water near-drownings; there is an increase in airway resistance and a decrease in lung compliance.

Assess, Monitor, and Document

Respiratory rate
Respiratory pattern, including depth
Work of breathing: retractions, nasal flaring
Breath sounds
Secretions: amount, description

Level of consciousness
Color
Arterial blood gases
Response to therapy: chest physical therapy, pulmonary hygiene

Anticipate

Alteration in respiratory status
  Atelectasis
  Pulmonary edema

Respiratory failure: hypoxia, hypercarbia, acidosis
Secondary drowning

CARDIOVASCULAR

Assess, Monitor, and Document

Heart rate
Rhythm
Blood pressure: arterial, central venous, pulmonary artery (if indicated), capillary wedge (if indicated)

Perfusion: peripheral pulses, color, skin condition, capillary filling
Cardiac output (if indicated): by thermodilution method

Anticipate

Alteration in cardiovascular status
Decreased cardiac output: increased heart rate, decreased arterial blood pressure
Decreased peripheral perfusion: weak pulses;

cool skin; mottled, dusky skin; poor capillary refill
Cardiac dysrhythmias
Cardiac arrest

FLUID AND ELECTROLYTE BALANCE

Assess, Monitor, and Document

Weight
Urine output, hourly
Urine specific gravity
Fluid intake: accurate administration of par-

enteral fluids (use infusion pump if available)
Serum electrolytes
Urine electrolytes

Anticipate

Alteration in fluid and electrolyte status
Fresh water aspiration: hypervolemia, hyperkalemia, hyponatremia

Salt water aspiration: hypovolemia, hypernatremia
Syndrome of inappropriate secretion of antidiuretic hormone (SIADH)

NEUROLOGIC

The central nervous system can be profoundly affected by the sequence of pathophysiologic changes that occur in a near-drowning episode. Cerebral edema with resultant increased intracranial pressure must be anticipated.

Assess, Monitor, and Document

Level of consciousness: lethargy, stupor, coma
Headache
Vomiting
Blood pressure: arterial
Pulse rate
Pupillary response
Reflex response
Motor response

Posture
Seizures (if applicable)
Intracranial pressure (if available): subarachnoid bolt, ventricular catheter, epidural monitor
Response to medical management: hyperventilation, fluid restriction, osmotherapy (mannitol), steroids, therapeutic hypothermia, barbiturate coma

Anticipate

Alteration in neurologic status
Increased intracranial pressure: seizures,

coma, respiratory arrest, cardiac arrest, posthypoxic encephalopathy

TEMPERATURE

Hypothermia, a common associated occurrence, may be protective as cerebral oxygen requirements are decreased and blood is preferentially shunted to the brain and heart.

Assess, Monitor, and Document

Temperature: thermocouple probe if profoundly hypothermic

Anticipate

Hypothermia

RENAL

The kidneys are a target organ system in terms of their sensitivity to hypoxia.

Assess, Monitor, and Document

Urinary output: amount (hourly), description, specific gravity, dipstick for blood and protein, urine electrolytes and osmolality

Serum electrolytes, BUN, creatinine, osmolality
Status of hydration: weight, blood pressure

Anticipate

Alteration in renal function
Acute renal failure: acute tubular necrosis (weight gain, increased blood pressure, decreased urine output)

Secretion of antidiuretic hormone: weight gain, decreased urine output (specific gravity > 1.015, decreased serum osmolality, increased urine osmolality, decreased serum sodium)

RESPONSE OF CHILD

Assess, Monitor, and Document

Developmental level: verbal, motor, psychosocial, cognitive
Perception of accident

Behavioral response: fearful, anxious, tearful
Response to nursing interventions

Anticipate

Emotional crisis
Inability to cope

RESPONSE OF FAMILY

Assess, Monitor, and Document

Behavioral response: anxious, fearful, verbal, angry
Perception of events surrounding accident: feelings of guilt
Level of understanding of child's condition

Expected outcome
Educational needs related to environmental safety
Response to nursing interventions

Anticipate

Inability to cope
Family crisis

Need for education related to environmental safety
Need for referral: social service, psychiatric

MIND SET

Assess

Respiratory status
Cardiovascular status
Fluid and electrolyte balance
Neurologic status

Temperature
Renal status
Response of child and family

Anticipate

Alteration in respiratory status
  Hypoxia
  Acidosis
  Respiratory arrest
Alteration in cardiovascular status
  Hypoperfusion
  Cardiac arrest

Alteration in neurologic status
  Posthypoxic encephalopathy
Alteration in body temperature
  Hypothermia
Alteration in renal function
  Acute renal failure: acute tubular necrosis
Emotional distress
Family crisis

ENDOCRINOLOGIC

CHAPTER
31

Syndrome of Inappropriate Secretion of ADH

CHARLES A. SKLAR, M.D.

The synthesis and release of the antidiuretic hormone (ADH) arginine vasopressin is regulated by both osmotic and nonosmotic stimuli. Under normal circumstances, ADH release occurs when the body is attempting to conserve free water in order to combat hyperosmolality or hypovolemia. Occasionally, ADH secretion may be appropriate for one regulatory factor but excessive or inappropriate with regard to another (e.g., water retention in response to intravascular volume depletion that results in hyponatremia). When the synthesis and release of ADH cannot be accounted for by any known physiologic stimulus, it is referred to as the syndrome of inappropriate secretion of antidiuretic hormone (SIADH). The following discussion deals with the pathophysiology, differential diagnosis, and therapy of SIADH.

PATHOPHYSIOLOGY

The underlying defect in SIADH, regardless of the specific etiology, is continued release of ADH when there is hyponatremia, hypo-osmolality, and normal or increased plasma volume. The excess and inappropriate secretion of ADH causes most of the filtered water to be reabsorbed from the kidneys back into the circulation. The subjects become progressively water-intoxicated and hypotonic with continued ingestion of water. They have circulating levels of ADH that do not suppress at the normal threshold osmolality and are incapable of producing a dilute urine. Ultimately, patients with SIADH develop an expanded circulatory volume secondary to water overload. Because the body cannot correct the volume problem by a water diuresis, other less efficient mechanisms are activated, including diminished aldosterone production and the elaboration of a putative natruretic or "third" factor, both of which promote sodium excretion via the kidneys. Obviously, loss of large amounts of sodium in the urine only worsens the pre-existing hyponatremia. It is important to note that although patients with SIADH develop an expanded circulatory volume, they do not form edema, which is generally a manifestation of total body excess of both sodium and water.

As a consequence of the aforementioned sequence of events, patients with SIADH present with the following laboratory profile: subnormal plasma concentration of sodium, with a concomitant hypo-osmolality of plasma; urinary osmolality, that is inappropriately elevated relative to plasma osmolality; high urinary sodium concentration; and no clinical or biochemical evidence of intravascular volume depletion.

Patients with SIADH become symptomatic as the plasma concentration of sodium falls. Few, if any, problems are encountered until the serum sodium drops below 125 mEq per L. Early symptoms include anorexia, nausea, and vomiting. When the sodium concentration slips below 120 mEq per L, one may observe more serious signs of cerebral edema, such as confusion, stupor, convulsions, or coma. Clinical symptoms are more likely to occur when the level of sodium falls acutely as opposed to situations in which the hyponatremia develops over a prolonged period of time.

A wide variety of abnormalities and path-

243

ologic processes can lead to episodes of SIADH (Table 31–1). Most commonly, SIADH in the pediatric population occurs in association with infections of the central nervous system (bacterial meningitis) and tumors of the hypothalamic region, following neurosurgical intervention, and in patients on positive pressure ventilators. Not uncommonly, transient episodes of SIADH are noted in individuals receiving vincristine, cyclophosphamide, or the anticonvulsant carbamazepine. Ectopic production of ADH by a malignant tumor has been described during childhood but is an extremely rare cause of SIADH.

DIFFERENTIAL DIAGNOSIS

Significant hyponatremia (plasma sodium less than 130 mEq/L) and hypotonicity (plasma osmolality less than 270 mOsm/kg) can result from a variety of disorders. Differentiating SIADH from other pathologic states associated with hyponatremia is critical, because the pathophysiology and treatment will differ greatly. At the outset, it is important to establish that the patient's hyponatremia truly reflects a hypo-osmolar state. Spurious hyponatremia can occur, for instance, when lipid and/or protein displace sodium and water from plasma. The sodium concentration is normal when measured in plasma water (after exclusion of lipid or protein), and plasma osmolality remains normal. Occasionally, hyponatremia and

Table 31–1. Disorders Associated with SIADH

Central Nervous System
  Infections
  Trauma
  Neoplasms
  Guillain–Barré syndrome
Intrathoracic
  Infections
  Positive-pressure ventilation
  Pneumothorax and atelectasis
  Asthma
Drugs
  Vincristine
  Cyclophosphamide
  Carbamazepine
  Clofibrate
  Phenothiazines
  Chlorpropamide
  Acetaminophen
  Indomethacin
Ectopic Production of ADH
  Oat cell carcinoma of lung
  Pancreatic carcinoma
  Lymphoma
  Acute lymphocytic leukemia
  Thymoma

increased plasma osmolality coexist. This generally indicates the presence of an impermeable solute such as glucose or mannitol which increases plasma osmolality and causes free water to move from the intracellular to the intravascular compartment. In this situation, plasma sodium concentration is genuinely reduced but reflects a redistribution rather than an excess of total body water.

All the various clinical conditions that result in hyponatremia and hypotonicity of plasma have excess retention of water, either absolute or relative. Even though the plasma concentration of sodium is low, *total body sodium* may be high, low, or normal. Assessment of the status of the intravascular and extracellular fluid volumes provides a convenient means by which the clinician can indirectly determine total body sodium and allow for a useful grouping of the various abnormalities that can cause hypo-osmolality.

Hyponatremia associated with decreased total body sodium implies that sodium losses exceed water losses. This results in hypovolemia, loss of extracellular fluid volume, and an inadequate intravascular volume. Clinically, these patients are dehydrated, hypotensive, and tachycardic. Because of the hypovolemia, the body mobilizes a variety of compensatory mechanisms, including increased aldosterone and ADH production, to restore the circulatory volume to normal. Because maintenance of fluid volume takes precedence over maintenance of fluid tonicity, ADH production and water retention will continue despite hypo-osmolality of plasma. Hypovolemic hyponatremia generally results from fluid loss via the gastrointestinal tract (e.g., viral gastroenteritis) or from renal salt wasting (e.g., mineralocorticoid deficiency, diuretic therapy, intrinsic renal disease). Less commonly, loss of fluid into a "third space" (e.g., burns, peritonitis) results in hypovolemic hyponatremia. In general, the aforementioned conditions can be easily differentiated from SIADH by history and routine clinical and biochemical parameters. When the site of salt and water loss is extrarenal, the urine sodium concentration will be very low (less than 10 mEq/L), which will further aid in excluding SIADH as the etiology.

Hyponatremia can be associated with conditions in which total body sodium and fluid are increased. The hallmark of these disorders is the presence of peripheral edema. The common underlying pathology is that of a reduced effective blood volume, which is responsible for activating renal and hormonal mechanisms to conserve salt and water. Hyponatremia in these states is generally mild unless excessive fluid intake combined with sodium restriction occurs simultaneously. Congestive heart failure (CHF), hepatic cirrhosis, and the nephrotic syndrome are the most common causes of hypervolemic hyponatremia. The presence of edema and the very low urine sodium concentration help to differentiate these disorders from SIADH.

Plasma hypo-osmolality associated with normal intravascular fluid volume and total body sodium is seen in relatively few pathologic situations. SIADH is by far the most likely diagnosis, and its features and causes have been previously delineated. Rarely, water intoxication resulting from excessive oral intake or intravenous (IV) administration of hypotonic fluids can result in isovolemic hyponatremia.

In contrast to that in patients with SIADH, the urine osmolality will be lowest in pure water intoxication, because these patients have retained the capacity to suppress ADH when hypo-osmolality and volume expansion are present. Finally, both hypothyroidism and cortisol deficiency can lead to an isovolemic form of hyponatremia that may be difficult to differentiate from SIADH. For this reason, assessment of thyroid and adrenal function is mandatory before a diagnosis of SIADH can be established.

In addition to the routine clinical (e.g., skin turgor, edema, body weight) and biochemical (e.g., BUN, hematocrit) indices of a patient's state of hydration, determination of the plasma level of uric acid may aid in the differential diagnosis of hyponatremia. A recent report indicated that most patients with SIADH have marked hypouricemia (mean = 2.9 mg/dl), whereas those subjects with hyponatremia resulting from other causes had normal to elevated uric acid levels (mean = 7.7 mg/dl). Until recently, reliable determinations of ADH levels were restricted to only a few research laboratories. At the present time, many medical centers and commercial laboratories are able to measure plasma concentrations of ADH. Rarely, however, will this information add significantly to the clinical diagnosis of SIADH. Furthermore, "inappropriately" elevated ADH levels will be present in most disorders associated with hyponatremia and decreased or ineffective intravascular volume.

TREATMENT

The cornerstone of therapy for SIADH is fluid restriction. Limiting fluid intake to an amount equal to total fluid losses (urine output and insensible fluid losses) prevents progressive water intoxication and progressive hyponatremia. Fluid intake must be more severely restricted when patients are already hypo-osmolar and hyponatremic in order to permit negative water balance to occur. Asymptomatic patients with a serum sodium less than 125 mEq per L should be restricted to as little fluid as possible.

When patients present with acute, life-threatening symptoms, more aggressive measures are needed to rapidly raise the plasma sodium concentration. We have found the combination of IV furosemide and hypertonic saline to be a safe and reliable method of rapidly correcting hyponatremia. A single IV bolus of furosemide (0.5 to 1.0 mg/kg) is given, followed by hourly determinations of the urine sodium and potassium concentrations. The electrolyte losses are replaced hourly with 3 percent saline plus appropriate amounts of potassium chloride. In general, this protocol results in a significant elevation in plasma sodium within several hours.

Although most forms of SIADH are transient, occasionally chronic forms are encountered. Many patients will tolerate chronic fluid restriction, in which case no other therapy is necessary. For those unable to cooperate with such a program, several drugs are available. Demeclocycline and lithium interfere with the action of ADH and induce a nephrogenic diabetes insipidus. Although demeclocycline appears to be the safer of the two drugs, neither has been used extensively in pediatric patients. Several recent articles report encouraging results with single daily doses of furosemide in subjects with chronic SIADH. The major drawback to this therapy is the necessity of providing both sodium and potassium supplementation to compensate for urinary losses.

CASE PRESENTATION

A 7½-year-old male presented to the emergency room with a 1-day history of increasing anorexia, nausea, and somnolence. While in the emergency room, he experienced a generalized tonic clonic seizure, lasting approximately 90 seconds. History revealed that the patient had a known seizure disorder, with the first seizure occurring at age 2 years. The details of his initial evaluation were unknown, but the patient had been placed on phenobarbital at that time. After 1 year of continuous phenobarbital treatment, the patient remained seizure-free and the mother discontinued his medication. The patient was apparently doing well without any seizures until 1 month prior to admission. At that time, he experienced a generalized tonic clonic seizure. After evaluation at a local emergency room, he was placed on Dilantin. One week later, he developed an urticarial rash over his trunk and extremities. His local physician discontinued the Dilantin, and the patient was then placed on carbamazepine. The remainder of his history was negative, including any recent trauma, infections, or known cardiac, liver, or renal disease.

Examination

Physical examination revealed an afebrile, healthy-appearing youngster, with stable vital signs and height and weight at the 25th percentile. He was hydrated and had normal skin turgor and no edema. The patient was lethargic but responsive. The results of his examination were otherwise unremarkable.

Test Results

Initial laboratory data revealed a plasma Na of 119 mEq/L and plasma osmolality of 250 mOsm/kg; K, Cl, CO_2, Ca, and glucose were normal. A simultaneous urine specimen had an osmolality of 850 mOsm/kg with a Na concentration of 58 mEq/L. Subsequent results showed a plasma BUN of 11 mg/dl, creatinine of 0.6 mg/dl, uric acid of 2 mg/dl, and a normal CBC.

Therapy consisted of an initial IV bolus of furosemide (1 mg/kg), which resulted in a prompt diuresis. Hourly determination of urinary Na concentration revealed a loss of approximately 25 mEq of Na per hour, which was replaced as 3 percent NaCl. Within 4 hours, his plasma Na was 127 mEq/L, and the patient was alert and oriented. He was then placed on fluid restriction such that his total intake was less than his total urine output. Over the next 24 hours, his plasma Na rose to 133 mEq/L. Futher evaluation revealed a normal CT brain scan and normal thyroid and adrenal function. His SIADH resolved over the next 72 hours, and at the time of discharge, the patient was taking ad lib oral fluids, with normal electrolytes and appropriate urinary osmolalities.

Problem List

Seizures

Although this patient had a known seizure disorder, presumably caused by idiopathic epilepsy, he was found to have significant hyponatremia at the time of his most recent seizure. This case illustrates the importance of screening for metabolic derangements in all patients who present with a documented seizure, even when an etiology has been previously established. Failure to investigate the possibility of a superimposed metabolic problem would have led to inappropriate therapy and perhaps repeated episodes of seizure activity. It is important to remember that in patients with seizure disorders, metabolic disorders such as hypoglycemia and hyponatremia will lower the seizure threshold and precipitate a convulsion.

Hyponatremia

Initial testing documented a hyponatremia with concurrent hypo-osmolality. The patient appeared to be well hydrated, without clinical or biochemical evidence of intravascular volume depletion or renal or mineralocorticoid insufficiency. The inappropriately high urine osmolality and sodium and the low plasma uric acid level indicated SIADH as the cause of the hyponatremia. After normal thyroid and adrenal function was verified, the patient fulfilled all the critical criteria to establish the diagnosis of SIADH. The SIADH was most probably caused by carbamazepine (Tegretol). The initial therapy was aimed at rapidly increasing the plasma Na concentration, because the patient was acutely symptomatic. When the Na level reached a safer level, more conservative treatment (fluid restriction) was instituted.

SUGGESTED READING

Decaux, G., Waterlot, Y., Genette, F., et al.: Inappropriate secretion of antidiuretic hormone treated with furosemide. Br. Med. J. 285:89 1982.

Forrest, J.R., Cox, M., Hong, C., et al.: Superiority of demeclocycline over lithium in the treatment of chronic syndrome of inappropriate secretion of antidiuretic hormone. N. Engl. J. Med. 298:173, 1978.

Hautman, D., Rossier, B., Zohlman, R., and Schrier, R.: Rapid correction of hyponatremia in the syndrome of inappropriate secretion of antidiuretic hormone. Ann. Intern. Med. 78:870, 1973.

Kaplan, S.L., and Feigin, R.: Syndromes of inappropriate secretion of antidiuretic hormone in children. In Barness, L.A. (ed.): Advances in Pediatrics, Vol. 27. Chicago, Year Book Medical Publishers, Inc., 1980, p. 247.

Robertson, G.L., Aycinema, P., and Zerbe, R.L.: Neurogenic disorders of osmoregulation. Am. J. Med. 72:339, 1982.

Nursing Process for Patient Care:
Syndrome of Inappropriate Secretion of ADH

The inappropriate secretion of antidiuretic hormone causes excessive water reabsorption from the kidneys, with resultant plasma hyponatremia and hypotonicity. The focus of attention is, therefore, on the altered fluid and electrolyte balance and its effect on the neurologic status of the child.

FLUID AND ELECTROLYTE BALANCE

Assess, Monitor and Document

Weight (daily)
Fluid intake
Urine output
Urine specific gravity

Urine osmolality
Urine sodium
Serum sodium
Serum osmolality

Anticipate

Alteration in fluid and electrolyte balance
Water intoxication: overhydration, hyponatremia, hypotonicity

NEUROLOGIC

Neurologic symptoms appear as the serum concentration of sodium decreases below 125 mEq/L.

Assess, Monitor, and Document

Nausea
Vomiting
Level of consciousness
Pupillary response
Reflex response

Muscle tone
Blood pressure
Pulse
Respiratory rate and pattern

Anticipate

Alteration in neurologic status
Seizures

Increased intracranial pressure
Coma

RESPONSE OF CHILD AND FAMILY

There are a variety of causes of SIADH. Most often, it occurs in association with infections of the central nervous system and following surgery on tumors of the hypothalamic region. These episodes are usually transient and are managed by fluid restriction. The response of the child and family to the underlying problem is important, because assessment parameters and intervention strategies are modified with the appearance of SIADH.

Assess, Monitor, and Document

Behavioral response: anxious, disappointed
Expected outcome
Ability to cope with this problem

Response to nursing interventions
Ability to cope with medical regimen

Anticipate

Emotional distress
Difficulty in compliance with fluid restriction

MIND SET

Assess

Fluid and electrolyte balance
Neurologic status
Response of child and family

Anticipate

Alteration in fluid and electrolyte balance
Water intoxication
Alteration in neurologic status

Cerebral edema
Emotional trauma
Family crisis

32

Diabetes Insipidus

CHARLES A. SKLAR, M.D.

In healthy people, water balance is regulated by a finely tuned homeostatic mechanism that maintains plasma osmolality within a narrow range. Despite almost constant changes in fluid requirements imposed by a variety of dietary and environmental factors, the osmolality of plasma and the concentration of sodium rarely fluctuate more than a few percent. This remarkable stability of plasma tonicity is a consequence of the body's ability to rapidly adjust both the intake and output of water, an ability governed by the hypothalamic centers controlling thirst and the synthesis of the antidiuretic hormone (ADH), arginine vasopressin. Whereas thirst ensures adequate intake of free water, ADH production and release serve to prevent the loss of water through the kidneys. Abnormalities in the synthesis, release, or action of ADH result in the syndrome of diabetes insipidus, which is characterized by the inability to produce a concentrated urine despite progressive hyperosmolality of plasma. In this chapter, the pathophysiology, differential diagnosis, and therapy of diabetes insipidus are discussed. Emphasis is directed toward the clinical management of acute forms of this syndrome.

PHYSIOLOGY OF NORMAL WATER METABOLISM

Antidiuretic Hormone (ADH)

ADH is synthesized by neurons in the supraoptic and paraventricular nuclei of the hypothalamus. Following its synthesis, ADH, along with its carrier protein neurophysin I, is transported via the neurohypophyseal tract to the posterior pituitary, where it is stored. A variety of factors, both physiologic and pathologic, influence the secretion and release of ADH into the circulation. The major physiologic regulators of ADH release include the osmolality of plasma and the hemodynamic sta-

tus of the patient. Although additional factors such as stress, anxiety, and pain are capable of influencing ADH secretion, they appear to have only a minor role in the control of normal water homeostasis. The most important determinant of ADH release on a minute-to-minute basis would appear to be plasma osmolality. Osmoreceptors located in the hypothalamus in close proximity to the nuclei that synthesize ADH are capable of sensing minor changes in osmolality and convey the information via nerve signals. When plasma osmolality is at or below approximately 280 mOsm per kg, ADH levels are uniformly suppressed, permitting a maximal diuresis of free water. Above this threshold osmolality, ADH release is in direct proportion to the osmotic stimuli, so that maximal plasma concentrations of ADH are achieved at a plasma osmolality of approximately 290 mOsm per kg. As the concentration of ADH increases, the osmolality of urine increases and the flow rate decreases, thus enabling the body to conserve free water. It should be noted that the osmoreceptors are solute-specific. Sodium, which normally contributes greater than 90 percent of plasma osmotic activity, is a very potent stimulus, whereas urea and glucose have little effect in activating osmoreceptors, despite their ability, under pathologic circumstances, to increase the total osmotic pressure of plasma.

The second important physiologic modulator of ADH secretion involves the hemodynamic status of the individual. Both blood volume and pressure exert an influence on ADH release via baroreceptors located in the left atrium and carotid sinus. Although changes in osmotic pressure as small as 1 to 2 percent can alter ADH release, hemodynamic changes of about 10 percent or greater are required before ADH secretion is significantly affected. Nonetheless, acute drops in blood pressure and/or volume as occurs after significant hemorrhage can be a potent stimulus for ADH release.

After it has been released into the circulation,

ADH mediates its major biologic function by attaching to receptors along the distal tubules and collecting ducts of the kidney. Activation of these ADH receptors results in an increase in the intracellular concentration of cyclic AMP, which causes the tubules to become permeable to water, allowing reabsorption of water from the tubular lumen to the hypertonic interstitium of the renal medulla. This results in the formation of a concentrated urine of diminished volume. In the absence of ADH, the tubules remain impermeable to water and the dilute urine presenting to the distal nephrons is excreted basically unchanged.

Thirst

The strong, deep-seated desire to drink is controlled by hypothalamic thirst centers, which are near but distinct from the hypothalamic centers of osmoreception and ADH synthesis. Thirst appears to be regulated primarily by plasma osmolality. The activation of thirst, however, takes place at a higher osmolality than that required for stimulation of ADH release. An intact thirst center is of paramount importance in maintaining normal water balance. As long as one is able to perceive and respond to the sensation of thirst, normal water homeostasis is generally maintained, even if ADH function is deficient.

PATHOPHYSIOLOGY OF DIABETES INSIPIDUS

The causes of diabetes insipidus can be grouped into two broad categories. Central or neurogenic diabetes insipidus encompasses all disorders in which the underlying defect involves the synthesis and/or release of ADH, whereas nephrogenic diabetes insipidus includes a variety of disease states in which the ability of the kidney to respond to ADH has been altered.

CENTRAL DIABETES INSIPIDUS

Most cases of central diabetes insipidus in a pediatric population are the result of an acquired problem, although congenital forms of ADH deficiency also occur. Patients with congenital defects in ADH synthesis may also demonstrate associated deficiencies of anterior pituitary hormones. Both familial and sporadic cases of congenital ADH deficiency have been described.

A wide variety of diseases and insults to the central nervous system can lead to acquired diabetes insipidus. Parapituitary tumors account for a large proportion of the cases and include such entities as craniopharyngioma, hypothalamic germinomas, gliomas, and hamartomas. Infiltrative processes such as histiocytosis X and leukemia can result in central diabetes insipidus when they invade and disrupt the hypothalamus. Trauma, both surgical and accidental, frequently results in ADH deficiency and diabetes insipidus. It should be noted that postoperative central diabetes insipidus can be seen following neurosurgery, even when the site of intervention is distant from the hypothalamic–pituitary region. Although in many cases the diabetes insipidus may be transient, permanent forms frequently occur, especially when the surgeon is attempting removal of lesions located within the suprasellar area. Inflammatory processes and vascular malformations, on rare occasions, have also resulted in neurogenic diabetes insipidus.

NEPHROGENIC DIABETES INSIPIDUS

Renal unresponsiveness to the action of ADH generally results from some underlying metabolic or kidney disorder in which the ability of ADH to exert its full biologic activity has been secondarily impaired. Hypokalemia and hypercalcemia cause damage to the distal tubules of the kidney, rendering them relatively unresponsive to ADH. A variety of primary renal disorders are characterized by the inability to produce a concentrated urine; this is frequently encountered in patients with medullary cystic disease, renal tubular acidosis, postobstructive nephropathy, and cystinosis and in the nephropathy seen in patients with sickle cell disease. Several pharmacologic agents have the ability to interfere with ADH action at the level of the renal tubules, causing a picture of nephrogenic diabetes insipidus. Among the agents described, lithium, demeclocycline, and amphotericin B are those most likely to be seen in a pediatric or adolescent population.

A rare, congenital form of renal unresponsiveness to ADH exists. This is generally inherited as an X-linked disorder and presumably is the result of an absent or abnormal ADH receptor. Patients with this disorder usually present in early infancy with failure to thrive, unexplained fevers, and extreme degrees of polyuria.

DIFFERENTIAL DIAGNOSIS

When evaluating children with symptoms of polyuria/polydipsia, several etiologic possibilities must be kept in mind. Aside from defective synthesis/release of ADH and end-organ resistance to ADH, two other conditions will result in excessive urine output. In the first situation, endogenous ADH is suppressed as a result of a physiologic stimulus such as inordinate fluid intake or intravascular volume expansion. Patients who have the first group of disorders include compulsive water drinkers and those who receive excessive IV fluid (e.g., colloid, blood) during surgery. In patients exhibiting the second group of disorders, polyuria occurs because of an osmotic diuresis that is capable of overriding the antidiuretic effect of ADH. The most common example of the latter is polyuria due to glycosuria in untreated patients with diabetes mellitus. Other agents capable of inducing an osmotic diuresis include mannitol and radiologic contrast material.

The initial screening evaluation of the polyuric patient should include a complete urinalysis to determine the presence of protein, blood, glucose, and casts, and specific gravity. Routine blood studies of electrolytes, calcium, BUN, creatinine, and glucose will enable the clinician to rule out serious renal disease and metabolic disturbances that could account for the clinical symptoms. The plasma concentration of sodium is of critical importance, because a value in the low or low normal range suggests a primary disorder in fluid intake, whereas a value above 145 mEq per L associated with a dilute urine establishes the diagnosis of diabetes insipidus. Further testing would be required to ascertain whether the abnormality was due to faulty synthesis/release of ADH or to renal unresponsiveness to the hormone. Because most patients with diabetes insipidus will be able to compensate for the chronic loss of water from the kidneys by fluid intake, screening blood studies will fail to establish the diagnosis in most affected subjects.

If the initial screening studies do not pinpoint an obvious cause for the polyuria, a more definitive test of the ability to concentrate urine should be performed. Although several types of testing have been described, the water deprivation test is the one most often used in clinical pediatric practice. The purpose of this test is to cause an increase in plasma osmolality that will result in maximal or near maximal stimulation of ADH release. If the patient is normal, water deprivation will result in the formation of a highly concentrated urine (> 800 mOsm/kg or specific gravity > 1.018). The 7-hour water deprivation test as described by Frasier and colleagues is generally adequate for differentiating between normal patients and those with significant concentrating defects. Normal patients will have a ratio of urine osmolality to serum osmolality greater than or equal to 1.5 at the end of the 7-hour test. A final urine to serum ratio of less than 1.5 is diagnostic of diabetes insipidus. In order to discriminate between patients with central diabetes insipidus and those with a nephrogenic variety, one must administer vasopressin exogenously and determine the change in urine osmolality. Classically, the water deprivation test has been terminated by the administration of the short-acting preparation aqueous vasopressin, 5 U subcutaneously; patients with central diabetes insipidus will demonstrate an increase in urine osmolality of approximately 200 percent, whereas patients with nephrogenic diabetes insipidus will fail to show any significant change in urine osmolality following vasopressin injection. Patients with partial forms of diabetes insipidus may, on occasion, present a more difficult diagnostic problem in that they may be able to concentrate their urine sufficiently to satisfy the previously outlined criteria. In such instances, a more prolonged water deprivation study may be required in order to unequivocally establish the diagnosis. Several precautions must be kept in mind whenever one is subjecting a small child to a water deprivation test. Because many of these children have an extremely limited capacity to conserve water, dangerous degrees of dehydration can occur if they are not observed carefully. The test should always be started in the morning, and the patients should be monitored continuously, including hourly determination of body weight and urine volume. After a subject has lost 5 percent of his body weight, the study should be terminated.

Whenever the physician has established a diagnosis of diabetes insipidus, a rigorous search for the underlying cause must be undertaken. Patients with clear-cut ADH deficiency *must* undergo an extensive neuroradiologic evaluation in order to rule out the presence of a neoplasm or infiltrative process. Failure to uncover a parapituitary lesion on initial evaluation does not exclude the possibility of central nervous system pathology. Careful follow-up, with periodic re-evaluation, is essential, because many lesions may not become apparent until several years after the symptoms of diabetes insipidus develop.

TREATMENT

In patients with ADH deficiency and a normal sensation of thirst and with no complications, therapy consists of simply hormonal replacement. The drug of choice is the new vasopressin analogue, 1-desamino-8-D-arginine-vasopressin (DDAVP). It possesses a long duration of action (8 to 24 hours) and is essentially devoid of vasopressor activity. DDAVP is administered via nasal insufflation at a dose of 5 to 20 μg per day, given once or twice daily. This agent restores urine volume to normal and, if administered properly, prevents nocturia. The other long-acting vasopressin preparation, Pitressin Tannate in Oil, is rarely used, because it has an unpredictable duration of action (12 to 48 hours) and must be given as an intramuscular injection.

Several short-acting preparations are also available, including aqueous vasopressin and lysine vasopressin. These drugs are effective for periods of 2 to 6 hours and are ill suited for chronic treatment. They do, however, have a place in the management of more acute forms of the syndrome such as occurs following cranial surgery.

Diabetes insipidus following cranial surgery may be permanent, transient, or cyclic, with intermittent periods of normal or even excess ADH production. Additional difficulties are encountered because most patients are unable to take fluids orally and are thus unable to regulate the amount of fluid they receive. Successful management of these patients requires meticulous attention to their fluid balance, the use of a vasopressin preparation, and a logical but flexible approach to IV fluid therapy. Although these individuals could theoretically be managed without the use of vasopressin, such a therapeutic approach is untenable from a nursing point of view and places the patient at risk for a variety of complications. Because the duration of the symptoms is usually uncertain, the use of a short-acting vasopressin preparation is preferred. We have found aqueous Pitressin, given either subcutaneously or as a continuous IV drip (0.5 mU/kg min), to be an excellent choice. Its brief duration of action allows for periodic reassessment of endogenous ADH function and avoids prolonged periods of antidiuresis, which may be unnecessary or even contraindicated. After the diagnosis of permanent diabetes insipidus has been established, the use of a longer-acting preparation (e.g., DDAVP) is more appropriate.

Fluid therapy involves decisions regarding both the amount and the type of fluid to be administered. Daily maintenance fluid requirements depend primarily upon both insensible losses and urine output. Postoperative patients will have a very unpredictable urinary loss of fluid, whereas insensible fluid losses can be anticipated with a fair degree of accuracy. Our general policy is to write initial fluid orders to cover insensible losses (400 to 600 ml/m²/day) and to replace urinary losses every 2 to 4 hours with additional IV fluid. Insensible losses are replaced by 0.25 percent normal saline (NS), whereas urinary losses should be replaced by 5 percent dextrose in water (D5W). This regimen has proved to be very safe and generally prevents the problem of water intoxication, which too often occurs when patients have a prolonged antidiuresis due to either overzealous vasopressin therapy or intermittent phases of inappropriate ADH secretion. When patients are awake and alert and a normal thirst mechanism is operative, IV fluids should be discontinued and free access to liquids should be allowed.

The previously outlined regimen, although based on physiologic criteria, represents only an "informed" guess as to what the patient will require. Frequent assessment of the patient's fluid and electrolyte status is absolutely essential in order to decide whether the therapy being administered is adequate. Strict recording of intake and output, urine specific gravities on each voided specimen, twice-daily determination of body weight, and plasma electrolytes will help ensure that the patient is receiving optimal therapy.

A variety of non-vasopressin agents have the ability to amplify or stimulate production of ADH and are useful in patients with partial ADH deficiency. Among the available agents, chlorpropamide, clofibrate, and carbamazepine are used most often.

The therapy of nephrogenic diabetes insipidus must rely on measures that reduce urine volume independent of ADH. Dietary restriction of both sodium and protein will reduce obligatory free water excretion and urine output. The use of the diuretic hydrochlorothiazide (3 mg/kg/day) will enhance proximal tubular reabsorption of fluid, causing a decrease in urine volume. Adequate potassium supplementation is necessary when hydrochlorothiazides are used. Patients with nephrogenic diabetes insipidus will always require a high water intake 24 hours per day.

CASE PRESENTATION

An 11-year-old female presented with a several-month history of decreased visual acuity and frontal headaches. A visual field deficit in the left eye was verified, and a subsequent CT brain scan revealed a large, cystic suprasellar mass consistent with a craniopharyngioma. There was no history of seizures, change in growth velocity, polyuria, or polydipsia.

Examination

Initial physical examination revealed normal vital signs, height and weight at the 50th percentile, and bilateral pale optic discs. The patient was prepubertal. The remainder of her physical examination was unremarkable.

Preoperative evaluation demonstrated normal electrolytes with a serum sodium of 135 mEq/L, a urine osmolality of 850 mOsm/kg after an overnight fast, and normal thyroid and adrenal function. In preparation for surgery, the patient was given pharmacologic doses of glucocorticoids (methylprednisolone, 1 gm/day, orally) in an attempt to reduce cerebral edema. The patient underwent a frontal craniotomy, and "complete" resection of the tumor was accomplished.

Her postoperative course was complicated by the development of polyuria (550 ml/hr) immediately following the surgical procedure. Her serum sodium was 153 mEq/L 1 hour postoperatively; a simultaneous urine sample had an osmolality of 150 mOsm/kg. Urine osmolality increased to 995 mOsm/kg after a single dose of aqueous vasopressin. The patient was maintained on an IV Pitressin drip and IV fluid until she was able to take oral fluids. She subsequently was switched to intranasal DDAVP twice daily and maintained normal fluid and electrolyte balance.

Problem List

Suprasellar Mass

The presence of a mass lesion in the hypothalamic-pituitary area raises the possibility of both anterior and posterior pituitary hormone deficiencies. Under optimal circumstances, a complete hormonal evaluation should be performed to assess the integrity of the pituitary-adrenal, thyroid, and gonadal axes as well as the status of growth hormone and ADH secretion. It is of critical importance to ascertain the patient's ability to produce cortisol whenever an invasive procedure such as surgery or angiography is contemplated. A patient with adrenocorticotropic hormone (ACTH) deficiency will not tolerate a stressful procedure unless supraphysiologic doses of glucocorticoid (3 to 5 times the daily production rate) are administered. It is also important to note that when ACTH-cortisol deficiency and ADH deficiency coexist, the symptoms of diabetes insipidus may be minimal; when glucocorticoid therapy is instituted, the diabetes insipidus will be "unmasked" and the symptoms of polyuria/polydipsia will become apparent.

When the diagnosis of ADH deficiency has been established, appropriate therapy to ensure positive water balance, which generally requires the use of a long-acting vasopressin analogue such as DDAVP, must be initiated. If the patient requires general anesthesia, all medical personnel involved must be alerted to the problem so that adequate IV fluids are provided and appropriate monitoring takes place. In general, a maintenance dose of DDAVP administered prior to the procedure will provide adequate protection from excess fluid loss and will minimize the danger of dehydration.

Glucocorticoid Therapy

Administration of pharmacologic doses of potent glucocorticoids such as methylprednisolone and dexamethasone is common in patients with intracranial mass lesions, because these agents have proved to be effective in decreasing peritumoral cerebral edema. The doses generally used are equivalent to 100 to 200 times the physiologic replacement dosage of cortisol. Thus, there is no need to provide any additional steroid coverage to these patients with suspected or proven ACTH deficiency during surgical or radiologic procedures.

Important and not infrequent complications of the usage of large doses of glucocorticoids are the development of glucose intolerance, hyperglycemia, and glycosuria. Such complications can result in an osmotic diuresis and polyuria–mimicking diabetes insipidus or in the exacerbation of diabetes insipidus if both situations occur simultaneously.

Polyuria

Polyuria in the immediate postoperative period can be due to a variety of causes. Careful attention to urine volume, urine osmolality, urine specific gravity and plasma sodium and osmolality will greatly assist in elucidating the cause of the polyuria. The following disorders frequently result in postoperative polyuria:

1. *Diuresis secondary to intraoperative fluid overload.* Administration of excessive parenteral fluid during surgery will result in a transient phase of diuresis. This is an appropriate response to re-establish normal water balance. Urine will be dilute (specific gravity < 1.005), and plasma sodium and osmolality will be normal to decreased. When the excess fluid has been excreted, urine volume will decrease and urine specific gravity and osmolality will increase. At no time will plasma osmolality exceed the normal range.

2. *Solute diuresis.* This may be secondary to hyperglycemia and glycosuria, which result from such factors as stress and glucocorticoid administration or osmotic diuretics (e.g., mannitol), which are frequently given during neurosurgical procedures. A solute diuresis generally results in a voluminous urine output, with urine specific gravity in the range of 1.010 or greater and normal to slightly low plasma concentration of sodium. One should test the urine for the presence of glucose whenever polyuria develops in the postoperative period.

3. *Acquired nephrogenic diabetes insipidus.* Metabolic derangements ($\uparrow$Ca, $\downarrow$K), drugs, and ischemic insults to the kidney can result in postoperative nephrogenic diabetes insipidus. This diagnosis is generally suspected on the basis of the clinical setting, an abnormal urine sediment, and biochemical evidence of azotemia. The failure of exogenous vasopressin to alter the symptoms establishes the diagnosis of renal unresponsiveness to ADH.

4. *Central diabetes insipidus.* Polyuria secondary to ADH deficiency commonly occurs following neurosurgical procedures. It results in large volumes of dilute urine (specific gravity <1.005 and osmolality <200 mOsm/kg) and normal to elevated plasma concentrations of sodium. Administration of vasopressin results in prompt improvement, with a decrease in urine volume and an increase in specific gravity and osmolality.

In this case, the polyuria was clearly secondary to central diabetes insipidus. The patient responded well to aqueous vasopressin and IV fluid replacement. When it became evident that her diabetes insipidus was permanent, the patient was switched to intranasal DDAVP, which permitted good control of her fluid and electrolyte problem.

SUGGESTED READING

Bode, H.H.: Disorders of the posterior pituitary. *In* Kaplan, S.A. (ed.): Clinical Pediatric and Adolescent Endocrinology. Philadelphia, W.B. Saunders Company, 1982, p 49.

Frasier, S.D., Kutnik, L.A., Schmidt, R.T., and Smith, F.G., Jr.: A water deprivation test for the diagnosis of diabetes insipidus in children. Am. J. Dis. Child. 114:157, 1967.

Freidenberg, G.R., Kosnik, E.J., and Sotos, J.F.: Hyperglycemic coma after supraseller surgery. N. Engl. J. Med. 303:863, 1980.

Lee, W.N.P., Lippe, B.M., La Franchi, S.H., and Kaplan, S.A.: Vasopressin analog DDAVP in the treatment of diabetes insipidus. Am. J. Dis. Child. 130:166, 1976.

Miller, M., Moses, A.M., and Streeten, D.H.P.: Recognition of partial defects in antidiuretic hormone secretion. Ann. Intern. Med. 73:721, 1970.

Robertson, G.L., Aycinena, P., and Zerbe, R.L.: Neurogenic disorders of osmoregulation. Am. J. Med. 72:339, 1982.

Shucart, W.A., and Jackson, I.: Management of diabetes insipidus in neurosurgical patients. J. Neurosurg. 44:65, 1976.

Sklar, C.A., Grumbach, M.M., Kaplan, S.L., and Conte, F.A.: Hormonal and metabolic abnormalities associated with central nervous system germinoma in children and adolescents and the effect of therapy: report of 10 patients. J. Clin. Endocrinol. Metab. 52:9, 1981.

Timmons, R.L., and Dugger, G.S.: Water and salt metabolism following pituitary stalk section. Neurology 19:790, 1969.

Nursing Process for Patient Care:

Diabetes Insipidus

Polyuria in the postoperative period may be the result of antidiuretic hormone (ADH) deficiency. It commonly occurs following neurosurgical procedures. Polyuria may also be due to other causes, including fluid overload, osmotic diuretics, metabolic derangements, and ischemic insults to the kidney.

Careful attention must be given to urine volume, urine osmolality, urine specific gravity, serum sodium, and serum osmolality. The fluid and electrolyte balance of the child is of prime importance.

FLUID AND ELECTROLYTE BALANCE

Assess, Monitor, and Document

Urine output
Urine specific gravity
Urine osmolality
Serum sodium

Serum osmolality
Fluid intake: thirst, weight (twice daily)
Response to pharmacologic management: vasopressin preparation

Anticipate

Alteration in fluid and electrolyte status
Dehydration

NEUROLOGIC

Because the underlying etiology of diabetes insipidus is related to the central nervous system, this system must be continuously assessed and monitored.

Assess, Monitor, and Document

Level of consciousness
Pupillary activity
Reflexes
Muscle tone
Blood pressure

Pulse
Respiratory rate and pattern
Intracranial pressure (if available)
Status of operative site (if operative procedure is performed)

Anticipate

Alteration in neurologic status
Increased intracranial pressure

RESPONSE OF CHILD AND FAMILY

Assess, Monitor, and Document

Behavioral response: anxious, concerned, disappointed
Expected outcome

Ability to cope
Response to nursing interventions

Anticipate

Emotional distress

MIND SET

Assess

Fluid and electrolyte balance
Neurologic status
Response of child and family

Anticipate

Alteration in fluid and electrolyte balance
Polyuria
Dehydration

Emotional distress
Family crisis

Diabetic Ketoacidosis

MICHAEL TRAISTER, M.D.

Diabetic ketoacidosis (DKA) is defined as the presence of hyperglycemia (serum glucose greater than 300 mg/dl), ketonemia (ketones strongly positive in the serum), and acidosis (pH less than 7.30 and/or serum bicarbonate less than 15 mEq/L). It is always associated with glycosuria, ketonuria, and dehydration. DKA is a true medical emergency, the treatment of which requires an understanding of its pathogenesis, careful attention to therapeutic details, and close cooperation between medical and nursing personnel. The estimated mortality of DKA is approximately 1 percent.

It has been estimated that ketoacidosis is the initial presenting manifestation of diabetes in children in approximately 20 to 25 percent of cases. The remaining patients present with a subacute course (3- to 4-week history) of polyuria, polydipsia, polyphagia, and loss of weight but fall short of frank acidosis. Most patients with type I (juvenile) diabetes develop a bout of ketoacidosis some time in their lives, owing to either poor control, noncompliance, or loss of existing control as a result of a coincidental infection.

ETIOLOGY

The etiology of type I diabetes is believed to be multifactorial, a combination of genetic, autoimmune, and viral influences. Although genetic clustering of diabetes has been well recognized, the inheritability of diabetes does not follow simple mendelian genetics. The argument in favor of a genetic predisposition was strengthened by the discovery that certain human lymphocyte antigen (HLA) types, including HLA B8, HLA Bw15, and HLA Dw4, have an increased frequency of developing type I diabetes.

An autoimmune basis for diabetes has been suggested for many years. Patients dying in acute DKA were found to have lymphocytic infiltrates in their pancreatic islet cells similar to infiltrates found in known autoimmune diseases. Patients with type I diabetes have an increased frequency of autoimmune disorders such as Hashimoto's thyroiditis, Addison's disease, hypoparathyroidism, pernicious anemia, and myasthenia gravis. Islet cell antibiodies can be seen in patients with newly diagnosed diabetes.

Viral infection has been implicated as a trigger mechanism for diabetes. Until recently, most of these observations were made based upon epidemiologic studies. Mumps, rubella, and Coxsackie B viruses were those viruses most often associated with diabetes. Patients with congenital rubella infection have been found to have an increased incidence of diabetes, although the onset of disease is many years later. In 1979, a Coxsackie B4 virus varient was isolated from the pancreas of a child who died acutely in DKA as the initial presentation of the disease. Pathology of the pancreas revealed lymphocytic infiltrates and beta cell necrosis. Antibody neutralization titers to this variant Coxsackie B4 virus rose significantly during the hospital course. After being isolated from the pancreas, the virus was then passed in genetically susceptible mice, with resulting beta cell necrosis and hyperglycemia. Antibody staining in the mouse pancreas revealed viral antigens in the beta cells. Autoimmunity and/or viral infection probably acts as a trigger in a genetically predisposed patient to "cause" diabetes.

PATHOPHYSIOLOGY

A deficiency of insulin ultimately leads to hyperglycemia, dehydration, and ketoacidosis. The mechanism for this is briefly summarized in Figure 33–1.

Glucose is used as the primary source of energy for cells. All cells require insulin for glucose uptake, with the exception of those of the central nervous system and red blood cells. Hy-

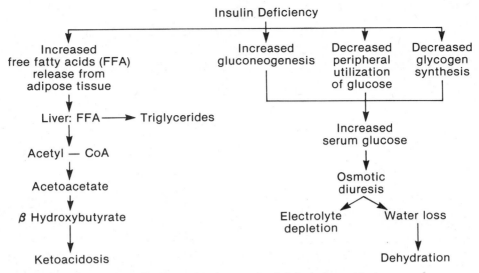

Figure 33-1. Summary of pathogenesis of diabetic ketoacidosis.

perglycemia occurs in diabetes as a direct consequence of insulin deficiency. Lack of insulin results in decreased peripheral utilization of glucose, especially in skeletal muscle and adipose cells, an inhibition of glycogen synthesis in the liver, and stimulation of gluconeogenesis, also in the liver. The resultant hyperglycemia increases the osmolality of the extracellular fluid, thus causing water to leave the cells. For each 18 mg per dl of glucose, the plasma osmolality is raised by 1 mOsm per L. Dilution of the serum electrolytes occurs. As the serum glucose rises, the ability of the renal tubules to reabsorb glucose is overwhelmed. When the renal threshold of approximately 180 mg per dl is exceeded, an osmotic diuresis occurs, resulting in loss of water and electrolytes. In the presence of acidosis, vomiting will also contribute to sodium and chloride loss and will prevent the patient from drinking enough to keep up with renal loss. Dehydration eventually occurs.

Acidosis is the result of hepatic overproduction and decreased peripheral utilization of ketone bodies, beta-hydroxybutyrate, acetoacetate, and acetone. The organic acids, beta-hydroxybutyrate and acetoacetate, are dissociated at the body's pH. When the body's buffering capacity and respiratory compensation are overwhelmed, acidosis occurs.

Free fatty acids (FFA) are mobilized from triglyceride stores in the peripheral adipose tissue. Trigger for release of these FFA is a lipase that is activated during starvation and exercise and in untreated diabetes. Carried in the plasma, the FFA are brought to the liver and other tissues. In the liver, the FFA may be esterified to

form triglycerides or may be oxidized to acetyl-CoA. In diabetes, as opposed to fasting and exercise, the pathway of oxidation of FFA to acetyl-CoA is dramatically increased. Acetyl-CoA utilization for both fatty acid synthesis and oxidation in the Krebs cycle is impaired, resulting in a large increase in acetoacetate and beta-hydroxybutyrate synthesis. As previously mentioned, there may be an additional underutilization of ketone bodies in the periphery.

CLINICAL PRESENTATION

Clinical recognition of the signs and symptoms of ketoacidosis is based upon an understanding of its pathogenesis. Acidosis is clinically manifested as deep and/or rapid respirations as the body attempts to increase minute ventilation to compensate for the low pH. Nausea, vomiting, and abdominal pain are also manifestations of systemic acidosis. The breath will frequently have a sweet, acetone odor.

Hyperglycemia and the ensuing osmotic diuresis present as polyuria, followed by polydipsia. Dehydration is evidenced by flushed, dry skin, dry tongue and mouth, and a rapid pulse. Headache, lethargy, and a decrease in visual acuity may be the result of dehydration and/or central nervous system acidosis.

Any suspicion of DKA should prompt the physician to test the urine for the presence of glucose and ketones. If present, serum should be drawn for determination of at least pH, glucose, and ketones to confirm the diagnosis. After the diagnosis of DKA has been established, appropriate and careful treatment should be instituted without delay.

TREATMENT

Prior to 1975, treatment of DKA in children was accomplished by using insulin doses given primarily subcutaneously. Most authors recommended 0.5 to 2.0 U insulin per kg of body weight every 2 to 4 hours. One half of the initial dose was given intravenously, the other half subcutaneously. The dose of insulin was gradually decreased over the first 24 hours of therapy. The dose of insulin was based upon the height of glucose concentration and clinical assessment of the severity of ketoacidosis.

In the late 1970's, the management of DKA was revolutionized by the introduction of continuous IV infusion of low doses of insulin. Rationale for this therapy was based upon the observation that maximum glucose transport will occur at serum insulin levels of 200 μU per ml. Higher levels of insulin will not decrease the serum glucose faster. The relatively high serum levels of insulin achieved in the "high dose" subcutaneous method will not lower the serum glucose any faster than using lower doses. Thus, the concept of insulin resistance in ketoacidosis may be factitious. The fact that sensitivity to insulin does not decrease in an acidotic patient was also realized.

The serum half-life of insulin is approximately 3 to 5 minutes. Thus, an IV bolus of insulin will be followed by a rapid fall in insulin concentration to basal levels by 25 minutes. Absorption of subcutaneous insulin may be erratic or delayed in a dehydrated patient. Advantages of the low-dose constant infusion are:

1. The constant infusion frees the physician from making empirical decisions regarding the dose, frequency, and route of insulin administration.

2. There is a predictable fall in serum glucose. It has been shown that the serum glucose will fall at a linear rate of approximately 75 to 100 mg per dl per hour. In the first hour of treatment, the glucose falls at a slightly higher rate, presumably because of rehydration. By extrapolating, the physician may anticipate normoglycemia.

3. There is lower risk of hypoglycemia. Because the half-life of insulin is short, serum insulin levels can be quickly changed by altering the infusion rate. Serum glucose levels should not significantly decline after the infusion is discontinued.

4. The serum insulin levels are more physiologic, approximating levels in normal nondiabetics. The serum insulin levels do not exceed the maximum effective level.

Studies have compared the effectiveness of the low-dose constant infusions with the "high-dose" subcutaneous method in children. It was concluded that both methods are equally effective. The low-dose group had a lower incidence of hypokalemia. Serum ketones may, however, persist longer when a low-dose constant infusion is used.

Management Problems

Dehydration

The first step in the treatment of DKA should be the stabilization of the circulatory system with ensurance of an adequate intravascular volume. A clinical estimation of the state of hydration should be made using pulse, blood pressure, and hematocrit. These parameters should be followed hourly, more frequently if the patient is hypotensive. The patient's weight should be noted and followed daily. Urine specific gravity will be elevated as a result of the presence of glucose and other solutes and will not be a useful parameter in assessing dehydration in DKA.

Fluid deficits usually range between 5 and 15 percent. Most moderately ill patients are considered to be 10 percent dehydrated. All fluids should be given intravenously via a large bore IV catheter. It is best to keep the patient NPO. Ice chips may be given for patient comfort. A nasogastric tube should be inserted in all unconscious patients and in patients with significant vomiting or paralytic ileus.

The initial IV fluid should be normal saline (NS), given at a rate of 20 ml per kg of body weight, over the first hour. (If the blood pressure is low, 5 percent albumin at 10 ml/kg should be added.) This should re-expand and stabilize the vascular compartment. Accurate urine output should be recorded on the flow chart (Fig. 33–2). If necessary, a Foley catheter should be inserted. This is usually necessary only in unconscious patients.

Over the first 24 hours of treatment, fluids should be given to cover maintenance, ongoing losses, and half the deficit. The other half of the deficit should be corrected over the second 24-hour period. Calculation of maintenance fluids must take into account an increased respiratory rate and/or presence of fever. As long as the serum glucose exceeds the renal thresh-

DIABETIC KETOACIDOSIS FLOW CHART
Department of Pediatrics
New York University Medical Center

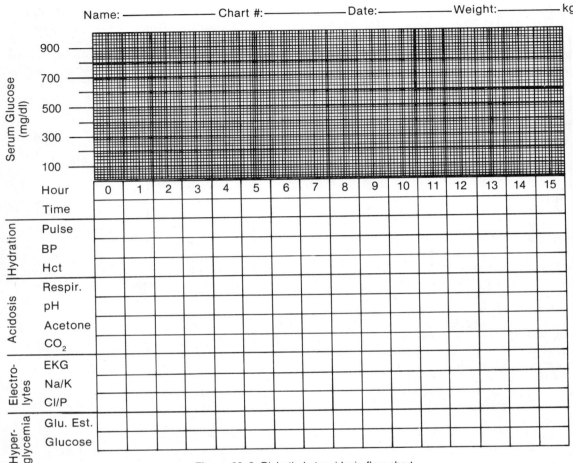

Name: —————— Chart #: —————— Date: —————— Weight: ————— kg

Figure 33–2. Diabetic ketoacidosis flow chart.

old for glucose, the osmotic diuresis will cause the ongoing losses to be a significant volume, which must be replaced. Functionally, the rate of fluid administration will be limited by the size of the IV catheter. Occasionally, a second IV may need to be started to deliver necessary fluids. The initial hydrating solution should be non–glucose-containing, either Ringer's lactate or one half NS.

The rate of fluid administration should be modified as needed according to blood pressure, pulse, hematocrit, and serum electrolytes. There should be rapid stabilization of blood pressure within the normal range and a smooth decline of both pulse and hematocrit to within normal limits.

Hyperglycemia

After securing the IV catheter and drawing an initial set of blood tests, insulin (regular,

purified pork) should be given intravenously. An initial dose of 0.1 U per kg of insulin administered by IV push is recommended. Following this bolus, a continuous infusion of 0.1 U per kg per hour of insulin should be started. The insulin infusion is made by adding 1 ml of U–100 purified pork regular insulin to a 500 ml bag of NS. The resulting solution contains 0.2 U of insulin per ml. A new Volutrol and tubing should be filled with this insulin solution, and the first 50 to 100 ml should be flushed through the system and discarded. Insulin in solution adsorbs to plastic surfaces, resulting in lower insulin concentrations than anticipated. Albumin added to the insulin solution reduces this adsorption to insignificant quantities. Preparing and flushing the infusion tubing system as suggested, however, makes the addition of albumin unnecessary. The insulin solution should be delivered via a reliable pump, piggybacked as close to the IV site as

	Hour	0	1	2	3	4	5	6	7	8	9	10	11	12	13	14	15
	Time																
Output / Urine	Volume (ml)																
	Clinitest (%)																
	Acetest																
Input / IV / Po	Type of solution																
	Volume (ml)																
Insulin	Type																
	Units																
	Route																
	Bolus dose																
	IV rate (ml/hr)																

NOTES: _____

Figure 33–2. *Continued*

possible. A fresh solution should be made every 4 to 6 hours.

Hourly blood tests should include serum glucose. Bedside estimates of glucose, using either reagent strips (Visidex, Ames or Chemstrip bG, Bio-Dynamics) or a reflectance photometer (Glucometer, Ames or Stat-Tek, Bio-Dynamics), are obligatory, because it may take hours to obtain results of laboratory glucose determinations. The concentration of serum glucose should fall at a linear rate of 75 to 100 mg per dl per hour. For the first hour, the rate may decline slightly more. If the serum glucose does not fall as expected, recheck the insulin infusion to ensure that it was constituted correctly and that it is being delivered at the prescribed rate. Rarely, the insulin rate may need to be increased to 0.2 U per kg per hour before the serum glucose falls as predicted.

The serum glucose may be plotted versus time. Extrapolation enables the physician to anticipate normoglycemia. Non–glucose-containing fluids and insulin infusion are continued until the serum glucose falls below 180 mg per dl and the urine is negative for sugar. At this time, glucose should be added to the hydrating solution (D5W/½ NS is suggested) and the insulin infusion should be adjusted down-

ward to 0.025 to 0.05 U per kg per hour to maintain a steady state of insulin and glucose so that the serum glucose remains constant. A suggested guide for this is 2 to 4 gm of glucose per U of insulin infused. Frequent blood sugar determinations and insulin infusion adjustments may be necessary to achieve this steady state. Any suspicion of hypoglycemia, either clinical or laboratory, should prompt the discontinuation of the insulin infusion.

The insulin infusion may be discontinued when the blood glucose is less than 180 mg per dl *and* the acidosis is corrected (pH > 7.30 and serum ketones negative). Urine ketones will persist for 24 to 48 hours. It should be expected that normoglycemia will be achieved earlier than complete correction of acidosis. After the infusion has stopped, oral feeding and subcutaneous insulin should begin immediately, because the half-life of serum insulin is short. If correction of hyperglycemia and acidosis is completed in the middle of the night, it is prudent to continue the glucose–insulin infusions until morning.

Ketoacidosis

Ketones in the blood may be detected by using an Acetest tablet (Ames). The nitroprusside reaction of the Acetest tablet will react primarily with the acetoacetate, less so with the acetone, and not at all with beta-hydroxybutyrate. Normally, the beta-hydroxybutyrate/ acetoacetate ratio is approximately 3:1. This increases to about 8:1 in DKA. Acetest tablets, therefore, tend to underestimate the degree of ketosis.

After measuring the hematocrit it is convenient to break the hematocrit tube and place one drop of serum onto the Acetest tablet. After 2 minutes, compare the color of the pill to the standard color provided by the manufacturer. The test is read as negative, small, moderate, or large. Some clinicians prefer to dilute the sera and then report the results as positive to a 1:2 or 1:4 dilution. It is usually unnecessary to do this.

Correction of ketoacidosis can be accomplished by the administration of adequate fluids and insulin. In the presence of insulin, the ketone bodies, acetoacetate, and beta-hydroxybutyrate are oxidized in the Krebs cycle to carbon dioxide and water. Thus, endogenous bicarbonate is produced.

IV sodium bicarbonate is occasionally used to rapidly correct the serum pH. Arguments against the use of bicarbonate include the following:

1. Mental function correlates with cerebrospinal fluid (CSF) pH and not with serum pH in patients with systemic acidosis. Treatment with sodium bicarbonate, although correcting the serum pH, may result in CSF acidosis and clinical worsening of the patient's mental status. This "paradoxical" CNS acidosis is explained by the relative impermeability of the blood–brain barrier to HCO_3 compared with CO_2. The carbon dioxide diffuses into the CSF and dissociates, causing a drop in pH.

2. Administration of bicarbonate to increase the serum pH will shift the oxyhemoglobin dissociation curve to the left, diminishing oxygen release to the tissues. In DKA, this would compound the left shift of the oxyhemoglobin dissociation curve already caused by decreased levels of red blood cell 2,3-DPG.

3. Rapid correction of acidosis will accelerate potassium entry into the cells and, therefore, may precipitously produce life-threatening hypokalemia.

4. It is believed that full correction of acidosis according to the calculated base deficit may overcorrect and result in alkalosis.

Arguments in favor of the use of bicarbonate include the following:

1. It has been shown that bicarbonate treatment in DKA does not significantly effect oxygen transport of red cells.

2. Very low serum pH decreases myocardial contractility and increases the risk of cardiac dysrhythmias.

3. As the pH falls below 7.1, the minute ventilation does not continue to rise; it falls, thus reducing the effectiveness of respiratory compensatory mechanisms and possibly increasing the severity of the acidosis.

In balancing the arguments in favor of and against the use of bicarbonate, it is recommended that sodium bicarbonate be reserved for severe acidosis (pH less than 7.1). With pH in the range of 7.1 to 7.2, the physician may judiciously use bicarbonate as long as he or she keeps in mind the arguments just stated. With a pH above 7.2, bicarbonate therapy is not indicated. Bicarbonate should be given in a dose of 1 to 2 mEq per kg as a slow drip over 1 to 3 hours, added to the hydrating solution of ½ NS. Bicarbonate is a hypertonic solution and should never be given by IV push.

Electrolytes

POTASSIUM BALANCE

In ketoacidosis, there is a deficiency in total body potassium. However, initially, the serum potassium is normal or elevated. Only rarely is the serum potassium below normal. In these rare situations, life-threatening hypokalemia may occur early in the course of treatment. When there is total body depletion, normal or elevated serum potassium levels occur as a consequence of both intravascular contraction secondary to dehydration and systemic acidosis, which causes potassium to exit from cells. As rehydration begins and acidosis is corrected, the serum potassium falls. This decline may be due to

1. Dilution secondary to rehydration.

2. Continued potassium loss in the urine.

3. Correction of acidosis with re-entry of potassium into the cells.

4. Increased potassium uptake by the cells as a result of insulin–glucose-mediated cellular uptake.

It is imperative to assess the serum level of potassium immediately upon diagnosing DKA. Both hyperkalemia upon presentation and hypokalemia during treatment may occur. Because a delay in obtaining results of electrolytes is common, an EKG rhythm strip or an EKG lead II should be performed initially and followed hourly to assess serum potassium levels. With more severe acidosis or with the use of bicarbonate, this monitoring is even more important.

The earliest manifestation of hyperkalemia is the presence of a tall, narrow, tented T wave.

Later, the QRS complex widens. The P wave eventually becomes wide and flattened, and ectopic rhythms with intraventricular block occur. In hypokalemia, the T wave is broadened, flattened, or even inverted. A U wave may be seen. The QT_c interval is prolonged, and there is ST segment depression. Eventually ectopic beats, both supraventricular and ventricular, occur.

If hypokalemia is suspected, correction of hyperglycemia and acidosis should proceed slowly and liberal amounts of potassium should be given. If toxic hyperkalemia with widening of the QRS is seen, potassium should be withheld from the hydrating solution. During the treatment of DKA, 20 to 50 percent of the intravenously administered potassium is lost in the urine. This fact must be taken into account when determining the amount and rate of potassium supplementation.

After the initial bolus of NS (20 ml/kg) and the establishment of urine flow, potassium should be added to the IV-hydrating solution in a dose of 2 to 4 mEq per kg every 24 hours. Usually, the final concentration is about 40 mEq (30 to 60 mEq) of potassium per L of hydrating solution. This dose may be increased or decreased based upon serum potassium level and/or EKG rhythm strip.

Sodium

Low serum sodium is to be expected in ketoacidosis. The serum sodium concentration is usually found to be reduced or normal despite water loss in excess of electrolytes. Hyponatremia may be protective by countering the hyperosmotic effects of hyperglycemia and thereby keeping the total serum osmolality normal or only slightly elevated. As the serum glucose falls, the serum sodium should rise to maintain the serum osmolality. Failure to do this may result in a significant hypo-osmolar state, with overexpansion of the intracellular space and perhaps cerebral edema. The low serum sodium, however, may be factitious due to hyperlipidemia, which may accompany poor diabetic control. This may be determined simply by visual inspection of the serum for turbidity.

The initial hydrating solution should be NS or Ringer's lactate, followed by ½ NS. This combination of solutions will provide adequate sodium.

Phosphorus

In DKA, there is a deficiency in phosphorus as a result of increased tissue catabolism, impaired cellular phosphorus uptake, and increased renal excretion of phosphorus. The serum concentration of phosphorus is usually normal initially but tends to fall within the first hours of therapy.

Phosphorus deficiency results in decreased erythrocyte 2,3-DPG concentration and thus a decreased oxygen–carrying capacity of the red cells. With acidosis, the oxyhemoglobin dissociation curve is shifted to the right, increasing the release of oxygen to the tissues. Decreased erythrocyte 2,3-DPG shifts the curve to the left or back to the pre-acidotic position. With correction of the pH but without correction of the red cell 2,3-DPG, the curve is shifted to the left, decreasing the release of oxygen to the tissues. Without phosphorus supplementation, it takes 72 to 96 hours to restore erythrocyte 2,3-DPG in adults. Phosphorus given during treatment of DKA accelerates 2,3-DPG restoration to within 12 to 24 hours. In children, however, erythrocyte 2,3-DPG concentrations return to normal in 24 hours, even without phosphate therapy.

It is now recommended that phosphorus be given intravenously, as potassium phosphate in DKA. Usually one half of the potassium is given as KCl and the other half is given as KH_2PO_4. Serum calcium and phosphorus should be monitored, because hypocalcemia and hyperphosphatemia may occur following potassium phosphate administration. There is evidence, however, that even with phosphorus supplementation, the serum phosphate level will fall 24 to 36 hours into therapy.

Infection

Intercurrent illness is a common trigger for loss of control and the development of ketoacidosis. All patients in DKA should have a "sepsis work-up," including blood culture, urine culture, and throat culture. Chest x-ray examination should be performed if the physical examination reveals rales or unequal breath sounds or if the respiratory rate is disproportionate to the degree of acidosis. Spinal tap should be performed in cases in which meningitis is clinically suspected. Careful inspection of the optic fundi is essential prior to the spinal tap. In addition to the routine cerebrospinal fluid (CSF) studies, CSF pressure and pH (compared with simultaneous serum pH) are recommended. Leukocytosis with a shift to the left is common in DKA and, therefore, is a poor indicator of infection. Antibiotics should be prescribed only if a bacterial infection is clinically suspected.

Cerebral Edema

A fortunately rare, however, unpredictable complication of the treatment of DKA is cerebral edema. Cerebral edema occurs in the first 3 to 24 hours of therapy, even as biochemical parameters are improving. Unexplained fever may be seen. The patient develops decreased mental status, which leads rapidly to coma. The mortality rate is high. Cerebral edema is treated with fluid restriction, mannitol, and/or steroids and/or diuretics. Results of therapy are disappointing.

The mechanism for the development of cerebral edema is unknown. Hyponatremia, excessive fluid administration, and a rapid decline in serum glucose have been implicated.

CASE PRESENTATION

D.B. is a 14-year-old male with known type I diabetes mellitus for 4 years. The insulin dose (purified pork) prescribed is 14 U of NPH (neutral protamine Hagedorn) and 6 U of regular in the morning and 7 U of NPH and 3 U of regular in the afternoon. However, D.B. admits that he frequently "forgets" to take the afternoon injection.

Three days prior to admission, D.B. developed an "upper respiratory infection" for which his mother gave him Tylenol elixir and a cough syrup. Over the next 2 days, D.B. experienced unusually excessive thirst and hunger. His urine output increased; he became nocturic. His urine tests, which are usually negative to 2 percent, were consistently 5 percent, acetone negative. On the day of admission, D.B. complained of abdominal pains and headache. Anorexia ensued, and he began vomiting. His breathing became rapid and labored, and his urine revealed large acetone. His mother brought him to the hospital.

Examination and Test Results

In the emergency room, physical examination revealed a thin, short 14-year-old male.

Vital signs: BP = 100/60 mm Hg; pulse = 160 beats/min; RR = 36 breaths/min, T = 38°C; weight = 40 kg.

HEENT: erythematous throat with exudate, dry tongue.

Neck: bilateral tender cervical adenopathy, without palpable thyroid.

Chest: breath sounds equal; no adventitious sounds.

Heart: regular rhythm, no murmur.

Abdomen: soft, no tenderness or organomegaly.

Skin: dry, flushed.

Neurologic: lethargic but easily arousable by verbal stimulation.

Laboratory tests in the emergency room: *Blood*: Visidex (Ames) glucose estimated at 800 mg/dl; hematocrit = 55 percent; serum acetone = moderate; venous pH = 7.05. *Urine*: Clinitest (2-drop method) = 5 percent; Acetest = large. *EKG lead II*: normal sinus rhythm, normal to slightly high T waves.

A diagnosis of DKA was made. Serum electrolytes, including glucose and phosphorus, were drawn. An IV was begun with NS. A low-dose constant insulin infusion was started. The patient was admitted to the ICU.

Problem List

Dehydration—Intake and Output (I&O)

D.B. is estimated to be 10 percent dehydrated, based upon an elevated pulse rate of 160 beats/min and an elevated hematocrit of 55 percent.

An initial bolus of 800 ml (20 ml/kg) of NS is given, followed by ½ NS at a rate of 150 ml/hr. This covers maintenance and one half the dehydration. Ongoing losses (i.e., urine volume) should also be replaced.

Hyperglycemia

The serum glucose is estimated to be 800 mg/dl. Four units (0.1 U/kg) of purified pork regular insulin are given by IV push, followed by 4 U (0.1 U/kg) per hr. The serum glucose is checked hourly.

As the serum glucose approaches 180 mg/dl, D5W/½ NS is used as a hydrating solution, and the insulin drip is lowered to 1 or 2 U (0.025–0.05 U/kg) per hr.

When the serum glucose is under 180 mg/dl *and* when the acidosis is corrected, the continuous infusion is discontinued.

Ketoacidosis

Serum ketones and venous pH are followed hourly. Bicarbonate is used because the venous pH is 7.05. After the initial bolus of NS is completed, 1 ampule (44.5 mEq, or about 1 mEq/kg) is added to the ½ NS hydrating solution and infused over the next few hours.

Ketonuria is expected to persist for 1 or 2 days, well after the serum is cleared of ketones and the pH has returned to normal.

Potassium Balance

An EKG rhythm strip performed in the emergency room revealed normal to slightly elevated T waves compatible with a normal to slightly elevated serum potassium. The serum potassium will fall as the acidosis and hyperglycemia correct.

Potassium, 40 mEq/L of hydrating solution, half as KCl, half as KH_2PO_4, should be infused after the initial NS bolus.

Sodium Balance

A low serum sodium is expected in DKA. As the patient is hydrated, the sodium balance should rise to normal.

Phosphorus Balance

The serum phosphate is normal initially but will fall within 24 hours of initiation of therapy. One half the potassium supplementation is given as the phosphate salt. Serum calcium and phosphorus are followed periodically.

Infectious

A throat culture, blood culture, and urine culture are obtained. In view of the erythematous pharynx and fever, a streptococcal tonsillitis is a strong possibility.

Cerebral Edema

Mental status is checked hourly. Any decrease in the state of consciousness during therapy may indicate the onset of cerebral edema.

SUGGESTED READING

Kaufman, I.A., Keller, M.A., and Nyham, W.Z.: Diabetic ketosis and acidosis: continuous infusion of low doses of insulin. J. Pediatr. 87:846, 1975.

Kreisberg, R.A.: Diabetic ketoacidosis: new concepts and trends in pathogenesis and treatment. Ann. Intern. Med. 88:681, 1978.

McGarry, J.D., and Foster, D.U.J.: Regulation of ketogenesis and clinical aspects of the ketotic state. Metabolism 21:471, 1972.

Sperling, M.A.: Diabetes mellitus. Pediatr. Clin. North Am. 26:149, 1979.

Traisman, H.S.: Management of Juvenile Diabetes Mellitus, 3rd ed. St. Louis, The C.V. Mosby Co. 1980.

Nursing Process for Patient Care:
Diabetic Ketoacidosis

The definition of diabetic ketoacidosis (DKA) includes the presence of hyperglycemia (serum glucose greater than 300 mg/dl), ketonemia (ketones strongly positive in the serum), and acidosis (pH less than 7.30 and/or serum bicarbonate less than 15 mEq/L). Assessment parameters, therefore, reflect the presence of these alterations and their subsequent effect on normal body function. Anticipation of potential life-threatening abnormalities is a key component in the nursing management of children with DKA.

HYPERGLYCEMIA

Hyperglycemia occurs in diabetes as a result of insulin deficiency. There is decreased utilization of glucose, and the serum concentration increases.

Once the renal threshold (approximately 180 mg/dl) is exceeded, glycosuria will result.

Assess, Monitor, and Document

Serum glucose (use flow sheet)
Urine glucose (use flow sheet)

Associated signs of hyperglycemia: polyuria, polydipsia

Anticipate

Hyperglycemia
Glycosuria

Polyuria
Polydipsia

FLUID BALANCE

The osmotic diuresis that occurs as a result of hyperglycemia causes loss of water and electrolytes. Dehydration occurs when the child's intake is unable to keep up with the renal losses.

Assess, Monitor, and Document

Weight
State of hydration: mucous membranes, skin turgor, tears
Urine output
Blood pressure

Heart rate
Fluid intake: accurate administration of parenteral fluids (use infusion pump, if available)

Anticipate

Dehydration: dry mucous membranes, flushed, dry skin, decreased blood pressure, tachycardia

Headache
Lethargy

ACID–BASE BALANCE

The normal acid–base balance in the blood is disrupted by the pathophysiologic changes that take place when there is an insulin deficiency. Ketonemia, ketonuria, and acidosis are present.

Assess, Monitor, and Document

Presence of ketones in blood and urine
Serum pH
Associated clinical manifestations of acidosis
  Deep and/or rapid respiratory rate
  Nausea

Vomiting
Abdominal pain
Sweet, acetone odor on breath
Altered level of consciousness: lethargy
Headache

Anticipate

Ketoacidosis: ketonemia, ketonuria

ELECTROLYTE ABNORMALITIES

The three key electrolytes affected by ketoacidosis are potassium, sodium, and phosphorus. The serum potassium level is of concern because of the potential for serious dysrhythmias. Although potassium may initially be normal or increased, the serum concentration decreases with therapy. Low serum sodium is to be expected. Of importance is the association between hyponatremia and cerebral edema. In DKA, there is usually a deficiency in phosphorus. Phosphorus deficiency results in a decreased oxygen–carrying capacity of the red cells and affects the oxyhemoglobin dissociation curve.

Assess, Monitor, and Document

Serum: potassium, sodium, phosphorus
EKG lead II rhythm strip
Response to pharmacologic management

Anticipate

Hypokalemia
   EKG changes: broadened, flattened and/or inverted T waves; U wave may be seen; depressed ST segments; ectopic activity (supraventricular, ventricular); ventricular fibrillation

Hyponatremia
   Cerebral edema: altered level of consciousness, headache, seizures
   Phosphorus deficiency

NEUROLOGIC

An alteration in the neurologic status can occur as a result of the treatment of DKA. Cerebral edema, although rare, can occur within the first 24 hours of therapy.

Assess, Monitor, and Document

Headache
Vomiting
Level of consciousness
Pupillary activity

Reflexes
Blood pressure
Heart rate
Respiratory rate and pattern

Anticipate

Cerebral edema
   Headache
   Vomiting
   Altered level of consciousness
   Increased blood pressure

Decreased pulse
Decreased respiratory rate and pattern
Seizures
Coma

RESPONSE OF CHILD

Assess, Monitor, and Document

Developmental level: verbal, psychosocial, cognitive, fears
Behavioral response: anxious, fearful, disappointed, calm, compliant

Educational needs: disease process, diet, insulin, urine/blood testing, activity
Response to nursing care plan

Anticipate

Emotional distress
Inability to cope

RESPONSE OF FAMILY

Assess, Monitor, and Document

Behavioral response: anxious, fearful, disappointed
Level of understanding of disease process and child's condition
Expected outcome
Ability to cope

Educational needs related to discharge: diet, insulin administration, activity, signs and symptoms of ketoacidosis and insulin shock and management of same.
Response to nursing interventions

Anticipate

Family crisis
Inability to cope

Educational needs related to discharge planning
Referral: social service

MIND SET

Assess

Hyperglycemia
Fluid balance
Acid–base balance

Electrolyte status
Neurologic status
Response of child and family

Anticipate

Hyperglycemia
Glycosuria
Dehydration
Acidosis: ketonemia, ketonuria
Electrolyte alterations: hypokalemia, hyponatremia, phosphorus deficiency

Cerebral edema
Alteration in mental status
Emotional distress in child
Family crisis
Educational needs of child and family

Hyperthyroidism

RAPHAEL DAVID, M.D.
LILY LEW, M.D.

Hyperthyroidism is not a common disorder of childhood; however, a peak incidence is observed during adolescence. A serious and potentially life-threatening complication, thyroid storm, necessitates intensive measures to change the course of an otherwise fatal outcome. Although the etiology of Graves' disease has not been fully established, there is evidence that autoimmunity plays an important role in this disease as well as in other thyroid disorders, notably Hashimoto's thyroiditis. The genetics of these disorders indicate a familial predisposition favoring the female sex. Recently, from histocompatibility studies, it has been shown that certain antigens (HLA-types B8 and DW3) were associated with a predisposition to Graves' disease, not necessarily the same HLA types in different ethnic populations. Associated disorders include diabetes mellitus, collagen vascular disease (e.g., lupus), and Down's syndrome.

In Graves' disease, an "abnormal" stimulator of the thyroid gland appears to have usurped the role of TSH (thyroid-stimulating hormone), its normal pituitary tropic hormone. Thus, the regulation of thyroid hormone synthesis is disrupted, and the feedback control system involving the pituitary and hypothalamus is shut off. Hence, serum levels of TSH are typically low and cannot be stimulated with the hypothalamic releasing hormone TRH (thyrotropin releasing hormone). The nature of this new stimulator is an IgG, referred to as thyroid-stimulating antibody or thyroid-stimulating immunoglobulin (TSAb or TSI). Its presence in the serum of patients with Graves' disease is determined by assays that measure its ability either to stimulate adenylate cyclase in normal thyroid tissue or to inhibit TSH-binding to thyroid membranes. These assays have yielded positive results in approximately 70 to 80 percent of patients with Graves' disease.

Thyrotoxicosis primarily results from an over-production of thyroxine (T_4) and triiodothyronine (T_3) by the thyroid gland, acting in an environment of increased sensitivity to catecholamines. Thus, patients with Graves' disease may show signs and symptoms that are attributable either directly to the thyroid hormones themselves or to a heightened sympathomimetic activity. Thyroid hormones exert multiple and diverse physiologic functions and are vital for normal growth and development. Heat production, basal metabolism, and oxidative cellular processes are all dependent upon thyroid hormone action. These and other metabolic effects are accelerated in thyrotoxicosis. The role of emotional or physical stress as a precipitating factor in Graves' disease has been debated for years. Such an event may antedate the clinical onset of the disease. More uniformly, it will act as the trigger for the rather sudden and catastrophic complication of Graves' disease, thyroid storm.

The diagnosis of Graves' disease is generally not difficult. Except in the relatively uncommon variant known as T_3 toxicosis (in which only serum T_3 is elevated; T_4 normal), in the classic form of the disorder, total serum T_4 as well as T_3 are elevated. The T_3 resin uptake is also elevated. The latter is an important adjunct in diagnosis, because it aids in the interpretation of an abnormal total T_4 value. For example, an elevated T_4 resulting from a high level of circulating thyroxin-binding globulin (TBG) will be accompanied by a low T_3 resin uptake and, therefore, a normal free T_4 index. High TBG levels occur during pregnancy and when taking contraceptive estrogen-containing pills. As mentioned previously, serum TSH is typically undetectable in Graves' disease and the presence of TSAb confirms that an abnormal stimulus exists underlying the excessive thyroid hormone secretion. The radioiodine uptake by the gland is elevated.

CLINICAL MANIFESTATIONS

The usual onset of hyperthyroidism is fairly insidious. Prominent among the early symptoms are emotional lability and a poor attention span, which leads to difficulties in school. The child appears flushed and fidgety, has fine tremors of the hands, experiences palpitations, and perspires easily. The hyperactivity is often accompanied by fatigue and weight loss. The eye signs in children are usually less frequent and less serious than those encountered in adults, but they can be troublesome. A stare with or without true exophthalmos may be present. The stare is due to lid retraction resulting from excessive sympathetic stimulation, whereas exophthalmos is caused by tissue infiltration behind the eyeglobe. Other serious eye manifestations, although rare in children, are ophthalmoplegia and chemosis.

Tachycardia and systolic hypertension with a wide pulse pressure are classic findings. Although cardiovascular manifestations are potentially the most serious, the occurrence of congestive heart failure (CHF) is rare in children. The thyroid gland is enlarged in most cases. The goiter is characteristically boggy, smooth, somewhat rubbery, and more or less symmetrical. A bruit may be heard.

Undoubtedly, the most serious complication of Graves' disease, fortunately rare, is the so-called *thyroid crisis* or *thyroid storm*, which may have a fatal outcome. It usually occurs in a patient who is either untreated or whose treatment is poorly controlled, and most frequently, a precipitating or "triggering" factor can be identified. Thus, when these two conditions prevail, the likelihood of thyroid storm should be kept in mind. The precipitating factor is an acute stressful event, such as surgery, infection, or trauma.

In thyroid storm, a severe hypermetabolic state exists and, in essence, all signs and symptoms of hyperthyroidism are exaggerated. A high fever develops, owing to an inability to dissipate the tremendous heat production. The manifestations are life-threatening and disparate, affecting mainly the central nervous system (CNS) and the cardiovascular and gastrointestinal systems. One of several symptom complexes may predominate, which could elude the physician because of its nonspecific character. Although blood levels of thyroid hormones are elevated in thyroid storm, the fact that in some cases they are no higher than they were prior to the crisis shows that other factors are involved in the pathogenesis of the crisis. It is likely that these factors are somehow related to beta-adrenergic influences and a "stress" that the patient suddenly seems unable to tolerate. Abrupt decompensation, therefore, occurs. The patient appears agitated, restless, and tremulous. Mental confusion, even delusion, and other psychotic reactions may occur. The cardiovascular system is taxed to the point of threatened CHF. Severe tachycardia is recorded, and the danger of peripheral vascular collapse may be imminent. Gastrointestinal symptoms, including nausea, vomiting, and abdominal pain, can at times simulate a surgical disorder.

TREATMENT

Thyroid storm can most effectively be prevented by diagnosing and adequately controlling Graves' disease in its early stages. When a thyrotoxic crisis has become apparent, immediate therapy is mandatory. The plan of action should address itself to three main issues: 1) Stopping the release of thyroid hormone as quickly as possible with iodide, 2) counteracting the severe sympathetic activity and attempting to control the tachycardia with a beta-adrenergic blocker (usually propranolol), and 3) using supportive measures in an effort to sustain cardiac action and vascular tone with parenteral fluids, antipyretics, amines, digitalis, and glucocorticoids. Steroids are useful not only against stress but also in reducing levels of circulating thyroid hormones. Antithyroid medications, such as propylthiouracil (PTU) or methimazole are started immediately, but their blocking effects will not be realized for days; thus, they cannot be relied upon to achieve a rapid reduction in circulating thyroid hormones. Despite all measures, a successful outcome is not always attained, and the mortality rate is a significant factor; in adults, it is said to be approximately 20 percent. Without any treatment, however, the mortality rate is 100 percent.

CASE PRESENTATION

A 10-year-old Oriental male with hyperthyroidism was admitted to the ICU in thyroid storm. The diagnosis of hyperthyroidism was made 2 months prior to admission, and the patient had been treated with methimazole, 5 mg P.O., every 6 hours. He had a total weight loss of 10 pounds over 8 months, slept poorly, sought cool spots in the house, and was hyperactive. Because of the objectionable taste of methimazole, the patient took the medication sporadically. Several days prior to admission, the mother noted a worsening of the child's restlessness. He hardly slept and was having loose stools. He looked ill and had a temperature of 102° to 103° F. The intestinal symptoms were attributed to the medication; thus, all therapy was stopped by the parents. He was brought to the hospital because of rapid deterioration and a further increase in temperature.

Examination

On admission, the patient was incoherent and restless, with a pulse of 300 beats/min, blood pressure of 160/100 mm Hg, and a temperature of 106° F. The skin was flushed, and the patient was diaphoretic. His eyes were rolling, but no seizure activity was observed. There was no exophthalmos, the thyroid gland was moderately enlarged (about 3 times normal size), and a bruit was heard. There was no heart murmur; the rhythm was regular. Respirations were 30 breaths/min. His lungs were clear. The abdomen was soft and without visceromegaly. There was no evidence of CHF.

Initial Therapy

IV fluids and oxygen by mask were administered. A nasograstric (NG) tube was inserted. Stat doses of the following medications were given: PTU, 150 mg NG; acetaminophen, 400 mg NG; propranolol, 10 mg NG and 2 mg IV. The patient was then placed on a hypothermia blanket. His temperature continued to rise to 108° F. He began to convulse. Diazepam, 5 mg IV, was given, and the seizure stopped. Sodium iodide (NaI), 1 gm over 24 hours by continuous IV drip, was started 1 hour after the first dose of PTU.

Serum electrolytes revealed: Na = 143 mEq/L, K = 5.6 mEq/L, Cl = 118 mEq/L, CO_2 = 10.5 mEq/L, and BUN = 34 mg/dl. Arterial blood gases on supplementary oxygen revealed: pH = 7.31, Pa_{O_2} = 134 mm Hg, and Pa_{CO_2} = 34 mm Hg. The hematocrit was 40 percent, the WBC was 9,000/mm³, with differential of 67 segmented polymorphonuclear leukocytes, 30 lymphocytes, and 3 monocytes; platelets were adequate. Serum T_4 was 19 µg/dl (normal 5.5–11.5), T_3 (RIA) was 478 ng/dl, (normal 90–240 ng/dl), and antithyroglobulin antibody titer was 1:1600. Blood and urine cultures were negative. A chest x-ray film showed no remarkable findings. Further treatment consisted of PTU, 150 mg NG q4h; propranolol, 20 mg NG q6h; dexamethasone, 2 mg NG q6h; saturated solution of potassium iodide (SSKI), 5 drops NG q4h; and acetaminophen, 400 mg NG q4h p.r.n. for fever. Pulse and temperature gradually returned to normal within 2 days. SSKI, steroid, and propranolol were gradually tapered and discontinued after 7 days. His mental status improved progressively. On Day 14 of hospitalization, PTU was reduced to 100 mg P.O. q8h. At the time of discharge, he was euthyroid clinically and biochemically.

Problem List

Hyperthyroidism

The appropriate management for a severe thyroid crisis is always medical therapy. The immediate aim of therapy is to inhibit thyroid hormone release and to block the adrenergically mediated effects of peripheral thyroid hormone action. These goals are accomplished by the prompt administration of NaI and propranolol. However, at least 1 hour prior to starting NaI, a dose of PTU must be given to block the organification of iodine within the thyroid gland. PTU is preferred to methimazole because of its additional effect of inhibiting the peripheral conversion of T_4 to T_3. Large doses of PTU (150–200 mg P.O. or NG q4h) or methimazole (15–20 mg P.O. or NG q4h) must be given; there are no IV preparations available. Iodide may be given as either Lugol's solution or SSKI (5 drops P.O. or NG q6h) or sodium iodide (1–2 gm/day IV).

Hydrocortisone is also administered in large doses (300 mg/day IV). Alternatively, dexamethasone (2 mg IV or NG q6h) may be used. Dexamethasone not only inhibits the release of hormone from the thyroid gland and peripheral conversion of T_4 to T_3 but also provides additional glucocorticoid support; thus, it synergizes the action of PTU and iodide.

Propranolol is the drug of choice to block the adrenergic effects of thyrotoxicosis. It also decreases the cardiac output and helps to correct supraventricular dysrhythmias. Propranolol is contraindicated in patients with asthma and CHF. The dose may be given orally (40–80 mg q6h) or intravenously. IV propranolol may be repeated every 4 hours (total dose: 1–2 mg q10 min, maximum 10 mg) or the drug may be given P.O.

In summary, medical therapy includes thionamide, iodide, steroid, and propranolol to prevent synthesis, release, and peripheral conversion of T_4 and to diminish the adrenergic effects. Clinical improvement should be noted within 12 hours, biochemical evidence of improvement should be evident by 24 hours, and recovery may be expected within a week. At this time, the use of iodide, propranolol, and steroids is tapered and then discontinued. Maintenance therapy consists of either PTU or methimazole.

Pyrexia

Pyrexia is a prominent feature. An antipyretic such as acetaminophen 10 mg/kg NG or per rectum q4h p.r.n. should be used. Aspirin should be avoided, because it is believed to displace T_4 from its binding proteins and possibly exacerbate the hyperthyroidism. Other measures used to decrease the temperature include a hypothermia blanket, ice packs, wet packs, and fans. Meanwhile, a source of infection should be excluded.

Dehydration

High fever, vomiting, and/or diarrhea will invariably cause dehydration. An assessment of the degree of dehydration should be made.

Initial IV fluid should consist of glucose solution containing saline to be given at a rate of 20 ml/kg of body weight over the first hour. Over the next 24 hours, fluid calculation would include deficit, ongoing losses, and maintenance requirements. Half of the fluids are given in the first 8 hours, and the remainder are given over the next 16 hours. If hyponatremia is present, sodium should be included in the deficit portion of the calculation. Fluid should also contain large quantities of glucose and vitamin B complex.

A NG tube should be inserted in all patients who are unconscious or who have significant vomiting; it also facilitates the administration of medication.

Cardiovascular

Tachydysrhythmia with or without CHF may be an important clinical feature in thyroid storm. CHF is rare in children. The marked tachycardia is disproportionate to the fever. An EKG will confirm the tachycardia and dysrhythmia. The latter can be sinus or ectopic in origin. Arterial blood gases may reveal slight acidosis. When there is no evidence of CHF, the drug of choice for the treatment of tachycardia is propranolol. Propranolol can be given intravenously (1–2 mg bolus); it is effective within 2 to 10 minutes and can be repeated after 10 to 15 minutes (maximum 10 mg). The duration of action is 3 to 4 hours. However, oral administration is the preferred route (40–80 mg P.O. or NG q6h). Propranolol aggravates bronchospasm in asthmatics and exacerbates CHF, because it decreases cardiac output and force of contraction. A specific beta-adrenergic blocker, such as atenolol 100 mg P.O. q12h, may be used in asthmatics.

When there is evidence of CHF, digoxin, diuretics, and oxygen therapy are required.

Central Nervous System

The spectrum of CNS manifestations can range from hyperactivity with increased irritability to lethargy and coma. If CNS symptoms are the predominant features, a neurologic or psychiatric diagnosis may be incorrectly made. The mental status is an important parameter for assessing the effectiveness of therapy. Therefore, sedation should be used with caution.

Seizures, fever, and lethargy may suggest an underlying infectious process. Thus, a lumbar puncture is indicated. Diazepam is given intravenously to control the seizures (0.3–0.75 mg/kg IV q15min, maximum 10 mg).

Gastrointestinal

Vomiting and diarrhea may be severe, resulting in pronounced dehydration. Dehydration must be assessed and corrected (Dehydration).

When jaundice is noted, it is an ominous sign. The abdominal complaints and findings may mimic those of an acute abdomen. A surgical consultation may be necessary.

Precipitating Factor

An intercurrent illness, usually an infection, is the most common precipitating factor. Appropriate cultures and studies should be obtained. Antibiotics are not warranted unless a source of infection is identified.

SUGGESTED READING

Austin, J.W., et al.: Medical grand rounds: thyroid storm. South. Med. J. 71 (2): 195, 1978.

Barnes, H.V., and Blizzard, R.M.: Antithyroid drug therapy for toxic diffuse goiter (Graves' disease): thirty years experience in children and adolescents. J. Pediatr. 91 (2): 313, 1977.

Braverman, L.E.: Thyroid storm. In Current Therapy in Endocrinology, 1983–1984. St. Louis, The C.V. Mosby Co., 1983, pp. 65–69.

Galaburda, M., Rosman, P.N., and Hadow, J.E.: Thyroid storm in an 11-year-old boy managed by propranolol. Pediatrics 53: 920, 1974.

Hayek, A.: Thyroid storm following radioiodine for thyrotoxicosis. J. Pediatr. 93 (6): 978, 1978.

Hellman, R.G.: The evaluation and management of hyperthyroid crises. Crit. Care Quart. 3: 77, 1980.

How, J., Khir, A.S.M., and Bewsher, P.O.: The effect of atenolol on serum thyroid hormones in hyperthyroid patients. Clin. Endocrinol. 13 (2): 299, 1980.

Lamphier, T.A.: Current status of diagnosis and treatment of thyroid storm. Md. State Med. J. 29 (6): 67, 1980.

Larsen, P.R.: Salicylate-induced increases in free triiodothyronine in human serum. J. Clin. Invest. 51: 1125, 1972.

Mackin, J.F., Canary, J.J., and Pittman, C.S.: Thyroid storm and its management. N. Engl. J. Med. 291 (26): 1396, 1974.

Mazzaferri, E.L.: Thyroid storm. Hosp. Medicine. November 1979, Vol. 15 No. 11, pp. 7-22.

Nursing Process for Patient Care:

Hyperthyroidism

The signs and symptoms of thyrotoxicosis result from increased production of T_3 and T_4 and heightened sensitivity to catecholamines. A hypermetabolic state is produced.

The effects of severe hyperthyroidism on other organ systems can be significant. These systems must be assessed and monitored to prevent the catastrophic sequelae of thyroid storm.

METABOLIC STATE

Assess, Monitor, and Document

Temperature: perspires easily
Activity: fidgety, fine tremors of the hands, fatigue
Weight

Eyes: stares, exophthalmos, ophthalmoplegia
Laboratory data: T_3, T_4
Response to pharmacologic management

Anticipate

Thyroid storm

THYROID

The thyroid gland itself may be enlarged. The nurse should include the thyroid gland in her physical assessment process. The goiter is usually symmetrical, smooth, rubbery, and boggy. A bruit may be heard.

Assess, Monitor, and Document

Size
Appearance

Characteristics
Presence of bruit

Anticipate

Enlarged thyroid gland

CARDIOVASCULAR

The cardiovascular status of the child can be altered significantly. The potential outcome may be congestive heart failure (CHF) and peripheral vascular collapse.

Assess, Monitor, and Document

Heart rate
Rhythm
Quality
Perfusion

Blood pressure
Respiratory rate
Breath sounds

Anticipate

Alteration in cardiovascular status
  Tachycardia
  Dysrhythmia

Elevated blood pressure: wide pulse pressure
Congestive heart failure
Peripheral vascular collapse

NEUROLOGIC

Assess, Monitor, and Document

Level of consciousness
Orientation
Motor responses

Reflexes
Behavior: emotional lability

Anticipate

Alteration in neurologic status
  Restlessness
  Agitation
  Tremulousness
  Confusion

Delusion
Psychosis
Seizures
Coma

GASTROINTESTINAL

Assess, Monitor, and Document

Pain: location, intensity
Nausea

Vomiting: amount, color, consistency
Diarrhea: amount, color

Anticipate

Alteration in gastrointestinal function

FLUID AND ELECTROLYTE BALANCE

Fluid and electrolyte balance are closely related to the degree of abdominal distress. Vomiting and diarrhea along with the fever can lead to dehydration.

Assess, Monitor, and Document

Weight
State of hydration: thirst, mucous membranes, skin turgor
Urine output (including specific gravity)

Fluid intake: accurate administration of parenteral fluids (use infusion pump if available)
Laboratory data: electrolytes

Anticipate

Alteration in fluid and electrolyte balance
  Dehydration

RESPONSE OF CHILD

Assess, Monitor, Document

Developmental level: tasks, fears
Degree of distress

Ability to cope
Response to nursing interventions

Anticipate

Emotional distress

RESPONSE OF FAMILY

Assess, Monitor, and Document

Behavioral response: shock, fearful, angry, guilty

Level of understanding of disease and child's condition

Expected outcome

Ability to cope

Response to nursing interventions

Anticipate

Family crisis

Inability to cope

MIND SET

Assess

Metabolic state

Thyroid status

Cardiovascular status

Neurologic status

Gastrointestinal system

Fluid and electrolyte balance

Emotional response of child and family

Anticipate

Thyroid crisis
  Fever
  Agitation
  Confusion

Congestive heart failure

Peripheral vascular collapse

Emotional distress

Family crisis

Adrenal Insufficiency and Steroid Withdrawal

LILY LEW, M.D.

RAPHAEL DAVID, M.D.

Adrenal insufficiency can culminate in one of the most dramatic crises, which, unless quickly recognized and promptly treated, will almost invariably result in a fatal outcome. In most instances, a state of chronic adrenal insufficiency antedates the acute crisis, and the latter is often precipitated by an intercurrent illness or other stressful situation. What may not be as widely appreciated is that there are various forms of adrenal insufficiency stemming from different pathogenetic mechanisms. Also, the symptoms of chronic insufficiency can be both subtle and nonspecific, hence the delay in diagnosis. To appreciate the spectrum of clinical manifestations, it is first necessary to review some of the basic mechanisms that regulate the adrenocortical secretion of three major hormones: cortisol, aldosterone, and the adrenal androgen, dehydroepiandrosterone (DHA).

Cortisol, the principal glucocorticoid of the zona fasciculata, is the most important hormone in terms of its life-sustaining capacity. Its secretion is under the control of pituitary ACTH (adrenocorticotropic hormone). Diminished cortisol secretion can occur in three situations: 1) hypothalamic–pituitary disease affecting ACTH secretion (secondary adrenal insufficiency), usually caused by suprasellar lesions, such as craniopharyngioma; 2) disorders of the adrenal cortex per se (primary adrenal insufficiency), such as Addison's disease, congenital adrenal hyperplasia (CAH), and selective cortisol deficiency such as occurs in the syndrome of ACTH unresponsiveness; and 3) withdrawal of glucocorticoid therapy too abruptly in patients receiving chronic steroid treatment. In these patients, the adrenals are atrophied and cannot recover soon enough to meet the endogenous demands for cortisol, especially in conditions of stress.

The effects of cortisol insufficiency are mainly circulatory in nature and result in an inability to maintain a normal blood glucose level. Hemodynamic changes include diminished cardiac output and renal perfusion. Vascular tone is decreased, leading to a fall in blood pressure and eventually to circulatory collapse.

Aldosterone is the principal mineralocorticoid secreted by the zona glomerulosa and is under the control of the renin–angiotensin system. Aldosterone is not significantly influenced by ACTH; therefore, lesions of the pituitary or hypothalamus do not generally affect aldosterone secretion, a fact that is frequently overlooked. Aldosterone deficiency results in hyponatremia due to salt wasting, hyperkalemia, and metabolic acidosis; blood urea nitrogen (BUN) and creatinine levels are also elevated. The most serious and potentially life-threatening effects are those of excessive potassium retention, particularly with respect to cardiac function. Thus, the electrocardiogram (EKG) is a useful adjunct in assessing the electrical behavior of the myocardium. Aldosterone deficiency occurs in Addison's disease, in the salt-losing forms of CAH, and in selective enzyme defects of aldosterone synthesis (e.g., 18–hydroxylase or methyl oxidase). In the latter familial syndrome, however, cortisol secretion remains intact.

Adrenal androgens, the most abundant being DHA, are secreted by the zona reticularis. Its physiologic significance is not known; therefore, DHA deficiency does not appear to be of clinical importance. Low levels are seen in Addison's disease, in hypopituitarism with ACTH deficiency, and in patients receiving suppressive doses of glucocorticoid. The assay of plasma DHA or its sulfate provides a sensitive indicator of adrenal function when basal cortisol levels are at the lower limit of the normal range. This, however, is not a reliable test in prepubertal children, because their adrenal androgen secretion is normally low.

TESTS OF ADRENAL FUNCTION

Cortisol

Basal levels of plasma cortisol are maximal during the early morning hours; therefore, it is customary to assess cortisol secretion at about 8:00 or 9:00 A.M. However, because resting levels can be near or even within the normal range in adrenal insufficiency, the best way to rapidly evaluate the capacity of the adrenals to secrete cortisol is with the ACTH test. A simple method consists of administering synthetic ACTH[1-24] (cosyntropin, Cortrosyn), 0.25 mg intravenously as a bolus, and measuring plasma cortisol before and 60 minutes after the injection. In this test, the response is considered normal if the increment in plasma cortisol is either at least 10 μg per dl or the level exceeds 20 μg per dl. A blunted response may be due to either primary or secondary adrenal insufficiency. Plasma ACTH measurements can help resolve the problem, because ACTH is elevated in the former instance. The metyrapone test is also helpful in evaluating ACTH reserve, as is the insulin-induced hypoglycemic stress test. However, the latter test should be avoided in patients with suspected Addison's disease, because they are very sensitive to insulin.

Aldosterone

The serum electrolyte pattern is generally characteristic in Addison's disease and other aldosterone deficient states so that actual measurement of plasma aldosterone is not usually necessary. Aldosterone levels may even be normal though inappropriate when hyponatremia and salt wasting are evident, which may be misleading. It is generally more helpful to measure plasma renin activity, which should be uniformly elevated in aldosterone deficient states. Urinary sodium and potassium excretion can be assessed rapidly and may provide an aid to diagnosis.

Clinical

The principal manifestations of acute adrenal insufficiency may vary according to the underlying pathology, as discussed previously. For example, in Addison's disease, which involves the destruction of all three zones of the adrenal cortex, symptoms of both cortisol and aldosterone deficiency can be observed. These symptoms include severe weakness, hypotension, variable hypoglycemia, dehydration due to salt wasting, and possibly signs of potassium excess. In addition, nonspecific symptoms, predominantly gastrointestinal (e.g., anorexia, vomiting, and abdominal pain), may occur. Fever is often present, which may result in confusion at times and cause difficulties in determining the existence of an underlying infection, which might have precipitated the adrenal crisis. Vascular collapse and shock may be imminent. In cases of long-standing adrenal insufficiency, the typical hyperpigmentation of the skin and mucous membranes can be seen.

In CAH (salt-losing forms), there is also ambiguity of the external genitalia in the female. The male may have an enlarged phallus and a hyperpigmented scrotum.

The clinical manifestations of secondary adrenal insufficiency (e.g., in hypothalamic–pituitary lesions) or of abrupt steroid withdrawal are limited to those of cortisol deficiency and, as previously described, are mainly circulatory with or without hypoglycemia. Serum electrolytes, specifically potassium, are usually normal. It should be noted, however, that in ACTH deficient states, there is a tendency to retain water, which can result in dilutional hyponatremia.

Finally, one should be aware that a precipitating event may have triggered the adrenal crisis; thus, every effort should be made to search for an underlying infection using the appropriate tests, including blood and urine cultures and a spinal tap if there are signs of meningitis or meningococcemia.

GUIDELINES FOR THERAPY

The mainstay of therapy in acute adrenal insufficiency is the prompt administration of parenteral aqueous soluble glucocorticoid (e.g., hydrocortisone hemisuccinate) in large "stress" doses (approximately 300 mg/m²/day of body surface area), along with IV saline and glucose solutions. A blood sample for cortisol assay should be drawn prior to the administration of hormone, although therapy should not await the result of this analysis. IV hydrocortisone should be continued around the clock, preferably in four divided doses. If salt-losing signs are present, mineralocorticoid therapy should be started with daily intramuscular (IM) desoxycorticosterone acetate, DOCA, (1 to 3 mg intramuscularly once daily) and as soon as possible changed to oral 9α-fluoro-hydrocortisone, Florinef (0.05 to 0.1 mg once daily). If serum potassium is very high and fails to respond to hormonal replacement, which is an unusual occurrence, potassium exchange resins may be given. Parenteral fluids (isotonic saline and glucose) are essential in sustaining the circulation, in correcting the dehydration, and in restoring blood sugar levels to normal. The metabolic acidosis will generally respond to this regimen and to mineralocorticoid replacement. Bicarbonate is seldom necessary. Improvement will be observed within hours, and if there is no underlying infection or other manifestations of "stress," maintenance steroid therapy in physiologic doses (hydrocortisone 20 to 25 mg/m²/day) can be started within a day or two. In the event of continuing infection and fever, stress doses of glucocorticoid (3 to 5 times physiologic doses) should be maintained until recovery becomes apparent; the steroid may then be tapered to a replacement dose within a few days.

Steroid Withdrawal

Suppression of the hypothalamic–pituitary axis occurs in all patients who receive pharmacologic doses of glucocorticoid for more than 2 or 3 weeks. This in turn results in adrenal suppression and eventually atrophy, which is reversible when therapy is discontinued. However, adrenal responsiveness does not return immediately; therefore, a state of adrenal insufficiency exists for a variable period of time. This condition becomes most apparent when there is an intercurrent illness or other stressful situation, such as trauma or surgery, in which the demands for cortisol cannot be met by the adrenal glands. Although the time for complete adrenal recovery to take place—that is, for a normal ACTH reserve to be restored—is variable, studies with the metyrapone test have shown that this may take up to 1 year. Therefore, in patients treated for longer than 3 weeks, steroids should be tapered slowly; and for a period of 1 year after therapy has been discontinued, patients should be treated with steroids during stressful conditions unless tests (e.g., metyrapone or insulin tests) have shown that ACTH reserve was normal. Periodic ACTH tests are also helpful in this respect.

Tapering of steroids in patients treated for only 2 or 3 weeks is probably unnecessary or may be achieved very rapidly within a day or two. For patients who have received more prolonged therapy, the following guidelines are offered. Initial reduction of steroid to physiologic doses may be accomplished progressively within approximately 2 or 3 weeks. At this point, it is more practical to substitute hydrocortisone for the more potent synthetic analogues generally used for pharmacologic treatment. Hydrocortisone, 20 to 25 mg per m² per day, is given for 1 week; thereafter, the dose is tapered gradually over approximately 4 to 5 weeks and is finally withdrawn. During the last few weeks of treatment, hydrocortisone may be given in a single daily dose, preferably in the morning. Monthly determinations of basal A.M. plasma cortisol levels with periodic ACTH tests, as previously mentioned, are recommended in order to assess the recovery of the pituitary–adrenal axis.

CASE PRESENTATION

A 28 month old Indian male was brought to the emergency room in a lethargic, cold, and sweaty condition.

He was born at term to a gravida I para 0; his birth weight was 6 pounds, 8 ounces; he was 20 inches long. The parents were nonconsanguineous. The neonatal period was uneventful. He was hospitalized at 8 months of age for dehydration secondary to gastroenteritis and at 11 months of age for a seizure with fever. The child was taken to India at 15 months of age to live with his grandparents. The grandmother noted that he developed an increasing craving for salty foods and added salt to his meals. One week prior to admission, the child returned to his parents. The mother did not recognize her child because he appeared darker, thinner, and less active. He was evaluated by the pediatrician, who advised stopping "junk foods" such as potato chips and popcorn. One day later, he vomited after eating and became lethargic, cold, and clammy. He had no known illnesses and was on no chronic medication.

Examination and Test Results

On physical examination, he appeared small for his age, lethargic, limp, and glassy-eyed. Vital signs were: T = 100°F; pulse = 132 beats/min and regular; RR = 34 breaths/min and regular; and BP = < 60 mm Hg. The skin was dark, cool, and clammy. The mucous membranes were dry. HEENT examination results were unremarkable. The thyroid was not palpable. The heart had a regular rhythm without any murmur, and the lungs were clear. The abdomen was flat, soft, and had no masses. The genitalia were normal (Tanner I). No neurologic deficit was elicited.

The Dextrostix was between 20 and 40 mg/dl. An EKG revealed a sinus tachycardia with slightly peaked T waves. CBC revealed a hematocrit of 38 percent; WBC of 10,500/mm³, with differential of

43 segmented polymorphonuclear leukocytes, 49 lymphocytes, and 8 eosinophils. Urine specific gravity was 1.027, pH was 6, and dipstick was negative. No reaction was seen with 10 percent ferric chloride. Serum electrolytes were as follows: $Na = 126$ mEq/L, $Cl = 96$ mEq/L, $CO_2 = 18$ mEq/L, $K = 8$ mEq/L, serum urea nitrogen $= 30$ mg/dl, creatinine $= 0.7$ mg/dl, glucose $= 52$ mg/dl, and $Ca = 4.5$ mEq/L. Blood was drawn for cortisol, 17-OH progesterone, plasma renin activity, aldosterone, and DHA-sulfate.

A presumptive diagnosis of adrenal insufficiency was made. IV fluid therapy, consisting of 5 percent dextrose in NS was initiated at 20 ml/kg/hr. A Stat dose of hydrocortisone hemisuccinate, 50 mg, was given intravenously as a bolus, followed by DOCA, 2 mg IM. A continuous infusion of hydrocortisone hemisuccinate was started to run at 50 mg every 8 hours.

Subsequently, radiologic studies of the chest and abdomen did not reveal any calcifications.

Problem List

Adrenal Crisis

When adrenal crisis is suspected, treatment should not be delayed or withheld to establish the diagnosis. Therapy consists of correcting the hormonal deficits of glucocorticoid and mineralocorticoid. Glucocorticoid therapy involves the immediate IV injection of hydrocortisone hemisuccinate (Solu-Cortef), 100–125 mg/m² of body surface area, followed by an IV infusion of 200–300 mg/m² over the next 24 hours. Mineralocorticoid therapy is given in the form of desoxycorticosterone acetate (DOCA), 1–3 mg IM once daily. After 1 to 2 days of parenteral therapy, the glucocorticoid can be tapered to maintenance oral dosage, provided that satisfactory improvement has occurred.

Maintenance treatment consists of oral hydrocortisone, 20–25 mg/m² per day in three divided doses, and oral 9α-fluoro-hydrocortisone (Florinef), 0.05–0.1 mg/day in a single dose, along with a liberal (ad lib) salt intake.

Dehydration

Significant dehydration may be present. Vomiting aggravates the situation. When hypotension is present, aggressive fluid therapy is necessary. IV fluid containing glucose and sodium chloride is infused at 20 ml/kg/hr initially. In the meantime, the degree of dehydration is estimated, and the appropriate amount of fluid and electrolyte composition is administered. Initially, K is withheld as long as serum K concentration is elevated. If shock is present, colloid solutions may be required. The blood pressure, urine output, and weight are useful guides in assessing the effectiveness of fluid replacement.

Electrolyte Imbalance

The abnormalities commonly found in adrenal insufficiency are hyponatremia, hyperkalemia, hypoglycemia, and metabolic acidosis. Hypercalcemia occurs less commonly. Hypertonic saline is rarely indicated unless the serum sodium level is critically low. Hyperkalemia usually responds to volume expansion and hormone replacement (glucocorticoid and mineralocorticoid). With extreme hyperkalemia and severe electrocardiographic changes, Kayexalate may be administered by rectum. Hypoglycemia is usually corrected with glucose infusion and hormone replacement. Hypercalcemia requires no specific therapy.

Infection or Other Precipitating "Stress"

Appropriate measures should be undertaken to identify an existing infection and to initiate specific antibiotic therapy.

SUGGESTED READING

Bondy, P.K.: The adrenal cortex. *In* Bondy, P.K., and Rosenberg, E. (eds.): Metabolic Control and Disease, 8th ed. Philadelphia, W.B. Saunders Company, 1980, pp. 1457–1464.

Bongiovanni, A.M.: Glucocorticoid therapy. *In* Rudolph, A.M. (ed.): Pediatrics, 17th ed. Norwalk, Connecticut, Appleton-Century-Crofts, 1982, pp. 1505–1509.

Byzny, R.L.: Withdrawal from glucocorticoid therapy. N. Engl. J. Med. 295(1):30, 1976.

Chamberlin, P., and Meyer, W.J.: Management of pituitary–adrenal suppression secondary to corticosteroid therapy. Pediatrics 67(2):245, 1981.

Job, J.C., and Chaussain, J.L.: Job, J.C., and Pierson, M. (eds.): The Adrenals. *In* Pediatric Endocrinology. New York, John Wiley & Sons, Inc., 1981, pp. 291–302.

Leisti, S., and Perheentupa, J.: Two-hour adrenocorticotropic hormone test: accuracy in the evaluation of the hypothalamic–pituitary–adrenocortical axis. Pediatr. Res. 12:272, 1978.

Migeon, C.J.: Adrenal cortex. *In* Rudolph, A.M. (ed.): Pediatrics, 17th ed. Norwalk, Connecticut, Appleton-Century-Crofts, 1982, pp. 1487–1498.

Nursing Process for Patient Care:

Adrenal Insufficiency and Steroid Withdrawal

Adrenal insufficiency may result from intrinsic disease of the adrenal gland or the hypothalamic–pituitary axis or may occur following withdrawal of exogenous steroids after prolonged use. The major consequence of adrenal insufficiency, with its fluid and electrolyte disturbances, is hemodynamic in nature.

CARDIOVASCULAR

The child's cardiovascular status can be profoundly altered by cortisol insufficiency. Vascular tone and cardiac output are affected.

Assess, Monitor, and Document

Heart rate
Rhythm
Blood pressure: arterial, central venous
Peripheral perfusion: capillary filling, skin condition, color

Level of consciousness
Urine output (including specific gravity)

Anticipate

Alteration in cardiovascular status
  Shock: increased cardiac rate, decreased blood pressure, poor peripheral perfusion
  Restlessness, agitation

Decreased urine output
Cyanosis
Cardiac arrest

FLUID AND ELECTROLYTE BALANCE

The child's fluid and electrolyte balance can be altered in response to aldosterone insufficiency. The characteristic findings are hyponatremia, hyperkalemia, metabolic acidosis, and dehydration.

Assess, Monitor, and Document

Weight
Urine output (including specific gravity)
Skin condition
Condition of mucous membranes
Fluid intake: accurate administration of par-

enteral fluids (use infusion pump if available)
Serum electrolytes, glucose, pH
Response to steroid and fluid management

Anticipate

Alteration in fluid and electrolyte status
  Dehydration: decreased weight, decreased urine output, dry mucous membranes, poor skin turgor

Electrolyte disturbances: hyponatremia, hyperkalemia (cardiac dysrhythmias, elevated T waves), hypoglycemia
Metabolic acidosis

RESPONSE OF CHILD

Assess, Monitor, and Document

Developmental level: cognitive, verbal, fearful, tasks
Behavioral response: fearful, anxious, compliant

Response to nursing interventions

Anticipate

Emotional distress
Disruption in normal growth and development

RESPONSE OF FAMILY

Assess, Monitor, and Document

Behavioral response: anxious, verbal
Level of understanding of child's condition
Educational needs for long-term management
  of child

Response to nursing interventions

Anticipate

Family crisis
Educational needs related to long-term care
  requirements

MIND SET

Assess

Cardiovascular status
Fluid and electrolyte balance
Response of child and family

Anticipate

Alteration in cardiovascular status
  Shock
Alteration in fluid and electrolyte balance
  Dehydration
  Hyponatremia

Hyperkalemia
Hypoglycemia
Metabolic acidosis
Emotional distress
Family crisis

METABOLIC

CHAPTER 36

Reye's Syndrome

DOUGLAS MACGREGOR, M.D.
SOL S. ZIMMERMAN, M.D.

Reye's syndrome, an acute encephalopathy associated with fatty infiltration of the viscera, is a relatively rare entity that has received widespread notoriety because of its high mortality rate and its recent link to the use of aspirin. Although the etiology remains obscure and the therapy empiric, the mortality rate has declined from 80 to 20 percent, over the course of the 20 years since it was first described. This decline is due in part to heightened awareness of the syndrome and, therefore, earlier diagnosis and intervention.

EPIDEMIOLOGY

Reye's syndrome has been described in children and adolescents, with peak incidences at 4 and 11 years of age. Reports of cases in adults are uncommon. The exact frequency of occurrence is unknown, but data from the Center for Disease Control suggests that there are 600 to 1200 cases annually. This is probably an underestimate, because noncomatose patients with this syndrome are frequently unrecognized and unreported.

The geographic distribution in the United States reveals a consistently high incidence in several mountain, West North Central, and East North Central states. There is a striking pattern of increased incidence in rural and suburban areas, with relative sparing of urban communities.

Reye's syndrome has been reported in all socioeconomic and ethnic groups. The overall incidence in blacks and whites reflects their respective proportions in the general population, as does the incidence in males and females. However, over half the case reports in children younger than 1 year of age are in blacks. Most of these children are from urban families of lower economic standing. Although there are no clear-cut boundaries, Reye's syndrome frequently presents in one of two different settings: an older, white, middle class suburban child, or a black, urban infant.

ETIOLOGY

Whereas the epidemiology of Reye's syndrome is well described, the etiology remains unknown. Possible mechanisms of injury have been examined, but, as yet, none explain both the clinical spectrum of the disease and the histologic findings. It seems that a variety of factors may act in concert to produce the disease. At the present time, etiology must be discussed in light of infectious, environmental, and genetic factors. Any one or a combination may play a role.

The association of Reye's syndrome with a preceding viral illness is well described. Although many viruses (parainfluenza, Epstein–Barr, coxsackie, ECHO, mumps, rubella, adenovirus, herpes simplex, polio, and reovirus) have been implicated in Reye's syndrome, influenza A and B and varicella are most frequently associated with subsequent disease. The severity of Reye's syndrome does not correlate with the type or severity of the preceding illness.

It is possible that an unidentified environmental agent predisposes people to the effects of a viral illness. Similar forms of encephalopathy may serve as models for Reye's syndrome. Udorn's encephalopathy is caused by aflatoxin, a metabolite of Aspergillus found in grains and nuts. Hepatic histopathology, however, differs from that in Reye's syndrome. Jamaican vomiting sickness results from ingestion of hypoglycin A, which is found in the unripe ackee nut. Serum and urine organic acids, however, are different from those seen in Reye's syndrome. Due to the rural and suburban distribution of the disease, the possible role of insecticides has been considered but not proved.

Several recent studies have suggested a link between aspirin use and subsequent development of Reye's syndrome. Diagnosed patients have a greater history of salicylate use and higher serum levels of salicylate than do control groups. It should be emphasized that although a consistent epidemiologic association between Reye's syndrome and the use of aspirin has been established, there is no proof of causality. However, the existing evidence is such that the Center for Disease Control, the American Academy of Pediatrics, and the Surgeon General have advised that aspirin be avoided in the treatment of influenza and varicella.

Host factors may be important in the development of this syndrome. Congenital defects of the urea cycle occur, presenting as vomiting, lethargy, and coma in association with hyperammonemia. These can be differentiated from Reye's syndrome by liver biopsy, protein loading, and column chromatography (see Chapter 37, Inborn Errors of Metabolism). It is possible, however, that a group of children exist who have partial urea cycle defects but who are in a compensated state until stressed by some exogenous factor. A relatively low familial incidence and low recurrence rate argue against a genetic etiology.

Clearly, our understanding of the cause of Reye's syndrome is still in its infancy. More than likely, the final answer will involve several agents that affect the host and result in a final common pathway of functional impairment.

PATHOPHYSIOLOGY

Reye's syndrome is a multisystem disorder. A complete understanding of the pathophysiology must unify the inciting event with known histologic alterations, biochemical abnormalities, and subsequent deterioration of physiologic function.

Histologic changes have been described in cardiac and skeletal muscle, kidney, and pancreas, but most of the attention has been directed toward liver and brain. The liver is large, pale, and yellow. Hepatocyte cytoplasm reveals small droplets of fat, giving it a foamy appearance. The nuclei remain central in location.

There is minimal inflammation and no necrosis or cholestasis. The brain shows evidence of cerebral edema and myelin blebs, with no inflammation of parenchyma or meninges.

Mitochondria have received special attention and may be the primary target of the disease. The mitochondria appear swollen, with matrix expansion and deformity of the outer membrane. There is glycogen depletion, proliferation of smooth endoplasmic reticulum, and increase in the number of peroxisomes. Dense bodies are absent. These changes are transient and revert to normal as early as 2 months following clinical recovery.

Mitochondria are altered not only morphologically but also functionally. Under normal conditions, nitrogenous wastes are disposed of via the urea cycle, which consists of five enzymes, three located in hepatocyte cytoplasm (argininosuccinic synthetase, argininosuccinic lyase, and arginase), and two located in mitochondria (ornithine transcarbamylase and carbamyl phosphate synthetase). In patients with Reye's syndrome, cytoplasmic enzymes have normal levels of activity, whereas mitochondrial enzyme activity is severely diminished. Ornithine transcarbamylase activity is virtually absent, and carbamyl phosphate synthetase has less than 30 percent of normal activity in most patients. These alterations in enzyme activity, like the histologic changes of the mitochondria, are transient. Hyperammonemia, a hallmark of the disease, results from this derangement of the urea cycle and the existence of a catabolic state.

Many biochemical abnormalities have been found in patients with Reye's syndrome. Undoubtedly, most are the consequences of the disease process; some may contribute to it. Several factors have been suggested as playing an important role in the etiology of clinical manifestations. Serum from affected patients has been found to inhibit isolated mitochondrial respiration. The so-called "Reye's syndrome factor" was subsequently isolated and found to be uric acid, but this does not seem to be a likely cause of the widespread dysfunction.

Hyperammonemia appears to play a central role in Reye's syndrome. Ammonia levels are consistently elevated early in the course of the illness. The early elevation correlates with the acute symptoms of vomiting and ataxia. If coma occurs, the onset usually coincides with the peak serum ammonia level. Ammonia concentration then declines to normal levels within 24 to 48 hours, regardless of the clinical condition. The degree of hyperammonemia, compared with other biochemical abnormalities, correlates most closely with disease severity and mortality. There is a significant increase in mortality when the blood ammonia rises above 300 mcg per dl. Tissue uptake studies show that brain levels of ammonia are actually higher than blood levels. There is much evidence that suggests that many of the clinical changes of Reye's syndrome may be caused by ammonia itself. Vomiting, alteration in mental status, increased intracranial pressure, and tachypnea are seen in both Reye's syndrome and congenital ornithine transcarbamylase deficiency. In experimental models, both respiratory rate and intracranial pressure are linearly related to ammonia levels.

Elevation of fatty and organic acids is another biochemical abnormality seen in patients with Reye's syndrome. In a small series of eight patients, disease severity correlated better with the concentration of the short chain fatty acids, proprionate, butyrate, and isobutyrate than with serum ammonia. The fatty infiltration of the liver in Reye's syndrome is the result of hepatic damage and consequent impairment of fatty acid metabolism combined with increased lipolysis of adipose stores. Experimental models have attempted to reproduce the manifestations of the syndrome by infusing various fatty acids; indeed, intravenous (IV) octanoate in the laboratory animal results in hyperventilation but no change in mental status. Interestingly, coma is more readily produced by infusions that combine fatty acids and ammonia. Carbamyl phosphate synthetase activity drops and ammonia rises still further. The implications of the fatty and organic acidemia for patients with Reye's syndrome remain unclear. Exchange transfusions and peritoneal dialysis fail to lower levels. Theoretically, infusions of glucose and insulin should help to decrease fatty acid levels by blocking their release from adipose tissue, but in clinical practice, such therapy has proved ineffective.

CLINICAL PRESENTATION

Reye's syndrome usually presents in a child between the ages of 5 and 15 years, either during or while recovering from a viral illness. The average time from onset of the initial illness to hospitalization is 6 to 7 days. The interval is usually shorter when varicella is the prodromal illness. More than 90 percent of patients with Reye's syndrome develop episodes of persistent vomiting and hyperventilation. Subsequently, there are behavioral changes ranging from irritability to aggression, alternating with con-

fusion and lethargy. The rate and degree of progression of this encephalopathic phase is variable. Some patients exhibit minimal neurologic involvement, whereas others rapidly lapse into coma, often with seizures. The system of neurologic staging described by Lovejoy is presented in Table 36–1.

The encephalopathy is usually of 24- to 96-hour duration after which there is gradual improvement in neurologic status and general recovery of organ function in patients who survive. A small group of patients remain comatose for a very prolonged period, and their prognosis for complete neurologic recovery is poor.

Children younger than 1 year of age present somewhat differently. The preceding illness is frequently milder and more often diarrheal in nature. Vomiting may be minimal. The more serious nature of Reye's syndrome may be announced by seizures or apneic episodes.

PHYSICAL EXAMINATION

At the time of presentation, physical findings characteristic of the prodromal illness are usu-

Table 36–1. Criteria for Stages in Reye's Syndrome: Clinical, Laboratory, and Electroencephalographic (EEG) Manifestations

Stage I Drowsiness, lethargy, vomiting; normal blood ammonia, increased liver enzyme activity; grade 1 EEG
Stage II Disorientation and combativeness; hyperventilation, tachycardia, pupillary dilation, purposeful response to painful stimuli, hyperactive reflexes, bilateral Babinski signs; elevated blood ammonia, increased liver enzyme activity; grade 2 or 3 EEG
Stage III Deepening coma, persistent hyperventilation, tachycardia, evidence of upper midbrain involvement (loss of ciliospinal reflex, pupillary dilation with active constriction to light, generalized increase in body tone, decorticate posturing in response to painful stimuli and bilateral Babinski signs); elevated blood ammonia and increased liver enzyme activity; grade 3 or 4 EEG
Stage IV Deepening coma, persistent hyperventilation, tachycardia, further rostral-caudal progression of brainstem dysfunction with evidence of mid- to lower midbrain involvement (progressive loss of doll's head maneuver and response to ice water calorics, pupillary dilation with sluggish constriction in response to light, increased body tone with decerebrate rigidity and decerebrate posturing in response to painful stimuli and bilateral Babinski signs); improving hepatic dysfunction; grade 3 or 4 EEG
Stage V Cessation of spontaneous respiration, loss of all superficial and deep reflexes, lack of response to painful stimuli, and absence of pupillary response to light, doll's head maneuver and ice water calorics; minimal hepatic dysfunction; grade 5 or electrocerebral silent EEG

From Lovejoy, F.H., Jr., and Smith, A.L.: Reye's syndrome. *In* Hoekelman, R.S., Blatman, S., et al. (eds.): Principles of Pediatrics, Health Care of the Young. New York, McGraw-Hill, Inc., 1978.

ally waning. The patient is generally afebrile. Hyperventilation is commonly evident. Hepatomegaly is found in less than 40 percent of the older children but is almost uniformly present in patients younger than 1 year of age. Jaundice is absent. Irritability, lethargy, combativeness, or coma reflects the general neurologic status. Focal neurologic signs are absent unless intracranial pressure has become markedly elevated.

LABORATORY FINDINGS

Laboratory evaluation reveals abnormalities consistent with the multisystem nature of this disease. Serum glutamic–oxaloacetic transaminase (SGOT), and serum glutamic–pyruvic transaminase (SGPT) are markedly increased, but the degree of abnormality does not correlate with the severity of the disease. Serum ammonia levels are almost always elevated at the time of initial presentation, returning to normal over a 2- to 5-day period. Prolongation of prothrombin time is evident in most patients, although clinical signs of a bleeding diathesis are uncommon. In contrast to other liver function tests, bilirubin is usually normal, differentiating Reye's syndrome from the encephalopathy associated with fulminating hepatitis. Serum glucose is generally normal except in patients younger than 1 year of age when hypoglycemia is prevalent. Increases in blood urea nitrogen (BUN) and creatinine, if present, are the consequence of dehydration. Both serum carbon dioxide tension and bicarbonate level are decreased, the former secondary to hyperventilation and the latter as the result of organic acidemia. Arterial pH, however, is often normal, but it is dependent upon which aspect of the mixed acid–base disorder predominates. Serum amylase is elevated when pancreatitis occurs in association with Reye's syndrome. Other frequently found chemistry-related abnormalities include increased uric acid, creatine phosphokinase, and lactic dehydrogenase and decreased calcium and phosphate.

Complete blood counts are nonspecific, and platelet counts are normal. Cerebrospinal fluid (CSF) is unremarkable with regard to cell count and chemistries unless hypoglycemia is present and the CSF glucose is decreased as a consequence.

A percutaneous liver biopsy is often performed to firmly establish the diagnosis of Rey's syndrome, especially in atypical or recurrent cases and in patients younger than 1 year of age. Routine hemotoxylin–eosin-stained sections reveal swelling of hepatocytes, minimal inflammatory response, rare cell necrosis, and little, if any, cholestasis. Staining for lipid with Sudan black or oil red O reveals diffuse distribution of small fat droplets.

The electroencephalogram (EEG) is abnormal at the time of presentation, even in the early stages, revealing low voltage and slow wave activity. The degree of EEG abnormality corresponds to the severity of clinical involvement.

DIFFERENTIAL DIAGNOSIS

Infection, metabolic disorders, poisoning, drug overdose, pancreatitis, and fulminating hepatitis may present with an encephalopathy similar to that of Reye's syndrome. A lumbar puncture should be performed in all patients with acute changes in sensorium to evaluate the possibility of central nervous system infection. The presence of normal CSF protein and glucose (except in the hypoglycemic patient) and the absence of pleocytosis distinguish Reye's syndrome from meningitis and encephalitis. In young children, various combinations of hypoglycemia, hyperammonemia, elevated transaminases, and metabolic acidosis may be seen in a number of inborn errors of metabolism, including urea cycle disorders, isovaleric acidemia, glycogen storage disease, hereditary fructose intolerance, and carnitine deficiency. Although family history, occurrence of hyperbilirubinemia, and presence of abdominal organomegaly and other physical signs are helpful in differentiating these entities, additional evaluation in the form of liver biopsy, enzyme determinations, substrate challenges, or column chromatography is most often necessary to make a specific diagnosis. Ingestion of toxins such as lead, chlordane, methyl bromide, and isopropyl alcohol and overdoses of such drugs as salicylates and acetaminophen may be identified by history, high index of suspicion, and toxicology screen. Pancreatitis may present with alteration in mental status but is usually diagnosed by abdominal examination and the laboratory finding of hyperamylasemia. As noted previously, the absence of significant hyperbilirubinemia and jaundice differentiates Reye's syndrome from acute, fulminating hepatitis.

TREATMENT

Early recognition is essential, because prognosis correlates with the degree of neurologic impairment at the time of initial presentation. Although Reye's syndrome is a multisystem disease, the target organ that is principally responsible for morbidity and mortality is the central nervous system. When the diagnosis is established or suspected, the child should be admitted to a hospital with the capacity for intracranial pressure monitoring and intensive care nursing. Determination of the stage (Lovejoy classification) of severity is important in guiding the therapeutic regimen. General supportive measures alone may suffice for patients in the early stages (I and II), but the addition of specific treatment modalities for reduction of intracranial pressure will be required for those in the advanced stages (III, IV, and V). Patients in Stage II who have serum ammonia levels in excess of 300 mcg per dl are often treated as if they were in Stage III.

When a disease process has an unknown etiology and is characterized by numerous metabolic disturbances, the therapeutic approach is often directed at normalization of measured biochemical parameters. Historically, exchange transfusion, peritoneal dialysis, hemodialysis, and hypothermic total body "washout" have been used on this basis. To date, none of these procedures has been shown to be more beneficial than a combination of general supportive care and reduction of elevated intracranial pressure. Initial reports of improved outcome with these procedures may be attributed to general intensive care support or possibly to lack of consistent staging.

General Supportive Measures

Close monitoring of fluid and electrolyte status is mandatory. Because of the potential for emesis and depression of level of consciousness, the patient is made NPO. Fluids are administered at a reduced rate of 2/3 to 3/4 maintenance, with a goal of maintaining serum osmolality between 300 and 310 mOsm per kg. Beginning with patients in Stage II, more aggressive monitoring is required. A central venous line should be placed and a Foley catheter should be passed. Central venous pressure (CVP) should be kept at less than 5 cm of H_2O, while ensuring adequate tissue perfusion and urine output. Glucose is usually given as a solution of 10 percent dextrose, with the intention of maintaining serum glucose in the range of 150 to 200 mg per dl. Possibly due to a fundamental defect in oxidative metabolism, conventional rates of glucose administration (100 to 150 mg per kg per hr) may not be adequate to achieve these serum concentrations.

As much as 600 mg per kg per hr of glucose may be given to patients with Reye's syndrome and not produce renal spillage. The use of insulin in conjunction with the administration of glucose in an effort to maximize substrate utilization has not been shown to be more efficacious than glucose infusion alone. Provision of adequate energy substrate (glucose) becomes more important as the disease progresses. The electrolyte composition of the infusate should be sodium, 4 mEq per kg per day, and potassium, 4 to 6 mEq per kg per day, with half the potassium requirement given in the form of phosphate. Calcium supplementation is often necessary and is administered in the form of calcium gluconate, 200 mg per kg per day.

Coagulation studies should be obtained at regular intervals. Vitamin K, 1–5 mg IV, should be given on a daily basis. If there is prolongation of the prothrombin time or clinical evidence of a bleeding diathesis, fresh frozen plasma, 10 ml per kg, may also be required to restore hemostasis.

Hyperammonemia is managed by administering lactulose via a nasogastric tube in a dose of 0.5 gm per kg per hr until passage of loose stool occurs; the dose is then reduced to 0.25 gm per kg q6 to 8h. An alternative to lactulose is neomycin, 100 mg per kg per day, given nasogastrically (NG) in four divided doses. Specific attempts to lower ammonia by infusing ornithine, citrulline, or glutamine–arginine have not been shown to be clinically efficacious.

Temperature, often elevated on a central basis, should be maintained in the normal range by use of sponge baths and hypothermia blankets. Salicylates should not be used. The safety of acetaminophen in this condition is unknown.

Efforts should be made to keep the patient quiet and comfortable; agitation contributes to increases in intracranial pressure. Procedures such as lumbar puncture and placement of an arterial catheter should be preceded by administration of short acting sedatives and the use of local anesthetics. Similarly, chest physiotherapy, turning, and suctioning may require premedication.

Specific Therapy Directed at Increased Intracranial Pressure (Stages III, IV, and V)

Patients with Reye's syndrome classified in Stage III or higher should be electively intubated. Endotracheal intubation itself may exacerbate an already elevated intracranial pressure; therefore, it should be preceded by IV administration of thiopental, 4 mg per kg, and either succinylcholine, 1 mg per kg, or pancuronium, 0.1 mg per kg. Muscle paralysis is maintained, if necessary, and the patient is mechanically hyperventilated to achieve a Pa_{CO_2} in the range of 25 to 30 mm Hg. Sedation and analgesia are continued, because pain and anxiety raise intracranial pressure, even in the iatrogenically paralyzed patient. The patient should be kept with the head elevated to 30 to 45 degrees and in the midline position to facilitate cerebral venous drainage.

An intracranial pressure monitoring device should be placed over the nondominant hemisphere. Any coagulopathy should be corrected prior to placement. Selection of intraventricular catheter, subarachnoid bolt, or epidural monitor is dependent upon the clinical circumstance and the preference of the neurosurgeon. The goal of therapy is reduction of intracranial pressure to less than 20 mm Hg (preferably less than 15 mm Hg), with maintenance of cerebral perfusion pressure greater than 50 mm Hg. Modalities of treatment include hyperventilation, fluid restriction, use of osmotic and loop diuretics, hypothermia, and barbiturate-induced coma. These treatment modalities are discussed in detail in Chapter 12, Increased Intracranial Pressure. The use of corticosteroids to reduce intracranial pressure in Reye's syndrome has not been shown to be effective; this might be anticipated from the cytotoxic, rather than vasogenic, nature of the cerebral edema in this condition.

Although attention is appropriately directed at the management of elevations in intracranial pressure, it is important not to lose sight of other potential problems. Renal failure, gastrointestinal hemorrhage, the syndrome of inappropriate secretion of antidiuretic hormone (S–IADH), and pancreatitis are recognized complications that may occur. Initial temperature elevations are almost always of central origin, but the potential for bacterial superinfection in a host with multiple indwelling catheters is such that fever should be presumed to be of infectious origin. Appropriate cultures should be obtained, and suspected infection should be treated aggressively. Nutritional needs should not be overlooked; hyperalimentation consistent with the hepatic state should be administered.

PROGNOSIS

Mortality has clearly declined from initial reports of 80 percent to recent figures of 20 per-

cent. Morbidity, however, has been much more difficult to gauge. The biochemical and histologic abnormalities that characterize the illness are completely reversible and usually resolve fully. Hepatic function is usually restored to normal within 2 weeks of the acute illness. Neurologic examination generally reveals complete recovery. Psychometric testing, however, may reveal perceptual deficits, which may adversely influence school performance. The degree of encephalopathy during the clinical course of Reye's syndrome appears to correlate with the occurrence of neuropsychologic sequelae.

CASE PRESENTATION

This was the first hospital admission for a 10-month-old female who presented to the pediatric emergency room with lethargy and fever.

She was in her usual state of good health until 2 weeks prior to admission, at which time she suffered a 5-day course of diarrhea that resolved without consequence. On the day of admission, she was described by her parents as being irritable. While standing in her crib, crying, she fell over the rail and landed on the floor. Subsequent to this fall, she was lethargic and difficult to arouse.

Upon arrival in the emergency room, she was arousable with some difficulty and cried irritably when awake.

Examination and Test Results

Her vital signs were remarkable for a temperature of 103.4°F. Her liver was palpable 3 cm below the right costal margin. The neurologic examination was remarkable for the alteration in mental status, semi-purposeful response to pain, and sluggish pupillary responses.

The initial laboratory data revealed a normal CBC, coagulation profile, serum glucose, sodium, potassium, BUN, creatinine, and bilirubin. Serum transaminases were both elevated, with an SGOT (serum glutamic–oxaloacetic transaminase) of 414 mU/ml (N1 7–40) and an SGPT (serum glutamic–pyruvic transaminase) of 597 mU/ml (N1 3–36). A toxicology screen was negative. Her serum ammonia level was 279 mcg/dl. An amino acid screen was unremarkable. A lumbar puncture revealed acellular CSF with normal protein and glucose. Skull x-ray examination revealed a 3-cm linear fracture of the parietal bone. A cerebral CAT scan, obtained to evaluate the possibility of intracranial hemorrhage, was normal.

Based upon the clinical and laboratory findings, the diagnosis of Reye's syndrome was made. The child was admitted directly to the pediatric ICU. Her neurologic status was categorized as Stage II by the Lovejoy classification.

Problem List

Neurologic

Neurologic signs were evaluated hourly to assess progression of the disease. The head of the bed was elevated to 30 degrees to facilitate cerebral venous return. The pediatric neurosurgeon was notified of the potential need for an intracranial pressure monitoring device.

Metabolic

Because of the patient's young age and complicated presentation, a liver biopsy was performed. The tissue obtained was pale and yellow. Lipid accumulation and glycogen depletion, both of a mild degree, were evident. Electron microscopy revealed the mitochondrial changes characteristic of Reye's syndrome.

Serum glucose was maintained at a concentration greater than 150 mg/dl by infusing dextrose at a rate of 450 mg/kg/hr. Serum osmolality was followed every 8 hours.

Hyperammonemia was treated by the NG administration of lactulose in a dose of 0.5 gm/kg/hr. This dose was continued until the passage of loose stools, at which time the dose was decreased to 0.25 gm/kg q6h.

Serum electrolytes, including calcium and phosphate, were monitored every 4 to 6 hours.

Fluid Balance

Upon admission to the ICU, a central venous line was established and a Foley catheter was passed. Fluids were administered at a rate of 3/4 maintenance. Care was taken to ensure the continued delivery of glucose at the mg/kg/hr rate required to maintain the desired serum concentration. Urine output averaged 1 ml/kg/hr, with a specific gravity in the 1.020–1.025 range. Serum osmolality was 300 mOsm/kg.

Hematologic

Vitamin K, 1 mg, IV, was administered following admission to the ICU and prior to the liver biopsy. Fresh frozen plasma was kept available. Coagulation studies were obtained every 8 to 12 hours.

Infectious

Cultures of CSF, blood, and urine were obtained. A chest x-ray film was unremarkable. Because of the acute febrile state, antibiotic coverage was instituted, pending culture results. The fever was treated with the use of a hypothermia blanket. No antipyretics were administered.

The child remained in Stage II of the Lovejoy classification throughout Day 1 of hospitalization. The serum glucose and the coagulation profile remained within normal limits. On Day 2, the serum ammonia declined to the normal range. Clinically, the child showed improvement over the course of 48 hours and went on to a full recovery.

SUGGESTED READING

Boveke, McA., et al.: The hepatic lesion in Reye's syndrome. Gastroenterology 69:685, 1975.

Corey, L., Rubin, R.J., Bregman, D., and Gregg, M.B.: Diagnostic criteria for influenza B-associated Reye's syndrome: clinical vs. pathologic criteria. Pediatrics 60:702, 1977.

Corey, L., Rubin, R.J., and Hattwick, M.A.W.: Reye's syndrome: clinical progression and evaluation of therapy. Pediatrics 60:708, 1977.

DeLong, G.R., and Glick, T.H.: Encephalopathy of Reye's syndrome: a review of pathogenetic hypotheses. Pediatrics 69:53, 1982.

DeVivo, D.C., Keating, J.P., and Haymond, M.W.: Reye's syndrome: results of intensive supportive care. J. Pediatr. 87:875, 1975.

Huttenlocher, P.R.: Reye's syndrome in infancy. Pediatrics 62:84, 1978.

Lovejoy, F.H., Smith, A.L., Bresnan, M.J., et al.: Clinical staging in Reye's syndrome. Am. J. Dis. Child 128:36, 1974.

Marshall, L.F., Shapiro, H.M., Rauscher, A., and Kaufman, N.: Pentobarbital therapy for intracranial hypertension in metabolic coma: Reye's syndrome. Crit. Care Med. 6:1, 1978.

Surgeon General's advisory on the use of salicylates and Reye's syndrome. MMWR 31:289, 1982.

Trauner, D.A.: Treatment of Reye's syndrome. Ann. Neurol. 7:2, 1980.

Reye's Syndrome

Reye's syndrome is a multisystem disorder whose primary target organs are the liver and the brain. Hyperammonemia and encephalopathy represent the physiologic dysfunction of these organ systems. Of significance is the degree of central nervous system (CNS) impairment as determined by the Lovejoy classification method. Assessment parameters and treatment modalities will be determined according to the stage of involvement.

NEUROLOGIC

CNS pathology accounts for most of the morbidity and mortality resulting from Reye's syndrome.

Assess, Monitor, and Document

Headache
Vomiting
Blood pressure
Pulse
Respiratory rate and pattern
Intracranial pressure (if indicated)
Level of consciousness: lethargy, stupor, coma

Pupillary response
Reflexes
Motor responses
Posture
Response to therapeutic modalities to reduce intracranial pressure

Anticipate

Increased intracranial pressure
Lovejoy Classification (see Table 36–1): progression through stages

RESPIRATORY

Respiratory involvement usually occurs in response to the degree of CNS dysfunction.

Assess, Monitor, and Document

Respiratory rate and pattern
Breath sounds

Color
Arterial blood gases

Anticipate

Alteration in respiratory status
Hyperventilation
Respiratory insufficiency: hypoxia, hyper-

carbia, acidosis
Respiratory arrest

METABOLIC STATE

Reye's syndrome is characterized by significant metabolic disturbances. These biochemical and associated histologic abnormalities are usually completely reversible and resolve completely.

Assess, Monitor, and Document

Laboratory data
    Serum: ammonia, glucose
    Electrolytes, including calcium and phosphate

Osmolality
Liver enzymes

Anticipate

Hyperammonemia
Elevated liver enzymes

FLUID AND ELECTROLYTE BALANCE

Assess, Monitor, and Document

Weight
Urine output (including specific gravity)
Urine electrolytes and osmolality
Fluid intake: accurate administration of parenteral fluids (usually 2/3 to 3/4 maintenance)
Serum electrolytes and osmolality
Central venous pressure

Anticipate

Alteration in fluid and electrolyte balance
  To manage increased intracranial pressure
Acute renal failure
Syndrome of inappropriate secretion of antidiuretic hormone (S–IADH)

HEMATOLOGIC

Assess, Monitor, and Document

Signs of bleeding
  Bruises
  Petechiae
  Oozing from puncture sites
  Gastrointestinal: stools, NG drainage
Coagulation studies

Anticipate

Alteration in hematologic status
  Bleeding: gastrointestinal hemorrhage
  Disseminated intravascular coagulation

INFECTIOUS PROCESS

Assess, Monitor, and Document

Temperature
Signs of infection
  Catheter insertion sites: warm, red, edema
  Foley catheter
  Urine: description
    Pulmonary status
Respiratory rate
Breath sounds
  Secretions: description
Laboratory evidence of infection
  White blood count
  Culture and sensitivities

Anticipate

Persistent temperature elevation
Clinical evidence of infection
Laboratory evidence of infection

RESPONSE OF CHILD

Assess, Monitor, and Document

Developmental level: verbal, motor, psycho-social, cognitive

Behavioral response: fearful, anxious, tearful, angry
Response to nursing interventions

Anticipate

Emotional distress

RESPONSE OF FAMILY

Assess, Monitor, and Document

Behavioral response: anxious, fearful, verbal, angry
Level of understanding of child's condition

Expected outcome
Response to nursing interventions

Anticipate

Inability to cope
Family crisis

MIND SET

Assess, Monitor, and Document

Neurologic status
Respiratory status
Metabolic status
Fluid and electrolyte balance

Hematologic status
Infectious process
Response of child and family

Anticipate

Alteration in neurologic status
  Increased intracranial pressure: progression through Stages I–V of the Lovejoy classification
Alteration in respiratory status
  Hyperventilation
  Cessation of spontaneous respiration

Alteration in metabolic status
Alteration in fluid and electrolyte balance
Alteration in hematologic status
  Bleeding diathesis
Presence of infectious process
Emotional distress
Family crisis

37

Inborn Errors of Metabolism

CLAUDE SANSARICQ, M.D.

In an intensive care unit (ICU), secondary metabolic derangements are commonly encountered, but true life-threatening, primary metabolic derangements are infrequently seen. Their rarity explains the common delay in their recognition and identification.

In this chapter, some of the more commonly diagnosed primary metabolic diseases will be reviewed and their pathophysiology and treatment will be discussed.

In 1908, in his "Croonian Lecture," Sir Archibald Garrold coined the term *inborn errors of metabolism* to describe the group of diseases resulting from a genetic defect at the molecular level. Implied in the definition was a characteristic failure or absence of an enzyme system affecting either the apoenzyme in its constitution or its cofactor. This reflected a direct error either in translation or transcription of the genetic code. At times, however, a regulator or repressor gene may be involved.

PATHOPHYSIOLOGY

The genetic error translates into a metabolic block that may affect catabolism as well as anabolism of proteins, carbohydrates, fatty acids, nucleic acids, minerals, vitamins, energy metabolism, the respiratory chain, and membrane transport. Actually, no sphere may be considered out of reach of these type of disorders. The block is responsible for several different events, leading to varied clinical manifestations. The block may be manifested by:

1. Accumulation of precursor products such as phenylalanine in phenylketonuria (PKU), the branch chain amino acids in maple syrup urine disease (MSUD), ammonia in disorders of the urea cycle, and organic acids in disorders of short-chain fatty acid metabolism.

2. Shifting of metabolism to minor pathways, with further accumulation of abnormal metabolites.

3. Deficiency of breakdown products essential to certain metabolic pathways. Striking examples are seen in the variant form of PKU whereby neurotransmitters such as dopamine and serotonin cannot be synthesized in the central nervous system (CNS) because of the lack of the cofactor tetrahydrobiopterin. This cofactor is essential to the hydroxylation of phenylalanine, tyrosine, and tryptophan. Its absence results in dire consequences for the CNS.

4. Activation of the coagulation cascade with subsequent thromboembolic phenomena as seen in homocystinuria.

5. Secondary inhibition of independent enzyme systems. Elevation of plasma ammonia is noted in the course of propionic acidemia, isovaleric acidemia, or methylmalonic acidemia. Inhibition of carbamyl phosphate synthetase I by these organic acids is responsible for this secondary metabolic abnormality.

6. Nonavailability or decreased availability of certain substances such as glucose in the case of glycogen storage disease. The subsequent shift to other energy sources, such as oxidation of fatty acids, explains the ketoacidoses seen under these circumstances.

7. Lack of a feedback inhibition system. An example of this is the accumulation of blood cholesterol that occurs in the absence of cell membrane receptors in type II hypercholesterolemia.

8. Accumulation of certain substrates or products within organelles such as the lysosome. Under the heading "lysosomal diseases" are mucopolysaccharidosis, Pompe's, Tay-Sachs', Gaucher's, and Niemann-Pick's diseases.

9. Failure of a membrane transport system as seen in cystinuria, Hartnup disease, and certain types of albinism.

10. Absence of certain carrier proteins such as seen in Wilson's disease.

11. Finally, another mechanism at work may involve bacterial action in the gut on unabsorbed substrates, which later are modified and

absorbed and cause changes in metabolism. One or more of these mechanisms may be operative in all the disorders that are reviewed here.

Four groups of primary metabolic diseases with acute onset necessitating admission to an ICU can be recognized: the hyperaminoacidemias, the organic acidemias, the hyperammonemias, and the hypoglycemias (see Table 37–1).

Group I: The Hyperaminoacidemias

This group of diseases comprises several entities in which the enzymatic block occurs in the first or second step of the degradative pathway of a particular amino acid. The offending substance is the amino acid itself or a closely related substance. They are very rare occurrences.

Phenylketonuria

Among the amino acidopathies, phenylketonuria (PKU) is the most commonly encountered. However, it is in only two rare variants of this disease that seizures and neurologic deterioration may occur in the undiagnosed infant and possibly result in admission to the ICU. In this instance, the cofactor for phenylalanine hydroxylase, the enzyme which catalyzes the conversion of phenylalanine to tyrosine, is missing (Fig. 37–1). This cofactor, tetrahydrobiopterin (BH$_4$), is also necessary for two other enzymes, hydroxyphenylacetate oxidase and tryptophan hydroxylase of tyrosine and tryptophan metabolism, respectively.

In the absence of BH$_4$, the clinical symptoms develop. The lack of two important neurotransmitters in the CNS, serotonin and dopamine, is responsible for the development of clinical signs, which consist of irritability, feeding dif-

Table 37–1. Primary Metabolic Diseases with Acute Onset

Group I: The Hyperamino Acidemias
  The PKU variant (tetrahydrobiopterin deficiency)
  Maple syrup urine disease and its variants
  Nonketotic hyperglycinemia
  Homocystinuria
Group II: The Organic Acidemias
  Propionic acidemia
  Isovaleric acidemia (sweaty feet syndrome)
  Methylmalonic acidemia
  β-methyl crotonyl acidemia
  Methyl acetoacetate methyl β-hydrobutyric acidemia
  Glutaric acidemia
  Pyroglutamic acidemia
  The multiple carboxylase deficiency
  Lactic acidosis, with pyruvate carboxylase deficiency
  Pyruvate dehydrogenase deficiency
Group III: The Hyperammonemias
  Carbamyl phosphate synthetase I deficiency
  Ornithine transcarbamylase deficiency
  Citrullinemia
  Arginosuccinic acidemia
  Arginase deficiency
Group IV: The Hypoglycemias
  Glycogenosis types I, III, and VI
  Galactosemia
  Fructose intolerance
  1,6-diphosphofructose-phosphatase deficiency
  Leucine sensitive hypoglycemia

ficulty, hypotonia, uncontrollable seizures, and an inexorable downhill course if treatment is not appropriately instituted. The symptoms do not usually develop before the age of 2 months. The diagnosis is made by plasma column chromatography, which reveals a definite, but variable, elevation in phenylalanine levels; tyrosine and tryptophan remain within the normal range. Urine studied by high pressure liquid chromatography (HPLC) shows an increase in neo- and sepiapterin and a decrease in biopterin. A liver biopsy reveals either absence of dihydrobiopterin synthetase or dihydropterin reductase. In both instances, tetrahydrobiop-

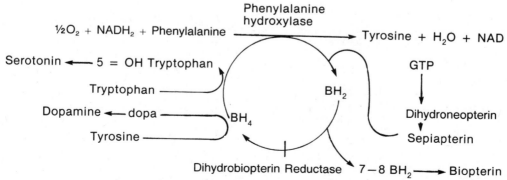

Figure 37–1. Biopterin metabolic pathways involved in the variant forms of PKU BH$_4$-tetrahydrobiopterin and BH$_2$-dihydrobiopterin.

terin will be missing. Recently, a screening procedure was developed that utilizes red blood cells collected on filter paper to study the reductase activity. This technique, in addition to the study of the pterins in the urine, allows for a definite diagnosis, eliminating the need for a liver biopsy.

Maple Syrup Urine Disease

The frequency of maple syrup urine disease (MSUD) has been estimated at 1:350,000 births but may in fact be even more rare. It has been noted in all ethnic groups and is probably the most commonly encountered primary metabolic disease in an ICU. It is an unusual disease because three amino acids are concomitantly affected by what appears to be the same enzyme defect. Normally, leucine, isoleucine, and valine, the branched-chain amino acids, are first transaminated before undergoing oxidative decarboxylation. This last step is the site of the enzymatic block in MSUD (Fig. 37–2). As a result of this defective decarboxylation, which requires thiamine, the branched-chain amino acids and their corresponding ketoacids accumulate in blood and tissues, causing the classic symptoms.

Progressive anorexia, with vomiting and irritability, is seen during the first week of life. The clinical signs quickly progress to lethargy, alternating periods of hypotonia, and stiffness leading to seizures, coma, respiratory failure and death. Acidosis may sometimes be seen as well as hypoglycemia. The typical odor of maple syrup can be found on the breath and in body secretions, including urine.

The odor of burnt or caramelized sugar is easily detectable in the urine, particularly if the specimen is warmed. This is the "nose test." An important diagnostic procedure, however,

is the dinitrophenylhydrazine (DNPH) test. A freshly voided urine specimen is mixed in equal volume with a 0.5 percent 2,4-DNPH in 2N HCl. Immediate clumping and precipitation of keto acids takes place, if present in large amounts, with enhancement of the maple syrup odor. If lesser amounts are present, a delay of up to 30 minutes in reading the results may be required before the test is declared negative. Drugs, such as antibiotics, may give a false-positive reaction; however, a control tube containing only 2N HCl would also show the same degree of clumping and precipitation. A 5 percent ferric chloride solution may give a bluish gray color when α keto acids are present. The diagnosis is confirmed by column chromatography of plasma, which shows elevation of the usual branched-chain amino acids in addition to allo-isoleucine, which is formed by enolization and transamination of excess keto-isoleucine.

Further evidence of plasma keto-acid elevations may be obtained by gas chromatography, but usually these are of the same magnitude as the amino acids. Determination of decarboxylase activity can be obtained from leukocytes or skin fibroblasts. The enzyme study is recommended, because the degree of remaining activity may allow the physician to recognize variant forms such as the intermediate, the intermittent, and the thiamine-responsive. The latter form may be totally correctable by addition of thiamine.

Homocystinuria

This autosomal recessive disease is characterized by a marfanoid habitus, ectopia lentis, thromboembolic phenomenon, malar flush with livido reticularis, telangiectasia, and osteoporosis. Mild to moderate mental retarda-

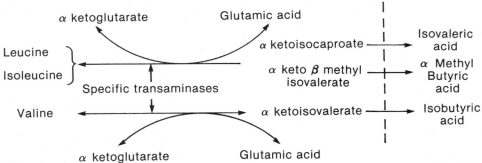

Figure 37–2. First steps in the degradative pathway of the branched-chain amino acids showing the block site in MSUD.

tion is seen in about 50 percent of the patients, and psychotic reactions are also reported. In an untreated patient, death due to thrombosis of large vessels and myocardial infarction is expected usually before the age of 25 years. Biochemically, the absence of cystathionine synthetase causes accumulation of methionine as well as homocystine and other derivatives (Fig. 37–3). Because of the high renal clearance of homocystine, large amounts are found in the urine, giving the disease its name. A B_6-dependent form is known and may be present in 50 percent of the patients. A rarer form involving the salvage pathway of methionine has been described, whereby N^5 methyltetrahydrofolate methyl transferase is inactive due to lack of its cofactors, methyl B_{12} and N^5 methyltetrahydrofolate. Patients with this disease may be admitted to an ICU because of thrombosis of cerebral or other major vessels and myocardial infarctions.

The diagnosis of homocystinuria is established by identifying a homocystine peak by column chromatography of the plasma. In the classical form, methionine is also elevated. A positive silver nitroprusside test in urine alkalinized with concentrated ammonium hydroxide is suggestive of the diagnosis.

Nonketotic Hyperglycinemia

The cleavage of the carboxyl group of glycine, involved in the synthesis of serine, by the enzyme serine hydroxymethyltransferase is defective in this disorder (Fig. 37–4). Serine hydroxymethyltransferase is normally present in large amounts in the brain and the liver. As a consequence, glycine accumulates in excessive amounts in the brain and cerebrospinal fluid (CSF). It is a potent inhibitory neurotransmitter at the synaptic level. Chronic exposure of neurons to high concentrations of glycine renders them insensitive to this inhibitory effect. The neurons are then predisposed to discharge excessively, leading to the intractable seizures that characterize the disease. Coma, respiratory failure, and death usually ensue in the first month of life. If the patient survives this period and can be weaned from a ventilator, he or she is usually hypotonic, blind, and mentally retarded. Acidosis is not a feature of this disease.

The diagnosis is established essentially by column chromatography of the CSF and plasma, which reveals a high glycine level. There is a greater degree of elevation in the CSF than that found in ketotic hyperglycinemia.

Management

In all the preceding disorders, the goals of treatment are: to remove the accumulated offending metabolites and prevent their reaccumulation; to supply any essential product that is deficient, because the enzymatic block cannot be corrected; to correct any secondary metabolic change that could be present, such as acidosis and hypoglycemia; to provide support in terms of calories, vitamins, fluid, electrolytes, and oxygen; and to control with medication any adverse symptoms such as seizures and thrombosis.

In the case of atypical phenylketonuria, the

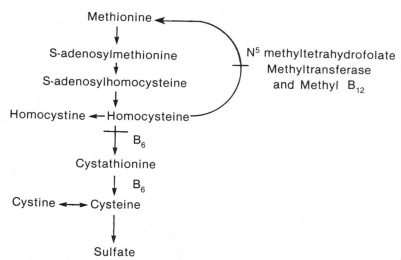

Figure 37–3. Simplified scheme of methionine degradation. The bars represent the site of the possible blocks in homocystinuria.

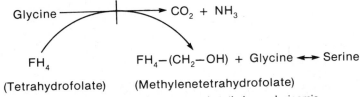

Figure 37–4. Enzymatic block in nonketotic hyperglycinemia.

essential task is to administer 10 mg of tetra-hydrobiopterin either orally or intramuscularly (IM). This constitutes a diagnostic test as well as a therapeutic maneuver. Phenylalanine levels are followed in the plasma. An abrupt drop establishes the diagnosis. Abatement of seizure activity will also be seen. Continuous treatment with this cofactor would be too expensive because of its limited availability. It is now produced only in Switzerland on a research basis. The possibility of using an available form of biopterin is currently being investigated. Treatment has, therefore, been limited to providing the patient with precursors of the neurotransmitters that he cannot synthesize, namely 5-hydroxytryptophan and dopa. Ten mg per kilogram of body weight of each compound is ordered in four divided doses around the clock. In addition, carbidopa is ordered at $^1/_{10}$ the dose of dopa. A controlled phenylalanine intake is also appropriate to maintain a normal plasma level of this amino acid.

For homocystinuria, a trial of vitamin B_6 at pharmacologic doses should be given. Up to 1000 mg per day has been used. Folate should also be given before reverting to an amino acid diet mixture in which methionine is given only at requirement levels while additional cystine is provided. The use of anticoagulants may be necessary in the therapy of embolic phenomenon. Management of cerebral or cardiac infarct should follow the routine protocols.

Patients with nonketotic hyperglycinemia may not benefit by any currently available medical therapy. Strychnine has been used, because it may reverse the actions of glycine at the synaptic level. This treatment has been a failure, because patients so treated remain profoundly retarded.

Maple Syrup Urine Disease

CASE PRESENTATION

Management of this disease will be illustrated by the following case:

A 10-day-old female infant was reported by the New York state screening test laboratory to have an elevated plasma leucine level. The parents, who were immediately alerted, brought the baby to the hos-

pital. She was the product of a full-term, uneventful pregnancy and a normal delivery. Birth weight was 7 lb. Apgar scores were 7 at 1 minute and 9 at 5 minutes. She had been on Similac since the initiation of feeding but quickly started vomiting and became irritable and anorexic. Upon the advice of the pediatrician, she underwent several changes in formula but with no success.

Examination and Test Results

Physical examination revealed a lethargic, dehydrated infant weighing 5.5 lb. She exhibited episodes of stiffness, opisthotonos, and rigidity, alternating with periods of relaxation. Moro's and grasp reflexes were absent, and pupils were dilated and nonreactive to light. A strong odor of burnt sugar was readily evident on her breath and in her secretions. The remainder of the physical was negative.

Laboratory investigations included the following: WBC = 15,300, hemoglobin = 17 gm %, hematocrit = 47.6 %, polys = 59, bands = 8, lymphs = 26, monos = 2, eos = 1, atypical lymphs = 4, and platelets = 529,000. Blood gases: pH = 7.28, PO_2 = 31 mm Hg, PCO_2 = 31 mm Hg, HCO_3^- = 14.3, and base excess = −10.5. Serum sodium = 138 mEq/L, potassium = 4.7 mEq/L, chloride = 105 mEq/L, HCO_3^- = 15.8 mEq/L, calcium = 4.7 mEq/L, and magnesium = 1.7 mEq/L. BUN = 8.7 mg/dl, creatinine = 1.3 mg/dl, glucose = 66 mg/dl, uric acid = 11 mg/dl, SGOT = 23, and SGPT = 28. Coagulation work-up was normal. A spinal tap showed clear fluid, no cells, a glucose of 47 mg/dl, and protein of 56 mg/dl. The urine was strongly positive to a 2,4-DNPH test, and plasma column chromatography revealed a leucine level of 69 mg/dl, an isoleucine of 11.2 mg/dl, a valine of 12.3 mg/dl, and an allo-isoleucine of 5.8 mg/dl, confirming the diagnosis of maple syrup urine disease.

The normal for these amino acids are 1.16 ± 0.27, 0.57 ± 0.18, 1.90 ± 0.39, and 0 mg/dl, respectively.

Problem List

Neurologic

The patient exhibited the typical encephalopathy described in maple syrup urine disease, that is, waxing and waning hypertonia, opisthotonos, dilated pupils, and disappearance of the primitive reflexes. Anticonvulsive therapy is not of much help, because only removal of the accumulated keto-acids can accomplish reliable seizure control.

Metabolic

The branched-chain amino acid elevation was impressive. Some degree of acidosis was present, with a venous pH of 7.28, a bicarbonate of 14.3, and a base excess of −10.5. An anion gap was not present. Hypoglycemia, though reported to be found in about 50 percent of the cases, was not present. However, the elevations of creatinine at 1.3 mg/dl and uric acid at 11 mg/dl are significant. The increase in creatinine is not a reflection of renal disease but is due to the presence of organic acids competing for elimination at the kidney level. This competition can also account for the uric acid elevation, although tissue breakdown and increased production of purines cannot be ruled out.

Correction of the acidosis requires the removal of the abnormal metabolites. Acutely, however, correction could be quickly achieved by IV administration of 8.4 percent sodium bicarbonate. Usually 3 mEq/kg are given, but the dose may be calculated from the base excess as follows: (base excess × 0.6 × kg) × 0.5. Additional amounts may be given as required.

Double volume exchange transfusion followed by peritoneal dialysis is the therapeutic regimen of choice in this case. Sufficient calories to prevent breakdown of tissue protein and reaccumulation of the acid must be provided. As the patient is dehydrated, the dialysate should not have a glucose concentration over 1.5 percent. The runs should be as frequent as every 15 minutes. The greater the gradient between plasma and dialysate, the greater the efficiency of the procedure, because equilibration is rapid. However, at low plasma levels, the efficiency is sharply reduced.

Fluid and Electrolyte Balance

The dehydration was the result of vomiting and poor feeding. Fluids should be administered to ensure a urine output of at least 0.5 to 1 ml/kg/hr. Adequacy of vascular volume must be established because peritoneal dialysis causes large fluid shifts and can contribute to an existing state of dehydration. Interpretation of urine output in the presence of continuous dialysis becomes more difficult; therefore, it is essential to monitor weight, central venous pressure, hematocrit, and the dialysis flow sheet at frequent intervals.

Nutritional

The rule in management of all metabolic diseases is to avoid a state of negative nitrogen balance at any cost. Appropriate amounts of calories (ideally 90–100 calories/kg) and essential amino acids must be provided. If feasible, glucose should be administered as a 10 percent solution. Intralipid should also be used beginning with 1 gm/kg, increasing to 2 gm/kg if tolerated. Small quantities of an amino acid mix, containing only essential amino acids except for the precursors of the offender (leucine, isoleucine, and valine), are prepared. Such a preparation is not yet available as an IV solution; therefore, it has to be given via a nasogastric (NG) tube in a volume not exceeding 10 ml q6h. The volume restriction is necessary because of the adynamic state of the intestine secondary to peritoneal dialysis. Too large a volume could cause regurgitation and aspiration. A reasonable starting dose of the amino acid mixture is 0.5 mg/kg, with progressive increases to 2 gm/kg. Addition of branched-chain amino acids will be calculated at their requirement level following normalization of their plasma levels.

Respiratory

The respiratory system is taxed by efforts to compensate for the metabolic acidosis. The patient tends to tire, and respiratory failure may occur spontaneously.

The burden of peritoneal dialysis, with the pressure it exerts against the diaphragm, may make a difficult situation worse. This patient did not require ventilatory assistance, because she was able to maintain normal blood gases.

Infectious

Prolonged peritoneal dialysis may increase the risk of infection by removing protective gamma globulin and perhaps introducing organisms in the peritoneal cavity. Thus, the prophylactic use of broad-spectrum antibiotics is of prime importance in the management of this patient. They may be administered via the dialysate or through the IV fluids (see Chapter 15, Acute Peritoneal Dialysis).

Course in the ICU

Seventy hours of dialysis were required to drop the elevated amino acids to normal limits. The neurologic status dramatically improved. Five hours after the start of dialysis, the pupils were reactive to light. Soon, the patient was crying. NG feeding started at 48 hours, and by day 9, the child was fed exclusively orally.

Group II: The Organic Acidemias

Disturbances of intermediary metabolism are responsible for accumulation of short-chain fatty acids and the acidosis encountered in the organic acidemias. The precursors of these organic acids are mainly the amino acids; the carbohydrates, to a certain extent, and the fats, to a lesser extent, are also evident. Characteristically, a defective enzyme in the degradative pathway of one or more amino acids is found. The most commonly encountered organic acidemias are propionic acidemia, methylmalonic acidemia, and isovaleric acidemia.

The precursors of propionic acid are methionine, isoleucine, threonine, odd-chain fatty acids, and the lateral chain of cholesterol. In the absence of propionic carboxylase, the conversion of propionic acid to methylmalonic acid (MMA) and succinic acid is no longer possible; thus, propionic acid accumulates in the blood and tissue (Fig. 37–5). In methylmalonic aci-

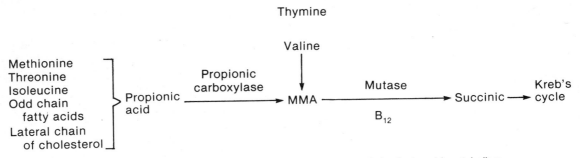

Figure 37-5. Schematic representation of propionic and methylmalonic acid metabolism.

demia, the site of the block is at the MMA mutase level, which uses vitamin B_{12} as a co-factor. MMA is not converted to succinic acid, and accumulation of both propionic acid and MMA are noted, because the propionic carboxylase reaction is reversible. In isovaleric acidemia, the precursor is leucine. The block is at the site of conversion of isovaleryl CoA to β-methylcrotonyl CoA, a reaction controlled by isovaleryl CoA dehydrogenase. The other organic acidemias are listed in Table 37–2, and the site of their enzymatic block is delineated in Figure 37–6.

Clinical Manifestations

The clinical manifestations of the organic acidemias are similar, and there are three classic presentations:

1. The neonatal form, which is usually severe and is seen a few days after feeding has been started.

2. The late onset form, which is seen mainly at the time of weaning when the protein intake increases.

3. The intermittent form, which manifests

Table 37-2. Organic Acidemias

Precursors	Accumulated Product	Missing Enzyme
Isoleucine	Methylacetoacetate Butanone	Methylacetoacetyl-CoA β-keto-thiolase
Isoleucine Methionine Threonine Odd-chain fatty acid Lateral chain of cholesterol	Propionic acid	Propionyl CoA carboxylase or pro-pionyl-CoA biotin synthetase
Isoleucine Methionine Threonine Odd-chain fatty acid Lateral chain of cholesterol Thymine Valine	Methylmalonic acid (MMA) Propionic acid	Methylmalonic CoA racemase or mutase Adenosyl B_{12} reductase
Leucine	Isovaleric acid methylcrotonyl-gly-cine (urine)	Isovaleryl CoA dehydrogenase methylcrotony CoA carboxylase
Lysine	Glutaric acid	Glutaryl CoA dehydrogenase Glutaconyl CoA decarboxylase
Glutathione	Proline Pyroglutamic acid	5-oxoprolinase
Various amino acids CHO as fructose galactose	Pyruvic acid Lactic acid	Pyruvate dehydrogenase Pyruvate carboxylase G-6 phosphatase 1,6-diphosphofructose-phosphatase

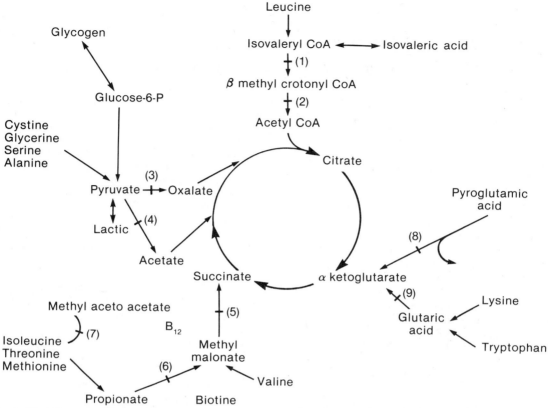

Figure 37–6. Organic acidemias. The bars represent the site of the enzymatic blocks. The numbers indicate the missing enzyme: (1) Isovaleryl CoA dehydrogenase, (2) β Methyl crotonyl carboxylase, (3) Pyruvate carboxylase, (4) Pyruvate dehydrogenase, (5) Methyl malonic mutase, (6) Propionyl CoA carboxylase, (7) α Methyl aceto acetyl CoA β ketothiolase, (8) 5 Oxoprolinase, and (9) Glutaryl CoA dehydrogenase.

itself during periods of stress, such as surgery and infection.

Vomiting is one of the most notable symptoms. Acidosis is present, in contrast to the alkalosis found with vomiting secondary to pyloric stenosis. The patient becomes dehydrated. Ketosis is also usually present, and in certain instances, specific odors may be elicited, identifying the metabolic error. A well-known syndrome characterized by the odor of sweaty feet or pungent cheese is isovaleric acidemia. A cat urine smell raises the possibility of β-methylcrotonyl acidemia. Tachypnea is a companion of the acidosis. If undiagnosed, this situation quickly progresses to coma, often with seizures, and death. If dehydration and acidosis are corrected, the patient quickly improves and may not show signs of illness, because he or she may spontaneously restrict protein intake. Eventually, another bout occurs. As a result of poor caloric and protein intake, failure to thrive may be seen. Mental retardation may be the consequence of repeated insults to the central nervous system. Floppiness is also a common feature.

Organic acidemias are rare. No accurate incidence statistics are available, but they may be as rare as 1:500,000. All are autosomal recessive.

Severe acidosis with an anion gap in the presence of vomiting is the first clue to the diagnosis, particularly if a fruity odor is detected in body secretions or on breath. Blood and urine should be immediately studied on column and gas chromatography for identification of the abnormal metabolites responsible for the acidosis. Propionic acid is detected in propionic acidemia, MMA, and in methylmalonic acidemia, and isovaleric acid in isovaleric acidemia.

Column chromatography will not reveal any elevation of the plasma levels of the precursors, but glycine may be higher than normal in the so-called ketotic glycinemias, that is, propionic and methylmalonic acidemia. When lactic and pyruvic acids also accumulate, alanine increases, because an equilibrium exists between these three compounds. Other laboratory findings may be hyperammonemia, hypoglycemia, hyperuricemia, hypocalcemia, and pancytopenia. Thrombocytopenia may be so marked as to suggest sepsis, especially in the neonatal period.

Management

The management is the same for all the preceding disorders. The following case history is presented as an example of management of organic acidemias.

CASE PRESENTATION

J.C., a 17-day-old black male, was transferred to our medical center in a deep coma.

The infant was the product of an uneventful pregnancy and a vaginal delivery. Birth weight was 8 lb. Apgar scores were 8 and 9. He was breast-fed and left the hospital on the fourth day of life. At 13 days of life, he began to feed poorly, became progressively lethargic, and developed a poor cry. By 16 days of life, he was stuporous and had poor urine output and a peculiar body odor. With severe dehydration, he was admitted to a local hospital. His weight had decreased to 6.5 lb.

A sepsis work-up was done, and the child was started on ampicillin and kanamycin. Multiple laboratory abnormalities were noted, including a WBC of 4,100 cells/mm³, with 5 percent polymorphonuclear neutrophiles and 95 percent lymphocytes, a hematocrit of 44.4 percent, a hemoglobin of 14.4 gm/dl, and a platelet count of 17,000. The blood pH was 7.31, with the following electrolytes: sodium = 152 mEq/L, potassium = 9.1 mEq/L, chloride = 115 mEq/L, carbon dioxide = 7 Eq/L, and calcium = 3.1 mEq/L. Serum glucose was 118 mg/dl, total protein was 6.5 gm/dl, and total bilirubin was 2.6 mg/dl. A coagulation profile was within normal range. Urinalysis was positive for large amounts of ketones, slight albuminuria, and microscopic hematuria. A spinal tap showed no cells, a glucose of 74 mg/dl, and a protein level of 158 mg/dl. The patient was hydrated, the hypocalcemia and acidosis were partially corrected, and he was transferred to our hospital.

Family History

The family history was significant in that a 19-month-old female sibling died in a state of severe acidosis, dehydration, and coma. Her body fluid emitted a peculiar odor, which was unidentified at that time. Her history was pertinent for multiple bouts of dehydration. During her last admission, she had a blood sugar of 186 mg/dl, an SGOT of 525 I.U., and an LDH (lactate dehydrogenase) of 595 I.U. These results led to a diagnosis of diabetic ketoacidosis (DKA), and she was unsuccessfully treated with insulin. The possibility of Reye's syndrome was also considered. An autopsy was unrevealing as to the cause of death.

Physical Examination and Test Results

Upon admission, the child was comatose and had intermittent tonic and clonic seizures. A pungent, cheesy odor was readily discernible from his breath and blood. The initial laboratory tests showed the following: ABG: pH = 7.55, PO_2 = 94 mm Hg, PCO_2 = 17 mm Hg, HCO_3^- = 15, and base excess of −3. Serum sodium = 148 mEq/L, potassium = 4.1 mEq/L, chloride = 118 mEq/L, HCO_3^- = 17 mEq/L, BUN = 14 mg/dl, creatinine = 1.1 mg/dl, Ca^{++} = 6.8 mg/dl, WBC = 1650, hemoglobin = 11.3 gm/dl, hematocrit = 32.5 percent, bands = 2, polys = 7, lymphs = 87, monos = 4, and platelets = 31,000. The ammonia level was 188 µg/dl. Plasma column chromatography showed an elevated glycine level, and gas chromatography revealed a level of isovaleric acid of 845 µgm/ml in the plasma and 700µg/ml in the CSF (normal: less than 1 µg/ml for blood and 0 in the CSF).

Problem List

Neurologic

Because of the normal spinal tap, the normal or elevated blood sugar level, and the extremely high concentration of isovaleric acid in the blood and CSF, the diagnosis of isovaleric acidemia with metabolic encephalopathy is undeniable.

Metabolic

The initial severe acidosis was treated by the infusion of bicarbonate and had shifted to a compensated state by the time of transfer. However, removal of isovaleric acid and reversal of acidosis should be accomplished by exchange transfusion and peritoneal dialysis, often in combination. Hemodialysis has also been used, but experience with this procedure in infants is limited, and it is not readily available in all medical centers. In this patient, double-volume exchange transfusion was performed, followed by peritoneal dialysis.

Elevation of ammonia up to 188 µg/dl was noted and was believed to be due to an inhibitory effect of the isovaleric acid on carbamyl phosphate synthetase I, the first enzyme of the urea cycle. This elevation of ammonia is of no clinical importance and will resolve with the removal of the isovaleric acid.

Fluid and Electrolyte Balance

Dehydration. The dehydration was severe and was partially corrected before transfer. Continuation of hydration, with at least one and a half times the volume of calculated maintenance, would be appropriate. A ¹/₅ normal sodium chloride solution would provide sodium maintenance. Sodium given as bicarbonate for correction of acidosis must be considered in maintenance calculations.

Hyperkalemia. Hyperkalemia is a companion of acidosis. Potassium leaves the cells and is eliminated as a diphosphate salt for formation of titratable acid. Any plasma excess can easily be removed by peritoneal dialysis (see Chapter 15, Acute Peritoneal Dialysis).

Hypocalcemia. Hypocalcemia is also a reflection of the acidosis. It was originally noted and appropriately corrected. Usually a dose of 200 mg/kg of a 10 percent calcium gluconate solution is administered IV. One should pay close attention to this problem, because tetany, seizures, and cardiac dysrhythmias can develop, further complicating the neurologic status.

Hyperosmolar State. The elevation of blood sugar level is not of particular significance here but theoretically could aggravate the neurologic status of the patient. It is believed to be the expression of stress and possibly the result of a larger amount of glucose than the body can immediately assimilate. Theoretically, this hyperglycemia could increase urine volume and contribute to dehydration. Adjustment of the IV glucose concentration to 5 or 2.5 percent should be considered.

Nutritional

In essence, the management at this point does not differ from that of Case History I except that the amino acid precursor to isovaleric acid is leucine. Therefore, only leucine should be removed from the amino acid mixture that is specially prepared for these patients. Commercially available preparations for the treatment of maple syrup urine disease called *MSUD-Aid* or *Milupa MSUD* could be used with addition of valine and isoleucine to meet the patient's requirements for these amino acids. At times, it is possible to offer a proprietary formula such as Similac or Enfamil, calculated to offer only 1.5 to 1.8 gm of protein/kg of body weight. Leucine supplementation to requirement level will be necessary after reduction of the patient's isovaleric acid levels to less than 1 mg/dl.

Respiratory

Respiratory assessment should not differ from that of patients with maple syrup urine disease. In this case, a ventilator was necessary.

Hematologic

Thrombocytopenia and neutropenia are known to occur in isovaleric acidemia. In this case, the thrombocytopenia was quite impressive (17,000) and suggested the possibility of sepsis or disseminated intravascular coagulation (DIC), both of which were ruled out. With supportive therapy, platelet transfusion, and removal of the isovaleric acid, the hematologic picture will normalize. Fortunately, this effect is temporary.

Infectious

Newborns are prone to sepsis. The neutropenia created by the action of isovaleric acid on the bone marrow may further endanger the neonate. Prolonged peritoneal dialysis enhances this possibility.

Coverage with broad-spectrum antibiotics is mandatory.

The treatment course is outlined in Figure 37–7.

Note: The use of glycine at the oral dose of 250 mg/kg has been advocated for enhancement of isovaleric acid elimination in the urine as isovalerylglycine. This procedure has been effective mainly as a prophylactic means during periods of stress or infection. Such an approach to therapy has no place in the management of the other organic acidemias such as MMA or propionic acidemia.

Group III: The Hyperammonemias

The urea cycle is outlined in Figure 37–8. In brief, six enzymes, including N–acetyl-glutamyl synthetase (N–AGA), carbamyl phosphate synthetase I (CPS I), ornithine transcarbamylase (OTC), arginosuccinic synthetase, arginosuccinic lyase, and arginase, are involved in the formation of this waste product of protein metabolism. The first three enzymes are mitochondrial; the others are cytosolic. Only the last four truly contribute to the urea cycle. Carbamyl phosphate is the product of the condensation of ammonia, bicarbonate, and adenosine triphosphate (ATP) in the presence of magnesium and N-acetyl glutamine. This latter substance is essential to the activation of the enzyme CPS I, which is also stimulated by arginase. CPS II, which exerts only $1/10$ of the activity of CPS I, utilizes glutamine as a source of ammonia and serves in the synthesis of pyrimidines. It is a cytosolic enzyme. Carbamyl phosphate reacts with ornithine to produce citrulline under the catalytic action of OTC. This compound combines with aspartic acid to form arginosuccinic acid, which yields fumarate and arginine. These two reactions are under the enzymatic action of arginosuccinic synthetase and lyase, respectively. Arginine is then split by arginase into urea and ornithine, thereby closing the cycle. The distribution of the different enzymes of the urea cycle can be seen in Figure 37–8.

Clinical Manifestations

The primary hyperammonemias seen in pediatric patients usually have two classical presentations. One is seen in the immediate neonatal period; the other is of delayed onset, but is usually seen not later than 9 years of age. The first clinical picture is associated with severe enzymatic deficiency interrupting any of the enzymatic steps of the cycle except the last one.

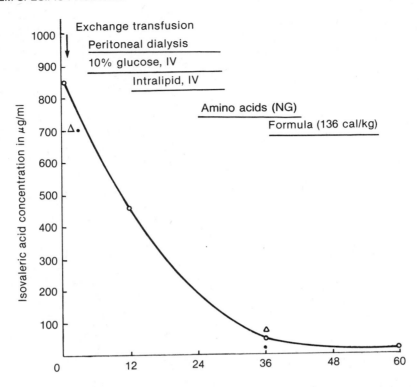

Figure 37-7. Effect of therapy on isovaleric acid concentration on serum (o), dialysate (•), and C.S.F. (cerebrospinal fluid; Δ).

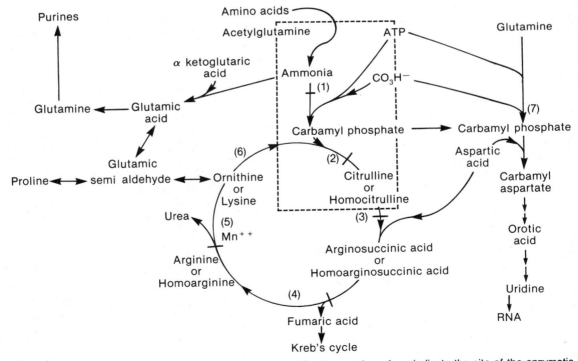

Figure 37–8. The urea cycle and some alternate pathways. The bars and numbers indicate the site of the enzymatic blocks: (1) Carbamyl phosphate synthetase (CPS I), (2) Ornithine transcarbamylase, (3) Arginosuccinic acid synthetase, (4) Arginosuccinic lyase, (5) Arginase, (6) Presumed defect of transmitochondrial membrane transport, and (7) Carbamyl phosphate synthetase (CPS II).

The delayed onset type of hyperammonemia presents when there is an increase in dietary protein or during periods of stress or infection. Patients with this type usually tend to avoid protein-rich food and often present with anorexia and failure to thrive. There is also a history of bouts of vomiting and dehydration, leading to lethargy, stupor, coma, and death. Neonatal retardation is one of the features encountered. Diffuse EEG abnormalities are mainly seen during a crisis. Among the various clinical syndromes, the picture varies only in a few aspects. Trichorexis nodosa is noted in about 50 percent of the cases of arginosuccinic acidemia. Hepatosplenomegaly may also be seen as a constant feature of the neonatal form of this disease. Pulmonary hemorrhage has been reported in citrullinemia, and a spastic diplegia with tiptoe walking has been noted in hyperargininemia. All hyperammonemias are autosomal recessive except OTC deficiency, which is transmitted through a dominant sex-linked mode of inheritance. In this last entity, males tend to die early in life and surviving females present with varied symptoms, depending on their remaining degree of enzyme activity.

Evidence of the clinical diagnosis may be suggested by the history and physical examination. Confirmation should be obtained by determination of plasma ammonia, electrolytes, blood gases, and column chromatography. In the presence of an elevated plasma ammonia concentration, that is, over 100 μg per dl in the newborn (normal: 30 to 50 μg/dl), acidosis, and an increased anion gap, the diagnosis is likely to be one of organic acidemia, such as propionic, methylmalonic, or lactic acidemia. In the absence of acidosis, column chromatography will be valuable in detecting either a deficit or an increase of certain products such as citrulline arginine or arginosuccinic acid. This latter amino acid is not normally identifiable in the blood. The flow chart (Fig. 37–9) will identify the site of the enzymatic block. Glutamic acid, glutamine, alanine, and sometimes lysine are usually elevated in all types of hyperammonemia. In addition, arginine is elevated in argininemia, citrulline, and arginosuccinic acid, and its anhydrides are elevated in arginosuccinic aciduria, and citrulline alone is elevated in citrullinemia. Further tests to delineate blocks in the initial steps of the cycle could include orotic acid analysis in blood and urine, paper chromatography for dibasic amino acids in urine, protein loads, and biopsy of liver and

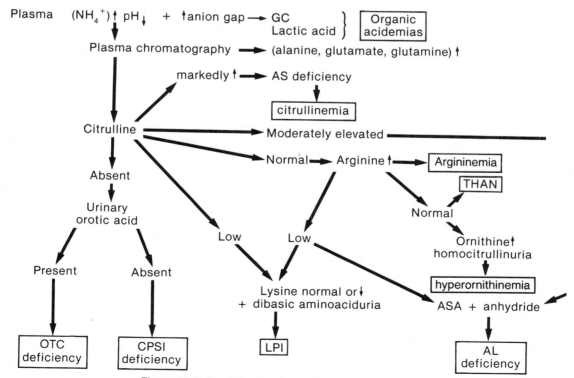

Figure 37–9. Flow chart for the study of hyperammonemia.

skin for enzyme determination (Table 37–3). Carbamyl phosphate is a precursor to orotic acid, uridine, and uracil synthesis. This is a key point for the differentiation of the first two steps of the urea cycle enzyme deficiency states from OTC deficiency. In this latter condition, production of orotic acid is considerably increased due to the leak from mitochondria of excess carbamylphosphate, which reacts in the cytosol with aspartic acid to produce carbamyl aspartate, the first step toward pyrimidine synthesis. By contrast, in CPS I and N-AGA synthetase deficiencies, there is no excessive production of orotic acid. The differentiation between these last two conditions can only be made by enzyme studies on liver biopsy specimens.

Dibasic aminoaciduria is described with argininemia, where it can simulate cystinuria. This can also be seen in ornithinemia and protein lysinuric intolerance (PLI), but in this last case, lysine is the predominant amino acid whereas cystine concentration is within normal range. Transient hyperammonemia of the newborn (THAN) may not reveal any specific abnormalities on plasma or urine chromatography, but increased production of orotic acid may be noted. Prematures and neonates with anoxia and respiratory distress and those receiving parenteral alimentation are at increased risk for this transient syndrome. Liver biopsy will show normal activity of the urea cycle enzymes. It is possible that delay in maturation or inhibition of N-AGA may be responsible for the accumulation of ammonia. The clinical evolution of the case with the development of complete tolerance for protein will confirm the diagnosis.

Table 37–3. Amino Acid Mixture for Treatment of Hyperammonemias

Amino Acid*	Arginase Deficiency	OTC Deficiency
L-Arginine	0	15.22
L-Aspartic acid	—	15.22
L-Cystine	4.9	3.41
L-Histidine	4.7	3.65
L-Isoleucine	13.0	9.13
L-Leucine	16.2	11.57
L-Lysine	13.5	7.98
L-Methionine	4.9	3.41
L-Phenylalanine	9.7	7.31
L-Threonine	9.7	6.7
L-Tryptophan	2.4	1.83
L-Tyrosine	9.7	6.7
L-Valine	11.3	7.92

*Measured in gm/dl

Management

The treatment of hyperammonemias should be aggressive and should be aimed at the rapid removal of ammonia while preventing further accumulation.

Again, peritoneal dialysis has been a very effective way of lowering plasma ammonia levels. A high degree of correlation exists between the plasma and dialysate ammonia level (r = 0.947882 p < 0.001; Fig. 37–10). However, when plasma ammonia levels are very high, a combination of double-volume exchange transfusion and peritoneal dialysis is recommended. Hemodialysis may be a quicker way to remove the ammonia, but it has been reported in only a few cases and is still being investigated.

Theoretically, drugs used to bypass the urea cycle should be effective. Phenylacetate, combining with glutamine to yield phenylacetyl glutamine, would eliminate as much as 2 moles of nitrogen and should be as effective as urea. Unfortunately, this drug may cause dizziness and nausea, even at the first dose. Sodium benzoate reacting with glycine is eliminated as hippurate and rids the body of 1 mole of nitrogen. However, it may inhibit the enzyme N-AGA, thus blocking the urea cycle. Sodium benzoate is contraindicated in the newborn period; it yields better results in older children. The use of lactulose to eliminate the intestinal content and prevent further absorption of ammonia made from the bacterial flora is an adjuvant that could be of help. The dose usually recommended is 0.2 to 0.4 gm per kg q 6–8 h.

CASE PRESENTATION

L.T. is a 4-year-old female, weighing about 30 lb and measuring about 35 inches, who was admitted to a local hospital with a chief complaint of altered state of consciousness.

The patient was well but unusually sleepy for the 2 days preceding admission. She complained of mild abdominal pain for which she was given a dose of two baby aspirin. She became irritable and lapsed into a state of lethargy alternating with combativeness. Although arousable, she was not able to follow commands. There was also the possibility that she might have consumed some berries that she had been found playing with the day before admission.

Past history included infrequent previous episodes of stupor. She had eaten very poorly all her life, refusing protein-rich foods such as meat, milk, eggs, and cheese.

Family History

The family history is relevant in that the mother avoided the same protein-rich foods and has mainly

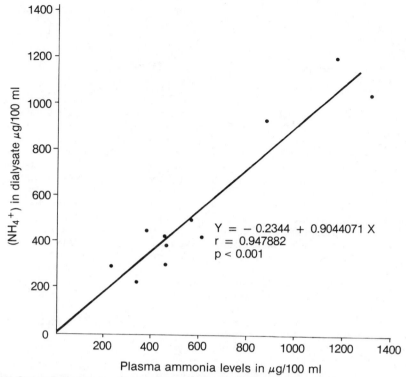

$$Y = -0.2344 + 0.9044071\ X$$
$$r = 0.947882$$
$$p < 0.001$$

Figure 37–10. Correlation between ammonia levels in plasma and dialysate in a patient with hyperammonemia.

been a vegetarian. She was found to have had hypofibrinogenemia during her pregnancies. The first male child of the family died at 2 days of age, with an unclear neurologic picture. A second brother has had a history of poor school performance and repeated episodes of vomiting, necessitating IV hydration. Another brother is normal. The father is healthy and well.

Examination and Test Results

The physical examination revealed an afebrile 4-year-old female who was at less than the third percentile of development for height and weight. BP = 90/60 mm Hg, P = 110 beats/min, RR = 24 breaths/min, and T = 98° F. She was comatose but responded to noxious stimuli. Her face appeared flushed, the pupils were dilated and nonresponsive to light, the corneal reflexes were present, and the discs were sharp. No focal neurologic signs were noted. There was no hepatosplenomegaly, and the remainder of the physical examination was within normal limits.

The laboratory investigations in the local hospital disclosed the following: hematocrit = 36 percent, WBC = 9,500, and platelets = 335,000. ABG: pH = 7.4, P_{CO_2} = 32, P_{O_2} = 100 mm Hg, HCO_3^- = 19.7, CO_2 = 20.7, and O_2 saturation = 97.6 percent, Na^+ 145 = mEq/L, K^+ = 3.9 mEq/L, Cl = 110 mEq/L, CO_2 = 24 mEq/L, Ca^{++} = 9.8 mg/dl, PO_4 = 4.5 mg/dl, total bilirubin = 0.6 mg/dl, glucose = 119 mg/dl, BUN = 13 mg/dl, creatinine = 0.5

mg/dl, LDH = 226 U, CPK (creatine phosphokinase) = 31 U, SGPT = 12 U, SGOT = 18 U, total protein = 6.3 gm, albumin = 4.3 gm, and ammonia = 194 μg. Coagulation profile: normal. Urinalysis: specific gravity = 1.035, positive for ketones and salicylate. Serum: ketone positive, but no salicylate detected. A spinal tap was normal, as was a cerebral CAT scan.

An infusion of D2.5W/0.45 percent NaCl, with 10 mEq of KCl for 500 ml was started at the rate of 30 ml/hr. Blood specimens were drawn for repeat tests, toxicologic survey, and gas and column chromatography. A challenge Narcan dose test was administered, with no effect. The patient rapidly improved with supportive therapy. She was responding to verbal stimuli by 10 hours after admission and was fully awake 4 hours later. The ammonia level on transfer was 154 μgm/dl and 139 μgm/dl the next day. All other laboratory data remained within normal limits. The toxicologic test was negative for toxic material, including atropine. The column chromatography study revealed elevation of glutamic acid, glutamine, and alanine.

Problem List

Coma

Coma presents a diagnostic problem. The age of the child, the clinical picture of flushed face and dilated pupils, the possible ingestion of berries, which could have contained atropine or atropine-like substances, and the quick progression to coma make acute intoxication a likely possibility. The child, however, had normal vital signs, was afebrile, and had a negative toxicologic screen. Morphine classically causes pinpoint pupils, but combined drug intoxication of the type seen with Lomotil was also ruled out by the Narcan test injection. The association of Reye's syndrome and aspirin ingestion, although seen in association with varicella or influenza, is currently being investigated. Such a diagnosis would not be of major concern here, however, although it was the provisional diagnosis at the local hospital. The absence of hepatomegaly, the presence of normal levels of hepatic enzymes, normoglycemia, and a normal coagulation profile make this diagnosis untenable. For the same reasons, the possibility of hepatitis is also rejected. An infectious encephalitis, although unlikely on clinical grounds, was ruled out by the spinal fluid examination, which revealed clear fluid with no pressure elevation and no increase in cell count, protein, and glucose. A traumatic or vascular lesion of the CNS was ruled out by the absence of focal signs, a normal spinal tap, and a normal CAT scan.

The remaining possibility is that of coma due to a metabolic encephalopathy not involving acid-base balance but related to ammonia elevation without hepatitis (see next section).

Persistent Elevation of Ammonia

The first ammonia level was 192 μgm/dl (normal: 30–50 μgm/dl), and it subsequently decreased to 154 μgm/dl and 130μgm/dl while the child was clinically improving.

Plasma column chromatography showed a striking elevation of glutamine, in the range of 25 mg/dl (normal: up to 15 mg/dl), and of alanine in the presence of a low arginine concentration and a normal citrulline. This pattern indicates a block in the metabolism of ammonia, either at the first or second step of the urea cycle. Further testing for urinary orotic acid elimination and later biopsy for determination of urea cycle enzyme activity would be necessary to firmly establish the diagnosis. The possibility of protein loading could also be considered. The child's attitude toward food points to a form of self-treatment often seen in these cases. The history of the mother's similar aversion to protein-rich food, the sex of the child, and the death of the first boy of the family at 2 days of age in a confused clinical picture favor the diagnosis of OTC deficiency, because it is known to be a sex-linked disorder.

Failure to Thrive

Although she was normal at birth, this child has been developing below the third percentile for height and weight. This is obviously the consequence of the discriminating anorexia she unconsciously developed as a conditioned reflex, a type of defense reaction. As a result, she could not regulate protein intake to meet her needs and a state of undernutrition or malnutrition slowly developed.

The diagnosis was eventually confirmed in the mother by administration of a protein load and in the child by study of orotic acid excretion in the urine and by liver biopsy, which showed a very low activity of OTC.

Management

In this case, the management was easy. The diagnosis was very difficult because of the atypical presentation and the rather low ammonia level. Only supportive therapy was called for, because at this level, there would not be a sufficient gradient to remove the ammonia by either exchange transfusion or peritoneal dialysis. Early administration of an appropriate amount of calories and reintroduction of a small quantity of protein, 0.5 gm/kg slowly increased to 1 gm/kg/day, are all that would be required at this stage. Amino acid composition of an appropriate diet is illustrated in Table 37–3. The use of sodium benzoate or phenylacetate would be unnecessary for the same reasons that were previously given.

Group IV: The Hypoglycemias

By definition, hypoglycemia is diagnosed when the blood sugar level is under 40 mg per dl in children, under 30 mg per dl in newborns, and under 20 mg per dl in premature infants. In asymptomatic patients, confirmation of low blood-glucose levels is required to avoid laboratory errors.

The etiology of the hypoglycemias are described in the following sections, and the pathways are illustrated in Figure 37–11.

Glycogen Storage Diseases

The clinical presentation of glycogen storage disease Types I, III, and VI is often indistinguishable and these three types are the only ones usually seen in an ICU. Hepatomegaly and stunted growth are prominent. Episodes of hypoglycemia, lactic acidosis, hyperlipidemia, hyperuricemia, and acetonuria are common.

Type I

Intolerance to fasting is most severe with Type I. The missing enzyme is G-6-phosphatase, the key enzyme in the degradative pathway of glycogen before free glucose is released into the circulation. As a consequence, glycogen remains in the cell and hypoglycemia ensues. Failure of this system causes the body to mobilize fatty acids as a source of energy, hence the production of ketones. Lactic acid production results from the shifting of metabolism to

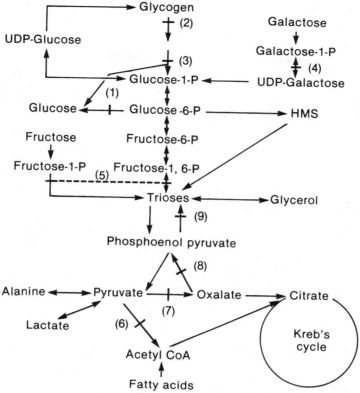

Figure 37-11. Pathway of the carbohydrate metabolism. The bars and numbers identify the enzymatic blocks referred to in the text: (1) Glucose-6-phosphatase, (2) Liver phosphorylase, (3) Amylo-1,6-glucosidase, (4) Galactose-1-phosphate uridyl transferase, (5) Fructose aldolase B, (6) Pyruvate dehydrogenase, (7) Pyruvate carboxylase, (8) Phosphoenol pyruvate carboxykinase (PEPCK), and (9) 1,6-Diphosphofructose phosphatase.

the hexose monophosphate shunt, with overproduction of reduced nicotinamide adenine dinucleotide phosphate (NADPH), which reduces pyruvate into lactate. Other mechanisms have been proposed, but this point requires further investigation.

Type III

In Type III, or Cori's disease, the missing enzyme is the debrancher (amylo-1,6-glucosidase). Partial glycogen degradation through the action of phosphorylase occurs, which is why children with this disease tend to tolerate a somewhat longer fasting period. Muscles and liver are usually equally affected, although in certain clinical variants, the muscle involvement may be less apparent.

Type VI

Type VI, or Hers' disease, involves only the hepatic phosphorylase, which is partially missing. There are different degrees of inactivation of this enzyme and, therefore, the clinical man-

ifestations are more variable. Type VI is compatible with a greater tolerance of fasting.

The glycogenoses can be suspected on physical examination, because hepatomegaly is usually prominent and xanthoma, lipemia retinalis, and failure to thrive are sometimes present. The diagnosis, however, can be confirmed by procedures such as tolerance to prolonged fasting, glucagon load test, galactose and fructose loads, and liver biopsy. White blood cells can be used to assay debrancher activity, and fibroblasts can be used for phosphorylase determination, but only liver, intestine, and kidneys, to a certain extent, contain G-6-phosphatase.

Leucine Sensitive Hypoglycemia

This disease is an exaggeration of a physiologic phenomenon, because certain amino acids may cause insulin release. Leucine appears to be very effective in this process. Onset is usually before the patient is 6 months of age, and hypoglycemia occurs in response to meals as well as to prolonged fasting. The patient presents with seizures caused by hypoglycemia. Mental retardation as a consequence of the frequency of the hypoglycemic episodes is common in these cases. No enzyme deficiency has been described as yet, but the likely cause of this disease is an abnormality in the receptor sites, either for insulin or for leucine.

The diagnosis is established with a leucine load administered orally (100 mg/kg); glucose, insulin, and growth hormone are measured at 15-minute intervals.

Fructose Intolerance and 1,6-Diphosphofructose-Phosphatase Deficiency

Fructose intolerance may cause episodes of vomiting, dehydration, acidosis, and failure to thrive, but rarely does the patient require admission to the ICU. Aldolase B is the defective enzyme. By contrast, the severe lactic acidosis and hypoglycemia characterize 1,6-diphosphofructose-phosphatase deficiency. The clinical picture closely simulates the presentation of Type I glycogen storage disease, and these patients often require care in an ICU.

The diagnosis is made by carefully loading the patient with fructose given orally (0.5 to 1.5 gm/kg) or intravenously (0.25 to 0.5 gm/kg). Simultaneous measurement of glucose, lactate, pyruvate phosphate, and uric acid should be carried out. Confirmation of the diagnosis is obtained by appropriate enzyme studies on skin fibroblasts or white cells.

Galactosemia

This entity is due to the absence of the enzyme galactose 1-phosphate uridyl transferase.

Screening tests for galactosemia in neonates are now being performed in at least 43 states. Early detection is, therefore, the rule. Nonetheless, several cases have been missed. The disease is so severe in the newborn period that the patient may be admitted to an ICU before the diagnosis is reported.

The symptoms may appear almost immediately after the first feedings and may quickly evolve. Vomiting, diarrhea, and poor feeding are the first manifestations reported by the patient's family. Such symptoms lead to repeated changes of formula by the pediatrician on the basis of a presumptive diagnosis of milk intolerance. Persistent jaundice, hepatomegaly, hypoglycemia, and sepsis are often present in this stage. Too often, the work-up is not ex-

tended beyond blood cultures and routine chemistries. In more severe cases, ophthalmologic examination may reveal oil drop changes and frank cataracts. Renal tubular acidosis, pseudotumor cerebri, hemolytic anemia, and liver failure with ascites may be part of the clinical picture, and death may occur before the true diagnosis has been determined.

Galactosemia is an autosomal recessive disease, with a frequency of 1:40,000 to 70,000 births. A family history is usually not elicited unless other siblings have been previously diagnosed. A positive urinalysis performed with Benedict's solution or clinitest in the presence of a negative glucose oxidase test (tape test) in a patient receiving breast milk or modified cow's milk should arouse suspicion of galactosemia. Other clues are persistent and/or worsening jaundice and the presence of cataracts. Such clues help to confirm the diagnosis while awaiting a definite determination of G-1-phosphate uridyl transferase activity and accumulation of G-1-phosphate in the red cells.

Management

HYPOGLYCEMIA

A 25 percent glucose solution is given by slow IV push. One to 2 ml per kg of body weight is administered within a 5-minute period, followed by a 15 percent glucose drip, which can be tapered to a 10 percent concentration, depending upon the patient's condition. Usually 9 to 11 mg of glucose per minute per kg is necessary to maintain a normal glucose level.

In glycogen storage disease, the use of corticosteroids is not recommended, because it will not increase the activity of missing enzymes and could, in fact, encourage further glycogen formation. In leucine-sensitive hypoglycemia, corticosteroid should not be used in therapy, because it could cause tissue breakdown and could increase plasma leucine levels. Glucagon, at a dose of 30 μgm per kg, administered subcutaneously or intravenously after a meal, could possibly have some effect in glycogen storage disease Types III and VI but not in the fasting state. In fact, this is the basis of differential testing used to identify the various types. Therapeutically, glucagon is not indicated for this group of diseases. In leucine-sensitive hypoglycemia, it could be used provided that precautions are taken to avoid the rebound phenomenon of hyperinsulin secretion and hypoglycemia usually seen 2 hours later. Diazoxide, at a dose of 5 to 20 mg per kg, has been very effective in controlling hypoglycemia seen in patients who are sensitive to leucine. Such a medication may have to be continued for 6 or more years before total remission occurs.

ACIDOSIS

Lactic acidosis is seen mainly in Type I glycogen storage disease and sometimes in galactosemia. It can be quite severe in fructose 1,6-diphosphatase deficiency. Correction can be achieved by IV administration of sodium bicarbonate calculated on the basis of the patient's actual base deficit. Large doses may be required, and one should not hesitate to order them.

JAUNDICE

When present, as seen in galactosemia, jaundice usually disappears after the appropriate dietary measures have been taken. If, however, the level approaches 20 mg per dl, exchange transfusion should be performed and repeated as often as necessary. For lesser levels, phototherapy may be sufficient.

COAGULATION ABNORMALITIES

As with liver failure, hypofibrinogenemia and prolonged prothrombin and thromboplastin times are seen in galactosemia and glycogen storage disease. They should be controlled by administration of fresh frozen plasma. Disseminated intravascular coagulation (DIC) may also complicate the picture when sepsis superimposes.

SEPSIS

Galactosemia may present as septicemia, meningitis, or urinary tract infection. Because of the frequent association of galactosemia with gram-negative organisms, antibiotic coverage is of prime importance in the acute phase.

DIET

In all the preceding situations, the diet calls for administration of glucose as the only car-

bohydrate capable of preventing acidosis and hypoglycemia except leucine-sensitive hypoglycemia. Obviously, breast-feeding and cow's milk are prohibited in galactosemia, whereas sucrose and fructose should be eliminated in fructose intolerance and 1,6-diphosphofructose-phosphatase deficiency. A formula such as Pregestimil, which provides glucose and starches as a source of carbohydrate, is excellent for the management of the glycogenoses and galactosemia.

In leucine-sensitive hypoglycemia, enough protein should be given to meet the needs of the patient. It should be equally divided throughout the day and preferably should be given in four meals to avoid a surge of insulin.

SUGGESTED READING

Cohen, R., Yudkoff, M., Rothman, R., and Segal, S.: Isovaleric acidemia: use of glycine therapy in neonates. N. Engl. J. Med. 299:996, 1978.

Cornblath, M., and Schwartz, R. (eds.): Hypoglycemia in the neonate. In Disorders of Carbohydrate Metabolism in Infancy, 2nd ed. Philadelphia, W.B. Saunders Company, 1976, pp. 155–205.

Curtius, H.C., Niederwieser, A., Viscontini, M., et al.: Atypical phenylketonuria due to tetrahydrobiopterin deficiency. Diagnosis and treatment with tetrahydrobiopterin, dihydrobiopterin, and sepiapterin. Clin. Chim. Acta 93:251, 1979.

Koch, R., et al.: Urea cycle symposium. Ped 68: Part I, pp. 271–289, Part II, pp. 446–459, 1981.

Krieger, I., and Tanaka, K.: Therapeutic effects of glycine in isovaleric acidemia. Pediatr. Res. 10:25, 1976.

Mudd, S.H., and Levy, H.L.: Disorders of transsulfuration. In Standbury, J.B., Wyngaarden, J.B., Frederickson, D.J., et al. (eds.): The Metabolic Basis of Inherited Disease, 5th ed. New York, McGraw-Hill, Inc., 1983, pp. 522–559.

Smith, I., Clayton, B.E., and Wolff, O.H.: New variant of phenylketonuria with progressive neurologic illness unresponsive to phenylalanine restriction. Lancet 1:1108, 1975.

Snyderman, S.E.: The therapy of maple syrup urine disease. Am. J. Dis. Child 113:68, 1967.

Snyderman, S.E., Sansaricq, C., Phansalkar, S.V., et al.: The therapy of hyperammonemia due to ornithine transcarbamylase deficiency in a male neonate. Pediatrics 56:65, 1975.

Winokur, P.A., Krishan, V., and Seshamani, R.: Isovalericacidemia: a case report. Pediatrics 61:902, 1978.

Nursing Process for Patient Care:

Inborn Errors of Metabolism

Children may be born with a wide variety of metabolic disorders. The effect of the metabolic derangement on total body function can be profound, with neurologic, respiratory, and cardiovascular manifestations. Independent of the specific defect, these inborn errors of metabolism share common features, which dictate monitoring and management.

METABOLIC STATE

The particular type of metabolic disorder accounts for the specific clinical presentation and management. Acidosis is a common problem to most of the inborn errors of metabolism.

Assess, Monitor, and Document

Specific metabolic defect
  Odor of body fluids and secretions: maple
    syrup, sweaty feet
  Arterial blood gases: pH, base deficit
Fluid and electrolyte balance
  Weight
  Intake: accurate administration of fluids
  Urine output: specific gravity
  State of hydration: observe (thirst, skin tur-
    gor, mucous membranes, fontanels,
    tears)
  Serum electrolytes
Nutritional status
  Caloric intake
Response to therapy
  Nutritional support
  Exchange transfusion
  Peritoneal dialysis

Anticipate

Alterations in metabolic status
  Acidosis
  Hypoglycemia
  Odor of body fluids and secretions: maple
    syrup, sweaty feet
Complications of therapy: exchange transfusion (thrombocytopenia, hypocalcemia), peritoneal dialysis (respiratory
  distress secondary to abdominal distention, infection)

NEUROLOGIC

Assess, Monitor, and Document

Level of consciousness
Pupillary response
Reflexes
Motor activity
Muscle tone
Posturing (if applicable)

Anticipate

Altered level of consciousness: lethargic, irritable, coma
Seizures

RESPIRATORY

The respiratory system can be affected by the underlying metabolic problem as well as by the therapy used to correct it. There is an increase in respiratory effort in an attempt to compensate for the metabolic acidosis. Respiratory failure may result from fatigue or progressive deterioration in neurologic status. The use of peritoneal dialysis to remove metabolites may further embarrass the respiratory system as pressure is exerted on the diaphragm by the fluid in the peritoneum.

Assess, Monitor, and Document

Respiratory rate
Respiratory pattern, including depth
Breath sounds

Color
Arterial blood gases

Anticipate

Alteration in respiratory status
    Tachypnea
    Hyperpnea

Respiratory insufficiency: restlessness secondary to hypoxemia

CARDIOVASCULAR

The cardiovascular system is assessed and monitored based upon its relationship to the child's fluid and electrolyte status. Rarely, the disease may affect the myocardium directly (myocardial infarction in homocystinuria).

Assess, Monitor and Document

Heart rate
Rhythm

Quality of pulses
Blood pressure: arterial, central venous

Anticipate

Alteration in cardiovascular status
    Hypovolemia
    Dysrhythmias

RESPONSE OF CHILD

Assess, Monitor, and Document

Developmental level: motor, psychosocial,
    cognitive
Developmental tasks: sense of trust
Behavioral response

Response to separation
Response to staff
Response to nursing interventions

Anticipate

Disruption in normal growth and development

RESPONSE OF FAMILY

Assess, Monitor, and Document

Behavioral response: anxious, fearful, verbal,
    angry
Level of understanding of the disorder and
    child's condition

Expected outcome
Educational needs related to discharge planning for home diet management
Response to nursing interventions

Anticipate

Inability to cope
Family crisis
Educational needs

MIND SET

Assess

Metabolic status
   Specific metabolic defect
   Fluid and electrolyte balance
   Nutritional status

Neurologic status
Respiratory status
Cardiovascular status
Response of child and family

Anticipate

Alteration in metabolic state
   Acidosis
   Dehydration
Alteration in neurologic function
   Hypotonia
   Seizures
   Coma

Alteration in respiratory status
Alteration in cardiovascular function
Disruption in normal growth and development
Family crisis

RENAL

CHAPTER

38

Acute Renal Failure

ROBERT G. SCHACHT, M.D.

The term *acute renal failure* (ARF) has been used to describe any clinical situation in which the biochemial indices of renal function, the blood urea nitrogen (BUN) and serum creatinine levels, rise. In this chapter, the recognition and management of those clinical events that occur when renal function deteriorates acutely and cannot be reversed rapidly by altering extrarenal factors will be discussed. It is during this period of time, when the kidneys are unable to maintain solute and water balance, that the physician must assiduously regulate the intake and output of these substances for the child.

RECOGNITION

The most frequent presentation of patients with ARF is that of a dramatic decrease in urine output (oliguria) associated with increased retention of nitrogenous waste products. This altered state of renal function typically lasts from a period of days to 3 or 4 weeks, and recovery is heralded by a sudden and often inappropriate increase in urine output (diuresis). A less commonly recognized presentation is that of non-oliguric renal failure in which the patient's usual urine output is unaffected and exceeds 400 ml per day (in the smaller patient, 1 ml/kg/hr). Despite near-normal urine output, azotemia occurs and persists for 7 to 10 days. Therefore, the clinician should place emphasis not on the quantity of urine excreted but on the recognition of those clinical events that might initiate a renal insult resulting in progressive azotemia.

After acute azotemia has been recognized, the clinician is then faced with a difficult diagnostic exercise in which he must differentiate between ARF and functional acute renal insufficiency (ARI). Utilizing the history, physical examination, and modest laboratory analyses, he must exclude those renal events that, if untreated, would progress to ARF (see Table 38–1).

OBSTRUCTIVE UROPATHY

The first and most important question to be asked is, Is obstruction of the urinary system the cause of azotemia? If so, is the obstruction at the level of the bladder neck urethra, or ureter? Because by definition, we are dealing with an acute deterioration in renal function in the pediatric patient, beyond the newborn period, certain disorders readily come to mind. Bladder outlet obstruction may occur with trauma to the perineum or pelvis, with infection or alteration of innervation to the bladder wall or sphincter. Malignancies or stone formation rarely present as an acute obstructive phenomenon in the otherwise healthy child. Obstruction at the ureteral level, must, by definition, be bilateral to cause renal failure and therefore is uncommonly seen in pediatric patients who do not have pre-existing renal disease. The exceptions are patients who have sudden release of uric acid during therapy for lymphoproliferative disorders or those who sustain bilateral papillary necrosis from severe bilateral pyelonephritis or sickle cell crisis.

The patient may have widely variable urine outputs or may be anuric. Biochemical tests reveal a severe hyperkalemic acidosis, with rising BUN and creatinine levels. In this clinical setting, the insertion of a bladder catheter may be both diagnostic and life-saving. Additional useful tests are nephrosonography, infusion

Table 38–1. Differential Diagnosis of Acute Renal Insufficiency (ARI)

Obstructive uropathy (post-renal)
  Bladder outlet: anatomic or functional
  Ureteral: always bilateral unless it occurs in a solitary
    kidney or in previously damaged kidneys
Decreased renal perfusion (pre-renal)
  Decreased effective circulating volume
    Hypovolemia
    Poor cardiac output
    Systemic vasodilatation
  Increased renal vascular resistance
  Renal vascular obstruction
Renal parenchymal disease (intrinsic)
  Glomerular
  Tubulointerstitial
  Vascular

pyelography, and unilateral retrograde pyelography.

DECREASED RENAL PERFUSION

Another question to be asked is, Are the kidneys being poorly perfused? Decreased effective circulatory volume is by far the most common disturbance seen in pediatric patients with ARI. The kidneys have the intrinsic capability of autoregulation, that is, altering arteriolar and glomerular resistances to maintain normal filtration pressure when renal blood flow is unfavorably changed. There are times when the renal vasculature cannot respond adequately to offset a hemodynamic insult and, consequently, the glomerular filtration rate falls. As glomerular filtration decreases, there is less filtration of nitrogenous waste products, marked salt and water reabsorption in the proximal tubule initiated by Starling forces, and avid sodium and water reabsorption distally following the release of aldosterone via the renin–angiotensin–aldosterone axis. Urea is reabsorbed with water; therefore, one can account for the urinary indices associated with pre-renal azotemia: 1) low urine output, 2) low sodium excretion: less than 10–20 mEq per L, 3) decreased fraction excretion of filtered sodium: less than 1 percent, 4) high urine osmolality: greater than 500 mOsm per kg per H_2O, 5) a high urine to plasma urea nitrogen ratio: greater than 8 and a high urine to plasma creatinine ratio: greater than 40. The patient may be hypovolemic, have poor cardiac output, or have marked systemic vasodilatation.

It is relatively easy to elicit the history and to see the physical findings of patients who are hypovolemic. When intravascular fluid is lost from the circulation via the gastrointestinal tract, the kidneys, or the skin by hemorrhage or by sequestration, the patient presents with orthostatic changes in the circulatory system, poor peripheral perfusion and tachycardia. Rapid intravenous (IV) infusion (within 30 min) of large volumes (20 ml/kg) of a fluid that will stay within the vascular space, that is, plasma, plasmanate, or Ringer's lactate, can be both diagnostic and therapeutic. Although intravascular resuscitation might be sufficient to correct inadequate urine output, most clinicians also administer a potent diuretic (furosemide 2–4 mg/kg) intravenously.

Although seen commonly in adult patients with congestive heart failure (CHF), impaired cardiac function as a cause of ARI is seen with increasing frequency in the pediatric population. In my own experience, post–open-heart surgical pediatric patients represent the majority of patients who present with nonoliguric renal insufficiency or failure and a significant number of those who present with oliguric renal failure. The exact nature of the event responsible for the observed renal impairment is difficult to discern, because open-heart surgical patients suffer multiple and varied insults. These physiologic aberrations include 1) varying degrees of impaired myocardial function from the surgical procedure and from the lesion requiring the procedure, 2) markedly elevated circulating levels of catecholamines and antidiuretic hormones, 3) hemolysis inherent to bypass procedures, and 4) infusions of pressor amines required to maintain adequate cardiac output. Whatever the initiating event, it is well accepted that persistent low cardiac output states are associated with an increased incidence and severity of renal functional impairment.

Patients suffering from burns and sepsis may have a decreased cardiac output from a circulating cardiotoxin. Finally, we should be aware of those drugs that we administer that lower cardiac output. If poor cardiac output is secondary to myocardial depression, the therapeutic regimen is directed at improvement in cardiac function. When the cardiac output is corrected, renal perfusion and function will normalize.

Even when a patient has adequate myocardial function and has not sustained a loss of volume, he or she may experience extreme vasodilatation from sepsis or drug administration. Conversely, increased renal vascular resistance that occurs during anesthesia, vasopressor amine administration, or the hepatorenal syndrome of liver failure may initiate progressive azotemia and eventually renal failure. Renal arterial obstruction is not seen in pediatric patients unless it is asssociated with major trauma.

RENAL PARENCHYMAL DISEASE

The pertinent question concerning renal parenchymal disease is, Is renal function impaired by glomerular, tubulointerstitial, or intrarenal vascular disease?

Primary diseases of the glomeruli and small blood vessels of the kidney may present with clinical courses that rapidly progress to renal failure. These pathologic states include hemolytic uremic syndrome, thrombotic thrombocytopenic purpura (TTP), Henoch–Schönlein purpura, membranoproliferative glomerulonephritis, post-streptococcal glomerulonephritis, endocarditis, vasculitis, malignant hypertension, cortical necrosis, and disseminated intravascular coagulopathy. Large vessel disease (i.e., renal artery thrombosis or embolism) and renal vein thrombosis are uncommon. When vascular and/or glomerular damage occurs, there is a reduction in glomerular perfusion pressure, which diminishes the glomerular filtration rate.

Acute tubular necrosis (ATN), frequently used synonomously with ARF, may result from either an ischemic or a nephrotoxic insult. When this insult is ischemic in nature and minor in degree, a transient cessation or diminution of renal function occurs. This transient aberration is termed *acute vasomotor nephropathy* (AVN) and generally is not associated with histologic damage to the nephron. Variability in the sensitivity of patients to decreases in renal perfusion is the rule; hence, even with transient ischemic changes similar to those responsible for acute vasomotor nephropathy, clinical and histologic manifestations of ATN may be initiated. Nephrotoxic agents, whether endogenous or exogenous in nature, have become increasingly important in the pathogenesis of acute renal failure. Endogenous release of pigments (hemoglobin or myoglobin), particularly into a volume-depleted patient following trauma, muscle injury, seizures, exercise, or coma, may initiate toxic ATN. Hypercalcemia and hyperuricemia are observed infrequently as the initiating insult.

The recognition of exogenous nephrotoxins has become increasingly important, because most of these agents are in the physician's diagnostic and therapeutic armamentarium.

Heavy metals (gold, lead, cadmium), hydrocarbons, antibiotics (aminoglycosides, penicillins, amphotericin, rifampin), antineoplastics (streptozotocin, nitrosoureas, *cis*-platinum), diuretics, analgesics (especially nonsteroidals), and contrast materials have all been associated with acute renal failure with and without the predisposing factors of volume depletion, preexisting renal disease, and diabetes. Although the precise mechanism (or mechanisms) by which nephrotoxins injure the tubules is unknown, the histologic insult is anatomically distinct. Tubular necrosis following an ischemic insult appears in an irregular anatomic distribution, whereas that resulting from nephrotoxin administration usually affects the proximal tubules.

PATHOGENESIS OF ACUTE RENAL FAILURE

Faced with the preceding myriad of pathologic events, which could initiate an episode of acute renal failure, one might simplify the classification into either hemodynamic or nephrotoxic etiologies, both of which occur with approximately equal frequency. Having thus categorized the insult, several factors must be evaluated that individually or in concert may not only initiate but also maintain the clinical features of ARF.

Hemodynamic Alterations Within the Kidney. There is abundant evidence that renal blood flow is both reduced and redistributed in nephrotoxic and ischemic renal failure. Arguments have been proposed with laboratory support that afferent arteriolar constriction occurs and that in some models of ARF, this decrease in blood flow alters the metabolism of the kidney. This metabolic derangement results in cell swelling, which then offsets filtration pressure.

Alteration in the Filtering Membrane. It is possible that following an ischemic or toxic insult there is a decrease in the surface area or in the permeability characteristics of the glomerular capillary.

Backleak of Glomerular Filtrate. The tubular backleak theory of ARF proposes that glomerular filtration continues, but the clinical insult has altered the integrity of the tubules such that glomerular filtrate leaks back from the tubules and returns into the peritubular vasculature.

Tubular Obstruction. This theory suggests

that the tubules are blocked by debris. It has been supported by demonstration of tubular casts in patients and hemoglobinuric renal failure.

The urinary indices of ARI (see page 314) differ markedly from those of established ARF which are: 1) a urinary sodium concentration greater than 40 mEq per L, 2) a urine osmolality less than 300 mOsm per kg H_2O, 3) a urine to plasma urea nitrogen ratio less than 3, 4) a urine to plasma creatinine ratio less than 20, and 5) a fractional excretion of filtered sodium greater than 1 percent.

Further examination of the urine may assist the diagnosis of acute renal failure. If the urinalysis is normal, that is, free of protein, sediment cells, and so on, one should consider prerenal or post-renal factors as operant in the initiation of ARF. When red blood cell (RBC) casts and/or proteinuria are found, glomerular or vascular disease should be considered. Pyuria with or without white blood cell (WBC) casts might indicate the presence of an interstitial nephropathy—when predominantly eosinophils: acute allergic interstitial nephritis; when polymorphs: infectious uropathy. Finally, the presence of epithelial or pigmented casts is highly suggestive of acute tubular necrosis.

When the diagnosis of renal failure has been established, the physician must support the patient until the illness has run its course, approximately 2 to 3 weeks in patients with oliguric renal failure and approximately 1 week in nonoliguric patients.

In the initial stage of acute renal failure there are typical daily increases in BUN of 10 to 20 mg per dl and in creatinine of 0.5 to 1.5 mg per dl. This phase is then followed in most patients by a gradual increase in glomerular filtration rate. The biochemical indicators begin to plateau, and there is a progressive increase in urine output. Some patients may develop an inappropriate diuresis. In this unusual clinical situation, glomerular filtration recovers more rapidly than tubular function, resulting in abnormal losses of solute and water and subsequent volume depletion. The clinician becomes aware of this by careful monitoring of the intake and output records and by recognition of an adverse change in the patient's clinical and biochemical status. The final phase of ARF is the recovery stage. Although the BUN and creatinine return to normal within a relatively short period of time, complete resolution to premorbid levels of filtration rate, blood flow, and tubular function may take months.

COMPLICATIONS

When the kidneys can no longer maintain their functions of excretion of nitrogenous waste products, and maintenance of fluid, electrolyte, and acid-base balance, a variety of biochemical and clinical complications become manifest. These derangements are less severe in the nonoliguric individual as there is usually a higher level of filtration rate and excretory rate. Conversely, it is obvious that the patient who is catabolic secondary to surgery, infection or malnutrition produces excess amounts of endogenous wastes, which can aggrevate his impaired biochemical status. The complications of ARF include:

1. Metabolic: acidosis, electrolyte disturbances
2. Cardiovascular: volume overload, dysrhythmias
3. Neurologic: coma, seizures
4. Hematologic: anemia, coagulopathy
5. Infectious
6. Gastrointestinal

Metabolic aberrations consist primarily of the development of acidosis and electrolyte abnormalities. An anion gap acidosis occurs in all patients with ARF secondary to retention of fixed acid. This is exaggerated in younger patients, who normally have a greater production of acid (2 mEq/kg/day) than adults (1 mEq/kg/day).

Uric acid levels exceeding 15 mg per dl observed during ARF are usually indicative of extensive cellular destruction.

Electrolyte disturbances in ARF are usually limited to hyponatremia, hypocalcemia or hypercalcemia, hyperkalemia, hyperphosphatemia and hyperuricemia. Hyponatremia results from the excess intake of water when there is an inability to excrete free water. Although uncommon, the serum sodium may be lowered sufficiently to initiate seizure activity. As phosphate intake or release continues in the presence of decreased renal clearance, hyperphosphatemia is observed. Hyperphosphatemia in concert with diminished renal production of 1,25-dihydroxyvitamin D may result in hypocalcemia. Hypercalcemia results from inappropriate administration of calcium to the patient with ARF or release with phosphate and uric acid from damaged muscles. Hyperkalemia may result from diminished renal excretion, from acidosis, catabolism, or inappropriate intake.

Cardiovascular complications include intravascular volume overload manifested by pulmonary edema and hypertension, dysrhythmias secondary to electrolyte disturbances and nitrogenous waste accumulation, and pericarditis. These complications are uncommonly seen in patients in whom early dialytic therapy is initiated.

The neurologic and gastrointestinal complications of ARF are generally ascribed to the accumulation of nitrogenous waste products or electrolyte imbalance. The patient may present with an altered sensorium, ranging from lethargy to coma and seizures. Neurologic manifestations tend to appear at lower levels of BUN in patients who have coexistent or pre-existent intracranial lesions, that is, postoperative cardiac patients who are hypoxic or postoperative neurosurgical patients. Nausea, vomiting, hiccups, and ileus are symptoms of uremia and may prevent patients from eating, thereby worsening their catabolic state. Hematologic aberrations consist of a normochromic, normocytic anemia, decreased marrow production of platelets, and impaired platelet function.

Decreased immune responses, catabolic states, and impaired white cell production contribute to the increased infection rate of patients with ARF. The presence of infection and its attendant complications and therapies are major risk factors in the management of uremic patients.

TREATMENT

Prevention

The hallmark of therapy for ARF is prevention; therefore, all initial efforts should be directed toward the diagnosis and remediation of those clinical events that can be reversed prior to the development of established ARF. Acute obstructive uropathy should be alleviated by catheter or nephrostomy drainage. Pre-renal insults may be ameliorated by providing an effective circulating volume. The patient who is volume-depleted requires intravascular resuscitation, with rapid infusions of a fluid (plasmanate, Ringer's lactate, saline) that will stay within the vascular space. These fluids (20 ml/kg) should be administered within a 30-minute time span. A second administration may be required to expand the patient's vascular space. Diuretics may be administered in conjunction with vascular expansion. My own preference is IV furosemide (a loop diuretic), 2 to 3 mg per kg, or mannitol (an osmotic diuretic), 1 gm per kg, given one time as a diagnostic test.

There is some evidence that a low-dose continuous infusion of dopamine, 2 to 3 mcg per kg per minute, may increase urine output by interfering with water reabsorption by the tubule or by lowering renal resistance. Obviously, low cardiac output syndromes or those associated with sepsis should have therapies directed at the initiating insult. If vasopressor amines are used in the treatment of low-output syndromes, one must be aware of their adverse effect in this clinical setting on renal vascular resistance.

Therapy

When the diagnosis of renal failure has been established, both general and specific guidelines for therapy must be considered. The general guidelines of therapy are supportive in nature and are directed at the prevention of accelerated catabolism, whereas specific therapies are developed to reverse or abate the complications of ARF.

General Principles

FLUID AND CALORIC MANAGEMENT

Fluid therapy, whether orally or intravenously administered, should be limited to 250 to 300 ml per m^2 (5–6 ml/kg) daily, plus urine output. The nonurinary output quantity is given as nonelectrolyte, high-caloric fluid and may result in a modest lowering of the serum sodium (see Complications). Obviously negligible in the oliguric or anuric patient, urinary losses of solute and water could be substantial in nonoliguric patients. It is my preference to replace these losses (spontaneous or diuretic induced) every 8 hours, having precisely determined the quantity and electrolyte composition of the urine. A general principle is to maintain as high a urine output as possible, thus decreasing the back diffusion of urea. It has been further suggested that such a manipulation of fluid balance would also favor the elimination of other uremic toxins that would otherwise contribute to morbidity. Patients should be carefully monitored for excess water losses, elevated temperature, gastroenteritis, and sweating and additional fluids should be given. The patient who presents with acute volume overload should initially receive less than 300 ml per m^2. A change in weight of approximately 0.5 to 1 percent per day in the absence of circulatory complications is indicative of adequate fluid management.

Caloric intake must approximate the patient's metabolic demands. In uncomplicated ARF, this may amount to 300 to 400 calories per m^2 per day (40–60 cal/kg/day); however, in hypermetabolic patients, these requirements may increase by several fold. Protein intake is limited to 0.5 to 1 gm per kg per day, orally or intravenously, and may now be offered as high biologic value protein (essential L-amino acid preparations). These preparations decrease the nonessential protein waste products and may allow the patient to reuse the nitrogen contained in urea as protein building blocks, which incorporate circulating electrolytes into newly formed cells, thus diminishing dialysis requirements. Administration of adequate amounts of carbohydrates will further diminish endogenous protein breakdown. When the oral route is unavailable or inadequate, IV alimentation is of paramount importance in the maintenance of caloric intake. The patient may receive 1 to 1.5 calories per ml via peripheral or central lines, and the daily prescription should contain carbohydrates, amino acids, lipids, and vitamins.

MONITORING

Accurate documentation of the patient's intake and output is essential if one is to develop a logical therapeutic plan. The patient should be weighed at least once daily, and clinical assessment of hydration may be reviewed in each 8-hour shift. Although serum electrolytes and acid–base determinants are obtained frequently (every 4–6 hours) during the first few days of ARF, they may be obtained twice daily as the renal insult stabilizes. There is usually no need to obtain a BUN, creatinine, complete blood count (CBC), or phosphate more frequently than once daily. The patient's serum solids can be evaluated every 3 to 4 days. Urine volume and electrolyte content should be recorded every 8 hours in patients with nonoliguric renal failure so that replacement fluid may be administered in addition to the required maintenance fluids. Obviously, in oliguric patients determination and replacement of urinary losses on a daily basis are required.

The use of an indwelling catheter should be avoided; if necessary, intermittent straight catheterization should be performed. A daily electrocardiogram (EKG) or rhythm strip may be of importance in the early detection of cardiac dysrhythmias or pericarditis. Of utmost importance is the careful review of these data

in a timely manner by the clinician. If all the aforementioned information is scattered throughout the chart and not placed in proper perspective, the documentation is an exercise in futility.

DRUG THERAPY

In the setting of ARF, the physician must carefully evaluate his or her therapeutic regimen. Pharmacologic agents, administered to ameliorate renal disorders and attendant complications, will be retained if their elimination is dependent upon glomerular filtration or the secretory capacity of the kidney. The medications per se, or their metabolites, can adversely affect the clinical course either by accumulation to toxic levels or by imposing an increased metabolic load to the patient. Obvious examples are digitalis, which is dependent upon glomerular filtration and tubular secretion for elimination, increased urea generated by steroid-induced catabolism, and sodium administered bound to antibiotics. Those agents not dependent upon renal elimination may have the potential for toxicity owing to altered metabolism, impaired function by the blood–brain barrier, decreased protein binding, or target organ failure coincident with the uremic state.

It is customary to offer the usual loading dose of medication to saturate the volume of distribution of the drug and then, depending upon its elimination characteristics, either prolong the interval between doses or diminish the dosage of the maintenance administration. Blood levels of the drug may be useful in guiding prolonged therapy (see Chapter 14, Clinical Pharmacology in the Critically Ill Child).

Specific Principles

METABOLIC

An anion gap acidosis, reflecting a net gain in nonvolatile acids, occurs as renal function is significantly decreased, that is, when the filtration rate decreases to 30 ml per minute. These fixed acids ordinarily result from the metabolism of exogenous or endogenous protein; however, incomplete combustion of fats and carbohydrates will add to the acid load of the patient. An initial compensation occurs that uses the buffer systems and the development of a respiratory alkalosis (alveolar hyperventilation). This latter compensatory mechanism must be kept in mind in those patients whose

CO_2 elimination is controlled by ventilatory assistance. Sodium bicarbonate or lactate (1–3 mEq/kg/day) given in multiple divided doses orally or intravenously should temporarily control the acidosis. This replacement/intervention is administered when the pH decreases below 7.2 to 7.25 and the serum bicarbonate is below 12 to 15 mEq per L. These limits usually reflect an increased workload (respiratory compensation) on the part of the patient, thereby increasing acid production and respiratory water loss. When volume overload or excess acid production secondary to uncontrolled catabolism becomes paramount, dialytic therapy should be instituted.

Electrolyte Disturbances

Serum sodium concentrations in ARF invariably reflect alterations in water balance, not in total body content of sodium. When unusual losses of water exist, hypernatremia will occur; conversely, too liberal administration of free water will cause hyponatremia. The oliguric patient who has no excess fluid loss usually exhibits a low serum sodium. Because the glomerular filtration rate is more depressed in this group of patients than in nonoliguric patients, a greater portion of the already depressed filtered load of sodium is reabsorbed proximally, limiting free water excretion and thus diluting the serum sodium. This same mechanism is operant to a lesser degree in patients with nonoliguric renal failure who have a substantial loss of sodium in the urine. Although the BUN may be significantly elevated in ARF, it should not alter plasma sodium concentration.

As the patient's sodium falls below 125 mEq per L, complaints of nausea and malaise are registered. Severe neurologic symptoms, lethargy, and obtundations become manifest as the sodium levels approach 110 mEq per L; seizures and coma may occur below this level. As mentioned previously, patients suffering from a coincidental or pre-existent cerebral insult may show neurologic complications with less deranged biochemical levels.

The general therapy for hyponatremia in ARF is water restriction. When large losses of sodium occur either spontaneously or are induced by diuretic therapy, sodium should be offered to the patient, keeping in mind the danger of intravascular volume expansion. When severe neurologic symptoms occur abruptly, acute sodium replacement may be required in addition to water restriction. One should not attempt to completely correct the plasma sodium but should raise it to an intermediate level. A useful formula is:

$$\text{sodium replacement in mEq}$$

$$= 0.3 \times \text{weight in kg} \times \text{desired}$$

$$- \text{observed plasma sodium.}$$

Thus, for a child weighing 10 kg who has seizure activity thought to be resultant from a plasma sodium of 105 mEq per L, an administration of 45 mEq of sodium would be required to raise the sodium concentration to approximately 120 mEq per L.

$$45 \text{ mEq} = 0.3 \times 10 \text{ kg} \times 120 \text{ (desired)}$$

$$- 105 \text{ (observed).}$$

The sodium should be administered as hypertonic saline, 2½ percent, to reduce the volume of administration; for example, 100 ml of 2½ percent solution as opposed to 300 ml of normal saline (INS). Concurrently, water should be restricted. This calculation is only a general estimate reflecting the amount of sodium required to return the plasma sodium toward normal. In practice, one begins the sodium replacement therapy and stops either when the seizures abate or when a reasonable plasma sodium is attained.

Hyperkalemia. After the plasma potassium concentration has been raised either by exogenous administration or endogenous release from tissue, this ion must be placed into cells or eliminated by the kidney. The fact that 98 percent of the total K^+ content of the body is contained within the intracellular compartment underscores its importance in multiple cellular functions. Furthermore, the gradient provided by the intracellular and extracellular potassium concentrations (160 mEq/L:4.5–5 mEq/L) profoundly influences the resting potential of muscle and nerve cells. When the plasma potassium is increased modestly, the resting potential is reduced and approaches the threshold potential of the cell, thereby increasing membrane excitability. More marked elevations can effect a depolarization block, with attendant paralysis. As the plasma potassium concentration is increased, there is an immediate attempt to store it in cells. This process is facilitated by the availability of insulin and is impaired (often reversed) in the presence of acidemia.

Renal regulation of potassium involves filtration, reabsorption, and secretion of the ion. The filtered load of potassium is almost entirely reabsorbed from the tubule by the time it exits the loop of Henle. Excretion, therefore, must be dependent upon distal tubular secretion of K^+. The tubular secretion rate for K^+ is dependent upon K^+ intake, aldosterone secretion, tubular flow rates, and the presence of poorly reabsorbable anions in the distal tubules, that is, sulfates and phosphates. As the plasma K^+ is increased, aldosterone is secreted, initiating a $Na^+ = K^+$ exchange favoring K^+ loss in the distal nephron. An increase in distal tubular flow, an increase in distal tubular delivery of sodium, or the presence of large negatively charged ions all promote K^+ secretion.

Hyperkalemia is frequently observed in ARF not only as a failure of excretion but also as a consequence of increased plasma load and decreased cellular storage. The clinical sequelae of hyperkalemia are muscular weakness and cardiac conduction abnormalities. As the plasma K^+ levels approach 6 mEq per L, peaked T waves and shortened Q-T intervals, representing rapid repolarization, are noticed. With further increases in plasma K^+, the QRS complex widens and flattens (electrical evidence of prolongation of depolarization) and ventricular fibrillation or standstill occurs. Potassium toxicity is enhanced when the patient is acidotic, hypocalcemia, or hyponatremic or if the rate of rise is rapid. Occasionally, one encounters pseudohyperkalemia during episodes of ARF. This aberration, observed with marked leukocytosis, thrombocytosis, or hemolysis during blood drawing, does not increase the plasma potassium concentration and, therefore, does not cause physiologic disturbance.

The treatment of true hyperkalemia (Table 38–2) is directed at decreasing the extracellular potassium load, promoting cellular storage, removing excess potassium from the body and/or reversing membrane excitability. The physiologic aberrations induced by elevation of plasma potassium will dictate the order in which the clinician applies the following therapies.

1. *Decrease the extracellular load of potassium by diminishing or eliminating oral and IV K^+.* Keep in mind that the potassium content of stored bank blood given in transfusions may offer an immediate and often intolerable load to the patient in ARF.

2. *Promote intracellular transport and storage of potassium by preventing tissue release (catabolism), by reversing acidosis, and by the administration of insulin.* Plasma potassium concentrations can be lowered rapidly by the administration of bicarbonate or insulin. These maneuvers may control hyperkalemia for short periods of time, preventing extrusion from and promoting K^+

Table 38–2. Treatment of Hyperkalemia

Recognize and monitor
Eliminate potassium intake and prevent catabolism
Antagonize membrane effect using IV calcium
Move potassium into cells
  Infuse bicarbonate
  Infuse insulin and glucose
Remove potassium from body
  Administer diuretics
  Administer cation exchange resins
  Dialysis

entry into the cells. For every 0.1 unit pH decrement, the plasma K^+ concentration may increase by 0.6 mEq/L per L as the cells accept hydrogen ions and secrete potassium. Therefore, reversal of acidosis by sodium bicarbonate administration (2–3 mEq/kg in 5–10 min) may drive K^+ into the cells. This manipulation is transient and offers an additional sodium load to the patient. Insulin facilitates the rapid entry of K^+ into cells within 30 minutes to 1 hour and maintains this effect for several hours. The usual dose of IV insulin is 0.1 mg per kg per hour, with a concurrent administration of 3 to 5 gm of glucose per U of insulin.

3. *Removal of potassium from the body can be accomplished using a diuretic, an exchange resin, or dialytic therapy.* Diuretics that usually effect an increased delivery of sodium to the potassium secretory sites of the distal nephron are of limited use in the treatment of excess K^+ in ARF. Nonoliguric patients usually have adequate tubular flow and distal delivery of sodium; therefore, K^+ secretion is relatively unimpaired. Distal delivery of salt and water in oliguric ARF patients is drastically reduced; therefore, any manuever that would increase filtration rate and decrease proximal reabsorption would favor K^+ excretion. Mannitol and carbonic anhydrase inhibitors, if otherwise tolerated, can deliver increased amounts of proximal tubular fluid to the distal sites where the more commonly used diuretics, furosemide and ethacrynic acid, can exert their effects.

Kayexalate (sodium polystyrene sulfonate) can be administered either orally or rectally. Each gram of this resin can bind 1 mEq of K^+, which is then eliminated by the alimentary tract, sodium being retained by the body. For mild degrees of hyperkalemia in patients who can be alimented, the resin is given orally (5 gm in 25 ml of water or sorbitol) several times a day. When administered rectally, the resin (10–20 gm mixed with sorbitol) must be retained for 30 minutes to 1 hour to be effective. It is my practice to repeat the enemas hourly until the plasma potassium reaches approximately 4 mEq per L and then administer it 3 to 4 times a day. Nausea, constipation, and sodium retention may limit the usefulness of this therapy.

4. *When immediate but short-term therapy for the pathophysiologic sequelae of marked potassium elevation is required, IV administration of 10 percent calcium gluconate (0.5 ml/kg) over a 2- to 3-minute period sould antagonize the membrane effect of K^+ excess.* As an increased Ca^{++} lowers the threshhold potential, membrane excitability is decreased. If this maneuver does not reverse the changes in T waves and in the QRS complexes, a second dose may be administered.

A suggested sequence of therapy for the functional correlates of severe hyperkalemia follows: (1) administer calcium, 0.5 ml per kg, to reverse membrane irritability, (2) administer bicarbonate, 2 to 3 mEq per kg, if tolerable, to reverse acidosis, (3) administer insulin, 0.1 U per kg, and glucose, 0.3 to 0.5 gm per kg, to promote cellular storage, (4) begin kayexalate therapy to remove potassium from the body, and (5) when all the aforementioned therapies fail to adequately control plasma K^+ excess, dialysis should be instituted.

Hyperphosphatemia. Hyperphosphatemia will occur as the filtration rate decreases and the dietary intake is constant or if cells release their content into the circulation. As plasma phosphate increases, the solubility product, that is, calcium times phosphate, is increased, favoring deposition of calcium phosphate in bone and soft tissue, thereby lowering serum calcium. This effect can be reversed by lowering the phosphate intake or by the administration of oral phosphate binder Amphojel or Basigel, 100 to 200 mg per kg per day. Magnesium gels should be avoided as renal elimination of magnesium is markedly altered.

Hypocalcemia. The hypocalcemia of ARF cannot be treated by calcium administration until the phosphate level is lowered or precipitation of calcium salts (metastatic calcification) will develop. When phosphate is controlled, oral administration of calcium, 50 mg per kg per day, may be instituted. In most cases, the episode of ARF resolves before significant disturbances in calcium metabolism can occur. Obviously the effects of parathyroid hormone offer little benefit in oligoanuric patients.

Uric acid levels may become markedly elevated during oliguric renal failure, because filtration rate and proximal tubular secretion are markedly altered. Therapy for hyperuricemia per se is rarely indicated and should be directed at removal of the acid (diuresis or dialysis). Allopurinol therapy is not indicated and may in fact be deleterious.

Cardiovascular Disturbances

Acute volume overload may occur in oliguric ARF if water intake is not curtailed or if previously mentioned medications administered to correct acid–base or electrolyte aberrations exceed the kidneys' excretory ability. Although diuretic therapy and fluid restriction are efficacious (see General Management), dialytic therapy may be required.

Hypertension. An uncommon but serious concomitant of ARF, hypertension is usually observed in patients with intravascular overload. Because the major determinants of blood pressure (BP) are the cardiac output (CO) and the systemic vascular resistance (SVR) (BP = CO × SVR), it follows that elevation of blood pressure occurs when an unopposed increase in either element develops. Rarely does the patient present with hypertension; rather, hypertension occurs with inappropriate administration of fluids when there is avid salt and water retention. The exception to this rule is patients whose episode of ARF is secondary to acute glomerulonephritis.

When hypertension is mild to moderate, therapy may be limited to a reduction of fluid intake with or without diuretic therapy. If diuretics are required, I have found those that have a more proximal site of action (furosemide, ethacrynic acid) to be more useful than those affecting sites in the distal nephron. If vascular overload cannot be ameliorated by diuresis, therapy is directed at prevention of fluid overload.

With dramatic elevation of blood pressure, specific antihypertensive therapies are required (see Chapter 20, Hypertension). The time-honored combination of reserpine and hydralazine (IM) is efficacious. IV Aldomet or hydralazine may be administered when control of blood pressure is required within minutes to an hour. IV nitroprusside, a potent vasodilator, would be my choice of drug in the rare patient presenting with hypertensive encephalopathy.

In review, the overwhelming majority of patients with ARF are normotensive, the exceptions being those with acute glomerulonephritis. Oliguric renal failure patients are at risk, once hospitalized, to develop vascular overload. Nonoliguric renal failure patients, by definition, have an inability to effectively conserve water and rarely show intravascular volume overload. Fluid restriction alone or coupled with diuretic therapy is therapeutic for most patients who develop hypertension during an episode of ARF. Vasodilatory agents are used when severe elevation occurs or when the patient becomes symptomatic. If medical management fails, dialytic and/or ultrafiltration therapies may be required.

NEUROLOGIC DISTURBANCES

Neurologic manifestations of ARF consist primarily of alterations in consciousness (lethargy, agitation, confusion, coma) or seizure activity. These neurologic events may be secondary to acute electrolyte disturbance (hypocalcemia or hyponatremia), acid–base disturbances (severe metabolic alkalosis or acidosis), accumulation of drugs that alter CNS function, hypertension, or the uremic state itself. The pathogenesis of seizure activity in ARF, however, is unknown. Current investigations suggest that calcium levels are elevated within the neural cells of those patients manifesting neurologic complications during chronic renal failure. These neurologic abnormalities can be reversed by dialysis and by correction of the metabolic aberration or ameliorated by anticonvulsant therapy. If seizure activity continues after initial correction of the metabolic disturbance, IV diazepam or rectal paraldehyde should be administered. If major seizure acitivity persists, an amytal drip should be used to suppress activity. Continued activity often suggests a primary neurologic disease whose presence is unmasked by the uremic state.

ANEMIA

Anemia, invariably present in ARF, may be due to a multiplicity of insults suffered by the patient, including diminished production of erythropoietin, bone marrow suppression, hemodilution, hemolysis, gastrointestinal bleeding and frequent blood sampling. Transfusion therapy should be withheld unless the patient is symptomatic or until the hematocrit falls below 20 percent. The complications of blood transfusions, that is, acidosis, hyperkalemia, and brisk elevation of blood pressure may be avoided by infusing fresh packed cells slowly. Although suppression of thrombocyte production or impaired function of platelets may be seen in ARF, clinically significant coagulopathies occur infrequently and are reversed by dialysis.

INFECTIONS

Infections not only complicate the course of patients in ARF but also continue to be the major cause of death. These dramatically ill patients frequently have disruption of normal anatomic barriers, which protect them from infection, have altered immune responsiveness, or have been treated with inappropriate antimicrobials. In examining those clinical events that initiate an episode of ARF, it is not uncommon to find a patient with surgical or traumatic wounds who is intubated and has an indwelling bladder catheter and IV lines. Hence, the common infections in ARF involve the urinary system, the respiratory system, and wound or line sepsis. Therapy is directed at prevention, using aseptic technique, continuous surveillance, and prompt appropriate therapy guided by cultures. Altered reactivity has been shown in both cellular and humoral responses. These alterations have not been consistent nor have they been correlated with the degree of impairment of renal function. The variable effects of impaired nutritional status, of catabolism, and of acute illness on the acutely uremic patient have been underscored but not specified. Inappropriate or prophylactic antibiotic therapy may permit the overgrowth of normal flora or the development of fungal infection. Infections impose dramatic metabolic loads on patients by increasing catabolism. The metabolic load is further increased, because the required antimicrobials that are administered are usually in the form of salts of weak acids (e.g., amikacin sulfate and sodium ampicillin).

THERAPY DURING THE RECOVERY PHASE

As the previously oliguric patient enters the diuretic phase of ARF, the management of fluids and electrolytes poses an important problem. It is during this phase that the patient begins to mobilize fluid retained during the acute insult. If the glomerular filtration rate improves more rapidly than tubular function, large volumes of water are filtered with inadequate tubular mechanisms for water conservation. This pathophysiologic imbalance allows the patient to become intravascularly depleted and theoretically could initiate another episode of ARF. [An improvement in the glomerular filtration rate of only 59 percent (4–5 ml/min) would result in an increased tubular load of water approximating 6.5 to 7 L/day [4–5 ml × 1440 min/day].] A useful practice is to offer the patient the equivalent of three quarters of his or her urinary water and electrolyte excretion each day while monitoring for signs and symptoms of dehydration. Urinary indices dependent upon tubular function may not be useful indicators of the patient's intravascular volume status.

Because the administration of pharmacologic agents dependent upon renal function for excretion was restricted during the acute insult, the dosage must be adjusted during the recovery phase.

Recent data suggest that the mortality rate in ARF in adults has not dramatically changed over the past 20 years; morbidity has dramatically decreased. In general, mortality figures relate to the underlying event initiating ARF. Hence, the postoperative, post-traumatic, or multiple organ failure states are associated with a higher mortality rate than that ascribed to the occurrence of renal failure in a medical illness.

There are indications that morbidity has dramatically decreased over the past decade. This decrease has occurred in association with improved diagnostic and monitoring facilities, with early institution of dialysis and with the advent of hyperalimentation.

CASE PRESENTATION

A 6-year-old female was admitted to the hospital for IV therapy to correct acute dehydration. Her mother stated that the child had refused solid foods for the past 5 days, began to vomit 2 to 3 times daily 3 days prior to admission, and, today, would tolerate only small sips of water or soda. For 2 days prior to admission, her daughter experienced watery, but not bloody, diarrhea. The mother stated that her child was increasingly lethargic, pale, and complained of intermittent headaches for several days. Her urine output had decreased markedly during the past several days.

Examination and Test Results

The patient's past history was noncontributory. When seen by her pediatrician the morning of admission, she was acutely ill and pale and weighed 2 lb less than she had 3 weeks previously, when she was examined for an illness characterized by myalgias, intermittent fever, and an upper respiratory infection. Examination results included weight = 42 lb, T = 100° F, P = 110 beats/min, RR = 25–30 breaths/min, and BP = 110/80 mmHg. She was pale and lethargic. Her mucous membranes were dry. Although tachypneic, her chest was clear to auscultation and percussion (A&P). Her precordium was active, and she was tachycardic without a murmur. Her abdominal examination was negative except for hyperactive bowel sounds. No other positive finding was observed.

The patient was catheterized for urine culture, and a small amount of concentrated urine was obtained. The specific gravity was 1.020 and the urine tested 2+ positive for protein and ketone, 1+ positive for

blood, and negative for nitrites. Appropriate IV fluids were administered to correct a 5–10 percent isotonic dehydration. Admission laboratory data revealed a Hct = 38 percent, with normal RBC morphology, WBC = 14,000, platelets = adequate, BUN = 72 mg/dl, creatine = 3.5 mg/dl, Na = 130 mEq/L K = 5.1 mEq/L, CO_2 = 14 mEq/L, Cl = 100 mEq/L, Ca = 8.2 mg/dl, phosphate = 6 mg/dl, uric acid = 14 mg/dl, U_{Na} = 7 mEq/L, U_K = 28 mEq/L, and Ucreatine = 150 mg/dl. Twelve hours after admission, there was no significant change in urine output, vital signs, or laboratory values. Fluids were increased by 20 percent, and within 10 hours, the patient's condition had deteriorated.

Vital signs were BP = 130/100 mm Hg, P = 120 beats/min, and RR = 32 breaths/min. The mucous membranes were moist. Lab values Hct = 28 percent, normal RBC morphology, BUN = 84 mg/dl, creatine = 4.7 mg/dl, Na = 134 mEq/L, K = 6.1 mEq/L, CO_2 = 14 mEq/L, Cl = 101 mEq/L, Ca = 7.6 mg/dl, phosphate = 6.2 mg/dl, and uric acid = 16 mg/dl. A central venous pressure was obtained at 20 cm H_2O. The diagnosis of ARF was made, and appropriate therapy was initiated. Subsequent laboratory data were positive for a change in antistreptolysin-O (ASLO) and C_3.

Problem List

Renal

This patient presented with marked renal functional impairment, which was clearly out of proportion to the historical and physical evidence of dehydration. Therefore, one should have considered a pre-existing or concomitant renal disease. Historically, the decrease in urinary output occurred prior to or concurrent with poor intake; her weight loss was documented at less than 5 percent. Physical examination revealed mild evidence of dehydration; however, the patient had an active precordium and tachycardia, subtle evidence of vascular congestion. Her blood pressure was modestly elevated, even on admission, and there was no evidence of a wide gap between systolic and diastolic recordings as one might observe in the hyperdynamic cardiac response to dehydration.

The urine analysis was positive for blood and protein. Such findings are uncommon in acute gastroenteritis; however, they may have been ascribed to the bladder catheterization procedure. Recent evidence suggests that the morphology of the red cell is markedly altered in glomerular bleeding, whereas it is unaffected in nonglomerular bleeding. Hence, a comment regarding microscopic findings, that is, morphology, presence of RBC casts, and so on, would have been helpful.

Finally, the clinical course of the patient dictated further investigations. When fluid therapy is properly calculated and administered for mild dehydration, clinical and biochemical improvement should be seen within several hours. In the protocol, the patient showed no improvement in 12 hours; therefore, fluid administration was markedly increased.

If a determination of central venous pressure had been obtained at this time, it would have been elevated, and instead of increasing fluids, either restriction of fluids or an attempt at diuresis should have been initiated.

SUGGESTED READING

Anderson, R.J., Linas, S.L., Berns, A.S., et al.: Nonoliguric acute renal failure. N. Engl. J. Med. 296:1134, 1977.

Balslov, J.T., and Jorgensen, H.E.: A survey of 499 patients with acute anuric renal insufficiency: causes, treatment, complications, and mortality. Am. J. Med. 34:753, 1963.

Boichis, H., and Winterborn, M.H.: Acute renal failure in childhood. Pediatr. Ann. 58, 1974.

Flamenbaum, W.: Pathophysiology of acute renal failure. Arch. Intern. Med. 131:911, 1973.

Maher, J.F.: Pathophysiology of renal hemodynamics. Nephron 27:215, 1981.

Nursing Process for Patient Care:

Acute Renal Failure

Acute renal insufficiency and failure may result from primary disease of the kidney, but in the intensive care setting, most often they are the consequence of nonrenal conditions such as shock and congestive heart failure (CHF). Early recognition of acute renal failure is of prime importance.

RENAL

The alteration in renal function is most often manifested by both a decrease in urine output and an increase in retention of nitrogenous waste products. Decreased urine output, although the most common presentation, is not a certainty, because nonoliguric renal failure does occur. Fluid and electrolyte balance must be closely monitored.

Assess, Monitor, and Document

Urine output
Fluid intake
Weight (at least daily)
Status of hydration: skin condition, mucous
  membranes, thirst

Laboratory data
  Serum: BUN, creatinine, electrolytes, pH,
    calcium, phosphate, uric acid
  Urine: volume, electrolytes
Response to therapy

Anticipate

Alteration in renal status
  Decreased urine output
  Fluid overload: weight gain, hypertension
  Laboratory data: acidosis, hyponatremia,

hyperkalemia, hypocalcemia or hypercalcemia, hyperphosphatemia, hyperuricemia

CARDIOVASCULAR

Assess, Monitor, and Document

Heart rate
Rhythm
Blood pressure: arterial, central venous

Respiratory rate
Breath sounds
Secretions: amount, description

Anticipate

Volume overload
  Hypertension
  Pulmonary edema: tachypnea, tachycardia,
    rales, rhonchi, increased secretions

Dysrhythmias

NEUROLOGIC

Assess, Monitor, and Document

Level of consciousness
  Degree of alteration: response to stimuli
  (verbal, tactile, motor)

Seizure activity
  Description: time of onset, type of activity,
    duration, treatment (if applicable)

Anticipate

Altered level of consciousness
  Lethargy
  Confusion

Coma
Seizures

GASTROINTESTINAL

Assess, Monitor, and Document

Nutritional intake: calories, protein, carbohydrates

Bowel sounds
Bowel movements: description

Anticipate

Alteration in gastrointestinal and nutritional
status

Inadequate nutritional intake
Paralytic ileus

HEMATOLOGIC

The hematologic consequences of renal failure include anemia, decreased production of platelets, and impaired platelet function.

Assess, Monitor, and Document

Clinical
  Skin: color, petechiae, ecchymosis
  Mucous membranes: color, bleeding
  Overt bleeding
Laboratory

Hematocrit
Hemoglobin
Red blood cell (RBC) count
Platelet count

Anticipate

Alteration in hematologic status
Anemia
Bleeding

INFECTIOUS PROCESS

Infection is the major cause of death in children with acute renal failure (ARF). Assessment of parameters suggesting an infection is essential.

Assess, Monitor, and Document

Temperature
Respiratory system: rate, secretions, breath
  sounds

Wound: description
Laboratory: white blood cell (WBC) count

Anticipate

Presence of infection
  Urinary tract
  Respiratory system

Wound
Peritonitis, if peritoneal dialysis is being performed

RESPONSE OF CHILD

Assess, Monitor, and Document

Developmental level: verbal, motor, cognitive,
  psychosocial

Behavioral response: fearful, angry, compliant
Response to nursing interventions

Anticipate

Emotional distress
Inability to cope

RESPONSE OF FAMILY

Assess, Monitor, and Document

Behavioral response: anxious, fearful, verbal, angry
Level of understanding of child's condition

Expected outcome
Response to nursing interventions

Anticipate

Family crisis

MIND SET

Assess

Renal function
Cardiovascular status
Neurologic status
Gastrointestinal status

Hematologic status
Infectious process
Response of child and family

Anticipate

Alteration in renal function
  Acute renal insufficiency
  Acute renal failure
Alteration in cardiovascular status
  Volume overload
  Dysrhythmias
Alteration in neurologic status

  Coma
  Seizures
Alteration in gastrointestinal status
Alteration in hematologic status
Infectious process
Emotional distress
Family crisis

Hemolytic–Uremic Syndrome

STEVEN J. WASSNER, M.D.

Few renal conditions are more easily recognized by pediatricians than the sudden occurrence of acute renal failure (ARF), hemolytic anemia, and thrombocytopenia in infants and children. Knowledge regarding this condition has increased significantly over the past three decades, and the hemolytic-uremic syndrome (HUS) is now recognized as the leading cause of ARF in infancy. The pathology of HUS has been well described, and patient survival has greatly improved since the high fatality rates reported in early studies. The explanations offered to explain the pathophysiology of HUS have generally been derived from post-mortem pathologic observations and occasional renal biopsy material, as well as analyses of alterations in blood chemistries and coagulation profiles. Although the pieces seem to fit into a logical and consistent framework, there have been few prospective studies performed wherein the course of the disease has been conclusively altered by therapy aimed directly at the presumed abnormality. It can be stated that our current knowledge is incomplete and that our hypotheses remain open to improvement.

ETIOLOGY

Any explanation of the etiology of HUS must also explain its predilection for certain age and population groups. Worldwide, the age incidence appears to be bimodal, with a major peak in infants younger than 1 year of age and a second but smaller peak in those 3 to 7 years of age. It is notable that the peak in infancy is more apparent in warmer, more southern latitudes, whereas the later peak has been reported to occur more often in northern latitudes. The frequent occurrence of a diarrheal or upper respiratory tract infection prodrome, as well as the seasonal and epidemic nature of involvement, suggests an infectious etiology, as does the syndrome's reported association with a wide variety of bacterial and viral infections.

An excellent prospective study by Koster and associates has identified shigellosis as one of the antecedents of this condition; however, no single agent has been shown to be responsible for most cases. The multiplicity of organisms isolated by various investigators may only relate to the appearance of HUS in infancy, when bacterial and viral diarrheas are common. The same may be said about the occasional reports relating HUS to immunizations in this period of life.

Kaplan and colleagues first called attention to the possible familial or genetic association of HUS. They collected data on 41 families with more than one affected sibling and noted in one subset that the same syndrome appeared in another family member within days or weeks of the index case. Patient survival was good, and relapses did not occur. In another subgroup, cases occurred more than 1 year apart, mortality was high, and relapses occurred in 6 out of 12 cases. Tune and associates examined siblings of index cases with HUS. In these clinically asymptomatic children, they detected some children with hematuria and/or mildly decreased renal function. Whereas it is possible that an infectious etiology is responsible for most cases, other cases are genetically determined or occur after infection in a predisposed host.

In addition to the epidemic and familial aggregation of HUS in children, a condition that is clinically indistinguishable has been described in postpartum women and in women receiving estrogen-containing medications. Thus, it seems probable that many different stimuli may initiate a set of responses that culminate in the clinical entity now recognized as HUS.

PATHOPHYSIOLOGY

A precise understanding of the pathophysiology of HUS is hampered by the lack of an appropriate experimental model. A similar but not identical condition appears to be the generalized Schwartzman reaction, as seen in rabbits. In that species, two injections of endotoxin, given 24 hours apart, lead to disseminated intravascular coagulation (DIC), renal endothelial damage, and deposition of fibrin, both in the kidneys and within other body organs. Rabbits may be protected against the development of DIC by administration of heparin at the time of the second endotoxin injection, but once the process has begun, it is of no benefit. In contrast to the Schwartzman reaction, organs other than the kidneys are less frequently involved in HUS, documentation of widespread fibrin deposition is unusual, DIC is not prominent, and endotoxemia has not been consistently shown. In the study noted previously, patients with shigellosis were followed prospectively and circulating endotoxin was demonstrated in 9 of 18 patients prior to their developing hemolysis and renal insufficiency (vs. the presence of endotoxin in only 3 of 61 patients who did not develop hemolysis). Interestingly, circulating endotoxin was found only before the development of hemolysis. These findings may explain the absence of endotoxemia in children studied after the onset of clinical HUS, but it is still not known whether the development of endotoxemia is always required for the development of this syndrome.

Current thoughts regarding the pathogenesis of HUS assign a central role to the renal lesion in the propagation of both the hemolysis and the thrombocytopenia. Renal biopsy and autopsy examinations confirm the presence of a thrombotic microangiopathy within the glomerular capillary membranes. Glomerular endothelial cells are swollen and detached from the glomerular basement membrane, whereas the glomerular capillary lumina are narrowed by the presence of both endothelial cells and fibrin deposits.

The development of anemia and characteristic red blood cell (RBC) morphology are thought to be due to the mechanical deformation and destruction of red cells passing through this abnormal meshwork of cells and fibers placed in an area of high blood flow. The diagnosis of the intravascular hemolytic anemia is confirmed by the presence of decreased hemoglobin levels (as low as 3 gm/dl), schistocytes, helmet and burr cells, and diminished plasma haptoglobin levels. Although jaundice is uncommon, pallor is frequently present. In spite of the presence of significant azotemia, the reticulocyte count is frequently high and the hemoglobin level generally returns toward normal by 2 weeks.

The thrombocytopenia seen in HUS is due to a combination of several factors: platelet aggregation at the site of renal endothelial damage and fibrin deposition; platelet destruction as a result of mechanical shearing forces and their subsequent removal by the spleen; and increased platelet aggregation due to the release of nucleotides from damaged RBCs. Platelet consumption is increased among infants with HUS, and the life span of infused platelets is diminished.

Recently, it has been proposed that patients with HUS lack a plasma factor necessary for the stimulation of vascular tissue prostacyclin production. Prostacyclin is a prostaglandin with potent vasodilatory and platelet antiaggregating properties. Whereas early reports suggested that the hematologic abnormalities of this syndrome responded rapidly to the administration of plasma, infusion of prostacyclin in a child with severe HUS did not result in clinical improvement.

TREATMENT

The first step in the treatment of HUS is the maintenance of a high state of alertness to those situations in which the condition is likely to occur. Because a diarrheal prodrome is so common, children with HUS are frequently given large volumes of replacement fluid and their lack of urinary output is often interpreted as an indication of continued volume depletion. Careful observation and repeated physical examination may detect signs of acute hemolysis and anemia, volume overload, or neurologic dysfunction. In this setting, detection of the characteristic RBC morphology and thrombocytopenia are diagnostic.

Twenty percent of patients may present with abdominal complaints. Patients have been admitted with initial diagnoses of ulcerative colitis, intussusception, or signs of peritoneal irritation. Only after admission and sometimes only postoperatively has the diagnosis become apparent.

Neurologic. Neurologic symptoms are common in patients with HUS and range from slight twitching and tremors to aphasias, hemiparesis, and focal or generalized seizures. These symptoms tend to be transient and not associated with significant residua. Seizures most often are the result of acute electrolyte abnormalities or hypertension, with or without volume overload. However, the possiblity of cerebral microthrombi leading to infarction should be kept in mind. Whenever a specific etiology is determined (i.e., hypo-osmolality, hypertension), definitive treatment should, of course, be directed toward its cause; seizures are an indication for early dialysis.

Anemia. The need to transfuse patients with HUS depends upon the degree of anemia present and the rapidity of the hemolytic process. Sufficient oxygen-carrying capacity must be maintained, so that the hemoglobin concentration is not allowed to drop below 7 to 8 gm per dl. Only fresh units of packed RBCs should be infused to minimize the risk of hyperkalemia. Volume overload and hyperkalemia may best be avoided by performing transfusions in conjunction with dialysis.

In the past, heparin administration was advocated as therapy for the presumed coagulopathy. More recently, both theoretical considerations and experimental studies have not documented any benefit of heparin in the acute stage. Proesmans has argued that there is a subset of patients with ongoing coagulopathy whose prognosis is poor and who might benefit from the early administration of heparin. Unfortunately, it is not currently possible to predict accurately which patients will benefit from heparin. Because more than 90 percent of children recover without the use of heparin and systemic anticoagulation incurs significant morbidity, the use of heparin cannot be generally recommended. Aspirin or dipyridamole, two drugs that interfere with platelet aggregation, have both been administered, but evidence supporting their use is equivocal. Finally, attempts have been made to speed the dissolution of fibrin thrombi through the use of streptokinase, infused either systemically or directly into the renal arteries. Neither method has been uniformly successful and neither is currently recommended.

Acute Renal Failure. The acute renal failure (ARF) seen in HUS is of the oligoanuric variety. As noted previously, recognition of the presence of this condition may occur only after the development of volume overload, hypertension, seizures, and/or hyponatremia. The hyponatremia is due to the excessive administration of hypotonic solutions and should be treated by volume restriction. Volume overload may lead to hypertension and possibly to congestive heart failure (CHF). Hypertension may also be due to hyperreninemia; thus, antihypertensive drugs are commonly required. Conservative management of ARF in these patients is complicated by ongoing hemolysis and thrombocytopenia, which may require transfusions of packed red cells or platelets. In addition, hemolysis releases the intracellular potassium of red cells and can rapidly lead to

dangerous hyperkalemia. Strict attention to volume and electrolyte status is therefore required. As in other forms of ARF, hypocalcemia is common and plasma calcium levels should be monitored. Finally, it is not surprising that metabolic acidosis is a common finding in this setting, bringing with it the added risk of further hyperkalemia.

Current criteria for peritoneal dialysis, including anuria of 24-hour duration, rapidly rising BUN, and persistent metabolic abnormalities, have resulted in a significant reduction in mortality rate. Dialysis facilitates management of hyperkalemia, acidosis, hypervolemia, and hypertension. It enhances the ability to provide calories either orally or intravenously, as well as through glucose absorbed during the dialysis. Although the institution of early dialysis has been associated with an improved survival among patients with HUS, it is unclear whether this is due to general improvements in the care of ARF or, as has been suggested, to a special role of dialysis in removing possible inhibitors of glomerular fibrinolysis.

Prognosis. The recovery of renal function in patients with HUS is related to the length of the oligoanuric period. Patients without oligoanuria or with short periods of decreased output, never requiring dialysis, have complete recovery of renal function. The percentage of patients with chronic renal failure increases as the duration of oligoanuria exceeds 14 to 21 days. With the exception of 5 to 10 percent of children whose initial insult is severe enough to lead to death or permanent renal failure in the acute stage, the prognosis for most patients is optimistic.

CASE PRESENTATION

An 18-month-old girl was well until 6 days prior to admission when she began vomiting and developed watery diarrhea. Over the next 2 days, she continued to have diarrhea but was able to tolerate oral feedings. Three days prior to admission, she was noted to become more active and alert and the diarrhea abated. On the day of admission, she vomited again and was seen by a physician, who noted mild dehydration and advised the parent to encourage fluids. The patient drank but did not void for the next 18 hours. At that time, she had a generalized seizure and was brought to the emergency room.

Examination and Test Results

Physical examination showed a well-developed, but pale and lethargic child. Blood pressure = 130/85 mm Hg, pulse = 170 beats/min, and weight =

13.5 kg (30 lb). There was good skin turgor, and no petechiae were noted. Bowel sounds were absent, there was diffuse abdominal tenderness, and the rectal examination revealed blood on the examining finger. The bladder was not palpated. The child was arousable only with difficulty, the reflexes were brisk, and no focal signs, tremors, or clonus were noted. Laboratory studies showed: hemoglobin = 8.8 gm/dl, hematocrit = 27 percent, platelet count = 74,000, WBC = 16,700, with 50 percent neutrophils, 22 percent bands, 25 percent lymphs, and 3 percent monocytes. Red cell morphology showed multiple schistocytes, spherocytes, occasional helmet cells, and many burr cells. The serum haptoglobin was not detectable. Serum electrolytes were: sodium = 125 mEq/L, chloride = 93 mEq/L, potassium = 4.2 mEq/L, and bicarbonate = 15 mEq/L. BUN = 81 mg/dl, creatinine = 5.4 mg/dl, calcium = 6.8 mg/dl, and phosphorus = 8.7 mg/dl. Abdominal x-rays showed nonspecific ileus. A cerebral CAT scan was normal. Phenobarbital was administered 4 hours after admission.

Peritoneal dialysis was immediately initiated. Four hours later, the hematocrit had decreased to 20 percent and the platelet count had decreased to 46,000. During dialysis, the child's weight decreased to 10.8 kg (24 lb) and her blood pressure decreased to 100/60 mm Hg. Plasma calcium and phosphorus levels became normal, and there were no further seizures. After 40 hours of dialysis, the child was alert and there was no further abdominal discomfort. The temporary dialysis catheter was removed, and the patient was transferred to the pediatric ward. She was placed on a low-protein diet, containing only 10 gm of protein/day, and fluid intake was restricted to 200 ml/day. Calcium, 250 mg q.i.d., was given orally to maintain the serum calcium. The child tolerated the dietary restrictions poorly, and over the next 3 days the BUN and creatinine rose to 127 mg/dl and 8.1 mg/dl, respectively. Hyperkalemia recurred and was treated with Kayexalate enemas. Because of continued anuria, on Day 6, a Tenkhoff peritoneal dialysis catheter was surgically placed and dialysis was reinstituted. While on dialysis, the infant was allowed a more liberal dietary intake and she began to show more interest in food. By Day 9, hemoglobin level rose to 9.5 gm/dl and the platelet count rose on 195,000. On Day 15, the patient urinated 190 ml, which had a specific gravity of 1.010, a pH of 6.5, 3+ protein, and 1+ blood. Urine output increased, and dialysis was stopped on Day 17. By Day 19, the child was urinating more than 1500 ml/day and her creatinine had decreased to 3.9 mg/dl. The patient was discharged from the hospital on Day 23. The infant's BUN and creatinine were normal by 4 weeks. On continued follow-up, she remains normotensive and is growing normally.

Problem List

Renal

This constellation of symptoms, along with the presence of a hemolytic anemia, thrombocytopenia,

and ARF, is characteristic of HUS. Management of ARF initially included fluid restriction to help correct the hyponatremia and hypertension. Frequent determinations of serum electrolytes are required to guard against the development of hyperkalemia. Whenever possible, a low-protein, high-calorie intake should be prescribed to limit the development of a catabolic state. Failure to correct electrolyte abnormalities or prevent the development of hypertension is an indication for dialysis.

Fluid and Electrolyte Balance

The continued presence of electrolyte abnormalities, and the development of hyperkalemia and anuria for more than 24 hours, led to the institution of peritoneal dialysis in this child. Because of the higher incidence of infection seen after 72 hours when a temporary dialysis catheter was used, the catheter was removed while the patient was still anuric. Currently, at our institution all children requiring peritoneal dialysis have Tenkhoff peritoneal dialysis catheters surgically inserted. These catheters can be maintained indefinitely, allowing better control of electrolyte abnormalities as well as more latitude in fluid administration.

Circulatory

Hypertension was treated with fluid removal during peritoneal dialysis. If necessary, pharmacologic treatment of hypertension can be started and is similar to the plan used in other forms of ARF (see Chapter 38, Acute Renal Failure).

Hematologic

Anemia was treated during dialysis with transfusions of freshly drawn packed RBCs to prevent further exacerbation of hyperkalemia and hypertension. The platelet counts were followed, but specific therapy was not required.

Gastrointestinal

Abdominal tenderness was evaluated with x-rays of the abdomen as well as frequent physical examinations. Oral intake was withheld until resolution of the ileus.

Neurologic

Most patients with HUS who seize, do so because of either electrolyte abnormalities or hypertension. With the correction of these problems, there were no further seizure episodes. In the postictal period, phenobarbital was administered to prevent further seizures. A follow-up EEG was normal, and the phenobarbital was tapered and discontinued.

SUGGESTED READING

Bale, J.F., Brasher, C. and Siegler, R.L.: CNS manifestations of the hemolytic uremic syndrome. Relationship to metabolic alterations and prognosis. Am. J. Dis. Child 134:869, 1980.

Fong, J.S., de Chadarevian, J.P., and Kaplan, B.S.: Hemolytic-uremic syndrome, current concepts and management. Pediatr. Clin. North Am. 29(4):835, 1982.

Giantonio, A., Vitacco, M., Mendilharzu, F., et al.: The hemolytic-uremic syndrome. Nephron 11:714, 1973.

Kaplan, B.S., Chesney, R.W., and Drummond, K.N.: Hemolytic-uremic syndrome in families. N. Engl. J. Med. 292:1090, 1975.

Kaplan, B.S., Thomson, P.D., and de Chadarevian, J.P.: The hemolytic-uremic syndrome. Pediatr. Clin. North Am. 23(4):761, 1976.

Kaplan, S., Katz, J., Krawitz, S., and Lurie, A.: An analysis of the results of therapy in 67 cases of the hemolytic uremic syndrome. J. Pediatr. 78(3):420, 1971.

Katz, J., Krawitz, S., Sacks, P.V., et al.: Platelet, erythrocyte, and fibrinogen kinetics in the hemolytic-uremic syndrome of infancy. J. Pediatr. 83(5):739, 1973.

ki-Muaka, P.B., Proesmans, W., and Eeckels, R.: The haemolytic uraemic syndrome in childhood: a study of the long-term prognosis. Eur. J. Pediatr., 136:237, 1981.

Koster, F., Levin, J., Walter, L., et al.: Hemolytic-uremic syndrome after shigellosis. Relation to endotoxemia and circulating immune complexes. N. Engl. J. Med. 298(17):927, 1978.

Lieberman, E.: Hemolytic-uremic syndrome. J. Pediatr. 80:1, 1972.

Perico, N., Scheipatti, A., Mecca, G., et al.: Prostacyclin and renal diseases. Clin. Nephrol. 18(3):111, 1982.

Proesmans, W., and Eeckels, R.: Has heparin changed the prognosis of the hemolytic-uremic syndrome? Clin. Nephrol. 2(5):169, 1974.

Tune, B.M., Groshong, T., Plumer, L.B., and Mendoza, S.A.: The hemolytic-uremic syndrome in siblings: a prospective study. J. Pediatr. 85(5):682, 1974.

Tune, B.M., Leavitt, T.J., and Gribble, T.J.: The hemolytic-uremic syndrome in California: a review of 28 nonheparinized cases with long-term follow-up. J. Pediatr. 82(2):304, 1973.

Nursing Process for Patient Care:

Hemolytic–Uremic Syndrome

This syndrome includes acute renal failure (ARF), hemolytic anemia, and thrombocytopenia. The focus is on the renal and hematologic systems. The impact of alterations of these systems on other major body systems, such as circulatory, gastrointestinal, and neurologic, must be understood in order to create a comprehensive mind set. Hemolytic-uremic syndrome (HUS) has two age peaks: infants younger than 1 year and children between the ages of 3 and 7 years.

RENAL

Assess, Monitor, and Document

Weight
Status of hydration
Urine output
Urine specific gravity
Blood pressure
Pulse
Breath sounds

Laboratory data
  Serum electrolytes: BUN, creatinine, osmolality
  Urine electrolytes and osmolality
Fluid intake: accurate administration of parenteral fluids (use infusion pump if available)

Anticipate

Acute renal failure
  Oliguria/anuria
  Hypervolemia
  Hypertension

Hyponatremia
Hyperkalemia
Hypocalcemia
Elevated BUN and creatinine

HEMATOLOGIC

The development of anemia and characteristic red blood cell (RBC) morphology are important factors in HUS. Of greater significance is the thrombocytopenia associated with this syndrome.

Assess, Monitor and Document

Serum hemoglobin and hematocrit
Platelet count
Presence of petechiae, bruises, and bleeding (overt and covert)

Child during transfusion (if needed)
Accurate administration and documentation of blood products (if required)

Anticipate

Alteration in hematologic status
  Anemia: pallor, fatigue, tachypnea, tachycardia

Bleeding

CARDIOVASCULAR

Assess, Monitor, and Document

Heart rate
Rhythm
Quality
Perfusion: peripheral pulses, skin color and condition

Blood pressure
Respiratory rate
Response to antihypertensive medications if required

Anticipate

Alteration in cardiovascular status
Congestive heart failure

Cardiac dysrhythmias: PVC's, ventricular fibrillation

NEUROLOGIC

Neurologic symptoms are common in children with HUS and are most often the result of the electrolyte abnormalities or hypertension.

Assess, Monitor, and Document

Level of consciousness
Orientation
Reflexes

Anticipate

Alteration in neurologic status
Seizures
Infarction

GASTROINTESTINAL

Assess, Monitor, and Document

Degree of abdominal discomfort
Abdominal girth
Presence of bowel sounds

Color, consistency, frequency of stools
Bleeding (overt or covert)

Anticipate

Alteration in gastrointestinal status
Abdominal distress: ileus, diarrhea
Bleeding

RESPONSE OF CHILD

Assess, Monitor, and Document

Developmental level
Degree of distress
Response to separation

Anticipate

Emotional distress

RESPONSE OF FAMILY

Assess, Monitor, and Document

Behavioral response: anxious, verbal
Level of understanding of child's condition

Expected outcome
Response to nursing interventions

Anticipate

Inability to cope
Family crisis

MIND SET

Assess

Renal status
Fluid and electrolyte balance
Hematologic status
Cardiovascular status

Neurologic status
Gastrointestinal status
Response of child and family

Anticipate

Alteration in renal status
  Acute renal failure
Alteration in hematologic status
  Anemia
  Bleeding
Alteration in cardiovascular status
  Congestive heart failure

Cardiac dysrhythmias
Alteration in neurologic status
  Seizures
Alteration in gastrointestinal status
  Abdominal distress
Emotional distress of child
Family crisis

GASTROINTESTINAL

Upper Gastrointestinal Bleeding

MARVIN E. AMENT, M.D.

Management of upper gastrointestinal bleeding is simple and logical. Before a history is taken, the physician must determine whether the patient is volume depleted and in shock and whether the patient must be stabilized. Following stabilization, efforts must be made to determine the source of the bleeding, stop it, and treat the patient so that further episodes do not occur. Surprisingly, most patients stop bleeding spontaneously. For those patients who do not, the type of intervention must be decided upon, with the idea of stopping the bleeding. Pediatric patients differ from adult patients in that the mortality from bleeding is not nearly as high because of the absence of cardiac, pulmonary, and renal disease in most patients who present with bleeding. Physicians must remember that accurate assessment of the severity of bleeding and vigorous and prompt resuscitation are the basic measures that must be taken in the management of bleeding.

PRESENTATION

Bleeding from the gastrointestinal tract may present in many ways. Hematemesis is bloody vomitus, either fresh and bright red or older and "coffee ground" in character. Melena is shiny, black or maroon-colored, sticky, sweet, and sickly smelling stool. It results from degradation of blood and must not be confused with the effects of exogenous stool darkeners such as iron, bismuth, or licorice. Frequently, stools that are dark green in color are mistaken for melena. The odor of melena is so characteristic that, once smelled, a physician is unlikely to forget it. Hematochezia is the passage of bright red blood from the rectum in the form of pure blood, blood intermixed with formed stool, or bloody diarrhea. In many instances, gastrointestinal blood loss is occult and is only detected by testing stool with a guaiac reagent. Finally, patients may present without any objective sign of bleeding but with symptoms of blood loss, such as dizziness, dyspnea, heart failure, and even shock. We have experienced patients going into shock from blood loss one or more hours before they have passed blood.

PATIENT ASSESSMENT

Vital Signs

Rapid assessment of the patient is critical when gastrointestinal bleeding is suspected (Table 40–1). The physician is faced with determining whether the bleeding is acute or chronic and whether the patient is unstable or stable. The first order of business is to objectively determine, with inspection of the stool or nasogastric aspirate, the presence of bleeding. Stabilization of the patient, however, should take precedence in patients who are obviously unstable. Vital signs are taken first, the patient's skin and mucous membranes are inspected for pallor or signs of shock, and blood is immediately sent to the laboratory for complete blood count, clotting studies, type and crossmatch, and routine chemistries if signs of blood loss are present. If transfusions are necessary, they can thus be given without delay. If the patient is hypotensive or has tachycardia, a venous line is established and volume expanded rapidly with normal saline (NS) in 5 percent albumin until vital signs are stabilized or until blood products become available.

Table 40–1. Steps in Management of Upper Gastrointestinal Bleeding

1. Establish stability of patient. Take vital signs:
   BP: supine, erect
   Pulse: supine, erect
   Respirations
2. If unstable, immediately place an Angiocath or scalp vein needle. Use the largest bore needle possible.
3. Infuse NS, 5 percent albumin in saline, or Ringer's lactate as fast as possible.
   Goal: 1 ml/kg/min
   Maintain this rate until vital signs stabilize.
4. Draw blood for CBC, PT, PTT, platelet count, electrolytes, BUN, creatinine, and type and cross-match.
5. If unsure of source of bleeding, examine oropharynx and nares before passing a nasogastric tube. Do a rectal examination if patient is shocky and has not passed blood or is stable and you wish to confirm history.
6. Transfuse whole blood as soon as it is available; replace it as quickly as possible.
7. Pass large bore orogastric tube, No. 34 French in children, to lavage stomach with iced saline or saline at room temperature.
8. Lavage for up to 1 hour.
9. If bleeding persists, do emergency endoscopy to identify the source.
10. If varices are present and if there is no other identifiable source, begin vasopressin infusion. Start with 0.1 U/min and increase to 0.4 U/min as necessary. Maintain for 24 hours before reducing dosage.
11. Sclerose varices electively, if possible, after 48 hours.
12. If an ulcer is identified with a bleeding vessel, consider electrocoagulation versus surgical therapy.
13. If gastritis is present, treat with maximal doses of antacids given hourly and cimetidine every 6 hours.

Presenting Manifestation

Hematemesis, melena, or hematochezia indicates an acute episode of bleeding, whereas occult bleeding is generally chronic. Hematemesis results from a combination of large amounts of blood filling the stomach plus the urge to vomit, which often accompanies vascular collapse. Thus, hematemesis generally indicates a more severe bleeding episode than melena, which occurs when bleeding is slow enough to allow time for degradation of the blood. However, there is great variation from person to person, and it would be unwise to assess the severity of bleeding solely on this basis.

Hematocrit

The hematocrit is typically used as a measurement of the magnitude of bleeding. Unfortunately, it reflects the actual amount of blood loss only after acute bleeding episodes. If a patient bleeds slowly and chronically, many liters of blood may be lost before the bone marrow iron stores are depleted and the hematocrit falls. At this time, a peripheral blood smear will usually reveal hypochromic and microcytic red blood cells (RBCs). The mean corpuscular volume (MCV) of these cells will be low. If blood loss is acute, the hematocrit will reflect the magnitude of the loss, but not immediately. The hematocrit may not change rapidly during the first few hours of hemorrhage, because proportionate reduction occurs in both plasma and red cell volumes. During this time, caution must be taken not to underestimate the severity of bleeding just because the hematocrit is normal. This is a frequent error in management. Hematocrit does not begin to fall until high-protein extravascular fluid enters the vascular space. This process begins shortly after bleeding occurs but is not complete for 24 to 72 hours. At this point, plasma volume is larger than normal and the hematocrit is at its lowest point. The MCV will be normal unless there has been prior chronic blood loss. The sequence is often modified by administration of exogenous fluids or blood and is not as pronounced in dehydrated patients.

Blood Pressure and Heart Rate

Frequent measurements of blood pressure and heart rate are the best ways to judge a patient's stability, regardless of the hematocrit. The blood pressure and heart rate depend upon the amount and the acuteness of blood loss and the extent of cardiac and vascular compensation. Postural hypotension may be the only physical finding early in the course of bleeding. Blood pressure is often maintained when the patient is recumbent but falls when the patient sits up. If it falls by greater than 10mm Hg, mild volume depletion is present. Tachycardia may not develop until blood loss is greater than 10 percent of blood volume. With greater blood losses, tachycardia and vasoconstriction develop compensatorily. Finally, in severe bleeding, recumbent hypotension occurs. It is at this point that vascular collapse has occurred and the patient is truly in shock. In these instances, the patient is ashen gray in color and diaphoretic and may have evidence of respiratory distress. Occasionally, patients experience a vasovagal reaction with bleeding, characterized by bradycardia, vasodilatation, and profound constitutional symptoms. Whether patients will show any of these findings depends upon their cardiac function, the status of their vascular system, their state of hydration, and whether or not their autonomic nervous system is intact. Heart rates over 120 beats per minute, a systolic blood pressure under 70 mm Hg, or a postural drop in blood pressure of 10 to 15 mm Hg reflects a blood loss of 20 percent or greater. Stable patients with chronic bleeding are evaluated electively, whereas those with acute bleeding or an unstable condition must immediately be resuscitated.

Resuscitation

Patients with significant acute bleeding or who are in an unstable condition should be admitted to an intensive care unit (ICU). However, venous access should be established as soon as possible whether the patient is in a clinic or in emergency room. Placing the patient in a reverse Trendelenburg position may distend or make visible neck veins in order to allow insertion of an Angiocath. Venous access is achieved with large-bore cannulas. The largest possible size compatible with the patient's veins should be used. Fluids are then started and are administered as rapidly as possible until the blood pressure is stabilized. NS and lactated Ringer's solution are the most commonly chosen fluids. If possible, placement of a central venous line to measure central venous pressure is useful in the fluid management of such patients, but this line should not be placed first if the patient is truly in shock. The administration of fluids should be begun, and then attempts to place a central line should be started. The obvious goals of therapy are to quickly improve the circulation of the remaining RBCs and to administer supplemental oxygen by nasal cannula or face mask to permit optimal red cell saturation. Vital signs, urine output, and electrocardiogram (EKG) are monitored frequently. A flow sheet on which the resuscitative measures and the patient's response to treatment are accurately documented should be at the patient's bedside.

Transfusion

Common sense dictates that patients who continue to bleed despite therapy, who have hematocrits less than 30 percent, or who have symptoms related to poor oxygenation should be transfused. For asymptomatic, stable patients with hematocrits above 25 to 30 percent, other factors must be considered: Is it likely that the hematocrit will drop further as vascular repletion occurs? From what hematocrit level could the patient withstand a recurrent episode of bleeding? Is bleeding acute or chronic? If transfusions are deemed unnecessary, iron supplements should be instituted as soon as possible. What should be transfused? Whole blood is transfused to improve oxygenation with red cells and to improve coagulation with plasma and platelets.

The relative necessity of fulfilling these goals varies among patients and determines the type of blood products transfused. Patients who are actively bleeding have a need for both and should be given whole blood or red cells reconstituted with fresh frozen plasma. Patients who have ceased bleeding and whose vascular volume has been replenished with saline or lactated Ringer's solution require predominantly RBCs. Administration of packed red cells to this type of patient not only spares the resource of blood banks but also reduces the volume of fluid transfused. This is an important factor in patients with marginal cardiac or renal function. Fresh frozen plasma is not required in most patients unless there is a disturbance of coagulation or massive bleeding. Patients with known cirrhosis should receive fresh frozen plasma after every second or third unit of packed RBCs. Platelets are used only with very large hemorrhages that constitute half or more of the blood volume. Supplemental calcium is usually necessary if patients use bank blood that is anticoagulated with calcium-binding agents. Blood should be replaced as rapidly as possible, because bleeding may be ongoing or may recur.

HISTORY AND PHYSICAL EXAMINATION

Historically, it is important to determine whether the patient has taken any medications that are ulcerogenic or known to cause acute gastritis just prior to the onset of the bleeding and whether the patient has a history of chronic liver disease, splenomegaly, or peptic ulcer disease.

On physical examination, it is important to examine the nose and nasopharynx, because hematemesis may be secondary to a posterior nasal hemorrhage. Similarly, examination of the abdomen may show either an enlarged cirrhotic liver with splenomegaly or splenomegaly alone secondary to portal vein thrombosis.

UPPER VS. LOWER GASTROINTESTINAL TRACT BLEEDING

As resuscitation is being carried out, the source of bleeding must be localized to the upper or lower gastrointestinal tract to direct further management. Hematemesis, either alone or in combination with other manifestations, indicates an upper gastrointestinal location, that is above the ligament of Treitz, as the source of bleeding. Melena occurs if enough hemoglobin in the gastrointestinal tract is oxidized to hematin or other hemochromes to blacken the stool. Melena can occur with as little as 100 to 200 ml of blood in an adult or as little as 1 to 2 percent of the blood volume lost acutely in children. Most patients with melena bleed from an upper gastrointestinal source. Bleeding colonic lesions may occasionally produce melena but only when three conditions are met: First, there must be enough blood degraded to blacken the stool. Second, bleeding must not be too brisk or hematochezia will ensue. Third, colonic motility must be sluggish to allow enough time for degradation to occur. Most colonic lesions either bleed in such small amounts that only occult blood is present in the stool or bleed so briskly that hematochezia occurs.

Hematochezia usually represents a lower gastrointestinal source of bleeding, although an upper gastrointestinal lesion may occasionally bleed so briskly that blood does not remain in the bowel long enough to become melena. Lesions of the small intestine may present as either hematochezia or melena, although small bowel lesions are an unusual source of gastrointestinal bleeding except for Meckel's diverticulum.

A nasogastric tube should be placed whenever the question arises as to the location of bleeding. A bloody aspirate confirms an upper gastrointestinal source, whereas a negative aspirate virtually excludes active upper gastrointestinal bleeding. Interpretation by the guaiac reaction of aspirates that are not grossly bloody should be cautious, because both false-positive and false-negative results may occur. Ten to 15 percent of postpyloric ulcers will bleed massively without reflux into the stomach, and the aspirate will be negative. Endoscopy is the only reliable way of detecting such occurrences, but other findings suggestive of upper gastrointestinal bleeding include hyperactive bowel sounds and elevation of the blood urea nitrogen (BUN) to 30 to 40 mg per dl. Such rises in the BUN occur after major upper gastrointestinal bleeding episodes and are the result of volume depletion plus absorbed blood products. Either factor alone will not result in elevation of the BUN.

ACUTE UPPER GASTROINTESTINAL BLEEDING

Mortality and Rebleeding

Ten percent of all patients with upper gastrointestinal bleeding die as a result. Mortality is much greater in patients over 60 years of age; however, death may occur in younger patients if they are improperly resuscitated. Of the lesions that bleed, esophageal varices account for a disproportionate number of deaths. This is no doubt secondary to the fact that these patients often have disrupted liver function and a disturbance in blood clotting mechanisms. Death from bleeding typically occurs in those patients who continue to bleed after admission to the hospital or who stop bleeding and then rebleed during the first 48 hours. Mortality in patients who cease bleeding is from 2 to 8 percent, whereas mortality from rebleeding ranges from 10 to 22 percent.

Medical Management

Bleeding must be stopped quickly without resorting to urgent surgery or other invasive therapy. Rebleeding, especially from esophageal varices, must be prevented. Measures designed to achieve these goals must be either empirical or specific. Empirical therapy is administered without a diagnosis in hand and must therefore be relatively safe and not require special expertise. Specific therapy, on the other hand, is usually more invasive or requires special skills in situations in which specific diagnosis is needed first.

Empirical Therapy to Stop Active Bleeding. Gastric lavage with iced saline is a time-honored empirical technique. In 90 percent of patients, gastric lavage at least temporarily causes bleeding to stop, regardless of the diagnosis. However, even if lavage were of no help in controlling the bleeding, it provides a good indication of the rapidity of bleeding and serves to cleanse the stomach for possible later endoscopy.

A large bore No. 34 to No. 36 French orogastric tube is placed in children when possible after removal of the smaller diameter nasogastric tube used for localization of bleeding. Aliquots of fluid, 500 to 1000 ml per 1.73 m², are instilled and then removed by gentle suction and gravity drainage. Iced saline is traditionally used because cold fluids reduce blood flow more effectively than room temperature fluids. On the other hand, cold fluids may impair coagulation. Some studies have indicated that room temperature tap water lavage may be as effective as iced saline lavage.

Lavage is continued until bleeding stops or until it becomes evident that other measures will be necessary. Most bleeding ceases during lavage. If the bleeding does not cease, several pharmacologic agents have been suggested for use in empirical therapy, the most widely used being agents to reduce gastric acidity. The rationale for such therapy is based on the following: First, peptic ulcers are a frequent cause of upper gastrointestinal bleeding. Second, pepsin, which promotes platelet disaggregation, is inactivated at high gastric pH. Third, there is in vitro evidence suggesting that blood coagulation is optimal when gastric pH is high.

Antacids have been studied only in patients with bleeding from acute gastritis. In one study, low doses of antacid either alone or with modest doses of cimetidine arrested bleeding in only one third of patients. A placebo-treated group was not used. In another study, antacids in doses sufficient to maintain gastric pH at 7 were reported to stop bleeding in 90 percent of patients with acute gastritis. There is no evidence, however, that this approach is better than the less intensive approach. Cimetidine has been evaluated versus placebo in two series of patients with continuing upper gastrointestinal bleeding of various causes, and in neither series was it successful. Dosages used were 7.5 mg per kg q6h or 1200 mg per m² per day. This dose may not raise gastric pH levels high enough to achieve inhibition of all secretion.

Some investigators have reported that somatostatin reduces gastric acidity more effectively than cimetidine and is more efficacious in stopping bleeding from peptic ulcers. These studies have involved relatively few patients and have been poorly controlled. It has been suggested that somatostatin may work by lowering portal venous pressure and might be useful in treating esophageal varices. There is some doubt, however, about the value of somatostatin in lowering portal pressure.

There are studies that attest to the value of the vasoconstrictor levarterenol in controlling ongoing bleeding, but these studies have not been controlled. Vasopressin is a vasoconstrictor agent that is effective in controlling bleeding from esophageal varices. If it is used intraarterially, a specific diagnosis should be made first, because arteriography requires special expertise. However, a low-dose constant infusion of vasopressin by vein is equally effective and can be instituted without the presence of a skilled angiographer.

In patients with evidence of cirrhosis and portal hypertension or portal hypertension alone, it is reasonable to try IV vasopressin empirically if bleeding continues. A starting dose of 0.1 U per minute is given and is gradually increased to 0.4 U per minute, if necessary. If bleeding ceases, this dose should be continued for 24 hours, after which it is tapered over the next 48 hours. If bleeding continues, sometimes increasing the dose to as much as 1.5 U per minute will work, although complications are more likely to develop.

There is no evidence that vasopressin is effective intravenously for nonvariceal lesions, and, therefore, it should not be used as empirical therapy in non-cirrhotic patients. It should be used with caution in patients with vascular disease or with a history of cardiac dysrhythmias. Thus, with the possible exception of vasopressin for patients with cirrhosis and portal hypertension or portal hypertension alone, there is no good empirical therapy for continued bleeding beyond gastric lavage. If bleeding continues, more specific and invasive measures will be needed. In this situation, the next step is to make a rapid specific diagnosis. Most patients cease bleeding, however, and immediate diagnosis is not as important. The next step for these patients is to institute empirical measures that might reduce the incidence of rebleeding. Neither cimetidine in a dosage of 7.5 mg per kg every 6 hours nor hourly antacids alone was better than placebo in the prevention of rebleeding from a variety of causes in a large United States study. The combination of the two medications reduced the incidence of rebleeding by one half compared with the placebo. In duodenal lesions specifically, rebleeding occurred in 6 percent of patients receiving the combination compared with 18 percent receiving placebo. These data suggest that a regimen producing intragastric pH levels higher than those achieved by cimetidine or antacids alone is more effective. Theoretically, the optimal regimen would be one that sustained gastric pH at 7.4 for 24 hours a day. To achieve this, it may be necessary to administer cimetidine as a constant IV infusion at a dosage of up to 1200 mg per 1.73 m^2 per hour in conjunction with hourly doses of potent liquid antacids by mouth or by tube. It is unknown, however, whether this regimen would be more effective clinically.

Diagnostic Approach

Patients who continue to bleed despite empirical therapy should promptly undergo endoscopy to find the particular lesion for which specific therapy is needed. For example, a patient with bleeding esophageal varices may require balloon tamponade, whereas a patient with a bleeding duodenal ulcer may need surgery. In cases in which endoscopy cannot be performed or selective vasoconstrictive therapy is required, arteriography is warranted. The approach to patients who cease bleeding is less straightforward but, as with patients who continue to bleed, often includes routine early endoscopy. The rationale is that making a prompt diagnosis will aid in the management of the patient.

Several controlled studies involving diverse patient populations suggest that at least in terms of objective measurements of outcome this is not the case. Routine performance of endoscopy in patients whose bleeding has ceased does not improve survival, reduce transfusion requirements, or shorten the hospital stay. Prior knowledge of the source of bleeding does not necessarily improve the outcome of patients who rebleed. There is at least one good explanation for these observations. A diagnosis is only as good as the therapy to which it leads, and for patients who cease bleeding, therapeutic options are limited. If the patient has bled from peptic ulcers, antacids, cimetidine, or ranitidine are currently used as therapy.

Whether or when to perform elective surgery is an unsettled issue. If bleeding has been from a Mallory-Weiss tear or from gastritis, antacids, cimetidine, or ranitidine are again the only therapy available. Sucralfate can also be used. Although some physicians choose variceal systemic shunts for patients who have bled from esophageal varices, there is little evidence that overall survival is improved. As a matter of fact, currently, physicians are more likely to sclerose the varices than perform a shunt procedure. There are other reasons for performing endoscopy. First, there are physicians who believe endoscopy should be performed routinely to select out patients with peptic ulcer in whom

there are "stigmata" of recent bleeding, that is, visible vessel or adherent clot. These patients may rebleed and require urgent surgery more often than patients without such findings. There is no evidence that these patients should be sent to surgery early because they have such lesions. Prophylactic electrocoagulation has been suggested as a means of preventing rebleeding from visible vessels. The evidence for using prophylactic electrocoagulation or argon laser photocoagulation to prevent rebleeding has not as yet been substantiated, nor has it benefited the patients in the short term. The incidence of rebleeding with esophageal varices is so high that some physicians have turned to prophylactic endoscopic variceal sclerosis, an old procedure that is experiencing a rebirth. If this approach is taken, patients with liver disease must first be examined endoscopically to ensure that no lesion other than varices is responsible for the bleeding episode; then the procedure may be performed. Many physicians believe that knowing the diagnosis has intangible worth; the patient may be better counseled if an accurate diagnosis has been made. It is difficult to refute such an argument, and it is unlikely that a controlled study will be done to settle the issue. It is difficult to suggest strict guidelines as to when endoscopy should or should not be performed in patients whose bleeding has ceased. At the least, controlled studies support the notion that if endoscopy is desired, it is not necessary to do it immediately. Rather, it can be safely postponed until regular elective endoscopy hours, when ancillary personnel are available.

CASE PRESENTATION

J.M., a previously healthy 6-year-old boy, was brought to the emergency room because of a 4-hour history of abdominal pain and three episodes of hematemesis. The patient was diaphoretic and pale and had nasal flaring.

Examination and Test Results

Vital signs: BP, recumbent = 80/50 mm Hg, erect = 60/30 mm Hg; P, recumbent = 100 beats/min, erect = 120 beats/min, RR = 40 breaths/min; T = 36.6°C; and weight = 25 kg (50 lb). The liver was not enlarged, but the spleen was palpable 4 cm below the left costal margin. The chest was clear, although respirations were labored and he had a gallop. A no. 22 Angiocath was placed in the external jugular vein following placement of the patient in a reverse Trendelenburg position. Five percent albumin *in saline* was begun and infused as rapidly as possible; 20 ml/kg was administered in 20 minutes. Blood was drawn for CBC, coagulation studies, electrolytes, and type and crossmatch. Recumbent BP, P, and RR were monitored every 5 minutes. At the end of 20 minutes, BP increased to 100/80 mm Hg, recumbent and 90/70 mm Hg, erect; tachycardia persisted; and RR decreased to 30 breaths/min. Hematocrit = 27 percent; hemoglobin = 9.0 gm/dl; WBC was 25,000, with a shift to the left. PT = 12/11.5; PTT = 34/31 and platelets = 250,000. Electrolytes were: Na = 140 mEq/L; K = 4.0 mEq/L; Cl = 101 mEq/L, and CO_2 = 20 mEq/L; SGOT = 40 IU/L; SGPT = 18 IU/L; and total bilirubin = 1.0 mg/dl.

Problem List

UGI Hemorrhage

The patient's history indicated that he had been a premature baby and had respiratory distress syndrome necessitating use of a ventilator and umbilical vessel catheterization. There was no history of peptic ulcer disease in the family or ingestion of ulcerogenic medications.

A presumptive diagnosis of esophageal varices secondary to portal vein thrombosis was made as a result of the splenomegaly and absence of evidence of liver disease.

Transfusion with whole blood was begun 1 hour following admission at a rate of 10 ml/kg/every 10 min for 20 minutes. A Pitressin infusion was begun at a rate of 0.1 U/min and was increased to a rate of 0.2 U/min when the patient vomited an additional 100 ml of blood and clots. No further bleeding occurred during the following 24 hours. Endoscopy was performed within 24 hours of admission and confirmed the varices. Pitressin dosage was gradually tapered in the second 24 hours after bleeding ceased. Endosclerosis of the varices was done in three separate sessions over a two-week period to prevent rebleeding.

SUGGESTED READING

Chojkier, M., and Conn, H.O.: Esophageal tamponade in the treatment of bleeding varices. Dig. Dis. Sci. 25:267, 1980.

Chojkier, M., et al.: A controlled comparison of continuous intra-arterial and intravenous infusions of vasopressin in hemorrhage from esophageal varices. Gastroenterology 77:540, 1979.

Clark, A.W., et al.: Prospective controlled trial of injection sclerotherapy in patients with cirrhosis and recent variceal hemorrhage. Lancet 2:552, 1980.

Gilbert, D.A., Saunders, D.R., Peoples, J., et al.: Failure of iced saline lavage to suppress hemorrhage from experimental bleeding ulcers. Gastroenterology 76:1138, 1979.

Hilsman, J.H.: The color of blood-containing feces following the instillation of citrated blood at various levels of the small intestine. Gastroenterology 15:131, 1980.

Himal, H.S., Perrault, C., and Mzabi, R.: Upper gastrointestinal hemorrhage: aggressive management decreases mortality. Surgery 84:448, 1978.

Johnson, J.H., Jensen, D.M., and Mautner, W.: Comparison of laser photocoagulation and electrocoagulation in endoscopic treatment of UGI bleeding. Gastroenterology 76:1162, 1979.

Luk, G.D., Bynum, T.E., and Hendrix, T.R.: Gastric aspiration in localization of gastrointestinal hemorrhage. JAMA 241:576, 1979.

Northfield, T.C., and Smith, T.: Hematemesis as an index of blood loss. Lancet 1:990, 1971.

Peterson, W.L., Barnett, C.C., Smith, H.J., et al.: Routine early endoscopy in upper gastrointestinal tract bleeding. N. Engl. J. Med. 304:925, 1981.

Ponsky, J.L., Hoffmann, M., and Swayngim, D.S.: Saline irrigation in gastric hemorrhage. The effect of temperature. J. Surg. Res. 28:204, 1980.

Simonian, S.J., and Curtis, L.E.: Treatment of hemorrhagic gastritis by antacid. Ann. Surg. 184:479, 1976.

Stellato, T., Rhodes, R.S., and McDougal, W.S.: Azotemia in upper gastrointestinal hemorrhage. Am. J. Gastroenterol. 73:486, 1980.

Winzelberg, G.G., McKusick, K.A., Strauss, A.W., et al.: Evaluation of gastrointestinal bleeding by red blood cell labelled in vivo with technetium 99m. J. Nucl. Med. 20:1080, 1979.

Nursing Process for Patient Care:
Upper Gastrointestinal Bleeding

Children admitted with upper gastrointestinal bleeding may present with a slow bleed, requiring continuous monitoring and diagnostic study, or with an acute bleed, in shock, requiring rapid fluid resuscitation. The significance of the bleed in terms of cardiovascular stability should be the major focus for the nurse.

CARDIOVASCULAR

Assess, Monitor, and Document

Level of consciousness
Blood pressure: arterial (recumbent, postural), central venous
Heart rate
Rhythm
Respiratory rate

Perfusion: peripheral pulses, capillary filling
Skin condition: color, temperature
Urine output
Laboratory data: hematocrit, hemoglobin
Response to therapy
Fluid intake: type, amount

Anticipate

Alteration in cardiovascular status
Shock
  Altered level of consciousness
  Postural hypotension
  Recumbent hypotension
  Tachycardia

  Tachypnea
  Poor peripheral perfusion
  Skin gray and cool
  Decreased urine output
Cardiac arrest

GASTROINTESTINAL

Assess, Monitor, and Document

Hematemesis: amount, description
Melena: amount, description
Hematochezia: amount, description
Response to therapy

Gastric lavage with iced saline
Pharmacologic agents: antacids, cimetidine, somatostatin, vasopressin

Anticipate

Alteration in gastrointestinal status
  Bleeding

  Rebleeding
Alteration in liver status

RESPONSE OF CHILD

The child who is actively bleeding can be very frightened by this experience. The visual presence of the blood and the intense activity associated with the treatment are factors that contribute to this response. The child's age and developmental level will also influence his or her behavior. Nursing interventions that serve to reduce the emotional distress generated by this experience must be developed and implemented.

Assess, Monitor, and Document

Developmental level: cognitive, verbal, motor, psychosocial, fears
Behavioral response: fearful, anxious, angry, compliant

Response to nursing interventions

Anticipate

Emotional distress

RESPONSE OF FAMILY

Assess, Monitor, and Document

Behavioral response: angry, fearful, verbal
Level of understanding of child's condition

Expected outcome
Response to nursing interventions

Anticipate

Inability to cope
Family crisis

MIND SET

Assess

Cardiovascular status
Gastrointestinal status
Response of child and family

Anticipate

Alteration in cardiovascular status
  Shock
Alteration in gastrointestinal system
  Hematemesis

Melena
Hematochezia
Emotional distress
Family crisis

41

Fulminant Hepatic Necrosis and Hepatic Coma

MARVIN E. AMENT, M.D.

Fulminant hepatic necrosis is an infrequent devastating form of liver disease, which, with its resulting hepatic coma, presents an overwhelming challenge to the pediatrician and support personnel who care for patients afflicted with it. The diagnosis of this condition is not difficult, but the medical support required for these patients can be complex. Mortality is high.

ETIOLOGY

Fulminant hepatic necrosis may occur as a consequence of a variety of hepatic injuries. During infancy, there is a greater chance of identifying the agent or factor responsible, whereas, in older children, diagnosis is often more difficult. Fulminant hepatic necrosis during early infancy is typically caused from disseminated Herpesvirus infection, viruses in the echovirus group (Types VI, XI, XIV, and XIX), viruses in the adenovirus group, and, in rare instances, the Epstein-Barr virus. Hepatitis B virus rarely causes severe hepatic failure in the first 2 weeks of life but more typically presents after the neonatal period. The metabolic causes of hepatic failure during the first weeks and months of life are quite rare but typically include tyrosinemia, congenital fructose intolerance, and galactosemia.

Infants with Zellweger's syndrome or cerebrohepatorenal syndrome, characterized by an enlarged liver and bilateral congenital glaucoma, cataracts, and epicanthi, may also have this condition. Patients with congenital heart disease in which there is low flow to the liver may be subject to hepatic necrosis secondary to insufficient flow to the organ, although this is uncommon. Other than in infancy, virus infections can be confirmed in only 30 percent of patients with fulminant hepatic necrosis. Although pediatric patients are routinely screened for hepatitis virus A and B, cytomegalovirus, and Epstein-Barr virus, children, unlike adults, are more likely to have non-A, non-B hepatotrophic viruses as the cause of fulminant hepatic necrosis and failure. Forty to 60 percent of adult patients with fulminant viral hepatitis are hepatitis B surface antigen positive. Patients who are immunologically compromised and who have undergone transplants may develop hepatic failure. Drug- or hepatotoxin-induced fulminant hepatic failure has been described. The agents most frequently associated are acetaminophen, isoniazid, aspirin, Depakene, indomethacin, halothane, fluothane, carbon tetrachloride, phosphorus, and plant toxins. Wilson's disease or copper storage disease has also been seen in association with hepatic necrosis.

Fewer than 1 in 1,000 icteric cases of presumed viral hepatitis develop hepatic necrosis. We have no knowledge why certain patients with viral-induced hepatitis develop massive hepatic necrosis and failure. Therefore, when considering the possibility of fulminant hepatic necrosis and hepatic coma, the possible causes should be thought of in the following order:

1. Infections
2. Poisons, chemicals, and drugs
3. Ischemia and hypoxia
4. Metabolic anomalies

Fulminant hepatic necrosis is infrequent in pediatric patients, and although survival rates for the condition are reported to be between 30 and 40 percent, these numbers are based upon a relatively small number of patients. The results in the pediatric population are reportedly better than those in adults, where only one of five patients with fulminant hepatic necrosis survives. One pediatric series reported only 1 survivor of 17 patients with the disease. On the continent of Europe and in Great Britain the three most common causes reported are viral hepatitis, acetaminophen overdosage, and drug- or anesthetic-induced disease.

PATHOLOGY

There is no definite relationship between certain hepatic morphologic features and the presence or absence of encephalopathy. Two types of pathological lesions have been described in fulminant hepatic failure. The Type I lesion is characterized by extensive necrosis and disappearance of hepatocytes. In massive hepatic necrosis, there are large confluent areas of hepatocellular necrosis involving adjacent lobules interspersed with areas of surviving hepatocytes. In diffuse hepatocellular necrosis, there is a patchy loss of hepatocytes throughout the lobule; in central lobular hepatocellular necrosis, there is a confluent loss of hepatocytes from the region of the lobule immediately adjacent to the terminal hepatic venule. The remaining hepatocytes may be swollen and vacuolated or shrunken with increased acidophilic staining of the cytoplasm in the presence or absence of nuclear material or acidophilic bodies. Large areas of confluent hepatocellular necrosis, sometimes called *multilobular necrosis* or *bridging necrosis,* may lead to condensation of the reticulum framework of the lobule. Rarely, there is surprisingly little hepatocellular necrosis. However, there may be a proliferation of bile duct–like structures and an inflammatory cell infiltrate of variable composition.

The Type II lesion is characterized by microvesicular fatty infiltration of hepatocytes, which cause swelling and pallor of the cells but do not typically displace their nuclei. This type of fatty infiltration is readily identified in sections specifically stained for fat. Fulminant hepatic failure due to the Type II lesion can occur in the presence of minimal histologic features of hepatocellular necrosis and is attributable to hepatocellular organal dysfunction. This type of lesion is most commonly seen with Reye's syndrome. It is also seen in tetracycline overdosage and fatty liver of pregnancy. Transaminase levels associated with the Type I lesion early in its course are typically quite high, in the range of 1000 to 4000 King-Armstrong units, whereas those associated with the Type II lesion are not as elevated; they are more typically in the range of 300 to 2000 King-Armstrong units. Patients may not be jaundiced, or may be only slightly so, when the hepatic failure is associated with acute hepatocellular steatosis. However, those who survive more than

a few days typically become jaundiced. Liver biopsy is not necessarily predictive of outcome. Patients who die from fulminant hepatic necrosis seldom show evidence of hepatic regeneration.

PATHOGENESIS

We have a poor understanding of why specific agents induce hepatocellular injury and impair hepatocellular function. We do not know why some patients have limited injury whereas in others it is massive. It is presumed that the mechanisms responsible for both mild and severe hepatocellular damage are similar; the severity of the lesion induced probably depends upon the magnitude of exposure to the agent and the susceptibility of the host to that agent. The role of the immune system in the mediation of necrosis of virus-infected hepatocytes is controversial. In studies of patients with hepatitis virus A, the amount of virus found in the liver was much larger in fulminant hepatitis virus A than in nonfulminant hepatitis virus A. The humoral response in these patients was apparently normal. In fulminant hepatitis virus B, the amount of viral antigen in the blood and the serologic responses to the infection seem to be similar to corresponding findings of nonfulminant acute hepatitis virus B.

Fulminant hepatic failure induced by certain drugs may be related to the metabolic activation by the hepatocyte of the agent. Hepatotoxicity of certain drugs may be caused by the production of metabolites or enzyme inducers, which may potentiate hepatotoxicity.

CLINICAL FEATURES

There are several clinical clues and laboratory tests that indicate that a patient is having an "atypical" course for a viral illness and that suggest that the condition is becoming fulminant. Patients with fulminant hepatic necrosis have persistent anorexia with general disregard for all types of food. They typically have jaundice, which becomes progressively deeper in color. They may have a relapse of the initial symptoms that caused their condition to be recognized in the first place, such as fever, nausea, vomiting and/or diarrhea. Typically there is a prolongation of the prothrombin time or a progressive prolongation, which does not respond to the administration of intramuscular vitamin K given daily for up to 3 days. Typically, one intramuscular or intravenous (IV) dosage of vitamin K of the appropriate dosage should improve the vitamin K–dependent clotting factors by 50 percent or more within 24 hours. Patients with fulminant hepatic necrosis typically have depressed serum albumin and fibrinogen levels and transaminase levels in excess of 3000 to 4000. Their bilirubin levels show progressive rise and are typically in excess of 20 mg per dl. Their livers, which initially may be enlarged, gradually shrink in size, although they fail to improve clinically. The patients may develop ascites and a respiratory alkalosis. Mentally, they may become confused, disoriented, and ultimately combative. They may become totally unresponsive to stimuli. Hypoglycemia, low BUN, leukocytosis, and thrombocytopenia are other features of the condition.

ENCEPHALOPATHY

There are four clinical stages of acute hepatic encephalopathy. In Stage I, the patient may be euphoric or depressed and appear mildly confused. The patient appears to be slow in thinking and is slow to react. The speech of the patient may become slurred, and his sleep pattern is disturbed. Patients such as this typically have a slight tremor and on electroencephalogram (EEG), no changes are seen. In Stage II, there is impending coma. There is an accentuation of the abnormalities seen in Stage I; the patient becomes drowsy and exhibits inappropriate behavior. Patients who formerly were trained for bladder and bowel control may become incontinent. These patients typically have a tremor and show generalized slowing on EEG. In Stage III, these patients sleep most of the time but are arousable. Their speech is not coherent, and they are confused. They usually have a tremor; they always have an abnormal EEG. In Stage IV, or deep coma, these patients may or may not respond to painful stimuli, and their tremor is absent; they always have an abnormal EEG.

It is most likely that the encephalopathy in fulminant hepatic failure is secondary to humoral toxins that are generated in severe hepatocellular disease. Fulminant hepatic failure is associated with changes in the concentration of a large number of compounds in plasma, cerebrospinal fluid, and the brain.

Several studies have excluded major roles for specific substances or classes of substances in the pathogenesis of the encephalopathy of fulminant hepatic failure. Acute ammonia intoxication in animals does not reproduce the clinical and neuropathologic changes of hepatic encephalopathy. Arterial plasma ammonia levels fail to correlate closely with the severity of encephalopathy in fulminant hepatic failure. The encephalopathy of fulminant hepatic failure may occur *before* any increase in blood ammonia. The severity of encephalopathy in fulminant hepatic failure does not correlate with plasma concentrations of individual amino acids, including those involved in the metabolism of neurotransmitters. There are several secondary factors that contribute to encephalopathy of fulminant hepatic failure. These factors, including hypoglycemia, hypoxemia due to cardiorespiratory failure and/or hemorrhage, cerebral edema, reduction of the affinity of hemoglobin for oxygen, decreased cerebral utilization of oxygen and glucose, and diminution of cerebral blood flow, may vary in extent in different patients. There are many similarities between hepatic encephalopathy of fulminant hepatic failure and that occurring in chronic hepatocellular disease, but the pathogeneses of the encephalopathies occurring in these two clinical settings are not necessarily identical.

CEREBRAL EDEMA

Cerebral edema is one of the most common and most serious extrahepatic complications frequently found in patients with fulminant hepatic failure. Its relationship to hepatic coma has not been clearly established. One quarter of the patients with cerebral edema show evidence of herniation of the cerebellar tonsil or the uncinate region of the temporal lobe. Therefore, cerebral edema of fulminant hepatic failure is not merely a terminal hypoxic event, but a definite neurologic complication of acute liver failure. A metabolic basis in the neuropathology of cerebral edema in fulminant hepatic failure has not been established. Three mechanisms may contribute to the development of cerebral edema: 1) a disruption of the blood–brain barrier, which is vasogenic in origin; 2) a failure of cellular osmol regulation; and 3) expansion of the extracellular space.

DISTURBANCE IN COAGULATION

Severe coagulopathy is associated with fulminant hepatic failure. This condition predisposes patients with fulminant hepatic failure to severe hemorrhage from the upper gastrointestinal tract. Two phenomena contribute to the coagulopathy of fulminant hepatic failure:

thrombocytopenia, and reduced plasma levels of liver-produced clotting factors. Half the cases of fulminant hepatic failure are associated with platelet counts of less than 100,000. The platelets that are present are typically smaller than normal.

Bleeding times are increased to a greater extent than would be expected from the degree of thrombocytopenia alone and correlate better with indices of abnormal platelet function such as in vivo aggregation associated with reduced platelet adenosine diphosphate (ADP) levels. Thrombocytopenia seen in fulminant hepatic failure is caused by: 1) bone marrow depression, 2) hypersplenism, 3) consumption by intravascular coagulation, and 4) adherence to components of extracorporeal hemoperfusion devices.

Both clotting factors and fibrinolytic factors are formed at reduced rates because of defective hepatic protein synthesis. Clotting factors synthesized in the liver are factors I (fibrinogen), II (prothrombin), V, VII, IX, and X. The degree of prolongation of prothrombin time (provided that vitamin K has been administerd parenterally) is regarded as a sensitive index of the severity of hepatocellular insufficiency, particularly of the protein synthetic capacity of the liver. Prolongation of the prothrombin time may precede clinical deterioration, including the development of coma. Normalization of prothrombin time tends to precede or accompany clinical improvement in fulminant hepatic failure. Because some clotting factors have short half-lives, impairment of synthesis of liver-produced plasma proteins occurs early in fulminant hepatic failure. This is why the prothrombin time rapidly becomes prolonged. Factor VII has been shown to decrease earlier in the plasma and to a greater extent and more consistently than those of other liver-produced clotting factors. Its decrease is secondary to its decreased rate of production. Factor V, being reduced in fulminant hepatic failure, indicates that damage has occurred independent of the vitamin K–dependent factors. The coagulopathy of fulminant hepatic failure is also associated with low plasma levels of plasminogen activator and plasminogen and increased plasma levels of fibrin/fibrinogen degradation products. Increased intravascular coagulation may be a direct consequence of necrosis of liver cells. The most common site of clinically overt bleeding is the upper gastrointestinal tract. Esophagitis and gastritis are common. Widespread petechiae often accompany fulminant hepatic failure and may reflect either vessel fragility or disseminated intravascular coagulation.

HYPOTENSION AND HYPOXEMIA

Hypotension occurs in most cases of fulminant hepatic failure. The basis for hypotension in most cases can be explained by hemorrhage, bacteremia, cardiac or respiratory abnormalities and/or the preterminal state. In the remainder of the patients, the cause of hypotension is not obvious. Cardiac output, peripheral vascular resistance, and the pulse rate tend to be decreased. Patients with fulminant hepatic failure can have hypotension in the presence of bradycardia, which indicates that there is some central vasomotor depression. In some instances, this can be secondary to cerebral edema. Increased capillary permeability and decreased peripheral vascular resistance secondary to endotoxemia have also been implicated in the pathogenesis of the hypotension.

Hypoxemia is typically present in fulminant hepatic failure. Hypotension accentuates the adverse effects of hypoxemia. Ventilation is impaired during prolonged periods of hypoxia, which is caused by depression of the respiratory centers. Pneumonia and pulmonary edema are respiratory complications of fulminant hepatic failure. Patients in stage IV coma have increased intrapulmonary arteriovenous shunting of blood, which contributes to the hypoxemia of fulminant hepatic failure and resolves with recovery. Respiratory arrest of central origin is a complication of fulminant hepatic failure. Clinical and radiologic evidence of pulmonary edema is seen in one third of cases of fulminant hepatic failure. This complication is not attributable to left ventricular failure or to renal failure. Much of the pulmonary vasodilatation seen in fulminant hepatic failure could be responsible for the edema. In some cases, there is inappropriate administration of sodium and fluids, especially when there is renal dysfunction. Hyponatremia, which is usually associated with an increase in total body sodium, is commonly present in fulminant hepatic failure. Hemodilution is often seen and is due to impairment of renal excretion of free water. The increased renal retention of sodium in patients with fulminant hepatic failure is frequently associated with clinically significant hypokalemia. Several factors may lead to hypokalemia, including inadequate potassium intake, vomiting, secondary aldosteronism, and, in some instances, the use of diuretics. Hypokalemia can exacerbate the encephalopathy of hepatic failure. Hypocalcemia and hypomagnesemia are also seen in this condition.

Hyperventilation, producing low carbon dioxide tension (PCO_2), is a common feature of fulminant hepatic failure and may lead to respiratory alkalosis. Hypokalemia is associated with an increased plasma concentration of bicarbonate and a metabolic alkalosis. If extensive tissue damage occurs secondary to massive hepatic necrosis, a metabolic acidosis may arise, with the accumulation of lactic acid, pyruvate, acetoacetate, citrate, succinate, fumarate, and free fatty acids. Progressive deterioration of liver function leads to an accumulation of citrate in the plasma. Lactic acid accumulation results in metabolic acidosis.

RENAL DYSFUNCTION

Renal failure is a common problem in fulminant hepatic failure and may be diagnosed when the glomerular filtration rate falls below 10 ml per minute per 1.73 m^2. Urinary output may be reduced to less than 400 ml per day per m^2, and serum creatinine may increase to more than 2 mg per dl. Azotemia with or without oliguria or anuria may develop. In rare instances, the renal failure is prerenal in origin. A spectrum of renal conditions from functional renal failure to acute tubular necrosis have been described in fulminant hepatic failure. Acute tubular necrosis is diagnosed when numerous granular and cellular casts are found in the urine, when the urine sodium concentration is more than 20 mM per L, and when the urine to plasma urea concentration ratio is less than 10. Functional renal failure of fulminant hepatic failure is characterized by normal urinary sediment and urinary sodium concentrations of less than 20 mM per L. The severity of liver cell failure does not correlate closely with the severity of renal failure. The serum creatinine concentration is a better index of the extent of renal failure than is the blood urea concentration, because fulminant hepatic failure may be associated with a marked decrease in the rate of urea synthesis by the Krebs–Henseleit cycle in the liver. Urea concentrations are typically less than 20 mg per dl in patients with fulminant hepatic failure.

HYPOGLYCEMIA

Thirty percent of patients with fulminant hepatic failure have severe hypoglycemia. It is more commonly seen in children than in adults. Abnormal hepatic glucose release is a major cause of the hypoglycemia. Massive necrosis of hepatocytes leads to depletion of the glycogen content of the liver and to impairment of gluconeogenesis. Changes in the serum concen-

trations of the hormones insulin and glucagon and the growth hormone may also contribute to the pathogenesis of the hypoglycemia. Hypoglycemic coma can occur independently of hepatic coma in acute hepatic failure. It can accentuate the coma of fulminant hepatic failure and cause additional brain damage, which may not be completely reversible.

CARDIAC DYSFUNCTION

Dysrhythmias occur in more than 90 percent of patients with fulminant hepatic failure who are in stage IV coma. Sinus tachycardia is the most common dysrhythmia, but a variety of others have been described. Patients with low arterial blood oxygen tensions, acidosis, and hyperkalemia are most subject to dysrhythmias.

PANCREATIC LESIONS

Morphologic evidence of acute pancreatitis is found in many patients who die of fulminant hepatic failure. This lesion does not seem to be related to the administration of corticosteroids, renal failure, or any particular pathogenesis of fulminant hepatic failure and is rarely diagnosed premortem.

SUSCEPTIBILITY TO INFECTION

Patients with fulminant hepatic failure have an increased risk of infection irrespective of corticosteroid treatment. The infections of the respiratory tract are promoted by the unconscious state, hypostasis, impaired reflexes, and inadequate respiration. IV and urinary catheters also predispose to infection. The sera of patients with fulminant hepatic failure contain a factor that inhibits the metabolic activity of the hexose monophosphate shunt.

PORTAL HYPERTENSION

Portal hypertension in fulminant hepatic failure is secondary to an intrahepatic block secondary to massive necrosis of liver cells. This contributes to the development of ascites.

CAUSES OF DEATH

Death is most commonly due to acute liver cell failure and one of its complications, which include hemorrhage from the gastrointestinal tract, cerebral edema with or without herniation of the cerebellum or temporal lobes, sepsis, renal failure, cardiac failure, cardiac arrest, respiratory failure, and acute pancreatitis. In some patients, the cause of death is multifactorial.

NATURAL HISTORY

It is not always possible to predict when a patient with acute hepatocellular disease will develop fulminant hepatic failure. However, progressively increasing prothrombin time and a decrease in serum C_3 concentration are ominous, often preceding the onset of encephalopathy. Fulminant hepatic failure typically occurs near the onset of acute hepatocellular disease. Encephalopathy may even precede the development of jaundice. Survival rates of 10 to 20 percent are most typically seen in series of patients with fulminant hepatic failure who have been in stage IV coma for a few hours. In pediatric patients, the survival rate appears to be better. Complete restoration of normal hepatic function and structure usually occurs in survivors of fulminant hepatic failure, even if they have been in deep coma and hepatocellular necrosis has been massive. Liver tests and histology of liver return to normal in 45 to 75 days after the onset of fulminant hepatic failure. Chronic active hepatitis has been described in 3 of 15 patients who survived fulminant hepatic failure; in 1 of the 3, cirrhosis also developed. It is generally thought that patients who survive fulminant viral hepatitis rarely develop chronic liver disease.

INDICES OF SEVERITY AND PROGNOSIS

There are no reliable criteria that enable the clinician to determine whether the patient will die or will regain consciousness and ultimately survive. Neither the duration of disease before the onset of coma nor the stage of encephalopathy on admission of the patient to the hospital correlates with the outcome. Mortality tends to be greater the deeper and more prolonged the coma. Survival is obviously greatest for those in lower stages of coma. Patients younger than 40 years of age, particularly children, tend to have better prognoses than older patients. This effect of age may be attributable to the superior capacity of the livers of young people to regenerate after severe insult. Small liver size or decreasing liver size tends to be

associated with a grave prognosis. Cardiac dysrhythmias other than sinus tachycardia are usually associated with a high mortality rate. Plasma ammonia, blood urea, plasma lactic acid, arterial blood carbon dioxide tension, serum aminotransferases, serum total bilirubin, blood sugar, serum alpha-1-antitrypsin, serum albumin, plasma concentrations of amino acids, cerebrospinal fluid glutamine level, total leukocyte count, and platelet count are unreliable indices of prognosis. The levels to which liver-synthesized clotting factors are depressed in fulminant hepatic failure correlate with the severity of the hepatic lesion. A progressively increasing prothrombin time in spite of the parenteral administration of vitamin K in the absence of variations in intravascular coagulation implies deteriorating hepatocellular function. A one-stage prothrombin time greater than 50 seconds with a control of 10 to 12 seconds or quick prothrombin indices of less than 30 percent of control is considered a bad prognostic feature but does not necessarily indicate a fatal outcome. Increasing concentrations of alpha-fetoprotein in sera in patients with fulminant hepatic failure has been interpreted as being indicative of active regeneration of hepatocytes after extensive hepatocellular injury. Measurable hepatic regeneration does not occur until the second week after hepatic insult, causing fulminant hepatic failure. However, increasing serum levels of alpha-fetoprotein do not necessarily imply ultimate recovery. Many patients with fulminant hepatic failure recover without elevation of the serum alpha-fetoprotein level.

DIAGNOSIS

Diagnosis of fulminant hepatic failure is based on the following criteria:

1. The absence of evidence of liver disease at least 8 weeks previously. Cutaneous stigmata of chronic liver disease; enlarged, hard liver; splenomegaly; and gross ascites at the time of developing encephalopathy are findings against fulminant hepatic failure.

2. The presence of clinical features compatible with hepatic encephalopathy, which may include changes in personality, episodes of antisocial behavior, impaired mental functions, character disturbances, nightmares, headaches, and dizziness. Violent behavior is common in children with hepatic encephalopathy. Convulsions may occur. Prominent motor abnormalities include asterixis, flapping tremor, paratonia, hyperactive stretch reflexes, and

decerebrate posturing. Patients may have psychiatric symptoms.

3. The presence of fetor hepaticus.

4. Routine biochemical and hematologic data indicative of hepatocellular dysfunction and hypofunction. The most important index of hepatocellular dysfunction is markedly elevated serum aminotransferase levels, at least in early cases. The most important index of hepatocellular hypofunction is markedly prolonged prothrombin time, which is not corrected by the parenteral administration of vitamin K.

GENERAL MANAGEMENT

Optimally, the urinary bladder should be catheterized, a nasogastric tube should be passed, and a venous catheter should be advanced to the supradiaphragmatic central vein or the right atrium. The nasogastric tube is aspirated regularly to detect upper gastrointestinal hemorrhage. Ideally, the patient should be placed on a bed that permits the body weight to be recorded. Formation of ammonia is minimized; other low molecular weight nitrogenous substances that are produced by the enteric bacterial flora should be inhibited from production by appropriate treatment. A high magnesium sulfate enema is administered twice daily with 1 percent dextrose. Sodium-free magnesium sulfate and neomycin in therapeutic dosages are administered every 4 hours via nasogastric tube. Lactulose may also be administered via nasogastric tube. There is some evidence that neomycin and lactulose together are superior to either alone in reducing the blood ammonia concentration in patients with chronic portal systemic encephalopathy. Proteins and amino acids are not given. Caloric intake is maintained by infusing hypertonic dextrose of 10 to 50 percent into a central vein, because concentrated solutions of dextrose can induce thrombophlebitis infused into peripheral veins. Supplemental vitamins other than vitamin K are usually given empirically. It is necessary to monitor the blood glucose concentration frequently, perhaps hourly, in order to detect hypoglycemia. Semiquantitative estimates with Dextrostix are useful as a screening test for hypoglycemia. In the initial few days of hepatic failure, the following laboratory tests should be done every 12 hours: hemoglobin; total leukocyte count and differential; platelet count; and plasma sodium, potassium, chloride, bicarbonate, and urea determinations. The following laboratory tests should be determined perhaps once a day or

every 2 days: prothrombin time; partial thromboplastin time; creatinine; plasma total and direct bilirubin; alkaline phosphatase; SGOT and SGPT; cholesterol; albumin; amylase; and fibrinogen and fibrinogen split products. A chest x-ray should also be obtained.

Because patients may need ventilatory support and hypoxia and/or hypercapnia may occur and influence intracranial pressure, measurements of arterial blood gases are necessary, despite the well-known hazards of obtaining arterial blood in patients with severe coagulopathies. Continuous EEG recordings seem to augment the accurate monitoring of the progress of a patient in fulminant hepatic failure. The changes seen on the EEG are not specific for fulminant hepatic failure but are similar to those seen with encephalopathy from other metabolic causes, such as hypoglycemia, uremia, and hypercapnea. The frequencies of the EEG wave forms of normal people are in the alpha range of 8 to 13 cycles per second. In hepatic encephalopathy, there is a slowing of the wave forms to as low as the delta range of 4 cycles per second. In advanced hepatic encephalopathy, there is a loss of amplitude of the wave forms. There is not always a close correlation between the severity of the encephalopathy as assessed clinically and electroencephalographically. The EEG may remain abnormal for weeks after the patient has regained full consciousness. Frequent EEG monitoring in fulminant hepatic failure may facilitate prompt changes in therapy. Dramatic increase in the abnormalities of the EEG trace is usually associated with sudden clinical deterioration. If hypoglycemia is found, its rapid correction with IV dextrose usually will lead to some improvement in the EEG tracing.

LIVER BIOPSY

There is no established place for liver biopsy in the management of fulminant hepatic failure. The procedure is precluded by the coagulopathy, but the information obtained is of little or no help to the clinician.

PRECAUTIONS FOR ATTENDING PERSONNEL

It is prudent to assume that blood and all excretions of a patient in fulminant hepatic failure are potentially capable of transmitting viral hepatitis. All attending personnel should wear protective gowns, gloves, and masks. Enteric isolation procedures are enforced, and all blood specimens should be clearly labeled as potentially infectious in order to protect laboratory personnel. It is necessary to ensure that everyone who comes in contact with the patient is made aware of the nature of the disease. Increased survival in patients with fulminant hepatic failure is probably secondary to the application of standard intensive care procedures. In the past several of these patients have died from cardiac and pulmonary problems that could have been eliminated by more careful monitoring and treatment. In addition to the conventional intensive care for an unconscious patient, monitoring the EKG, the EEG, and central venous pressure and frequent semiquantitative assessments of clinical neurologic status are essential. This requires the continuous presence of specialized medical, paramedical, and nursing personnel.

TREATMENT OF COMPLICATIONS

Hypoglycemia

When hypoglycemia occurs, the amount of dextrose being administered intravenously must be increased.

Fluid and Electrolyte Imbalance

Patients' fluid should be limited to two thirds to three quarters of maintenance. Total intake and output of fluids should be carefully recorded, and, if possible, the patient should be weighed twice daily. Correction of electrolyte abnormalities should be done. Hypokalemia and the effects of potassium deficiency detected on the EKG must be corrected promptly by adding appropriate quantities of potassium chloride to IV fluids. As much as 600 mEq of potassium per 1.73 m^2 may be needed, but usually about 120 mEq daily per 1.73 m^2 is adequate. Calcium and magnesium supplementation of the IV fluid may be necessary. Sodium chloride supplementation to IV fluids is not indicated in the presence of hyponatremia unless there is evidence of excessive losses of sodium from the body. There may be iatrogenic sodium and fluid overload resulting from the infusion of blood products such as fresh frozen plasma, particularly when renal function is impaired. Hyperkalemia may occur with renal failure. Dialysis may be used to correct sodium and fluid overload or hyperkalemia.

Acid-Base Balance

Any combination of the four major abnormalities of acid-base balance may occur in fulminant hepatic failure. Losses should be defined, and appropriate remedial action should be taken.

Respiratory Function

Normal indications for endotracheal intubation and assisted ventilation prevail in fulminant hepatic failure. Endotracheal intubation at the onset of stage IV coma has been advocated to prevent aspiration pneumonitis and to facilitate bronchial cleansing. Hypoxemia, anemia, or shock is an indication for administration of 100 percent oxygen by face mask. If arterial hypoxemia is not corrected by the simple measure or other appropriate measures, positive end-expiratory pressure ventilatory support is indicated. Correction of hypocapnia by augmenting the CO_2 content of inspired air is contraindicated. If pulmonary edema is detected, early ventilatory support and positive end-expiratory pressure is necessary to achieve an adequate arterial blood oxygen tension.

Renal Failure

Indications for dialysis include hyperkalemia with associated electrocardiographic changes, other severe electrolyte abnormalities, markedly increased plasma creatinine concentrations, severe refractory disorders of acid-base balance, and fluid overload, with increasing oliguria. Hemodialysis is more likely to be needed than peritoneal dialysis.

Sepsis

Patients in fulminant hepatic failure need frequent intensive microbiological monitoring, and the environment in which the patient is maintained should be kept as clean as possible. Daily cultures of blood, urine, and sputum are recommended. Appropriate use of antibiotics is advocated.

Cerebral Edema

The sudden deterioration of level of consciousness, the development of sluggish pupillary reflexes to light, absent ciliospinal reflexes, sudden changes in pulse rate and blood pressure unrelated to hemorrhage, and rapid deterioration of EEG tracings are suggestive of elevated increase in intracranial pressure. Intracranial pressure can be monitored directly by introducing a stable, drift-free intracranial transducer through either a right parietal or right temporal burr hole and attaching a transducer to a flat-bed recording system. An attempt to reduce intracranial pressure should be made, but current therapies of the cerebral edema of fulminant hepatic failure are not usually effective. The cerebral edema of patients with fulminant hepatic failure does not seem to respond to the use of corticosteroids in any form. It has been shown in animal models that they may be effective in reducing the severity of cerebral edema if given early in the course of fulminant hepatic failure. Vistaril, 1.5 mg per kg per day, IM has not induced appreciable clinical improvement in patients with fulminant hepatic failure and cerebral edema. The dose used did not alter plasma osmolarity, and higher doses can induce intravascular coagulation. Mannitol administered intravenously as a bolus of 40 to 80 gm per m² was shown to reduce the elevated intracranial pressures in patients with fulminant hepatic failure when the pressures were less than 60 mm Hg, but it had a variable and potentially deleterious effect on intracranial pressures when the intracranial pressures were greater than 60 mm Hg. Mannitol should not be administered without prior knowledge of intracranial pressure.

Hypotension

Hypotension should be treated promptly. Transfusions of fresh blood are given when hemorrhage is responsible for hypotension and, when possible, cardiorespiratory abnormalities are corrected. IV fluids are given to the extent necessary to normalize central venous pressure. There are no control data indicating that the administration of pressor amines such as dopamine improves the prognosis for hypotensive patients with fulminant hepatic failure. Cardiac dysrhythmias are treated with conventional methods (see chapter 18, Dysrhythmias).

Hemorrhagic Diathesis

The efficacy of hemostasis is improved to prevent hemorrhage. Vitamin K is given on a daily basis intramuscularly to ensure that a deficiency of this vitamin does not contribute to reduced plasma levels of clotting factors produced by the liver. Prophylactic infusions of concentrations of clotting factors are not advocated. All preparations of clotting factors are likely to contain activated factors that can exacerbate intravascular coagulation. It is important to reduce the likelihood of acid–pepsin-provoked hemorrhage from the upper gastrointestinal tract. Cimetidine given intravenously in a dosage of 7.5 mg per kg every 6 hours is effective in preventing upper gastrointestinal hemorrhage. However, some investigators have shown that hourly dosages of antacids are more effective in neutralizing acid. Therefore, we recommend the use of antacids on an hourly basis around the clock while the patient is in hepatic coma.

Fresh blood is richer in factor V and in platelets than stored blood. Fresh frozen plasma and fresh concentrates of platelets may also be infused in an attempt to achieve hemostasis. Because disseminated intravascular coagulation in fulminant hepatic failure is not usually severe, heparin is not indicated in the routine management of fulminant hepatic failure; heparin therapy itself may cause bleeding.

Delirium and Convulsions

When delirium occurs, it is best treated by good nursing care alone. Most often, episodes of delirium are brief and mild and are not accompanied by convulsions. Delirium that is severe and prolonged may necessitate drug therapy, especially when accompanied by convulsions. Opiates and barbiturates are contraindicated. Paraldehyde may cause lactic acidosis, and diazepam may precipitate respiratory failure; therefore, it is best to avoid using these drugs. It has been suggested that promethazine should be used. If one of these drugs is given, the dose must be the absolute minimum necessary to achieve adequate control of the delirium or convulsions. Individual titration of dosages is essential.

Specific Therapies

Rationale for the use of corticosteroids in fulminant hepatic failure is based on the assumption that their anti-inflammatory action will reduce hepatocellular necrosis, possibly by exerting a protective effect in cellular and somatic breakdown. This might apply irrespective of the cause of fulminant hepatic failure. Furthermore, if the hepatocellular necrosis is mediated by an immunological mechanism, that mechanism may be suppressed by corticosteroids. There are no definitive data supporting the existence of these potentially beneficial effects of corticosteroids in fulminant hepatic failure. At this time, liver transplantation does not have an established place in the management of fulminant hepatic failure.

Other Therapies

L-Dopa does not have an established role in the treatment of fulminant hepatic failure. Currently, there is also no established role for insulin and glucagon.

Exchange transfusion in children with fulminant hepatic necrosis has not proved to be particularly useful. Similarly, trials of hemoperfusion over charcoal, membrane hemodialysis, plasmapheresis, and plasma exchange have not usually been beneficial.

Fulminant hepatic failure in infants differs in several respects from that in children and adults. Bleeding tends to be a more prominent component of the clinical syndrome than does encephalopathy. Fulminant hepatic failure is often related to an inborn error of metabolism. Pathologically, massive necrosis of hepatocytes is unusual, so fulminant hepatic failure is typically attributed to functional failure of the organelles of hepatocytes. The prognosis for infants with fulminant hepatic failure is said to be better than that for children or adults, possibly because of a greater regenerative capacity of a very young liver, but also because effective therapies are available for a larger proportion of the diseases that cause fulminant hepatic failure in infancy.

CASE PRESENTATION

A previously healthy 4-year-old male was admitted to the intensive care unit (ICU) because of vomiting and lethargy of 24-hour duration. Seven days prior to admission he had a sudden onset of fever, cough, coryza, and myalgia. The fever subsided after 72 hours, and the other symptoms ceased 2 days before the onset of the vomiting. He had received only acetaminophen for control of fever.

Examination

Findings on physical examination included T = 37.6°C; BP = 100/80 mm Hg; P = 88 beats/min; RR = 16 breaths/min; wt = 21 kg (50 lb); height = 101.6 cm (40 in.).

He was somnolent but responded to his name and to simple questions appropriately.

Head: normocephalic. Ears: TMs not injected; good light reflexes. Nose: no discharge; mucosa boggy. Mouth: no tonsillar hypertrophy; mucosa of oropharynx injected. Eyes: pupils are equal and regular and react to light directly and consensually. Neck: full range of motion. Chest: clear to percussion and auscultation. Heart: no murmurs. Abdomen: liver percussed to a total height of 12 cm and was palpable 4 cm below the right costal margin. The left lobe was palpated 2 cm below the left costal margin. It was tender to palpation. The spleen was not enlarged. Bowel sounds were present and normal. Skin: nonicteric. Muscles and joints: no pathological findings. Neurologic findings: cranial nerves intact; reflexes increased in upper and lower extremities. There were no pathological finger or toe signs; response to painful stimuli was appropriate. A presumptive diagnosis of Reye's syndrome was made.

Laboratory Results

Hemoglobin = 12.0 gm/dl; hematocrit = 36 percent; WBC = 7.9×10^3; PMNs (leukocytes) = 70 percent; bands = 6 percent; lymphs = 20 percent; Eos (eosinophils) = 2 percent; basophils = 2 percent; urinalysis: specific gravity = 1.018; RBCs = 0; WBCs = 0; protein = 0; sugar = 0; bile = 0; sodium = 130 mEq/L; potassium = 4.0 mEq/L; chloride = 98 mEq/L; CO_2 content = 25 mEq/L; BUN = 18 mg/dl; creatinine = 0.8 mg/dl; total bilirubin = 1.5 mg/dl; direct bilirubin = 0.4 mg/dl; SGOT = 700 IU/L; SGPT = 420 IU/L; total protein = 6.2 gm/dl; albumin = 4.0 gm/dl; ammonia = 350 mcg/dl; prothrombin time = 15 sec/11 sec, Pt/cont; PTT = 47 sec/32 sec, Pt/cont; blood glucose = 50 mg/dl; serum osmolarity = 280 mOsm/L; urine osmolarity = 650 mOsm/L.

An IV infusion of D10W, with maintenance electrolytes, was started at a rate to provide three quarters of maintenance fluids, and 5 mg of vitamin K was given intramuscularly to ascertain whether the liver could respond by making clotting factors. The patient was given nothing by mouth, and a Silastic nasogastric (NG) tube was placed to give lactulose when he refused to take it by mouth. A dose of 1.0 gm was given four times a day, and magnesium citrate, 1 oz, was given with a similar frequency. Vital signs, except for temperature, were monitored hourly. Blood glucose was measured every 4 hours, and electrolytes were measured every 8 hours. Serum and urine osmolarity were measured daily, as were liver function tests and ammonia. An intracranial bolt to measure increases in intracranial pressure was not placed, because there were no signs of increased intracranial pressure. If increased intracranial pressure were present, such a device would have been used.

The patient remained stable for 24 hours, with a decrease in weight to 20.5 kg (48 lb) and a decrease in lethargy. Blood glucose increased to 70 mg/dl. SGOT, SGPT, and bilirubin did not change. Blood ammonia level decreased to 150 mcg/dl. PT and PTT did not change. Urine osmolarity = 620 mOsm/L, and serum osmolarity = 300 mOsm/L.

The liver remained enlarged. After 2 days, the liver decreased in size and liver function tests improved substantially. Serum osmolarity returned to normal, and blood ammonia returned to normal. Lactulose and magnesium citrate were discontinued, and oral feedings were reinstituted. The patient made an uneventful recovery, and the liver returned to normal size within 2 weeks, with no residual abnormalities in liver function tests.

SUGGESTED READING

Adkins, B.J., and Steele, R.H.: Death from massive hepatic necrosis in infectious mononucleosis. N.Z. Med. J. 85:56, 1977.

Adler, R., Mahnovski, V., Henser, E.T., et al.: Fulminant hepatitis. A presentation of Wilson's disease. Am. J. Dis. Child. 131:870, 1977.

Benhamou, J.P.: Common nonviral causes of fulminant hepatic failure. Am. J. Gastroenterol. 69:365, 1978.

Black, M., Mitchell, J.R., Zimuemia, H.J., et al.: Isoniazid hepatitis in 114 patients. Gastroenterology 69:289, 1975.

Dymock, I.W., Tucker, J.S., Woolf, I.L., et al.: Coagulation studies as a prognostic index in acute liver failure. Br. J. Hematol. 35:301, 1977.

Horney, J.J., and Galambos, J.J.: The liver during and after fulminant hepatitis. Gastroenterology 73:639, 1977.

Macdougall, B.R.D., and Williams, R.: H₂ receptor antagonists and antacids in the prevention of acute gastrointestinal hemorrhage in fulminant hepatic failure. Two controlled trials. Lancet 1:617, 1977.

Mathiesen, L.R., Skinog, P., Nielsen, J.O., et al.: Hepatitis type A, B, and non-A, non-B, in fulminant hepatitis. Gut 21:72, 1980.

Mitchell, J.J., Reigel, E.H., Cocke, D.R., et al.: Intracranial pressure: monitoring and normalization therapy in children. Pediatrics 59:606, 1977.

Mosley, J.W.: Viruses in the etiology of fulminant hepatic failure, Am. J. Gastroenterol. 69:365, 1978.

Mosley, J.W., Combes, B., Volwiler, W., et al.: Corticosteroids in fulminant hepatitis. N. Engl. J. Med. 295:898, 1976.

Opolon, P.: Liver biopsy and prognosis. Am. J. Gastroenterol. 69:368, 1978.

Plum, F., Fishman, R.A., Ware, A.J., et al.: Cerebral edema in FHF. Am. J. Gastroenterol. 69:360, 1978.

Rueff, B., and Benhamou, J.P.: Acute hepatic necrosis and fulminant hepatic failure. Gastroenterology 14:805, 1973.

Scheuer, P.J.: Liver Biopsy Interpretation, 3rd ed. London, Macmillan, 1980, pp. 60 and 80.

Sherlock, S., and Parbhoo, S.P.: The management of acute hepatic failure. Postgrad. Med. J. 47:493, 1971.

Stahl, J.: Studies of the blood ammonia in liver disease. Ann. Intern. Med. 58:1, 1963.

Trey, C.: The fulminant hepatic failure surveillance study. In Saunders, S.J., and Terblanche, J. (eds.): Liver. London, Pitman Medical 1973, p. 120.

Ware, A.J., D'Agnostino, A., and Contes, B.: Cerebral edema: a major complication of massive hepatic necrosis. Gastroenterology 61:877, 1971.

Wilkinson, S.P., Blendis, L.M., and Williams, R.: Frequency and type of renal and electrolyte disorders in fulminant hepatic failure. Br. Med. J. 1:186, 1974.

Williams, R.: Artificial liver support in fulminant hepatic failure. Bull. N.Y. Acad. Med. 51:505, 1975.

Zimmerman, H.J.: Serum enzymes—activities in the differential diagnosis of FHF. Am. J. Gastroenterol. 69:356, 1978.

Nursing Process for Patient Care:

Fulminant Hepatic Necrosis and Hepatic Coma

Hepatic

Assess, Monitor, and Document

Clinical clues: skin color, appetite, nausea/vomiting, level of consciousness
Laboratory data
  Prolonged prothrombin time
  Depressed albumin level

Depressed fibrinogen level
Elevated transaminase levels
Elevated bilirubin levels
Decreased blood glucose
Decreased platelets

Anticipate

Alteration in liver function
Progressive deterioration

NEUROLOGIC

Assess, Monitor, and Document

Encephalopathy
  Level of consciousness
  Motor responses: speech, presence of tremor, bowel and bladder control
  Electroencephalogram (EEG) changes
Cerebral edema
  Level of consciousness

Blood pressure
Pulse
Respiratory rate
Pupillary response
Reflexes
Intracranial pressure (if available)

Anticipate

Alteration in neurologic status
  Encephalopathy: progression from stages I–IV (deep coma, abnormal EEG)
  Cerebral edema: herniation (change in level of consciousness, increased blood pressure, decreased pulse, decreased respiratory rate, altered reflex responses)

HEMATOLOGIC

Assess, Monitor, and Document

Clinical signs of bleeding: overt, occult
Vital signs
Laboratory data

Coagulation profile: prothrombin time, bleeding time, clotting factors
Platelet count

Anticipate

Alteration in coagulation status
  Bleeding diathesis: clinical, laboratory (prolonged prothrombin time, decreased clotting factors, thrombocytopenia)

CARDIORESPIRATORY

Assess, Monitor, and Document

Blood pressure: arterial, central venous
Heart rate
Cardiac Rhythm
Peripheral perfusion
Respiratory rate

Respiratory pattern
Breath sounds
Secretions: amount, description
Arterial blood gases

Anticipate

Alteration in cardiorespiratory status
  Hypotension
  Bradycardia
  Hypoxemia

Pneumonia
Pulmonary edema
Respiratory arrest

RENAL

Assess, Monitor, and Document

Weight
Blood pressure
Urine output, including specific gravity
Laboratory data

Serum: BUN, creatinine, electrolytes, osmolality
Urine: electrolytes, osmolality
Fluid intake: amount, type

Anticipate

Acute renal failure
  Clinical: decreased urine output, hypertension, increased weight

Laboratory data: increased serum BUN, creatinine; alteration in serum electrolytes; alteration in urine electrolytes

FLUID AND ELECTROLYTE BALANCE

Assess, Monitor, and Document

Fluid intake
Urine output
Clinical parameters of state of hydration: weight, blood pressure, skin condition, mucous membranes

Laboratory data: glucose, electrolytes, hematocrit, pH

Anticipate

Overhydration
  Increased weight
  Increased blood pressure
  Hemodilution
Laboratory
  Hyponatremia

Hypokalemia
Hypocalcemia
Hypomagnesemia
Acidosis: metabolic
Hypoglycemia

INFECTIOUS PROCESS

Assess, Monitor, and Document

Temperature
Signs of infection: edema, redness, secretions (amount, description), urine (amount, description)

Laboratory data: white blood count, appropriate cultures

Anticipate

Presence of infection
Sepsis

PANCREATIC

Assess, Monitor, and Document

Clinical: abdominal pain, distention
Laboratory: serum amylase

Anticipate

Alteration in pancreatic function
Pancreatitis

RESPONSE OF CHILD

Assess, Monitor, and Document

Developmental level: cognitive, verbal, motor, psychosocial, fears
Behavioral response: fearful, combative, passive

Response to nursing strategies

Anticipate

Emotional distress

RESPONSE OF FAMILY

Assess, Monitor, and Document

Behavioral response: fearful, tearful, withdrawn, verbal, angry
Level of understanding of child's condition

Expected outcome
Coping mechanisms in operation
Response to nursing interventions

Anticipate

Family crisis
Inability to cope

MIND SET

Assess

Hepatic function
Neurologic status
Hematologic status
Cardiorespiratory status
Renal status

Fluid and electrolyte balance
Infectious process
Pancreatic function
Response of child and family

Anticipate

Alteration in hepatic function
  Clinical clues
  Laboratory tests
Alteration in neurologic status
  Encephalopathy
  Cerebral edema
Alteration in hematologic status
  Bleeding
Alteration in cardiorespiratory status
  Hypotension
  Hypoxemia

  Dysrhythmias
Alteration in renal function
  Acute renal failure
Alteration in fluid and electrolyte balance
Presence of infection
  Sepsis
Alteration in pancreatic function
  Pancreatitis
Emotional distress
Family crisis

42

Pancreatitis

HOWARD B. GINSBURG, M.D.

Historically, pancreatitis, a disease seen primarily in adults, is being recognized more and more frequently in the pediatric age group. Undoubtedly, this is in great part due to an increased awareness of pancreatitis by those rendering primary care to children. With more aggressive use of surgical and drug therapy and decreased mortality rates in critically ill newborns and children with chronic diseases, the actual number of children with pancreatitis may be increasing.

FUNCTION OF THE PANCREAS

The pancreas functions as both an endocrine and an exocrine organ. The endocrine function is mainly that of blood sugar control through the release of insulin into the blood stream. Insulin production in the islet cells of the pancreas often is not directly affected by pancreatitis. The acute inflammatory process associated with pancreatitis, however, can cause a transient islet cell dysfunction leading to temporary hyperglycemia. In most children, hyperglycemia is totally reversible when the acute pancreatitic episode subsides. Under certain circumstances, especially in those children with chronic recurrent pancreatitis, permanent damage can be done to the endocrine portion of the pancreas, causing diabetes mellitus, requiring chronic exogenous insulin administration.

The exocrine function of the pancreas includes the production of enzymes used in the digestion of food in the gastrointestinal tract. These enzymes include inactive precursors of trypsin, chymotrypsin, elastase, phospholipase, and carboxypeptidases A and B. In addition, active forms of alpha-amylase, lipase, ribonuclease, deoxyribonuclease, and phosphorylase are also produced by the pancreas. The proteolytic enzyme precursors are secreted into the gastrointestinal tract through the pancreatic duct and are activated in the small intestine by

enterokinase. Production and release of these enzymes is interdependent upon secretions from both the biliary tract and the stomach. Additionally, secretin, released in response to duodenal acid, stimulates the production of fluid and bicarbonate by the pancreas.

ETIOLOGY

Common to most forms of pancreatitis is autolysis of the pancreas by endogenous proteolytic enzymes. These enzymes are either released and activated within the pancreas or refluxed back into the pancreas from the duodenum in their activated forms, causing a severe local inflammatory response. In many instances, the actual initiating factor of autolysis remains a mystery.

Several broad etiologic classifications of pancreatitis in children have been recognized, including 1) traumatic, 2) drug induced, 3) obstructive, 4) infectious, and 5) idiopathic. Alcoholism and biliary tract disease, commonly the causative agents in adult pancreatitis, are rarely seen in children.

Penetrating or blunt abdominal trauma is probably the most common identifiable cause of pancreatitis in children. Direct damage to the pancreas itself causes release of proteolytic enzymes, which produce a local inflammatory response with subsequent fibrosis and possible obstruction of the pancreatic duct. Children with these symptoms are especially prone to the formation of pseudocysts. When the inflammatory response resolves and there is no further ductal obstruction, symptoms of acute pancreatitis usually resolve without development of a chronic recurrent process. Postoperative pancreatitis should probably be placed in this classification, because inadvertent damage to the pancreas during an operative procedure can cause similar injuries.

Drug-induced pancreatitis is most often seen

after steroid administration. Several theories have been suggested to explain the relationship between pancreatitis and steroid therapy. It has been reported that both volume and viscosity of pancreatic secretions increase with the administration of steroids, possibly leading to dilatation and relative obstruction of the pancreatic duct. Other possible etiologic factors associated with steroids include hyperlipemia, fluid and electrolyte imbalance, and intravascular coagulation. An underlying collagen vascular disease being treated by steroids may predispose to pancreatitis. No direct correlation has been found between the severity of the pancreatitis and the type, dosage, or duration of steroid therapy. Other drugs that have been implicated in causing pancreatitis include L-asparaginase, sulfonamides, thiazides, indomethacin, and isoniazid. Drug-induced pancreatitis seems to carry with it a significantly high mortality rate unless it is recognized early. It is still unclear whether discontinuation of the offending medication has any effect on the eventual outcome.

Direct obstruction of the pancreatic duct can lead to the onset of pancreatitis. This is not a common cause in children, although it is one that should always be considered. In contrast with what is seen in adults, obstructive causes in children are usually congenital in nature, including choledochal cysts, congenital stenoses of the pancreatic duct, annular pancreas, and intestinal duplications. Biliary tract disease with choledocholithiasis occurs to a lesser extent in children than in adults and can cause obstructive problems at the ampulla of Vater. In addition, Ascaris, the worm that causes mechanical obstruction of the pancreatic ducts, has been implicated in several reports of pancreatitis. Unless corrected, the obstructive causes of pancreatitis can lead to chronic recurrent pancreatitis, with eventual fibrosis of the gland. Fortunately, most of these problems can be surgically corrected.

Various infections, both viral and bacterial, have been associated with an increased frequency of pancreatitis. Probably most common among these is mumps, which can lead to both clinical pancreatitis and asymptomatic hyperamylasemia, associated with sialadenitis. Other viral agents as well as mycoplasma and generalized bacterial sepsis have been associated wtih pancreatitis.

Although certain specific problems such as cystic fibrosis and increased intracranial pressure may lead to pancreatitis, most of the remaining cases fall into a miscellaneous or idiopathic classification. No single compelling etiologic factor can be recognized in this group. There have been suggestions that severe dehydration and malnutrition can lead to pancreatitis, but this has not been a constant finding. Frequently, an otherwise healthy child with no prior unusual medical history will develop the signs and symptoms of acute pancreatitis. Most often, these cases are limited to a single acute episode.

ACUTE PANCREATITIS

Signs and Symptoms

The most common symptom associated with acute pancreatitis in school-age children is abdominal pain. The pain is usually described as constant and dull and most often is located in the midepigastric or periumbilical area. Not infrequently, the pain radiates to the back and is sometimes alleviated by the patient sitting in the knee–chest position. With fulminant pancreatitis, the child may present in a state of circulatory collapse, being pale, unresponsive, and hypotensive. Abdominal findings range from mild, localized epigastric tenderness to diffuse peritoneal signs, with rebound tenderness. In certain circumstances, the abdomen may be distended with evidence of ascites. Nausea and vomiting, along with hyperpyrexia and possible jaundice, are frequently associated findings.

Laboratory Findings

Hyperamylasemia is the single most consistent finding in acute pancreatitis. Although this elevation in amylase is not always present and the severity of the disease cannot be correlated with the degree of elevation, the diagnosis of pancreatitis can usually be made from a combination of positive clinical findings associated with hyperamylasemia. Because hyperamylasemia may be associated with other clinical conditions such as sialadenitis of mumps, the breakdown of amylase levels into its various isoenzymes may be important. The ratio of creatinine clearance to amylase clearance is a sensitive indicator of pancreatitis and can be used to differentiate true pancreatitis from hyperamylasemia secondary to renal failure. This is a simple test to perform, requiring only simultaneous spot serum and urine samples for creatine and amylase.

$$\frac{\text{Amylase clearance}}{\text{Creatinine clearance}}\,(\%) =$$

$$\frac{\text{urine amylase}}{\text{serum amylase}} \times \frac{\text{serum creatinine}}{\text{urine creatinine}} \times 100$$

The upper limits of normal range from 3 to 5.3 percent. Levels above this are diagnostic of pancreatitis. This test may also be important in patients with hyperlipemic serum when direct amylase determinations are inaccurate. Serum lipase determinations have proved unreliable and in most cases are not indicated.

Other chemical abnormalities that may or may not be present include hyperglycemia, hypocalcemia, hyperbilirubinemia, and an elevated white blood cell count. Various liver function tests such as LDH, SGOT, SGPT, and alkaline phosphatase may be elevated. Initially, because of third-space fluid loss, the patient may show signs of hemoconcentration, reflected in an elevated hematocrit. With progression to severe hemorrhagic pancreatitis, the hematocrit may drop dramatically secondary to retroperitoneal bleeding. Associated with the more severe forms of pancreatitis is significant fluid sequestration, metabolic acidosis, and renal failure.

Several radiologic findings are often present in pancreatitis. The abdominal film may reveal a sentinel loop, which represents local ileus from direct contact with the inflammatory mass. In addition, a colon cutoff sign has been described, denoting apparent partial obstruction of the midtransverse colon secondary to its proximity to the pancreas. Contrast studies may reveal a widened duodenal sweep or C-loop. This is caused by the acutely inflamed pancreas distorting the duodenum in its retroperitoneal portion. Recent experience with ultrasonography and CT scanning has increased the accuracy of diagnosis.

More invasive procedures such as transhepatic cholangiography and endoscope retrograde cholangiopancreatography (ERCP) may be useful in situations requiring specialized procedures. Transhepatic cholangiography may diagnose pancreatitis associated with biliary tract disease, particularly when associated with biliary tract obstruction. ERCP outlines the anatomy of the pancreatic duct. These two procedures, however, should be performed only by experienced personnel and only in circumstances in which either the diagnosis of pancreatitis has not been made by the more conventional methods or additional anatomic information is essential. They are most useful in defining the anatomy of the pancreatic and biliary systems in patients with chronic pancreatitis.

Recently, peritoneal lavage has begun to play an important role in both the diagnosis and management of pancreatitis. The presence of bacteria or blood in peritoneal fluid may indicate that surgical intervention is necessary. High fluid amylase levels are helpful in the diagnosis.

Management

Traditionally, the management of acute pancreatitis is nonoperative and depends upon allowing the gastrointestinal tract to rest. The patient is made NPO, and nasogastric suction is instituted, which significantly decreases any pancreatic stimulation. Fluid and electrolytes are monitored carefully. Accurate measurement of intake and output is critical, especially in the more severe forms of pancreatitis. Significant amounts of fluid may be sequestered and must be replaced. Replacement of calcium losses can be extremely important in preventing tetany. Other acute problems that require correction are metabolic acidosis and retroperitoneal blood loss. With persistent symptoms or complications of pancreatitis, total parenteral nutrition may be crucial.

Severe pain may be relieved by prescribing meperidine rather than morphine, which may cause constriction of Oddi's sphincter and consequently exacerbate the pancreatitis. Antispasmodics have been used in the past, but it appears that they have no direct influence on the pancreatitis itself. Some investigators suggest the standard use of antibiotics as part of the treatment protocol, but this procedure remains controversial.

Pulmonary findings are sometimes present, especially with severe pancreatitis. Resultant pulmonary insufficiency may necessitate the use of ventilatory assistance. Recent studies have revealed a possible beneficial effect from peritoneal lavage in patients with such advanced disease.

Surgical therapy in patients with acute pancreatitis should be undertaken with extreme caution. There is evidence that inadvertent surgical intervention may increase morbidity and mortality. Indications for surgical intervention include: 1) inability to differentiate between pancreatitis and other intra-abdominal catastrophes, 2) correction of an underlying cause of pancreatitis such as biliary tract disease, 3) continued clinical deterioration despite adequate medical management, and 4) evidence of pancreatic abscess requiring drainage.

CHRONIC PANCREATITIS

Although pancreatitis in children is most often limited to a single, acute episode, recurrent disease does exist. Chronic pancreatitis may be divided into three subgroups: 1) familial hereditary pancreatitis, 2) relapsing pancreatitis, and 3) chronic fibrosing pancreatitis. There are no distinct boundaries separating these classifications, and a great amount of overlap occurs. Indeed, a common finding in all three subgroups is obstruction, either complete or incomplete, of the pancreatic and biliary systems.

Hereditary pancreatitis was first described in 1952, and since then, a few cases have been added to the series. It appears that the disease is inherited as an autosomal dominant with incomplete penetrance. The presentation is usually one of recurrent bouts of abdominal pain, which may begin in early childhood. With continued episodes, pancreatic insufficiency often ocurrs. An exceedingly high number of abdominal carcinomas has been reported in association with this disease. These carcinomas are not limited to the pancreas; they may be seen in the colon and in other intra-abdominal organs. Other complications include diabetes mellitus, glucose intolerance, pseudocyst formation, and portal and splenic vein thrombosis. Aminoaciduria, hyperparathyroidism, and hyperlipidemia may be associated with hereditary pancreatitis.

Chronic relapsing pancreatitis and chronic fibrosing pancreatitis do not seem to have a familial incidence and are usually related to underlying congenital problems causing stricture of the ductal system. The causes include intestinal duplication within the pancreas, chronic biliary obstruction from calculous disease, congenital strictures, and traumatic damage to the pancreas. The symptoms of chronic pancreatitis are similar to those of hereditary pancreatitis, with chronic recurrent abdominal pain being the most common symptom. Patients with chronic pancreatitis may also develop malabsorption, steatorrhea, and glucose intolerance. Classical diabetes mellitus is uncommon; the islet cells seem to be spared, despite progressive fibrosis of the gland.

Diagnosis of chronic pancreatitis may be difficult, because the chronic recurrent pain is often mistaken for other intra-abdominal problems. Antecedent episodes of acute, fulminant pancreatitis are the exception rather than the rule. Hyperamylasemia may not be seen and, when present, amylase elevations may only be minimal. Occasionally, urinary amylase and amylase clearance are more sensitive than serum amylase. More recently, ultrasonography and ERCP have been used in making an early diagnosis. The abdominal ultrasound may reveal an enlarged C-loop and an irregularly enlarged pancreas. ERCP may be especially beneficial by outlining the anatomy of the pancreatic and biliary ducts and displaying evidence of obstruction. Often a simple abdominal flat plate will delineate calcifications within the pancreas and lead to a suspicion of chronic pancreatitis. Early diagnosis may be important in the outcome of the disease, because an anatomic obstruction corrected expeditiously will lead to significant symptomatic relief as well as prevention of further deterioration of the pancreas itself.

Management

Medical management of chronic pancreatitis includes many of the same procedures as management of acute pancreatitis. Each individual exacerbation should be treated with supportive care, including gastrointestinal decompression, IV hydration, and management of pain.

Recent experiences with surgical management of chronic pancreatitis have led to good results in some patients. Operative pancreatography enables significant strictures of the pancreatic duct not previously diagnosed by other means to be seen in detail. Local periampullary strictures can be treated by sphincteroplasty, enabling free drainage of pancreatic secretions into the duodenum. For patients with a single distal pancreatic duct stricture, distal pancreatectomy should be curative. More commonly, with multiple pancreatic duct strictures, the "chain of lakes" effect is found. Many of these cases are treated adequately by pancreaticojejunostomy, as described by Peustow. Correction of calculus disease by cholecystectomy and common duct exploration is crucial in preventing further bouts of recurrent pancreatitis.

Clearly, there is a broad spectrum of anatomic problems associated with chronic pancreatitis, and each must be treated individually. No single operative procedure can adequately treat the variety of abnormalities encountered with this problem. It is crucial to be selective not only of the operation chosen but also of those patients who undergo the operation. Not every child with recurrent pancreatitis has symptoms that are significant enough to warrant the possible hazards of operative intervention.

COMPLICATIONS

Pseudocysts

Pseudocysts are nonepithelized cystic masses originating from the pancreas and containing pancreatic fluid. In children, approximately 60 percent of pseudocysts occur after abdominal trauma, although they can occur after acute pancreatitis from other causes. The formation of a pseudocyst may occur at varying intervals after the initial trauma to the pancreas and is often accompanied by a triad of symptoms, including abdominal pain, vomiting, and fever. Often, a discrete abdominal mass can be palpated, although this is not a universal finding. Serum amylase levels are usually elevated and, indeed, a persistent hyperamylasemia after an acute bout of pancreatitis should make one suspicious of a pancreatic pseudocyst. Recently, both ultrasonography and CT scanning have significantly increased the accuracy of this diagnosis. In most cases, pseudocysts should be diagnosed preoperatively.

The initial treatment for pancreatic pseudocysts is observation and nasogastric decompression if the patient's clinical status is stable. It is unwise to attempt drainage of a pseudocyst if the wall is immature and thin, because surgery at this time is both difficult and dangerous. If a pseudocyst persists for 2 to 3 weeks, surgical intervention is indicated to prevent complications such as hemorrhage, perforation, intestinal obstruction, biliary obstruction, and abscess formation. At this point, the pseudocapsule will have matured to the point where surgical drainage is relatively safe. The actual operative therapy is determined by the position, size, and maturity of the pseudocyst. External drainage of the cyst leads to complications such as pancreatic fistulas and recurrent pseudocysts. Consequently, internal drainage seems to be the treatment of choice in most cases. It provides a reliable method of decompression of the cyst itself and is effective in relieving both signs and symptoms.

Diabetes Mellitus

Acute pancreatitis may lead to episodes of hyperglycemia because of the effect of the in-

flammatory response on islet cells. In most cases, this problem is transient and will only require temporary medical support. In cases in which diabetes is permanent, long-term insulin therapy is indicated.

Pancreatic Insufficiency

This complication is most commonly seen with chronic recurrent or chronic fibrosing pancreatitis. A gradual destruction of the pancreas will lead to malabsorption and steatorrhea. Although pancreatic insufficiency can be seen in acute pancreatitis, it is usually transient. However, in chronic pancreatitis with fibrosis and permanent pancreatic insufficiency, oral preparations of pancreatic enzymes may be required.

CONCLUSION

Pancreatitis in its acute form may be a fulminant, lethal disease. Early, accurate diagnosis will decrease the relatively high morbidity and mortality rate seen in children. On the other end of the spectrum, chronic pancreatitis is a progressive, debilitating disease with an ever-increasing list of complications occurring over the course of the disease. Accurate diagnosis of this problem may arrest the progressive nature of the disease and restore these children to normal, active lives. In both cases, diagnosis should be followed by appropriate medical and surgical therapy. Awareness of the multifactorial problems will render treatable an otherwise potentially devastating disease.

CASE PRESENTATION

A 17-year-old male was previously admitted to the hospital because of gastrointestinal bleeding, abdominal pain, night sweats, and weight loss. An abdominal mass was palpated in the left upper abdomen. He underwent exploratory laparotomy, at which time a large mass involving the retroperitoneum, duodenum, stomach, and pancreas was discovered and biopsied. The diagnosis of histiocytic lymphoma was made, and the patient was started on a course of chemotherapy that included vincristine, cytoxan, methotrexate, and prednisone. Response to this course was good, and the patient was discharged on prednisone, with outpatient chemotherapy planned.

Ten days after discharge, he began experiencing severe abdominal pain, which radiated to the back and was relieved somewhat by sitting. Several episodes of nausea and vomiting had occurred.

Examination and Test Results

Physical examination revealed the following vital signs: T = 98.8°F, BP = 178/72 mm Hg, P = 90 beats/min, and RR = 24 breaths/min. This thin, oriented male was in obvious pain. HEENT: several ulcers of the buccal mucosa. Chest: clear with some decreased breath sounds at left base. Cor: regular rhythm, no murmurs. Abdomen: generalized tenderness, which was greatest in left upper quadrant (LUQ), mild rebound tenderness; mass palpated in LUQ; bowel sounds hypoactive. Neuro: intact. Abdominal and chest x-rays were obtained as well as a CBC, electrolytes, liver function tests (LFTs), and serum amylase.

Laboratory data revealed a serum amylase of 1080 (normal 30–170); WBC = 11,000; hct = 32.3 percent; Ca = 9.0, and glucose = 125.

Problem List

Gastrointestinal

Abdominal x-ray examination revealed a questionable LUQ mass. A nasogastric (NG) tube was placed and attached to suction.

Intake and Output

The remainder of the electrolytes were normal, although the urine specific gravity was 1.030. The patient was kept NPO, and a Foley catheter was inserted. He was begun on IV fluids of D5 1/3 normal saline (NS), with 10 mEq of KCL/500 ml at 1½ maintenance.

Histiocytic Lymphoma

The patient was maintained on 100 mg of hydrocortisone. Abdominal symptoms resolved quickly with NG suction, although the amylase was persistently elevated. Ultrasound and CT scan revealed an enlarged pancreas, consistent with pancreatitis and a LUQ mass consistent with the original lymphoma. He was begun on IV hyperalimentation and kept NPO for 16 days. After that period, he tolerated a low-fat diet well and was discharged after 23 days of hospitalization. Amylase prior to discharge was 200.

Ten days after discharge, the patient was again admitted for repeated episodes of abdominal pain, nausea, and vomiting. Results of physical examination revealed T = 97.5°F, BP = 90/60 mm Hg, P = 90 beats/min, and RR = 20 breaths/min. He was a thin, cachectic male in abdominal distress. HEENT: mucous membranes dry. Chest: clear. Cor: regular rhythm, no murmur. Abdomen: soft, minimal left-sided tenderness, with LUQ abdominal mass palpated. Bowel sounds were high pitched. Abdominal and chest x-rays were obtained as well as CBC, LFTs, electrolytes, serum calcium and serum amylase.

Laboratory data revealed a serum amylase of 220; WBC = 2,900; and hct = 38.5 percent. Serum calcium was normal.

Final Assessment

Gastrointestinal

Abdominal x-rays revealed a dilated stomach and proximal duodenum, with scant amounts of air throughout the remaining intestine. The patient was placed NPO on NG suction.

Intake and Output

The urine specific gravity was 1.030, and the urine output was poor. He was placed on D5 1/3 NS, with 10 mEq of KCl/500 ml at 1½ maintenance. Strict intake and output were recorded.

Histiocytic Lymphoma

The patient was maintained on IV hydrocortisone. Despite IV fluids at 1½ maintenance, multiple fluid pushes were required before urine output improved. NG drainage was consistently high. Abdominal ultrasound and CT scan revealed a fluid-filled mass posterior to the stomach.

Seven days after admission, the patient was operated on for a pancreatic pseudocyst and a cystogastrostomy was performed. Immediately postoperatively, the serum amylase fell to normal levels. He quickly regained intestinal function and was discharged 10 days postoperatively. No evidence of recurrent lymphoma had been identified at the time of the operation.

SUGGESTED READING

Andorsky, M., Finley, A., and Davidson, M.: Pediatric gastroenterology 1/1/69–12/31/75: a review Part I. Hollow viscera and the pancreas. Am. J. Dig. Dis. 22:56, 1977.

Blumenstock, D.A., Mithoefer, J., and Santulli, T.V.: Acute pancreatitis in children. Pediatrics 19:1002, 1957.

Blumenthal, H.T., and Probstein, J.G.: Acute pancreatitis in the newborn, in infancy, and in childhood. Am. Surg. 27:533, 1961.

Buntain, W.L., Wood, J.B., and Woolley, M.W.: Pancreatitis in childhood. J. Pediatr. Surg. 13:143, 1978.

Eichelberger, M.R., Hoelzer, D.J., and Koop, C.E.: Acute pancreatitis, the difficulties of diagnosis and therapy. J. Pediatr. Surg. 17:244, 1982.

Fonkalsrud, E.W., Henney, R.P., Riemenschneider, T.A., and Barker, W.F.: Management of pancreatitis in infants and children. Am. J. Surg. 116:198, 1968.

Hendren, W.H., Greep, J.M., and Patton, A.S.: Pancreatitis in childhood: experience with 15 cases. Arch. Dis. Child. 40:132, 1965.

Kattwinkel, J., Lapey, A., Di Sant'Agnese, P.A., et al.: Hereditary pancreatitis: three new kindreds and a critical review of the literature. Pediatrics 51:55, 1973.

O'Neill, J.A., Jr., Greene, H., and Grishan, F.K.: Surgical implications of chronic pancreatitis. J. Pediatr. Surg. 17:920 1982.

Riemenschneider, T.A., Wilson, J.F., and Vernier, R.L.: Glucocorticoid-induced pancreatitis in children. Pediatrics 41:428, 1968.

Nursing Process for Patient Care:

Pancreatitis

Pancreatitis is most often seen in the pediatric critical care unit (CCU) as a result of trauma, obstruction, infection, drugs, and possibly inadvertent intraoperative damage. Nursing personnel must be aware of the high-risk population in order to anticipate its occurrence as a secondary diagnosis.

The primary system involved is the gastrointestinal system. The pancreas has both endocrine and exocrine functions. It is responsible for insulin production and, therefore, blood sugar control. It also produces enzymes used in the digestion of food.

GASTROINTESTINAL

Assess, Monitor, and Document

Pain
  Intensity: usually constant and dull
  Location: midepigastric, periumbilical, radiates to back
Nausea
Vomiting
Abdominal distention: measure abdominal girth

Nasogastric (NG) drainage: amount, color, consistency
Jaundice
Laboratory data: amylase, bilirubin, hct, liver function tests

Anticipate

Pain
Nausea
Vomiting
Abdominal distention: ascites
Jaundice
Hyperpyrexia
Abnormal laboratory data: elevated amylase, hyperbilirubinemia, elevated liver function tests

Retroperitoneal bleed
Pseudocysts: pain, vomiting, fever, persistent hyperamylasemia
Diabetes mellitus: hyperglycemia
Pulmonary insufficiency
Circulatory collapse: unresponsive, hypotensive

FLUID AND ELECTROLYTE BALANCE

Associated with pancreatitis, especially the more severe forms, is significant fluid sequestration, which may lead to hemoconcentration, metabolic acidosis, and renal failure. Chemical abnormalities may or may not be present but should be monitored.

Assess, Monitor, and Document

Daily weight
State of hydration: blood pressure, edema
Urinary output, including specific gravity
NG drainage: amount, color

Fluid intake: accurate administration of parenteral fluids (use infusion pump if available)
Laboratory data: glucose, calcium, pH, HCO_3

Anticipate

Fluid sequestration
  Decreasing urine output
  Increasing abdominal girth
Metabolic acidosis

Acute renal failure
  Decreased urine output
  Weight gain

RESPONSE OF CHILD

Assess, Monitor, and Document

Developmental level
Behavioral response: quiet, tearful, angry

Anticipate

Emotional crisis
Inability to cope

RESPONSE OF FAMILY

Assess, Monitor, and Document

Behavioral response: Angry, hostile, verbal
Level of understanding of illness and child's
  condition

Expected outcome
Response to nursing interventions

Anticipate

Family crisis
Inability to cope

MIND SET

Assess

Gastrointestinal system
Fluid and electrolyte balance
Response of child and family

Anticipate

Alteration in gastrointestinal status
  Gastrointestinal distress: pain, nausea,
  vomiting, abdominal distention, retroper-
  itoneal bleed, pseudocysts
  Diabetes mellitus
  Pulmonary insufficiency

Circulatory collapse
Alteration in fluid and electrolyte balance
  Acute renal failure
Emotional trauma
Family crisis

NEUROLOGIC

43

Management of Pediatric Head Trauma

JEFFREY H. WISOFF, M.D.
FRED J. EPSTEIN, M.D.

Head injuries are a common cause of morbidity and mortality in the pediatric population. Approximately 1 of 10 children will experience traumatic loss of consciousness during childhood. Annually, over 500,000 children are hospitalized following a head injury, with 3,000 to 4,000 deaths resulting; an additional 15,000 children will require prolonged inpatient care, often with poor outcome.

The goal of therapy in the head-injured child is preservation of function, prevention of secondary insults, physical rehabilitation, and psychosocial reintegration.

The medical and surgical therapies discussed in this chapter are only the first steps in the child's ultimate recovery. Social workers, psychologists, and psychiatrists continue the often lengthy rehabilitative process, providing support and guidance for the entire family unit.

Recent studies of severely head-injured children indicate that both morbidity and mortality can be dramatically reduced through aggressive medical and surgical management. Thus, a thorough understanding of several basic concepts in the management and pathophysiology of pediatric craniocerebral trauma is mandatory for all medical personnel engaged in the treatment of the head-injured child.

PATHOPHYSIOLOGY

A major concept in the management and pathophysiology of pediatric craniocerebral trauma is primary vs. secondary brain injury. The primary injury occurs at the moment of impact. The severity is directly proportional to the amount and kind of biomechanical stress transmitted to the cranium and brain. Forces produced by linear acceleration tend to create focal damage, that is, fracture and brain contusion. Rotational acceleration sets up shearing forces with the brain that disrupt function and anatomy diffusely, beginning at the surface of the brain and extending centripetally toward white matter, diencephalon, and brain stem, depending upon the magnitude of the initial injury. Physiologic dysfunction can occur in the absence of gross anatomic disruption, the dysfunction often far exceeding anatomic injury.

The secondary injury results from those events that exacerbate the effects of the primary injury. Systemic hypotension, hypercarbia, and hypoxia result in brain ischemia and edema; intra- and extra-axial hematomas result in local compression and, ultimately, herniation. Potentially reversible lesions are made permanent, and new lesions occur from ischemic and anoxic damage, thus leading to increased morbidity and mortality. The prevention and treatment of these secondary insults is a vital part of our current therapeutic regime.

A popular misconception is the belief that a comatose child with abnormal brain stem reflexes has suffered an irreversible brain stem injury. In fact, primary brain stem injury is a catastrophic event. Patients with such injuries usually die within 2 hours following the insult. These patients rarely reach the hospital alive. Children who present with skew deviation, impaired corneal reflexes, dilated pupils, and extension posturing (decerebration) usually have diffuse white matter injuries. The realization that these are not primary irreversible brain stem lesions has led to aggressive management to avoid or minimize secondary insults, early treatment of elevated intracranial pressure (ICP), and subsequent neurologic recovery in most children.

A third concept that is unique to the pediatric population is post-traumatic cerebrovascular hyperemia. The CAT scan shows diffuse swelling of the brain with loss of subarachnoid cisterns and slit ventricles, with a concomitant increased ICP. The pathophysiology appears to be a diffuse increase in cerebral blood volume. This is probably a unique response of the immature brain to the same biomechanical forces that create diffuse brain injury. This condition may respond well to medical therapy.

PHYSICAL EXAMINATION AND HISTORY

The goal of the neurologic examination in head trauma is to provide an estimate of the extent and location of the injury, a baseline status against which the progress of the disease can be measured, and a means to correlate current neurologic function and ultimate recovery.

Whenever possible, a brief history should be obtained; relatives, paramedics, police, or other witnesses often can provide useful information. Important points include the time, location, and mechanism of injury: direct blows to the head are more likely to cause extra-axial hematomas and fractures; acceleration/deceleration injuries usually result in diffuse white matter damage. A lucid interval suggests that relatively insignificant amounts of biomechanical force were initially applied to the brain and that a secondary insult such as diffuse brain swelling, intracranial hematoma, or systemic compromise is responsible for the patient's deterioration. In children, it is important to ascertain whether apnea or seizures have occurred.

The neurologic examination should be succinct and directed toward those areas that will provide maximal definition of the extent of the injury while being rapid enough to not delay treatment. The patient's level of consciousness is the single, most significant, indicator of the severity of the injury. Single-word terms such as *stupor* and *lethargy* should be avoided. A description of verbal responsiveness and the ability to follow various commands are more appropriate indications of the extent of the patient's injury.

In patients with impaired levels of consciousness, the Glasgow Coma Scale (GCS) provides a useful, easily reproducible examination. The scale consists of three parts: eye opening, motor response, and verbal response (Table 43–1). Extensive clinical data indicate that motor response correlates best with the extent of injury and outcome. One drawback of the GCS for young children is the difficulty in applying the verbal response parameters. Table 43–2 is a verbal scale modified for infants.

Further evaluation should include description of pupillary size and reaction to light, corneal responses, either oculovestibular or oculocephalic reflexes, and lateralizing motor responses. The gag reflex, heart rate, and presence of spontaneous ventilation should be evaluated to indicate function of the lower pons and medulla.

EMERGENCY MANAGEMENT

The treatment of head-injured children must begin at the accident site, with attention directed to ensuring an adequate airway and cardiovascular support. The most common secondary insults in head injury occur in the prehospital phase. These include hypoxemia, from aspiration and mechanical airway obstruction, and shock. The airway should be cleared manually. If experienced personnel are available, the posterior pharynx may be palpated for fracture dislocation of the body of C2. Secretions are aspirated, and an oral airway is inserted. The child can then be ventilated easily by mask. Most children will hyperventilate spontaneously and correct any hypercarbia after any airway obstruction has been removed. Occasionally, gentle cricoid pressure will help clear the airway. An oxygen mixture of 50 percent is administered to avoid hypoxemia. Failure of spontaneous ventilation is an extremely ominous sign. Intubation should not

Table 43–1. Glasgow Coma Scale

Eye Opening	4. Spontaneous
	3. To speech
	2. To pain
	1. None
Best Verbal Response	5. Oriented
	4. Confused
	3. Inappropriate
	2. Incomprehensible
	1. None
Best Motor Response	6. Obeys commands
	5. Localized pain
	4. Withdraws
	3. Flexion to pain
	2. Extension to pain
	1. None

Table 43–2. Glasgow Coma Scale (Infants)*

One Month	1. None 2. Crying to stimuli 3. Crying spontaneously 4. Blink when eyelashes touched 5. Throaty noises
Two Months	1. None 2. Crying to stimuli 3. Shuts eyes to light 4. Smiles when caressing 5. Babbles—single vowel sounds
Three Months	1. None 2. Crying to stimuli (moans) 3. Stares to response and looks at environment 4. Smiles to sound stimulation 5. Coos, chuckles, *vowels* in a prolonged way
Four Months	1. None 2. Crying to stimuli (moans) 3. Turns head to sound 4. Smiles spontaneously or stimulated, laughs when socially stimulated 5. Modulating voice and perfect vocalization of vowels
Five and Six Months	1. None 2. Crying to stimuli (moans) 3. Localizes general direction of sound 4. Discriminates family members 5. Babbles to people, toys
Seven and Eight Months	1. None 2. Crying to stimuli (moans) 3. Recognizes familiar voices and family 4. Babbles 5. "Ba," "Ma," "Da"
Nine and Ten Months	1. None 2. Crying to stimuli (moans) 3. Recognizes (smiles or laughs) 4. Babbles 5. "MaMa," "DaDa"
Eleven and Twelve Months	1. None 2. Crying to stimuli (moans) 3. Recognizes—smiles 4. Babbles 5. Words (specifically "Mama" and "Dada")

*Courtesy of Dr. Kenneth Shapiro, Department of Neurosurgery, Albert Einstein College of Medicine, New York, New York.

be attempted at the accident site. Lateral cervical spine x-rays should be obtained prior to intubation to exclude fracture-subluxation. If the airway is compromised and the possibility of a cervical spine injury cannot be excluded, an emergency tracheostomy may be indicated.

Systemic hypotension in patients older than 1 year of age is almost never due to head injury. Bradycardia and hypotension suggest cervical spinal cord injury, whereas the more usual tachycardia/hypotension is secondary to hypovolemic shock. Immediate treatment with large-bore IV lines and volume replacement with colloid and/or isotonic solutions is mandatory. Hypotonic solutions (i.e., D5W) should be avoided, because they decrease serum osmolality and secondarily increase cerebral edema. A diligent search for the source of hemorrhage includes peritoneal lavage in the comatose patient. Rarely, in infant and toddler patients, severe scalp bleeding or otorrhagia secondary to basilar skull fracture may cause hypovolemic shock.

The cornerstone of emergency room treatment is normalization of blood pressure, hyperventilation, and diuretic therapy. Two large-bore IV lines are inserted, and blood is drawn for CBC, electrolytes, amylase, coagulation profile, arterial blood gas, and type and crossmatch. If there is no evidence of hypovolemic shock, fluid management should be D5W/1/3 normal saline (NS) for children younger than 10 years of age and D2.5W/1/2 NS for older children, at two thirds maintenance rate. Mild dehydration with serum osmolality in the 300 to 310 mOsm range is desirable.

X-rays of the cervical spine (also chest and pelvis in multiple trauma) are obtained. If the gag reflex is present, a nasogastric (NG) tube may be inserted prior to intubation. (All unconscious patients require an NG tube.)

After stabilization of vital signs and neurologic evaluation, an endotracheal tube is inserted in all patients with a GCS score of 8 or less. If experienced personnel are available, muscle paralysis with pancuronium and sedation with sodium pentothal may be used to prevent bucking and catastrophic elevations of intracranial pressure. Paralysis and hyperventilation to a Pa_{CO_2} of 25 mm Hg are maintained until a CAT scan is obtained.

Simultaneous with hyperventilation, furosemide, 1 mg per kg, and mannitol, 1 gm per kg, are given as bolus injections. The use of steroids in head trauma is controversial. Some medical centers recommend dexamethasone, 1.5 mg per kg, or 5 to 6 mg per kg of methylprednisolone as an initial bolus, administered thereafter every 6 hours. These initial resuscitation and therapeutic maneuvers should be accomplished within 15 to 20 minutes of the patient's arrival in the emergency room. Infrequently, the patient remains unstable and will require emergency trephination, subdural taps, or craniotomy without a diagnostic study.

Whenever possible, a CT scan should be performed. CT provides the maximum diagnostic information in head trauma and supersedes the need for skull x-ray, ventriculography, or angiography. An initial scan through the lateral ventricles will identify any urgent surgical mass lesion. If the patient is stable, the entire cranium from the foramen magnum to the vertex is scanned. Bony lesions and fractures, extra- and intra-axial hematomas, cortical contusions, diffuse injuries, and the status of the ventricular system can be rapidly and accurately documented. If the CT scan is not available, metrizamide/air ventriculography through a ventricular catheter or angiography is the most rapid method of detecting mass lesions.

FRACTURES

Fractures are the most common neurosurgical injury following head trauma. One half of all linear fractures occur in the pediatric population. More than 50 percent of children younger than 1 year of age with significant head injury will sustain a linear fracture. In most children, a linear fracture is associated with no loss of consciousness. In the infant and toddler age groups, a large subgaleal hematoma or cephalohematoma may occur. These patients may be admitted to the hospital, and serial hematocrits must be obtained (these two patient populations may have hypovolemia secondary to head injury). Treatment is expectant. Aspiration of the hematoma is not advised.

In older infants, a linear fracture may result in a dural laceration with cyst formation and a growing fracture. In this situation, localized cerebral hernia and, ultimately, venous infarction of incarcerated brain may occur. Skull x-rays are repeated 2 months post trauma and again at 4 months to detect growing fractures.

Depressed fractures can be separated into neonatal "ping-pong" fractures and true traumatic depressed fractures. In newborns, these fractures are rare compared with the overall birth rate. They are usually associated with a prolonged or difficult labor in which the parietal or frontal bone is compressed against the sacral promontory. Depressed fractures are rarely a consequence of obstetric forceps. Small indentations will usually elevate spontaneously. Moderate or large depressions should be surgically elevated, because it is unlikely that they will resolve, and the cosmetic deformity can be quite noticeable.

In older children, depressed fractures that are compound, depressed more than the thickness of the skull, or cosmetically deforming should be elevated or débrided. Neurologic deficits are usually secondary to local cerebral trauma and are seen in less than half of these patients. Surgery is performed to prevent late onset of seizures (especially when the fracture is close to the motor cortex), relieve local mass effect, prevent infection (compound fractures), and improve cosmetic appearance. A CT scan is essential to delineate underlying cerebral contusion or hematoma, as well as the extent of the bony unjury. If the fracture crosses a major dural sinus, preoperative angiography may be indicated.

All patients receive loading doses of anticonvulsants prior to surgery. If the dura is intact and there is no evidence of contusion on CT scan, the anticonvulsants are not continued postoperatively. Although prophylactic antibiotic therapy is a controversial issue, most medical centers recommend perioperative antistaphylococcal antibiotics (oxacillin, 200 mg/kg/day). The principal goal of treatment in compound fractures is prevention of infection. At surgery, the bone is elevated and débrided, and dural lacerations are repaired. Jennet has shown that in compound fractures the bone fragments may be cleaned and replaced primarily, obviating the need for subsequent cranioplasty; the cause of infection is the delay of more than 24 hours from injury to surgery, not replacement of débrided bone. These children receive 7 to 10 days of postoperative antibiotics. Anticonvulsants are continued for at least 1 year.

Basal skull fractures occur in 6 to 14 percent of head injuries in children. Significant cerebrospinal fluid (CSF) fistulas rarely occur: CSF rhinorrhea in less than 1 percent, and otorrhea in 0.5 to 6 percent of pediatric head injuries. Eighty to 90 percent of CSF fistulas will heal spontaneously within 1 week of the injury. Treatment is expectant: bed rest in a position that minimizes or stops the rhinorrhea, and spinal drainage if the fistula persists beyond 3 to 4 days. Prophylactic antibiotics are not used; the natural incidence of meningitis is low, and the likelihood of selecting resistant organisms is high. Persistent fistulas require evaluation with metrizamide CT scanning or isotope scanning to localize the leak, followed by definitive operative repair.

HEMATOMAS

Epidural

Epidural hematomas occur in approximately 5 percent of moderately to severely injured children. They are rare in infants because of the firm adherence of the dura to the skull at the suture lines. The location tends to be more superior and posterior in the parieto-occipitotemporal region compared with the usual anterior temporal location in adults. Only 50 percent of such children have an associated skull fracture; CT scan is the diagnostic test of choice. The classic picture consists of a high-density biconvex, well-localized lesion adjacent to the inner table with an appropriate mass effect and shift.

The clinical presentation of the child with an epidural hematoma includes a blow to the head, occasionally of minor significance, with or without transient loss of consciousness, followed by a lucid interval, then increasing headache, obtundation, contralateral hemiparesis progressing to decerebration, anisocoria (with the dilated pupil ipsilateral to the hematoma), and bradycardia. Only 30 to 58 percent of patients have the classic lucid interval; 30 to 50 percent never lose consciousness.

An alternate syndrome of delayed signs and symptoms may occur with venous epidurals in the parietal area. Unlike a hematoma in the temporal fossa, which causes early herniation of medial temporal lobe and brain stem compression, a similar hematoma over the posterior convexity may cause symptoms later, because a greater degree of brain shift is necessary for brain stem compression. These children present 1 to 2 weeks following injury, with increasingly severe headache, nausea/vomiting, and papilledema. Drowsiness and bradycardia may be the forerunners of an acute decompensation. A high degree of clinical suspicion is necessary for the diagnosis.

If the child presents with a GCS score of 8 or less or deteriorates during initial evaluation, emergency resuscitation, including intubation, hyperventilation, and diuretics, is indicated. Usually, the child can be stabilized and a CT scan can be obtained. About 15 percent of the cases require emergency surgery without a diagnostic test. A dilated pupil ipsilateral to the hematoma is the most valuable indication. The definitive treatment of epidural hematomas is craniotomy and surgical evacuation of the hematoma. All children with any degree of preoperative obtundation have an ICP monitor inserted at the conclusion of the craniotomy and are monitored for at least 72 hours, the period of greatest risk for brain edema/hyperemia and consequent intracranial hypertension. The prognosis is excellent for most children; even the presence of bilateral fixed and dilated pupils does not preclude a good recovery.

Subdural

Acute subdural hematomas may occur as a result of birth injury, child abuse, or accidental impact injuries from motor vehicle accidents or falls. In neonates, distress usually occurs within 12 hours of birth, with signs of tentorial herniation, tense bulging fontanelle, subhyaloid hemorrhages, and respiratory distress. Difficult labor, breech presentation, and low Apgar scores have been associated with neonatal hemorrhage.

In infants younger than 1 year of age, acute subdural hematoma is often associated with child abuse. The child presents with acute coma or apnea, occasionally heralded by a seizure. When an impact injury occurs, there may be a lucid interval. Level of consciousness can vary from mild obtundation to deep coma, with decerebrate posturing or flaccidity. The fontanelle is tense and bulging, retinal hemorrhages are invariably present, pupils may be fixed and dilated, and often there are multiple bruises from abuse. Apnea is a particularly ominous sign.

Initial management includes hyperventilation by mask, then intubation. Mannitol and/or furosemide are given intravenously. As soon as the airway is secured, the subdural space is tapped bilaterally with an No. 18 or 20 gauge Angiocath catheter. Frequently, 5 to 10 ml. of bloody, nonclotting fluid under pressure is obtained from each side, with immediate relaxation of the fontanelle and improvement in neurologic status. The catheters are left in the subdural space and are connected to closed drainage. After they have stabilized, these infants receive a CT scan.

CT scan may show one of two pictures. A high-density crescentic lesion overlying one or both hemispheres with compression of the ipsilateral ventricle and shift is the classic appearance of an acute subdural hematoma. The other CT picture may be seen in infants with positive subdural taps. There is often only a very thin layer of blood over the convexities and in the interhemispheric fissure. Other CT findings include subacute or chronic isodense subdurals diagnosed by white matter buckling on high-resolution CT or by angiography. Occipital lobe infarction from acute herniation and compression of the posterior cerebral arteries may be seen during the acute phase.

Surgical evacuation of a large localized hematoma or a holohemispheric clot exceeding 5 mm in thickness is recommended. Often the CT will not reveal a significant surgical lesion (as just described). All patients are treated with ICP monitoring, hyperventilation, steroids, and furosemide. They are at significant risk for development of acute brain swelling (hyperemia) and must be carefully monitored, with elevated ICP vigorously treated to avoid secondary damage from intracranial hypertension. In the nonsurgical group, the subdural catheters are removed after 24 hours. Serial CT scans are mandatory to monitor reaccumulation of an acute hematoma or development of a chronic subdural hematoma. In infants treated conservatively, Bruce and associates at Children's Hospital of Philadelphia report less than a 10 percent incidence of delayed hematomas requiring trephination or subdural peritoneal shunting. The mortality rate in this population is low, approximately 5 percent; however, only 25 percent have normal development, and all show atrophy on subsequent CT.

Motor vehicle accidents and falls are the causes of most acute subdural hematomas in older children. In urban settings, direct blows to the head from assailants have become increasingly common among adolescents. Many of these children have associated cerebral contusion and laceration. More of these children have surgical lesions requiring craniotomy than do infants. Again, both surgical and nonsurgical patients are at high risk for subsequent intracranial hypertension. Medical control of ICP is essential to prevent secondary swelling and ischemia and to permit recovery. The mortality rate from uncomplicated acute subdural hematomas in children is about 10 percent, but with combinations of epidural, subdural, and cortical laceration, it may be 60 to 80 percent.

Intracerebral

Intracerebral hematomas occur in 6 percent of children who suffer severe head injury. CT scan is crucial for diagnosis and management. Occasionally, superficial hematomas causing regional mass effect and neurologic deterioration require surgical evacuation. Deep hematomas are treated nonoperatively by medical control of ICP and are followed with serial CT scans. Late effects of intracerebral hematomas include porencephalic cysts and a high incidence of seizures.

Diffuse Brain Swelling

Acute diffuse brain swelling, or "malignant edema," is the most common neurosurgical condition in pediatric head trauma, occurring in 50 percent of children with GCS scores of less than 8. The clinical presentation follows two distinct patterns. In the first pattern, the child sustains an injury of varying intensity but is awake and alert. Over a period of several minutes to hours, there is progressive obtundation, sweating, nausea/vomiting, bradycardia, and occasional focal neurologic signs. Further clinical deterioration may cease or progress to coma, with dilated pupils (often unilateral), and abnormal motor posturing. Intervention at this point is necessary to prevent a fatal outcome. Hyperventilation is instituted, and diuretics and anticonvulsants are administered. A CT scan is obtained. The classic appearance is that of diffuse cerebral swelling, with slitlike or absent ventricles and loss of CSF cisterns. No mass lesion is noted. After 48 to 72 hours, hyperventilation can be gradually tapered without elevations of ICP. Consciousness returns over the next few days. With adequate resuscitation and aggressive intensive care, a good to excellent recovery should be anticipated.

The other clinical pattern more closely resembles adult head injuries. Patients present in deep coma with no history of a lucid interval. These patients have usually sustained a greater diffuse cerebral injury at the time of impact. Examination will show decortication, decerebration or flaccidity, abnormal brain stem and pupillary reflexes, and bradypnea or apnea. Absence of spontaneous respirations is a particularly ominous sign. Emergency resuscitation, as previously outlined, is carried out, and a CT scan is obtained to rule out the possibility of an extra-axial hematoma.

Vigorous ICP management is essential (see Chapter 12, Increased Intracranial Pressure). An ICP monitor is inserted in all patients. Hyperventilation to a Pa_{CO_2} of approximately 25 mm Hg is maintained. Furosemide, 1 mg per kg q4h, is administered for ICP greater than 20 mm Hg. IV fluids are given at two thirds maintenance, and the head of the bed is elevated 30 to 45 degrees. The lesion that is being treated over the first 24 to 48 hours is cerebral hyperemia. Mannitol is not used during this period, because it increases blood volume and may increase the intracranial hypertension. After this phase, further rises in ICP may be secondary to true cerebral edema or, possibly, to multiple petechial hemorrhages not resolved on CT scan. Mannitol, 1 gm per kg IV bolus, followed by 0.25 to 0.5 mg per kg q6h may be used to maintain ICP less than 20 mm Hg. If ICP cannot be controlled or if serum osmolality rises above 320 mOsm, diuretic therapy is discontinued and barbiturate hibernation is begun.

After placement of a Swan-Ganz catheter and volume expansion with colloid, a loading dose of pentobarbital, 5 mg per kg IV, is given over 15 to 20 minutes and is followed by a continuous infusion varying from 2 to 5 mg per kg per hour. The aim of therapy is to maintain ICP less than 20 mm Hg. If the ICP is not controlled, the infusion may be increased until a flat line electroencephalogram (EEG) is obtained with serum barbiturate levels ranging from 3 to 5 mg per dl. If ICP continues to be high, further increases in barbiturates are unlikely to be beneficial. Reinstitution of mannitol and furosemide may be efficacious.

The use of barbiturates requires careful monitoring of the cardiovascular system with a Swan-Ganz catheter. Adolescents and young adults will often become severely hypotensive during induction of barbiturate coma, whereas younger children may have a paradoxical hypertension from peripheral vasoconstriction. Measurement of cardiac output, pulmonary wedge pressure, and central venous pressure is essential to guide the complex management of barbiturate cardiotoxicity with combinations of volume replacement, vasodilators, and inotropic agents (dobutamine or dopamine).

CONCLUSION

Aggressive medical management to avoid secondary brain injury, use of CT scanning to establish prompt, accurate diagnoses, and intensive therapy to counter intracranial hypertension have dramatically altered morbidity and mortality in pediatric head injury. Mortality rates in the most severely injured patients with decerebrate posturing or flaccidity (GCS 3–4) have gone from 44 to 100 percent, to 18 to 28 percent. The overall mortality rate for children with GCS 3 to 8 is only 3 to 14 percent. More important, a good to excellent outcome can be expected in 60 percent of children with brain contusion and in up to 90 percent of those with diffuse nonfocal injury.

CASE PRESENTATION 1—ACUTE SUBDURAL HEMATOMA

A 10-month-old boy fell off a kitchen chair, striking the left side of his head. Immediately after the fall, he was crying vigorously and moving all extremities. Over the next 20 minutes, he became progressively lethargic and his mother noted a strange periodic breathing pattern (i.e., Cheyne-Stokes). He was brought to the emergency room several minutes later. Examination revealed a comatose child, bulging tense fontanelle, dilated left pupil, and bilateral decerebrate posturing. A percutaneous left subdural tap yielded 15 ml of fresh blood; a right subdural tap was negative. He received mannitol (1 gm/kg) and lasix (1 mg/kg) and was then intubated. Following the subdural tap, the fontanelle was flat and the child began to move appropriately in response to pain. An emergency CT scan showed a left acute subdural hematoma and a left parietal linear skull fracture. A craniotomy was performed, and a 60 ml subdural hematoma was evacuated. Postoperatively, the patient had no focal neurologic deficits, but his development has been delayed.

CASE PRESENTATION 2—DIFFUSE CEREBRAL HYPEREMIA

A 12-year-old girl was involved in a high-speed motor vehicle accident. In the emergency room, she was comatose with small, minimally reactive pupils, bilateral decorticate posturing, and Cheyne-Stokes respirations. She received mannitol (1 gm/kg) and lasix (1 mg/kg) and was intubated. An emergency CT scan showed slitlike ventricles, an absence of subarachnoid cisterns, and no evidence of shift or focal intracranial mass. A subarachnoid pressure monitor (Richmond screw) was placed, with an initial ICP of 20 mm Hg. Using hyperventilation (PCO_2 = 25 mm Hg) and lasix every 4 hours, her ICP was maintained below 15 mm Hg. She required 7 days of ICP monitoring before she could be weaned from lasix and hyperventilation therapy. She made a gradual neurologic recovery; 3 months after her injury, she had no focal deficit; by 6 months, she was back in school. She required neuropsychological testing and therapy for difficulties with attention span and short-term memory. These problems had resolved by 2 years.

SUGGESTED READING

Bruce, D.A., Schut, L., Bruno, L.A., et al.: Outcome following severe head injury in children. J. Neurosurg. 48:679, 1978.

Bruce, D.A., Alavi, A., Bilaniuk, L., et al.: Diffuse cerebral swelling following head injuries in children: the syndrome of "malignant brain edema." J. Neurosurg. 54:170, 1981.

Bruce, D.A., and Schut, L.: Management of acute craniocerebral trauma in children. Contemp. Neurosurg. 10:1, 1979.

Cooper, P.R. (ed.): Head Injury. Baltimore, William & Wilkins, 1982.

McLaurin, R. (ed.): Pediatric Neurosurgery. Surgery of the Developing Nervous System. New York, Grune & Stratton, Inc., 1982.

Shapiro, K., and Marmarou, A.: Clinical applications of the pressure-volume index in the treatment of pediatric head injuries. J. Neurosurg. 56:819, 1982.

Management of Pediatric Head Trauma

Head trauma is a frequent cause of admission to the pediatric intensive care unit (ICU). Level of consciousness is the primary parameter in the assessment of the severity of traumatic head injury. Initial attention is directed toward establishing and maintaining adequate respiratory and cardiovascular support. Subsequent action is directed toward preserving cerebral function and preventing secondary insults. Morbidity and mortality can be dramatically reduced through aggressive management.

NEUROLOGIC

Accurate assessment and monitoring of the child's neurologic status is important. It provides an estimate of the extent and location of the injury and a baseline from which changes can be measured.

Assess, Monitor, and Document

Level of consciousness
  Description of verbal response
  Ability to follow commands
  Glasgow Coma Scale: eye opening, motor response, verbal response
Pupillary response: size, reaction to light
Reflexes: corneal, oculocephalic, gag

Posture
Blood pressure
Pulse
Respiratory rate and pattern
Intracranial pressure (ICP)
Seizures
Response to treatment of increased ICP

Anticipate

Increased ICP
  Headache
  Vomiting
  Altered level of consciousness
  Increased blood pressure
  Decreased heart rate
  Decreased respiratory rate and altered pattern

Altered reflexes: pupillary, oculocephalic, oculovestibular, corneal, gag
Posturing: decorticate, decerebrate
Seizures
Apnea
Respiratory arrest
Cardiac arrest

RESPIRATORY

The child's respiratory function must be preserved if secondary insults to the brain are to be prevented. The most common insults are related to the degree of hypoxemia caused by airway obstruction, aspiration, and apnea.

Assess, Monitor, and Document

Status of airway: patency
Secretions: amount, description
Endotracheal tube: patency, position
Breath sounds
Respiratory rate
Respiratory pattern, including depth

Color
Agitation
Restlessness
Arterial blood gases
Response to therapy: ventilatory support, paralysis

Anticipate

Alteration in respiratory status
  Airway obstruction
  Aspiration
  Apnea

Respiratory insufficiency: hypoxia, hypercarbia, acidosis
Respiratory arrest
Cardiac arrest

CARDIOVASCULAR

Assess, Monitor, and Document

Blood pressure: arterial, central venous
Heart rate
Perfusion: peripheral pulses, capillary filling, condition and color of skin, urine output (specific gravity)

Fluid intake
Response to therapy: volume replacement, pharmacologic management

Anticipate

Alteration in cardiovascular status
Shock: decreased blood pressure, increased pulse rate, poor perfusion, decreased capillary filling

Decreased urinary output

INTEGUMENTARY

The comatose child is at risk for developing pressure sores and infection from prolonged bed rest and immobility.

Assess, Monitor, and Document

Skin condition
Special attention to bony prominences, burr holes, and ICP insertion site (if applicable)
Skin care

Turning schedule
Use of adjuncts to care: egg-crate foam, sheepskin

Anticipate

Alteration in skin condition
Decubiti
Wound infection

RESPONSE OF CHILD

Assess, Monitor, and Document

Developmental level: verbal, motor, psychosocial, cognitive
Perception of events surrounding accident

Behavioral response: fearful, anxious, tearful, angry
Response to nursing interventions

Anticipate

Emotional crisis
Inability to cope

RESPONSE OF FAMILY

Assess, Monitor, and Document

Behavioral response: anxious, fearful, verbal, angry
Perception of events associated with the accident: feelings of guilt

Level of understanding of child's condition
Expected outcome
Response to nursing interventions

Anticipate

Inability to cope
Family crisis

Need for referral: social service, psychiatry,
rehabilitation

MIND SET

Assess

Neurologic status
Respiratory status
Cardiovascular status

Integumentary system
Response of child and family

Anticipate

Alteration in neurologic status
   Increased ICP
Alteration in respiratory status
   Respiratory insufficiency
   Respiratory arrest
Alteration in cardiovascular status

Hypotension
Shock
Cardiac arrest
Alteration in skin condition
Emotional distress
Family crisis

Pediatric Spinal Cord Trauma

JONATHAN GREENBERG, M.D.
FRED J. EPSTEIN, M.D.

The three primary goals of management of the acutely spinal cord–injured pediatric patient are: (1) preservation of neurologic function and prevention of further neurologic deterioration, (2) maximization of neurologic recovery, and (3) prevention of intercurrent non-neurologic complications that interfere with rehabilitation to the highest attainable functional level. Because the neurologic damage in spinal cord trauma can evolve so rapidly and can be so devastating, a thorough and systematic management is essential if disaster is to be averted.

ETIOLOGY

Injury to the spinal cord and nerve roots can occur whenever stress applied to the vertebral column is sufficient to overcome the bony, ligamentous, and soft-tissue physiologic limits of resistance and creep. High-speed acceleration, deceleration, or rotatory, shear, or compressive forces applied to the vertebral column can result in fracture or dislocation of bony structures and disruption of the stabilizing soft tissues. The disruption can result in instability and compression of intradural structures.

The highly mobile cervical spine, unprotected by rib, pelvic girdle, or heavy paraspinal support, is most susceptible to trauma. Much of the following material pertains to cervical spine trauma, although it is also applicable to thoracic and lumbar spinal injury.

Extension injuries result from acceleration trauma of sufficient intensity to overcome the resistance of the strap muscles of the neck and the anterior longitudinal ligament, an avulsion fracture of the anterior lip of a vertebral body. Occasionally, overextension can place traction on the vertebral arteries as they course through foramina between C6 and C2, resulting in spasm or occlusion, with severe neurologic sequelae. Small children may also be prone to

traction injuries of the cord in hyperextension, resulting in either stretching or even complete disruption of the cord over several segments because of the inherent elasticity differences of the supporting cartilaginous and soft-tissue structures, as opposed to the even more elastic neural supporting structures that allow for greater stretch. Rear-end automobile collisions are the paradigm of the extension injury. High-speed deceleration traction injuries may result in *avulsion of nerve roots* from the spinal cord itself, as in brachial plexus injuries sustained in motorcycle accidents.

Flexion injuries to the spine are more common than traction injuries. Acute decelerations of sufficient magnitude to disrupt the interspinous ligaments, jump or fracture the articulating facets of the laminae, and injure or rupture the posterior longitudinal ligament and ligamentum flavum produce instability of the neural arch surrounding dural structures. Massive compressive forces exerted during flexion can create compression or burst fractures of the vertebral bodies, the latter driving fragments directly into the dural tube, containing neural structures. Head-on motor vehicle collisions and diving accidents are characteristic injuries. Even in the absence of a bony injury, the relative looseness of the spinal cord, which, although partially tethered along its lateral aspects in the cervical and thoracic region by dentate ligaments, allows it to float free in the dural tube and may allow it to strike the posterior longitudinal ligament and vertebral body in sudden decelerations, resulting in severe neural damage. In the presence of a *congenitally narrowed spinal canal,* momentary acute buckling of the posterior longitudinal ligament and the ligamentum flavum and severe spinal cord compression can occur even in the absence of a bony fracture or dislocation; this entity has been seen in contact sports, especially football injuries.

Rotary injuries result in injuries to articulations of the bony neural arch, with dislocation of articulating surfaces, partial dislocation, and instability of the bony column. C1 and C2, which account for almost half the rotary motion of the neck, are particularly susceptible.

Relatively more stable than their cervical counterparts are the thoracic and lumbar vertebrae, which, by virtue of their greater bony (ribs, pelvis) and muscular (intercostals, paraspinals) support, are less susceptible to flexion and extension injuries. *Shear and flexion injuries,* the result of rapid horizontal or vertical decelerations, as in seat belt injuries or falls, respectively, can result in compression or burst injuries and ligamentous damage, with dural tube compression.

Finally, secondary spinal cord or root compression may result from epidural cord compression by an *epidural hematoma* arising from injury to the epidural venous plexus. The effects of this injury may be insidious, following the initial injury by several hours or days. *Intramedullary spinal cord hematoma,* the result of direct trauma, may expand and act as a mass compressing neural tissue and resulting in progressive neurologic deficit.

PATHOPHYSIOLOGY

Spinal cord injury can result from direct trauma to nervous tissue within the dural tube, from ischemia caused by a loss of local arterial blood supply or an obstruction of venous drainage, or from the secondary effects of ischemic injury to nervous tissue.

Direct trauma to the neurons, axons, and glial-supporting structures (knife or gunshot wounds, spinal cord stretch, contusion, disruption, or transection) or the interruption of the *arterial supply* or *venous drainage* to a region of the spinal cord with subsequent infarction of cord tissue produces obvious and often profound neurologic deficits. Spinal radicular artery compression or occlusion can result in spinal cord ischemia in *watershed regions* of blood supply to the cord. Systemic hypotension and underperfusion may mimic this condition or exacerbate its effect. *Metabolic effects* secondary to primary spinal cord trauma may adversely affect otherwise viable neural tissue adjacent to these traumatized areas.

Within minutes following spinal cord injuries, there is usually a pronounced decrease in spinal cord blood flow. Systemic factors, such as systemic hypotension and decreased cardiac output, and local factors, such as catechol-amines and possibly prostaglandins and free radical lipoperoxides, impair cellular metabolism. Free radical lipoperoxides liberated from damaged cell membranes both inactivate enzymes responsible for the maintenance of cellular integrity and catalyze further free radical reactions. They have also been implicated in the activation of synthesis and propagation of the vasospastic and thrombogenic prostaglandins, which can cause arterial vasospasm, microvascular platelet aggregation, and microvascular thrombosis. Cellular metabolic acidosis ensues, with a drop in cytoplasmic adenosine triphosphate (ATP) concentrations and a decreased extracellular calcium concentration, which is indicative of further cellular damage. Lysosomal aggregation and rupture releases hydrolases, which can cause further indiscriminate damage to local neural structures. The amount of time necessary for irreversible metabolic injury to occur in the spinal cord is not known, but it is probably within the range of minutes to several hours.

TREATMENT

Recognition is the key to optimal treatment of spinal cord trauma and to the prevention of further injury to compromised neural tissue. When a patient has multiple trauma or multiple medical problems, the diagnosis may be overlooked. It cannot be overemphasized, therefore, that a high index of suspicion is essential, not only because this knowledge will influence all subsequent management but also because it may prevent the loss of salvageable neurologic function through inadvertent manipulation.

For cervical spine trauma, initial treatment is *immobilization* in a soft cervical collar, with sandbags placed on either side of the neck. The vertebral column (especially for thoracic or lumbar vertebral trauma) should be supported on a rigid frame, with adequate shoulder and pelvic girdle support. The head should be supported in a neutral position during transport, but *under no circumstances, should manipulation be attempted without traction apparatus,* and then only by experienced personnel.

Recognition

History. The way in which the injury occurred provides important information as to the nature of the forces acting on the vertebral column and spinal cord. If possible, this information should be obtained from witnesses or from the patient on admission.

General Examination. Careful palpation of the spinous processes for evidence of a gap, indicative of subluxation or a rotatory deformity, should be done. Hyperextension injuries may be associated with anterior soft-tissue trauma and, occasionally, hematoma formation with tracheal deviation or compression. Paraspinal muscular spasm with torticollis may indicate facet injury with nerve root entrapment.

Neurologic Examination. *The initial neurologic examination is critical to adequate assessment of spinal cord trauma.* In the acute emergency setting, a brief examination may be made; a more detailed examination can be performed after stabilization. The neurologic examination should include: (1) voluntary motor function of major muscle groups in all extremities; (2) sensory function to pin and joint position sense; (3) rectal tone and perianal sensation, and the bulbocavernosus reflex; and (4) deep tendon reflexes.

The highest level at which normal neurologic function is present is designated the *cord level of injury.* Deep tendon reflexes ae usually lost in spinal shock, but partial injury may leave them partially preserved. Likewise, presence of sacral sparing (rectal tone, perianal sensation) may, because of the peripheral location of these fibers in the cord, have important prognostic implications if even minimal motor function exists in the lower extremities.

The continuum of spinal cord trauma ranges from subclinical (abnormal somatosensory evoked potentials only) to the full-blown complete cord syndrome. Accurate *recognition of the partial cord syndromes is crucial* because of the potential for recovery of function (Table 44–1).

Radiologic Examination. Even a grossly normal neurologic examination is no guarantee

against vertebral column instability, which can later result in subluxation with catastrophic consequences. For this reason, x-ray examination of suspected areas of injury is mandatory. Cervical spine examination is especially important in cases of major head trauma. In children, however, x-ray diagnosis is difficult, because their developing cartilaginous structures are radiolucent. Spinal cord injury may coexist with an x-ray that appears normal or shows only a loss of normal lordosis with prevertebral swelling; obversely, 20 percent of the children who are 7 years of age or younger will have a pseudosubluxation of C2 on C3 or C3 on C4 or C5 on x-ray examination without neurologic deficit.

General Resuscitation Considerations

Patients with spinal cord trauma may suffer from multiple injuries or from the systemic effects of spinal cord injury itself. Injured spinal cord tissue or borderline viability is further compromised by hypoxemia and ischemia, and implicit in neurologic resuscitation is the restoration of normal systemic oxygenation and perfusion. Special considerations however, pertain to the resuscitation of spinal cord–injured patients.

Ventilation. Patients with injury to the cervical and thoracic spine will experience a loss of intercostal and, rarely, with C4 or higher cervical spinal trauma, diaphragmatic function. Deterioration of pulmonary function, with only a small fraction of normal tidal volume, vital capacity, and inspiratory force, may result, mandating endotracheal intubation. Intubation should be performed *nasotracheally if at all possible,* with the head maintained in neutral position and *care taken not to manipulate the head.* If the nasotracheal route is inadequate or not available, a tracheostomy should be performed, although this procedure may interfere with subsequent surgical stabilization from an anterior approach. Patients who do not require intubation should nonetheless have their pulmonary functions, including arterial blood gas, followed conscientiously throughout hospitalization.

Perfusion. High level injuries to the spinal cord can result in loss of autonomic nervous system function, a reflex dysautonomia. Immediate effects, however, include a loss of vasomotor tone and sympathetic cardiac tone, the latter causing a decrease both in cardiac rate and contractility and, occasionally, heart block with ventricular ectopy. Loss of vasomotor in-

Table 44–1. Partial Cord Syndromes

Syndrome	Effect
Posterior cord	Loss of joint position sense and vibration
Anterior cord (anterior spinal artery syndrome)	Loss of motor function with preservation of joint position sense
Central cord	Relative weakness of upper extremities in relation to lower extremities
Partial cord (Brown-Séquard)	Ipsilateral motor weakness with contralateral loss of pin sensation
Cauda equina/root	Radicular distribution of pain, weakness; bowel and bladder impairment

nervation results in vasodilatation and a functional hypovolemia.

The cardiac effects can be treated initially with IV atropine followed by cardiotonic drips (dopamine, dobutamine; isuprel should be used with caution because of its beta-agonist vasodilator effect). Patients with severe or prolonged bradycardia may require temporary or permanent placement of transvenous pacemaker (this determination may require bundle of His studies). Agents such as terbutyline and aminophylline, in addition to their role in improving pulmonary function, also exert cardiotonic activity and improve cardiac contractility.

The functional hypovolemia may be treated with volume expansion. Because of the disruption of normal vascular-neural interfaces and edema of nervous tissue, isotonic isosmolar crystalloids (D5W–0.45 NS) or colloids should be used for volume maintenance after initial volume replenishment has been attained using standard solutions (RL, NS, PCs). A central venous or Swan-Ganz catheter may be necessary to adequately monitor filling pressures in the right atrium and pulmonary vascular bed and for following cardiac output.

Following initial fluid resuscitation, subsequent evidence of hypovolemia should prompt a search for other sources of intravascular loss (hemothorax, hemoperitoneum, retroperitoneal hematoma, and long bone fractures), which should be treated independently.

A Foley catheter should be placed not only for monitoring fluid resuscitation and renal function but also to prevent acute urinary retention with subsequent hemorrhagic cystitis or shock following drainage.

Spinal Cord Resuscitation

Primary pharmacologic treatment of spinal cord trauma remains controversial. Despite the absence of a controlled clinical trial, recent laboratory studies indicate that high doses of *glucocorticoids* and *naloxone* may be of benefit. Glucocorticoids have been shown to increase local spinal cord blood flow to injured areas, despite causing a transient reduction in systemic blood pressure. Proposed mechanisms of action, in addition to increasing blood flow, include stabilization of cell and lysosomal membranes, scavenging of free radials (aborting the prostaglandin cascade or mediating its effects), and prevention of intracellular calcium deposition. In experimental animals, naloxone, in high doses, has been shown to increase local spinal cord blood flow and systemic blood pressure, possibly on the basis of mediation or endogenous opiate effects on the central nervous system receptors. Hypothermia has also been suggested for decreasing the rate of spinal cord metabolism during periods of decreased perfusion, although this treatment is not often used.

Glucocorticoids. Doses of glucocorticoids on the order of 15 to 30 mg per kg of methylprednisolone, or its equivalent, administered within 45 minutes of a graded spinal cord injury in laboratory animals have been shown to result in statistically significant improvement in spinal cord function. Pharmacologic studies suggest that this initial loading dose, delivered over a few minutes, should be followed by doses of 5 to 15 mg per kg q1h to q6h and maintained for several days (maximum 10 days), with monitoring of neurologic function, unless there is no change in neurologic activity after 72 hours.

Naloxone. Current clinical research shows that initial loading doses of 4.0 mg per kg may be tolerated in adults, with a constant infusion of 3 mg per kg/hr thereafter. Applicability to children has not been shown, however, and the preservatives in commercially marketed ampules of 0.4-mg doses may have adverse toxic effects. Therefore, pending further study, caution should be used in administering this drug.

Realignment, Stabilization, and Decompression

Realignment of the vertebral column may result in decompression of the spinal cord, by stretching buckled ligamentum flavum and posterior longitudinal ligament, retracting bony fragments, and partially reducing fractures. Decompression of soft tissues and bony structures and reduction of the distortion of spinal cord vasculature may improve local blood supply to borderline regions of injured neural tissue. Realignment is accomplished only with *traction*, which should be applied slowly with serial x-ray correlation. Optimal traction for cervical spine injuries involves bony fixation of the traction apparatus in a line parallel to the axis of the vertebral column. Halo ring, Gardner-Wells, or Crutchfeld tongs, or, in very small children, epidural wires placed via burr holes are alternatives to traction. Traction will also accomplish the goal of *stabilization*, pending the ultimate goal of rigid stabilization and operative (if necessary) decompression.

Injuries to the thoracic and lumbar spine are

usually not amenable to conventional traction techniques, and operative decompression and internal fixation (wiring, plating, or Harrington rod placement with bone grafting) is the procedure of choice. Locked cervical facets with subluxation also require operative decompression.

In the absence of a neurologic or orthopedic surgeon familiar with the foregoing traction techniques, interim traction may be fashioned with a halter neck traction device, provided that care is taken to: (1) maintain the head in neutral position, and (2) maintain the axis of traction parallel to the axis of the vertebral column. Care must be taken not to overdistract the spinal cord, especially in the presence of damaged soft tissues and supporting structures; a rule of thumb is that the weight of traction applied should be no more than the weight of the head. Confirmation of decompression by *myelography* with free flow of contrast beyond the area of injury following reduction of vertebral deformity is mandatory; metrizamide myelography with concurrent CAT scanning provides additional information about the bony canal and spinal stability.

Prevention and Treatment of Complications

Post–Traumatic Reflex Dysautonomia

Autonomic fibers coursing through the spinal cord may be ablated in spinal cord trauma, resulting in severe and paroxysmal autonomic dysfunction, predominantly the result of interruption or damage to sympathetic fibers at the cervical level.

Cardiac dysrhythmias and impaired contractility, resulting from interruption of sympathetic fibers with unimpaired vagal tone, have been discussed previously.

Systemic hypotension or hypertension, also discussed previously, is especially prone to paroxysmal fluctuations because of the loss of autonomic homeostatic mechanisms. Severe postural hypotension may necessitate the administration of mineralocorticoid analogues such as fluorinef to increase plasma volume. Systemic hypertension, occasionally to frightening proportions, may require antihypertensives, of which hydralazine is most efficacious because of its beta-agonist effects.

Cutaneous vasomotor instability, with abnormal modulations of sympathetic and parasympathetic activity, may cause *profound sweating*, with fluid and heat loss or anhydrosis, with heat retention. Hypothermia or hyperthermia blankets, in addition to compensation for insensate fluid loss, should be used, providing that care is taken to protect anaesthetic areas of the skin that are in contact with the blankets from thermal damage.

Cervical and thoracic spinal cord injuries often cause a transient ileus, which necessitates nasogastric (NG) drainage for decompression and replacement of fluid and electrolytes. Severe ileus may cause diaphragmatic compression and hypoventilation if distended bowel is not decompressed. Later, a *hyperactive gastrocolic reflex* may lead to gastric dumping, which can mimic or obscure hyperosmolar damage to intestinal mucosa during subsequent attempts at nasogastric alimentation; this complicates the management of both the patient's nutritional and fluid balance.

A bowel regime is mandatory if constipation and obstipation are to be avoided. Failure to maintain bowel care risks intestinal obstruction, sepsis, and perforation of an abdominal viscus. The bowel regime should consist of stool softeners, evacuette suppositories, enemas, and, if necessary, digital disimpaction.

Depending upon the level of injury, spinal trauma may result in either a *hypotonic neurogenic* or a *spastic hypertonic bladder*. Initial treatment of the spinal cord injury patient includes Foley catheterization, with administration of chronic urinary antibacterial suppressant therapy. Usual medication includes ascorbic acid q6h and Mandelamine q6h. *Urinary tract infections* are frequent sequelae in catheterized patients. Routine Foley catheter changes as well as urinalyses and urine cultures should be performed. Suprapubic catheterizations are rarely necessary, and urinary diversionary procedures are discouraged.

Within several weeks of injury, the bladder function should be checked both by voiding pattern (overflow vs. spastic) and urinary residual (greater than 30 ml postvoid residual is abnormal). A voiding cystourethrogram may be necessary to characterize the nature of the lesion. Anticholinergics, such as Urecholine, are used for hypotonic bladders, whereas an alpha-adrenergic blocker (e.g., Dibenzyline) or an antispasmotic (e.g., baclofen) may be required for the spastic bladder.

Stress Ulceration and Viscus Perforation

Approximately 20 percent of spinal cord injury patients will develop stress ulceration with gastrointestinal hemorrhage, which can be massive. Severely injured patients are unable to respond to such insults with reflex tachycardia and increased vascular tone. Consequently, patients in the early post-injury phase should have their hematocrits and stool and NG guaiacs monitored frequently; and, an unexplained drop in blood pressure following initial fluid resuscitation should always prompt a search for occult bleeding.

Steroids have not been shown to increase the incidence of gastrointestinal hemorrhage in spinal cord–injured patients, including those on mini-heparin therapy. The pathophysiology of the hemorrhage is thought to be related to focal mucosa ischemia secondary to the initial sympathetic cascade at the time of trauma. Oral or NG antacid therapy, such as Mylanta (cathartic) or Amphojel (constipating), has been shown to be as efficacious as H_2 blockers (cimetidine, ranitidine) when used to titrate gastric pH at 4.0 or higher.

Abdominal viscus perforation and peritonitis are even more sinister and serious complications in patients being treated with steroids. *Because patients with high injury levels have no sensation, symptoms of peritonitis may be masked until fever and leukocytosis appear.* Even these late signs may be masked by glucocorticoids. Abdominal distention with fever of unknown origin should, therefore, prompt a search for possible intra-abdominal sepsis.

Pneumonia and Pulmonary Embolism

Pneumonia is prevented by a regime of vigorous pulmonary toilet and maintenance of good aeration, including tracheal suctioning, intermittent positive pressure breathing (IPPB) with expectorants (Bronkosol, SSKI, Mucomyst), and close monitoring of pulmonary functions. Although obvious cases of aspiration should be treated, many patients will inevitably become colonized with hospital organisms, and only true pneumonitis should be treated with the most specific antibiotics to avoid selecting out resistant organisms.

Pulmonary embolus may mimic pneumonitis but should always be kept in mind as a complication in the immobilized spinal injury patient. Ace wraps or TED stockings, together with early mobilization and vigorous physical therapy, are the keys to prevention. Low-dose heparin (mini-heparin) therapy has been advocated, but its efficacy has not been conclusively shown.

Decubiti (Pressure Sores)

Local ischemia secondary to direct pressure over bony prominences can result in a through-and-through necrosis of skin and subcutaneous elements, with subsequent breakdown and infection. Pressure points of Halo vests or thoracolumbar cases are not immune.

Prevention is the key to avoiding decubiti. Frequent turning, either manually or by the Roto-Bed (or similar device; *not* the circular bed or *Stryker Frame*), and minimizing focal pressure with an air or water mattress, clinitron bed, sheepskin, or foam posies are recommended methods. Decubiti should be treated with local débridement (mechanical and collagenase) and hyperalimentation.

Deformity

The development of scoliosis in patients recuperating from spinal injury, but nonetheless having residual deficit, should always be considered as a possible late complication. An orthopedic consultation should be arranged during hospitalization to determine whether spinal bracing will be needed.

CASE PRESENTATION 1

A 14-year-old boy was brought to the emergency room by the local volunteer ambulance corps following a swimming pool accident. Witnesses reported that the boy dove from the shallow end of the pool, striking his head on the bottom and losing consciousness. He was immediately dragged from the water and resuscitated by the lifeguard but was initially poorly arousable. His neck was in sandbags, and he was lying on a wooden board, wearing an oxygen mask.

On admission, he was poorly responsive, with skin pallor and some spontaneous thrashing movements of his arms but not his legs; he had an obvious frontal scalp contusion.

His vital signs were: BP = 70/40 mm Hg; P = 40 beats/min (regular); RR = 10 breaths/min; and T = 95°F.

Problem List

Neurologic

1. Probable cervical spine injury with shock.

Treatment: General resuscitation for shock; keep neck stabilized (sandbags, soft cervical collar); x-rays of cervical spine and head.

2. Impaired mental status, rule out cerebral concussion, secondary to hypoperfusion.

Treatment: Observe during resuscitation; CAT scan after initial medical stabilization if no improvement.

3. Neurologic deficit, secondary to Problem number 1.

Treatment: Methylprednisolone, 30 mg/kg IV push, over 1 minute, with 5 mg/kg IV q1–2h thereafter; naloxone, 2–4 mg/kg IV, and check for response; give antacids while on steroids; air mattress/water bed; sheepskin/posies.

Respiratory

1. Hypoventilation, probably secondary to neurologic problems; rule out cerebral concussion and aspiration.

Treatment: Nasotracheal intubation and suctioning; arterial blood gases (ABG), ventilator for respiratory support (suctioning may induce bradycardia/heart block).

Cardiac

1. Bradycardia, probably secondary to neurologic problems.

Treatment: EKG monitor; IV atropine; dopamine/ dobutamine drip on standby; transvenous pacemaker if necessary.

2. Hypotension, possibly secondary to neurologic and cardiac problems.

Treatment: Same as above; also, IV normal saline (NS) and serum albumin; Foley catheter, Ace wraps to both legs; Trendelenberg position p.r.n.

Gastrointestinal

1. Ileus, secondary to neurologic problems.

Treatment: NG tube for initial decompression and later for NG antacids and nutrition, daily bowel regimen (Colace, Dulcolax/Evacuette suppositories, enemas) to be written following recovery from ileus.

Hypothermia

1. Possibly secondary to neurologic problems or to exposure.

Treatment: Hyperthermia blanket.

The patient's color improves, and he awakens following resuscitation. He can now signal yes and no and follow simple commands. General physical examination reveals lower cervical spine tenderness and spinous process discontinuity. Neurologic examination reveals three fifths motor function of biceps, with a trace motor of triceps and the right iliopsoas. He has a pin sensory level at L3 but has diminished, but present, rectal sphincter tone and bilateral anal wink; his bulbocavernosus reflex is equivocal. He has weak biceps deep tendon reflexes only, and his toes are mute. Sensation is slightly greater on the left.

Admission C-spine x-rays reveal a compression fracture of the C5 vertebral body, with anterior subluxation of C5 on C6, bilateral jumped facets, and a 50 percent narrowing of the cervical canal. C7 is not seen, and repeat lateral C-spine is performed, revealing a normal canal at C6 and C7. Chest x-ray reveals bibasilar atelectasis and hypoaeration. Admission ABG is reported: pH = 7.28, PO_2 = 64 mm Hg, and PCO_2 = 48 mm Hg.

Neurologic

1. Cervical spine injury, with subluxation and narrowing of the canal, and spinal cord compression, with partial spinal cord injury; modified anterior spinal cord and Brown-Séquard syndromes.

Treatment: Cervical decompression with traction (neurosurgeon called) and patient placed in Gardner-Wells tongs with 20-lb traction; serial lateral C-spine x-ray films confirm reduction of dislocation; absence of block to CSF flow to be confirmed by myelography via (C1–C2 puncture).

Respiratory

1. Bibasilar atelectasis.

Treatment: Daily monitoring of pulmonary function following reinflation of lungs on respirator; sputums for culture if clinically indicated; IPPB with Bronkosol or Mucomyst; terbutaline, p.r.n.; serial ABGs.

2. ABG respiratory/metabolic acidosis.

Treatment: Same as above and continue resuscitation.

Twenty-four hours post-injury, the patient is placed in a Halo vest, with surgery for permanent fixation scheduled for later in the week. Four days post-injury, he develops a low-grade fever. NG aspirate and stool guaiac are negative. CXR reveals a left lower lobe (LLL) infiltrate. Urinalysis shows 5–10 WBCs. Urine culture grows 10^4 gram-negative rods. Physical examination reveals rales at left base, benign abdomen, and sacroischeal erythema.

Infection

1. LLL infiltrate.

Treatment: Pulmonary toilet, antibiotics for acquired hospital pneumonitis, sputum cultures, and gram stain; lung scan to rule out pulmonary emboli if appropriate (patient may require mini-heparinization or full anticoagulation if positive).

2. Incipient urinary tract infection (UTI).

Treatment: Periodic changing of Foley catheter; ascorbic acid, and Mandelamine (or other bacterial suppressant agents).

Skin Care

1. Incipient decubitus formation.

Treatment: Foam ring to support surrounding tissues; if skin breakdown progresses, local wound care, including collagenase and Debrisan; zinc sulfate P.O. (single dose is adequate), water bed, frequent turning and repositioning.

Following resolution of his medical problems, the patient underwent surgical fusion, followed by an extensive course of physical therapy and rehabilitation, with social service support for home care plans.

SUGGESTED READING

Demopoulos, H.B., Flamm, E.S., Pietronigro, D.D., and Seligman, M.L.: The free radical pathology and the microcirculation in the major central nervous system disorders. Acta Physiol. Scand. (Suppl) 492:91, 1980.

Flamm, E.S., Young, W., Demopoulos, H.B., et al.: Experimental spinal cord injury: treatment with naloxone. Neurosurgery 10(2): 227, .

Hall, E.D., and Braughler, J.M.: Effects of intravenous methylprednisolone on spinal cord lipid peroxidation and (Na+ + K+)-APTase activity. Dose-response analysis during 1st hour after contusion injury in the cat. J. Neurosurg. 57:247, 1982.

Hall, E.D., and Braughler, J.M.: Glucocorticoid mechanisms in acute spinal cord injury: a review and therapeutic rationale. Surg. Neurol. 18(5):320, 1982.

Pierce, D.S., and Nickel, V.H.: The Total Care of Spinal Cord Injuries. Boston, Little, Brown and Company, 1977.

Rothman, R.H., and Simeone, F.A.: The Spine. Philadelphia: W.B. Saunders Company, 1982, pp. 647–756.

Venes, J.: Spinal cord injury. In Pediatric Neurosurgery: Surgery of the Developing Nervous System (Section of Pediatric Neurosurgery of the American Association of Neurological Surgeons). New York, Grune & Stratton, 1982, pp. 333–343.

Young, W., and Flamm, E.S.: Effect of high-dose corticosteroid therapy on blood flow, evoked potentials, and extracellular calcium in experimental spinal injury. J. Neurosurg. 57:667, 1982.

Caring for patients with spinal cord injuries is a challenge. The approach to nursing management is sequential as the patient progresses from an acute to a chronic state. In the acute phase, concern is for adequate oxygenation, perfusion, preservation of neurologic function, and prevention of further neurologic deterioration. In the convalescent or chronic phase, concern is for maximization of neurologic recovery and prevention of sequelae associated with immobility. Anticipation of these complications is important, because the patient is unable to communicate associated symptoms related to the sensory loss.

NEUROLOGIC

Assess, Monitor, and Document

Motor and sensory levels (by report and physical examination)
Voluntary motor response and strength (differentiate from spasm)
Autonomic dysfunction: temperature, cardiovascular

Maintenance of cervical traction (where appropriate): weights, lines, tongs (insertion site)

Anticipate

Possible change in motor and sensory function: improvement, deterioration

RESPIRATORY

Special attention must be given to the respiratory status of the spinal cord–injured patient. Normal systemic oxygenation along with adequate perfusion must be maintained. Injury to the spinal cord at the cervical or thoracic level can result in a loss of diaphragmatic (C4 or higher) and intercostal function. Nurses must be aware of the potential for a deterioration of the pulmonary status.

Assess, Monitor, and Document

Respiratory rate
Respiratory pattern, including depth
Breath sounds
Color
Arterial blood gases
Response to pulmonary hygiene

Chest physical therapy: clapping, vibration, incentive spirometer, IPPB with expectorants
Suctioning
Secretions: amount, description

Anticipate

Alteration in respiratory status
    Deterioration in function related to injury
    Aspiration

Pneumonia
Pulmonary embolus

CARDIOVASCULAR

Severe paroxysmal autonomic dysfunction can occur as a result of high level cord injuries. Autonomic fibers are affected with subsequent vasomotor and cardiac alterations that may interfere with adequate tissue oxygenation and perfusion.

Assess, Monitor, and Document

Heart rate
Rhythm
Blood pressure: arterial, central venous
Perfusion: peripheral pulses, color of skin, capillary filling

Fluid intake
Urine output, including specific gravity
Response to therapy: volume replacement (pharmacologic intervention)

Anticipate

Alteration in cardiovascular status
  Cardiac dysrhythmias: bradycardia, heart block, ventricular ectopy
  Functional hypovolemia: decreased blood pressure (arterial, central venous), decreased urine output

Systemic hypotension
Systemic hypertension
Cutaneous vasomotor instability: sweating (fluid loss, heat loss), anhydrosis (heat retention)

GASTROINTESTINAL

Injury to the thoracic and cervical spinal cord often affects the gastrointestinal system. A transient ileus is a fairly common occurrence. Of concern is the fact that a distended bowel may contribute to hypoventilation by compressing the diaphragm. Constipation may be a significant problem, because it may lead to intestinal obstruction, perforation, peritonitis, and sepsis. A hyperactive gastrocolic reflex, which may damage intestinal mucosa, may follow later. This may affect both the nutritional and fluid management. Stress ulceration and gastrointestinal hemorrhage must also be anticipated.

Assess, Monitor, and Document

Nasogastric drainage: amount, description, hematest, replacement
Abdominal girth
Bowel sounds
Bowel movements: frequency, description, hematest

Temperature
Blood pressure
Hematocrit

Anticipate

Alteration in gastrointestinal status
  Paralytic ileus: abdominal distention, decreased bowel sounds
  Hyperactive gastrocolic reflex
  Constipation

Intestinal obstruction
Perforation
Peritonitis
Sepsis
Gastrointestinal hemorrhage

RENAL

Spinal cord injury will affect bladder tone. A hypotonic neurogenic or a spastic hypertonic bladder may result. Incorporated in the initial management regime is the insertion of a Foley catheter. Bladder function, along with the parameters indicative of a urinary tract infection, must be assessed.

Assess, Monitor, and Document

Urine output: amount, description (color, odor)
Laboratory data: routine urinalysis
Urine culture and sensitivities

Foley catheter care: frequency of change
Bladder function: voiding pattern, residual urine

Anticipate

Alteration in bladder function
  Hypotonic neurogenic bladder
  Spastic hypertonic bladder
Urinary tract infection

Temperature elevation
Change in color and consistency
Positive culture

INTEGUMENTARY

The condition of the skin is an important consideration in spinal cord trauma. Prolonged bedrest and associated immobility predispose the spinal cord injury patient to pressure sores and infection.

Assess, Monitor, and Document

Skin condition: special attention to bony prominences and pressure points of Halo vests

Skin care: turning schedule, adjuncts to care (egg crate foam, gel pad, water bolsters, Clinitron bed)

Anticipate

Alteration in skin condition
Decubiti

MUSCULOSKELETAL

Assess, Monitor, and Document

Active range of motion (where possible)
Passive range of motion
Proper body alignment

Adjuncts to care: braces and splints, foot board, sneakers, hand rolls

Anticipate

Alteration in musculoskeletal system
Atrophy

Contractures
Scoliosis

RESPONSE OF CHILD

The child who presents with a spinal cord injury is in a physical and emotional crisis. The physiologic changes are profound, because they involve multiorgan systems. The emotional effect is significant, because this injury permanently alters the life of the patient. The suddeness of this tragedy and the total loss associated with it contribute to the complexity of the patient's response. The physical and emotional needs are great and require knowledge, skill, and sensitivity of nursing personnel to meet them.

Assess, Monitor, and Document

Developmental level: psychosocial, cognitive, motor, verbal
Behavioral response: denial, depressed, angry
Level of understanding of condition and limitations

Perception of events surrounding accident
Expected outcome
Educational needs related to rehabilitation and home management
Response to nursing interventions

Anticipate

Profound emotional crisis
Need for referral: social service, psychiatrist, chaplain

RESPONSE OF FAMILY

Assess, Monitor, and Document

Behavior response: denial, despair, angry, hostile

Level of understanding of child's condition

Expected outcome

Educational needs related to rehabilitation and home management

Response to nursing interventions

Anticipate

Family crisis

Inability to cope

Educational needs related to rehabilitation and home management

Referral: social service, psychiatry, rehabilitation

MIND SET

Assess

Neurologic status

Respiratory status

Cardiovascular status

Gastrointestinal system

Renal status

Integumentary system

Musculoskeletal system

Response of child and family

Anticipate

Alteration in neurologic function

Alteration in respiratory status

　Respiratory insufficiency: pneumonia, pulmonary embolism

Alteration in cardiovascular function

　Cardiac dysrhythmias

　Systemic hypotension or hypertension

　Cutaneous vasomotor instability

Alteration in gastrointestinal function

　Ileus

　Intestinal obstruction

　Stress ulcer

　Perforation

Alteration in renal function

　Urinary tract infections

Alteration in skin condition

Alteration in musculoskeletal system

Emotional trauma

Family crisis

Referral services

　Rehabilitation

　Social service

Hypoxic–Ischemic Encephalopathy

REGINA R. DE CARLO, M.D.

Normal brain function requires an adequate, continuous supply of oxygen, because 90 percent of cerebral energy is the result of aerobic metabolism. The great dependence of the brain on oxygen can be seen by the fraction of total oxygen consumption attributed to cerebral metabolism, 25 percent in adults and approximately 50 percent in children younger than four years of age. Oxygen deprivation beyond a critically short margin of tolerance leads to irreversible damage of brain tissue.

The duration of hypoxia beyond which irreversible cerebral damage is said to occur shows some individual and age variability. However, it is commonly stated that the human brain is irreversibly damaged after 5 minutes of cardiac or respiratory arrest. The presence of other factors such as hypoglycemia, hypercapnia, and acidosis contribute to the adverse effect that oxygen deprivation has on neuronal tissue, and it is often the sum of these factors that determines the severity of outcome.

ETIOLOGY

Cerebral anoxia can result from a variety of causes, including drowning, hanging, high-altitude exposure, smoke inhalation, strangulation, foreign body aspiration, pulmonary infection, anesthesia accidents, shock, cardiac arrest, and poisonings (e.g., cyanide and carbon monoxide). These causes can be categorized into four basic mechanisms that result in cerebral hypoxia.

1. Insufficient blood oxygen saturation. This can result from any process that interferes with adequacy of inspired oxygen, ventilation, or capillary–alveolar gas exchange (e.g., high altitudes, anesthesia accidents, drowning, strangulation, or pulmonary infection).

2. Insufficient hemoglobin to provide adequate O_2 carrying capacity (e.g., severe anemia).

3. Insufficient blood flow to tissues so that the rate of oxygen delivery is slower than the rate of oxygen consumption (e.g., shock, cardiac arrest, or hyperviscosity syndromes).

4. Interference with oxygen utilization in cells by toxic agents (e.g., cyanide poisoning).

The underlying pathophysiologic changes brought about by any mechanism of cerebral anoxia are basically the same. In addition, if the brain is deprived of its primary energy source, glucose, similar changes result.

Autoregulatory control mechanisms, which attempt to maintain a relatively constant cerebral blood flow, ensuring delivery of substrate for normal cerebral metabolism (i.e., brain oxygen supply at an optimum level, 3.3 ml O_2/100 gm of brain/min), are present. Suboptimal oxygen content and increased carbon dioxide content in blood as well as local increases in organic acids cause cerebral arteriolar vasodilatation. This results in an increase in cerebral blood flow, with an ensuing increased delivery of substrate.

Prolonged severe hypoxia, however, interferes with cerebral autoregulation. A vicious cycle of decreased cerebral perfusion, tissue hypoxia, and tissue acidosis is established. The end result is damage to brain tissue.

Cerebral blood flow and oxygenation are dependent upon the relationship of systemic arterial pressure to intracranial pressure (ICP). The difference between mean arterial pressure (MAP) and ICP is called the *cerebral perfusion pressure* (CPP)—CPP = MAP − ICP. Therefore, either profound systemic hypotension or increased ICP decreases the CPP and interferes with the delivery of oxygen and substrate to brain tissue.

Optimally, CPP should be greater than 50 mm Hg. Therapeutic measures should be taken to keep ICP less than 15 mm Hg and MAP greater than 60 mm Hg to ensure adequate cerebral perfusion.

Hypoxia and acidosis via failure of the cerebral autoregulatory mechanism result in increased vascular permeability and cerebral edema. Cerebral edema increases ICP, which, in turn, reduces CPP and decreases O_2 and substrate delivery to the brain.

The areas of the brain most sensitive to anoxia are the occipital and parietal lobes of the cerebral cortex, the hippocampus, the caudate nucleus, and the Purkinje's cells of the cerebellum.

The duration and severity of hypoxia rather than the specific cause determine the development of neurologic signs. Mild degrees of hypoxia cause inattention, incoordination, and poor judgment. Clinically, this syndrome is completely reversible.

With severe hypoxia, consciousness is lost within seconds. If oxygenation is restored within 3 to 5 minutes, recovery is usually complete. Beyond this 3- to 5-minute period of severe hypoxia, permanent, often severe, damage to the brain is usual.

CLINICAL FEATURES

Encephalopathy

This is an alteration of mental status that ranges from mild confusion to stupor and coma. The degree of abnormality depends upon the duration and severity of hypoxia. Hypoxia can result in diffuse bilateral cortical dysfunction and/or brain stem dysfunction. The altered level of consciousness can be a result of damage to either or both areas. Clinically, the brain stem appears to be more resistant to hypoxia than the cerebral hemispheres. However, brain stem reflex abnormalities, which include abnormal pupillary response, absent or depressed corneal reflex, or absent oculocephalic reflex are common in the early post-resuscitation period. Intact brain stem function in the early post-resuscitation period (less than 6 hours) indicates a good outlook for recovery. At the other extreme, if any of these abnormalities persist for more than 24 to 48 hours after severe hypoxia, the outcome for survival is poor. If the child does survive, the degree of neurologic dysfunction is severe.

Seizure Activity

Seizures are frequent during the first 12 to 24 hours after the acute hypoxic episode. The most common types of seizure are either partial seizures, with elementary or complex symptoms or myoclonic seizures. Generalized seizures and tonoclonic type "shivering" can also be seen.

The seizures that occur are often difficult to control with anticonvulsants and are potentially injurious to posthypoxic patients. Seizures increase cerebral energy requirements and may contribute to cerebral hypoxia and edema by compromising respiratory effort.

Seizures, especially myoclonic seizures, often cease spontaneously in a few days.

Increased Intracranial Pressure (ICP)

Increased ICP is secondary to the cerebral edema that develops in the posthypoxic brain. Increased ICP can directly contribute to the depressed level of consciousness by pressure on the brain stem, as well as indirectly by decreasing CPP.

The duration of symptoms and the rate of recovery in general are variable and difficult to predict.

Delayed Posthypoxic Encephalopathy

This delayed response can occur after an interval of apparently normal behavior of 2 to 21 days following recovery from the hypoxic insult. Then, abruptly, the patient becomes irritable, inattentive, and confused. Some patients may become agitated. The deterioration may progress to coma or death or may arrest itself at any point. The exact cause of delayed posthypoxic encephalopathy is unknown.

TREATMENT

Treatment requires close observation, support of vital function, seizure control, and reduction of cerebral edema.

Respiratory Function

Centers for respiratory control are in the brain stem. As with other types of metabolic coma, abnormal respiratory patterns as well as absence of spontaneous respiration may occur. Arterial blood gases should be followed to ensure adequate oxygenation. Endotracheal intubation and mechanical respiratory support may be required to maintain adequate blood oxygenation in comatose patients.

Blood Pressure

Patients who have suffered hypoxic-ischemic insult to the brain must not be allowed to become hypotensive. MAP must be maintained at least 50 mm Hg above the mean ICP, a level that ensures adequate cerebral perfusion. The infusion of pressors may be required.

Careful attention must be paid to circulating fluid volume and central venous pressure, especially when drugs used to control cerebral edema are being administered. Medications such as mannitol and glycerol are osmotic diuretics that can lower blood pressure as a consequence of volume depletion.

Temperature Regulation

After severe hypoxia, patients may develop the inability to regulate body temperature. Either hypo or hyperthermia may result secondary to damage to the center for temperature control in the hypothalamus. It is important to realize that hyperthermia increases cerebral oxygen demand. Patients with impaired cerebral perfusion should be kept normal or hypothermic, because brain metabolism is decreased by one half at body temperature of 32 to 33°C (89 to 91°F). Hypothermia may, therefore, be protective.

Increased Intracranial Pressure (ICP)

Increased ICP is the result of cerebral edema that develops secondary to hypoxia. ICP monitoring is useful in deeply comatose posthypoxic patients. Either a subarachnoid bolt or an intraventricular cannula can be used to measure ICP. Therapeutic modalities can be adjusted accordingly to maintain a baseline mean ICP less than 15 mm Hg and to decrease the frequency of spontaneous-reactive pressure waves. Hyperventilation, hyperosmotic agents, and steroids are all useful in controlling ICP.

Hyperventilation is the most rapid means of decreasing ICP. It results in a lower PCO_2, which causes cerebral vasoconstriction and subsequent decrease in capillary pressure.

Hypertonic solutions such as mannitol and glycerol provide an osmotic gradient across the blood–brain barrier. They rapidly decrease brain swelling but their effect is short-lived. Their use requires careful monitoring of urine output, blood pressure, serum electrolytes, and serum osmolality.

Mannitol (20 percent solution), at a dose of 0.5 to 1.0 gm per kg, is given intravenously over 20 to 30 minutes and may be repeated at 4- to 6-hour intervals. An alternative is glycerol, 0.5 to 1.0 gm per kg per dose, given nasogastrically, with subsequent doses at 6-hour intervals. If glycerol is administered to an unconscious patient by the NG route, care must be taken because of the potential risk of aspiration. Glycerol, as a 10 percent solution, can be given intravenously in a dose of 1.0 gm per kg, but hemolysis has been reported as a consequence.

Steroids, especially dexamethasone, are reported to be effective in decreasing cerebral edema by decreasing vascular permeability via membrane stabilization. Dexamethasone, 0.25 to 0.5 mg per kg per day IV or IM, is given divided q6h. A loading dose equal to one third the daily dose can be given initially. It takes 12 to 24 hours for steroids to take effect.

Seizure Activity

Seizures that frequently develop in posthypoxic patients may be difficult to control.

Management includes anticonvulsants such as

1. Valium, 0.25 to 0.5 mg per kg given by slow IV infusion ×2 doses, 15 to 20 minutes apart. (No more than 10 mg per dose should be administered.)

2. Phenobarbital, 15 mg per kg IV loading dose, followed by 6 mg per kg per day maintenance dose.

3. Dilantin, 15 to 20 mg per kg IV as a loading dose, followed by 5 to 8 mg per kg per day maintenance dose. Blood pressure and heart rate must be monitored closely during IV administration of Dilantin.

Fluid and Electrolyte Balance

Fluid therapy should be directed toward maintaining normal electrolyte and acid–base balance. Overhydration should be avoided. The patient should receive one-half to two-thirds maintenance fluid. Close monitoring of fluid and electrolyte status is especially important when osmotic diuretics are used. One should also keep in mind that the syndrome of inappropriate ADH (see Chapter 31) and acute renal failure (see Chapter 38) can follow severe hypoxia.

General Care

Patients should be turned frequently to avoid decubitus formation and atelectasis. Care must be taken to avoid contractures by passive range-of-motion exercises.

Neurologic recovery depends upon the extent of damage, the specific areas of brain irreversibly damaged by the acute hypoxic event, and the ability to support vital function and interrupt the vicious cycle that can develop and lead to brain death.

CASE PRESENTATION

A 1-year-old female was admitted to the hospital for elective surgical excision of a giant hairy nevus located on her right shoulder. The child's intraoperative course was remarkable for a brief episode of ventricular tachycardia, which resolved spontaneously. The child was taken to the recovery room postoperatively.

Her vital signs were stable upon arrival. An arterial blood gas done in the recovery room following extubation was completely within normal limits. After 2 hours in the recovery room, the child continued to respond only to noxious stimuli. Her pupils were noted to be 3 mm and sluggishly reactive. The remainder of the physical examination was unremarkable.

Shortly, thereafter, the child had a generalized seizure of approximately 2 minutes duration. Phenobarbital, 15 mg/kg, was being given intravenously when a second, brief, generalized seizure occurred. Her neurologic examination remained nonfocal, and her brain stem reflexes were intact. She had several additional generalized seizures during the night, even though maintenance phenobarbital therapy had been instituted 8 hours after the initial, loading dose. For this flurry of seizures, she was given an additional 10 mg/kg dose IV. No further seizure activity occurred. The child did not regain consciousness, and 18 hours postoperative she was noted to respond to noxious stimuli by flexion of both upper extremities and extension of both lower extremities. She also developed bilateral upgoing toes. A CAT scan was interpreted as normal. An EEG revealed bilateral diffuse slow wave activity. A lumbar puncture was normal for opening pressure. Cerebrospinal fluid (CSF) cell count, glucose, and protein were all within normal limits.

The child showed no signs of neurologic improvement, and 3 weeks postoperative, a cerebral CAT scan revealed lucent areas in both basal ganglia. The child remained in a vegetative state.

SUGGESTED READING

Dougherty, J.H., Rawlinson, D.G., Levy, D.E., and Plum, F.: Hypoxic–ischemic brain injury and the vegetative state: clinical and neuropathologic correlations. Neurology 31:991, 1981.

Richardson, J.C., Chambers, R.A., and Heywood, P.M.: Encephalopathies of anoxia and hypoglycemia. Arch. Neurol. 1:178, 1959.

Robenson, J.C.: Physiology and pathology of acute hypoxia. Br. J. Anesth. 36:536, 1964.

Snyder, B.D., Ramirez-Lassepas, M., and Lippert, D.M.: Neurologic status and prognosis after cardiopulmonary arrest: I. A retrospective study. Neurology 27:807, 1977.

Snyder, B.D., Loewenson, R.B., Gummit, R., et al.: Neurologic prognosis after cardiopulmonary arrest: II. Level of consciousness. Neurology 30:52, 1980.

Snyder, B.D., Hauser, A.A., Loewenson, R.B., et al.: Neurologic prognosis after cardiac pulmonary arrest: III. Seizure activity. Neurology 30:1292, 1980.

Snyder, B.D., Gummit, R.J., Leppik, W.A., and Hauser, R.B.: Neurologic prognosis after cardiopulmonary arrest: IV. Brainstem reflexes. Neurology 31:1092, 1981.

Hypoxic–Ischemic Encephalopathy

The effect of oxygen deprivation on the brain can be profound, the degree of cerebral damage being dependent upon the duration and the severity of the hypoxemia. The magnitude of cerebral insult will be reflected in the development of various neurologic signs. Other organ systems may be affected by the initial hypoxia, the specific area of brain involved or the presence of generalized increased intracranial pressure (ICP).

NEUROLOGIC

Assess, Monitor, and Document

Level of consciousness
Pupillary response
Other reflex activity: corneal, oculocephalic
Posture: decorticate, decerebrate

Blood pressure
Pulse
Temperature
Respiratory rate and pattern

Anticipate

Altered level of consciousness: confusion, stupor, coma
Abnormal reflex activity
　Unequal or absent pupillary response
　Absent corneal reflex
　Absent oculocephalic response
Posturing: decorticate, decerebrate
Seizure activity
　Occurs frequently within the first 12–24 hours after the episode of acute hypoxia

Temperature instability
Increased ICP
　Increased blood pressure
　Decreased pulse
　Decreased respiratory rate
　Altered respiratory pattern
Decreased cerebral perfusion pressure (CPP)
Delayed posthypoxic encephalopathy

RESPIRATORY

The centers for respiratory control are in the brain stem. An increase in ICP can result in alterations in respiratory rate and pattern. Complete absence of spontaneous respiration can occur.

Assess, Monitor, and Document

Respiratory rate
Respiratory pattern

Breath sounds
Arterial blood gas results

Anticipate

Respiratory insufficiency
Respiratory arrest

CARDIAC

Effective cardiac output must be maintained to deliver oxygen and other substrates to the brain. The systemic arterial blood pressure is important, because it reflects the adequacy of tissue perfusion. Mean arterial pressure (MAP) must be monitored along with the ICP to evaluate the CPP.

Assess, Monitor, and Document

Blood pressure (mean)
Central venous pressure
Heart rate

Rhythm
Quality
Perfusion

Anticipate

Hypotension

FLUID AND ELECTROLYTE BALANCE

Assess, Monitor, and Document

Weight
Urine output, including specific gravity
Fluid intake: accurate administration of parenteral fluids (use infusion pump if available)

Central venous pressure
Response to pharmacologic management: mannitol, glycerol
Laboratory data: serum electrolytes, serum osmolality, urine electrolytes

Anticipate

Alteration in fluid and electrolyte balance
Volume depletion
Syndrome of inappropriate ADH

INTEGUMENTARY/MUSCULOSKELETAL

Assess, Monitor, and Document

Skin condition: dry, moist
Pressure points
Excoriated areas
Areas of breakdown

Nursing interventions: turn, position, proper body alignment, passive range-of-motion exercises
Posturing

Anticipate

Decubiti
Contractures

RESPONSE OF CHILD

Assess, Monitor, and Document

Developmental level: verbal, cognitive, motor, psychosocial

Behavioral response: fearful, passive
Response to nursing interventions

Anticipate

Emotional distress

RESPONSE OF FAMILY

The response of parents to a comatose, neurologically compromised child may be quite variable. It may range from anger and guilt to hope and despair. The nurse must assess the response of the parents and plan interventions to facilitate coping mechanisms and ease the emotional pain.

Assess, Monitor, and Document

Behavioral response: angry, guilty, fearful, despair, denial
Level of knowledge of child's condition

Expected outcome
Ability to cope
Response to nursing interventions

Anticipate

Inability to cope
Emotional distress
Family crisis

MIND SET

Assess

Neurologic status
Respiratory status
Cardiac status

Fluid and electrolyte balance
Integumentary and musculoskeletal system
Response of child and family

Anticipate

Alteration in neurologic status
  Encephalopathy
  Seizures
  Increased ICP
  Delayed posthypoxic encephalopathy
  Temperature instability
Alteration in respiratory status

Alteration in fluid and electrolyte balance
  Syndrome of inappropriate ADH
Alteration in integumentary/musculoskeletal
  integrity
Emotional trauma
Family crisis

Status Epilepticus

SOL S. ZIMMERMAN, M.D.
IRVING FISH, M.D.

Status epilepticus may be defined as a seizure or series of seizures lasting more than 30 minutes and during which consciousness is not regained. The seizures may be general or focal, but the generalized tonoclonic seizure is the most common and of greatest concern. Whereas individual seizures are infrequently associated with morbidity and rarely with mortality, status epilepticus has a case fatality rate of 5 to 15 percent. A much higher percentage of patients experience morbidity. Seventy-five percent of cases in the pediatric population occur in children younger than 3 years of age.

PATHOPHYSIOLOGY

At the cellular level, a seizure is the result of the abnormal discharge of a neuron or group of neurons. The epileptiform cell or group of cells have a threshold of depolarization below the usual 15 mv and discharge too readily. The impulse is propagated to surrounding cells, and a seizure results. In most circumstances, the cell membranes then restabilize and the seizure stops. When restabilization does not occur, status epilepticus is the consequence.

Because a generalized seizure implies large numbers of neurons discharging simultaneously, the metabolic activity of the brain increases substantially. Cerebral blood flow must increase to ensure adequate provision of oxygen and glucose. If the seizure is prolonged, the requirments may exceed the capacity to deliver substrate; the resulting oxygen debt can become sufficient to cause hypoxic encephalopathy. This is especially true in a brain already compromised by impaired circulation, edema, or tumor.

Other factors influence the metabolic status of the brain during the seizure state. Secretions accumulate in the pharynx, and respirations are frequently irregular and labored during the sei-

zure, further impairing oxygenation. Hyperpyrexia, either pre-existing or secondary to the seizure, increases cerebral metabolic requirements, aggravating the imbalance between supply and demand. In addition, the anticonvulsants used to treat status epilepticus may induce hypotension and decrease delivery of oxygen to the brain. Hypoxia leads to cerebral edema, which decreases blood flow. This results in a vicious detrimental cycle of events, which, if not terminated, can result in brain damage.

ETIOLOGY

The most common cause of status epilepticus is the sudden withdrawal of anticonvulsant medication in an epileptic. An adolescent may refuse to take his medication, the pre- or postoperative patient who is NPO may not have had parenteral substitution for his oral dose, and the barbiturate abuser may be unable to obtain drugs. Metabolic disturbances such as hypoxia, hypoglycemia, hypocalcemia, hypomagnesemia, water intoxication, uremia, and disorders of amino metabolism may have an etiologic role. Exogenous toxins such as lead are included in this group. Patients who have an underlying seizure disorder are more likely than nonepileptics to go into status as a consequence of metabolic dysfunction. Other etiologies include trauma, infection, tumors, vascular malformations, neurocutaneous syndromes, and degenerative diseases of the central nervous system (CNS). Although it is unusual, children younger than 2 years of age can go into status as a result of high fever unassociated with CNS infection.

Because 25 percent of status epilepticus episodes are secondary to acute processes that affect the CNS, efforts must be made to identify the etiology. It is not enough to simply treat seizures symptomatically by instituting an anticonvulsant protocol. Many etiologies may be life-threatening themselves, and in some cases, the associated seizures may be relatively refractory to the usual therapeutic regimen.

In obtaining the history, questions should be directed at determining the presence of a pre-existing neurologic deficit or developmental delay, the existence of a known seizure disorder; and the use of anticonvulsants, their doses, and the degree of compliance. The possibility of head trauma, CNS infection, substance abuse, and poisoning should be explored. All medical illnesses should be carefully noted.

Physical examination is directed at looking for signs of CNS infection, trauma, and increased intracranial pressure (ICP). Although the neurologic examination during status epilepticus may reveal only transient deficits, these may be useful in subsequent evaluation.

Diagnostic laboratory studies include complete blood count, arterial blood gases, urinalysis, and determinations of serum glucose, sodium, calcium, magnesium, and BUN. Serum transaminases, ammonia, and lead may be indicated. Blood and urine should be sent for a toxicology screen, and anticonvulsant levels should be obtained if the patient is a known epileptic. In neonates, column chromatography for evaluation of disorders of amino acid metabolism may be indicated. A lumbar puncture should be performed unless a mass lesion is suspected. If the patient is febrile, appropriate cultures of blood, cerebrospinal fluid (CSF), and urine should be obtained. Skull x-rays may identify fractures. A cerebral CAT scan is the procedure of choice for diagnosis of intracranial mass and hemorrhage.

Laboratory results often reveal leukocytosis, hyperglycemia, metabolic acidosis, and elevation of creatine phosphokinase (CPK). Increased white blood count and blood sugar are most often attributed to the stress response evoked by status epilepticus, but sepsis must be ruled out. Metabolic acidosis is the consequence of hypoxia and protracted tonic muscle contractions. Elevated CPK reflects the marked increase in muscle activity characteristic of prolonged seizures and may also result from soft-tissue injury, common during an epileptic episode.

TREATMENT

Initial management is directed at general supportive measures to ensure adequacy of ventilation and circulation. An oral airway should be placed, oxygen administered, and an IV line established. In the presence of hyperpyrexia, a hypothermia blanket may be necessary. The dehydrated patient should be returned to the euvolemic state, but fluid intake, in general, should be restricted to less than maintenance so as not to contribute to the potential for cerebral edema. If hypoglycemia, hyponatremia, or hypocalcemia is suspected, appropriate therapeutic measures should be undertaken. The electrocardiogram (EKG) should be closely monitored if calcium is infused.

Specific anticonvulsant measures are directed at stopping the current seizure and preventing recurrences. There are several medications that are commonly used, and it is the physician's responsibility to be aware of the onset and duration of action and the adverse effects of each. All the anticonvulsants have the potential to depress respirations and alter cardiovascular dynamics. The key to good management, therefore, is adequate preparation. The appropriate-sized laryngoscope and endotracheal tube for intubation, colloid and/or crystalloid for volume expansion, and pressor agents for reversal of hypotension should be at the patient's bedside.

Which is the best medication or sequence of medications is a controversial issue. Most often, the choice of drug is dictated by the clinical circumstance or is based upon personal preference. Irrespective of which anticonvulsant is chosen, there are two basic therapeutic principles: treat intravenously, and treat with adequate doses. The most common error in the management of status epilepticus is use of too low a dose of anticonvulsant.

Phenobarbital

Phenobarbital is commonly used as a first line antiepileptic, especially in children who have not received anticonvulsants previously. Because of its long half-life, phenobarbital not only treats the acute seizure but also establishes a brain concentration of drug that is effective in preventing recurrences. It is administered intravenously in a dose of 15-20 mg per kg over at least 5 to 10 minutes. If the seizure is not controlled in 20 minutes, a second dose of 10 mg per kg should be administered. It can be diluted in normal saline (NS) to any desired concentration prior to infusion. This dose of phenobarbital can cause respiratory depression and hypotension; therefore, vital signs must be closely monitored, even after cessation of the seizure.

Phenytoin

Phenytoin has onset of action within several minutes and a long half-life. It is, therefore, efficacious in the acute management of status and the long-term control of seizures. Advantages to its use include the relative absence of both sedation and respiratory depression. It is the drug of choice when the ability to monitor level of consciousness is essential. Phenytoin is administered intravenously in a dose of 15-20 mg per kg (maximum: 1000 mg). Bradycardia, dysrhythmias, and hypotension may result from rapid infusion. Delivery of medication, therefore, should not exceed a rate of 50 mg per minute. EKG and blood pressure monitoring must be performed during drug administration. Phenytoin should be infused directly into the vein or the most proximal site in the IV tubing to avoid dilution and subsequent crystallization.

Diazepam

Diazepam has very rapid onset of action, which is its major advantage. Because of its brief duration of action, however, additional doses may be required to control the seizure. Another medication must be added to provide long-term anticonvulsant effect. It is administered by slow IV infusion in a dose of 0.3 to 0.5 mg per kg, with a maximum of 10 mg. Diazepam may cause profound sedation, hypotension, and respiratory depression. This potential for cardiorespiratory depression is enhanced if phenobarbital has been given previously.

Paraldehyde

Paraldehyde has a slow onset of action. It may be useful if other agents have been unsuccessful in controlling the seizure. Although it can be given by nasogastric (NG) tube, rectally, or intramuscularly, the IV route is preferred in status epilepticus. Paraldehyde, as a 4 percent solution, is administered by slow IV infusion in a dose of 0.15 mg per kg. Because of its incompatibility with plastic, it must be drawn up in a glass syringe. Paraldehyde has the potential to produce pulmonary edema.

A frequently used regimen is the initial administration of diazepam for rapid seizure control with the addition of phenytoin for prolonged anticonvulsant activity. Another common approach is the initial administration of phenobarbital, which provides both short- and long-term anticonvulsant effect. If phenobarbital fails to control the seizure, phenytoin is added as the second medication.

There are rare circumstances in which the status fails to be controlled even by all the described medications in appropriate dosages. When all these anticonvulsants are used in combination, respiratory depression is almost a certainty and the patient will require intubation. The remaining therapeutic measures are either an amobarbital drip or general anesthesia.

Amobarbital is administered intravenously in a dose of 1.0 mg per kg every 30 seconds until the seizure stops. A continuous infusion is then begun at a dose of 0.5 to 1.0 mg per kg per hour. Because cardiovascular depression is a likely result, a dopamine drip should be prepared and kept at the patient's bedside. A long-term anticonvulsant must be given in conjunction with amobarbital to prevent recurrence of seizures.

Choice of general anesthetic agent and use of pancuronium or curare to induce muscle paralysis are at the discretion of the anesthesiologist. An EEG must be monitored to follow electrical activity, because the motor manifestations of a seizure may no longer be evident.

CASE PRESENTATION

A 5-year-old female with shunted hydrocephalus fell from the third rung of the monkey bars. She was witnessed to have a 1-minute loss of consciousness and was brought to a local emergency room. Her vital signs were normal and a neurologic examination was described as unremarkable. Because of a hematoma over the right parietal region, skull x-rays were obtained but no fractures were present. The child was admitted for observation, had an uneventful course, and was discharged the following day.

Two days later, the mother went to her daughter's room because she heard a "pounding" sound; she observed the child having a grand mal seizure. The girl was taken by ambulance to the emergency room. An oral airway was established by the paramedics, and oxygen was administered by nasal cannulae. Efforts were made to keep the child from injuring herself.

Upon arrival, the child was described as having a generalized tonoclonic seizure, with no focal neurologic signs. The airway was suctioned, and an IV catheter was placed. The seizure was now of 35 minutes duration. Her weight was estimated to be 20 kg (48 lb). Diazepam, 6 mg (0.3 mg/kg), was administered intravenously over 5 minutes. The seizure stopped 2 minutes later, and plans were made for transfer to the intensive care unit (ICU). Fifteen minutes later, just prior to transfer, the seizure recurred and a second dose of diazepam was given. Phenytoin, 400 mg (20 mg/kg), was given at a rate of 25 to 50 mg per minute, with close monitoring of blood pressure and EKG. The child was transferred to the ICU, and plans were made for an emergency CAT scan and further evaluation.

Diazepam was selected for rapid control of the seizure. All emergency room and ICU personnel should be aware of its brief duration of action and the frequent necessity for a second dose. An anticonvulsant with long-term effect must be given to prevent recurrences. Phenytoin was chosen because it does not cause sedation, and level of consciousness is a key factor in monitoring the post–head trauma patient.

SUGGESTED READING

Delgado-Escueta, A.V., Wasterlain, C., Treiman, C.M., et al.: Management of status epilepticus. N. Engl. J. Med. 306:1337, 1982.

Dodson, W.E., Prensky, A.L., DeVivo, D.C., et al.: Management of seizure disorders: selected aspects. Part I. J. Pediatr. 89:527, 1976.

Johnson, M.V., and Freeman, J.M.: Pharmacological advances in seizure control. Pediatr. Clin. North Am. 28:179, 1981.

Oppenheimer, E.Y., and Rosman, N.P.: Seizures and seizure-like states in the child: an approach to emergency management. Emerg. Med. Clin. North Am. 1:125, 1983.

Rothner, A.D., and Erenberg, G.: Status epilepticus. Pediatr. Clin. North Am. 27:593, 1980.

Nursing Process for Patient Care:
Status Epilepticus

The presentation of a child with status epilepticus requires rapid assessment and management in terms of airway, breathing, circulation, and seizure activity. The mind set that emerges focuses on the impact of the seizure activity on other organ systems and the child and family.

NEUROLOGIC

Assess, Monitor, and Document

Seizure activity
  Type: focal, tonoclonic
  Duration
  Response to pharmacologic management
Medication:
  Phenobarbital: side effects (respiratory depression, hypotension), long half-life. Observe for side effects even after cessation of seizure
  Phenytoin: side effects (bradycardia, dysrhythmias, hypotension), monitor EKG and blood pressure during infusion

Diazepam: side effects (profound sedation, hypotension, respiratory depression). The potential for cardiorespiratory depression is enhanced if phenobarbital has been given previously
Level of consciousness
Pupillary activity
Reflexes
Movement of extremities
Blood pressure
Pulse
Respiratory rate and pattern

Anticipate

Recurrent seizures
Side effects of medications: respiratory depression, hypotension, dysrhythmias
Cerebral edema
  Altered level of consciousness
  Altered pupillary response

Increased blood pressure
Bradycardia
Decreased respiratory rate
Altered respiratory pattern
Hypoxic encephalopathy
  Altered level of consciousness

RESPIRATORY

Assess, Monitor, and Document

Status of airway
Respiratory rate and pattern
Breath sounds

Color
Arterial blood gases
Response to pharmacologic management

Anticipate

Airway obstruction
Respiratory insufficiency
Respiratory arrest

CARDIOVASCULAR

Assess, Monitor, and Document

Heart rate
Rhythm
Blood pressure

Anticipate

Bradycardia
Dysrhythmias
Hypotension

RESPONSE OF CHILD

Assess, Monitor, and Document

Developmental level: verbal, motor, cognitive, fearful

Behavioral response: anxious, fearful, upset over loss of control

Response to nursing interventions

Educational needs of child related to discharge and management

Recurrent seizures

Administration of medications

Anticipate

Emotional distress

RESPONSE OF FAMILY

Assess, Monitor, and Document

Behavioral response: anxious, fearful, angry, disappointed

Ability to cope

Educational needs related to discharge and home management

Recurrent seizures

Administration of medications

Response to nursing interventions

Anticipate

Family crisis
Inability to cope

Educational needs related to discharge and home management

MIND SET

Assess

Neurologic status
  Seizure activity
Respiratory status

Cardiovascular status
Response of child and family

Anticipate

Seizure recurrence
Alteration in respiratory function
  Decreased respiratory rate
  Accumulation of secretions
  Cumulative action of pharmacologic agents
Alteration in cardiovascular status
  Tachycardia
  Bradycardia
  Hypotension
  Dysrhythmias

Hypoxia
Cerebral edema
Hypoxic encephalopathy
Emotional distress
Family crisis
Educational needs of child and family related to seizures

Guillain–Barré Syndrome

RICHARD M. HANSON, M.D.
REGINA R. DeCARLO, M.D.

Guillain-Barré syndrome (GBS) is an acute, self-limited, monophasic inflammatory neuropathy, the hallmark of which is an acute, symmetric ascending, areflexic paralysis, with little sensorineuropathy. The pathogenesis is thought to be an immunologic reaction directed at the myelin of the peripheral nervous system.

EPIDEMIOLOGY

GBS is without geographic or seasonal predilection and has a worldwide incidence of 0.6 to 1.9 cases per 100,000 population. An age range from 8 months to 70 years, with a linear correlation between age and attack rate, has been documented. A 30 percent male predominance and a 50 to 60 percent higher attack rate for whites has been recorded.

Retrospective review reveals the historical presence of an antecedent viral syndrome in half the patients. The illness appears 2 to 3 weeks prior to the onset of GBS and is usually upper respiratory or diarrheal in nature. Although a specific virus has not been identified, reports implicate Epstein-Barr, cytomegalic, and hepatitis viruses as involved in the triggering mechanism. There is little evidence suggesting influenza A or B as an etiologic determinant. An exception was the increased incidence of GBS seen shortly after the introduction of the 1976–1977 influenza vaccination program. In subsequent immunization years, however, no increased occurrence was noted, suggesting the possibility that variability in vaccine preparation, rather than the actual vaccine, was the significant factor in the earlier outbreak. Mycoplasma infections, surgical manipulation, and myeloproliferative disorders, especially Hodgkin's disease, have all been associated with GBS.

CLINICAL PRESENTATION

The characteristic feature of GBS is the ascending areflexic paralysis. The clinical picture is variable, ranging from a minimal paraparesis to a complete quadriplegia. Symmetric involvement is the rule; persistent monoparesis is not consistent with the diagnosis. Ascending paralysis describes an initial involvement of the lower extremities, which is followed by upper extremity, trunk, and, finally, cranial paresis. Involvement of the brachiometric muscles (those innervated by cranial nerves) is not uncommon, with approximately one half of the cases exhibiting facial diplegia. Other cranial nerves are less commonly involved, presenting as dysarthria or dysphagia. The Miller-Fisher variant of GBS involves the oculomotor nerves and presents as ophthalmoplegia associated with limb ataxia and areflexia. Aside from this presentation, it follows the usual temporal course and has the typical laboratory profile.

Because of the rapid progression of the paralysis, muscle atrophy and fasciculations are not seen. Complete areflexia is the usual finding, but the presence of proximal hyporeflexia does not preclude the diagnosis.

Although 30 percent of patients with GBS initially complain of paresthesias, this complaint is transient. A sensorineuropathy may be present in some cases, but rarely is a discrete pin level found. Bladder function is preserved, although transient urinary retention may be seen early in the illness.

Autonomic dysfunction is a common occurrence in GBS but seldom lasts more than 2 to 3 weeks. Autonomic dysfunction manifests as tachycardia, bradycardia, labile blood pressure, and episodic diaphoresis, pallor, and flush. Involvement of the nonmyelinated small nerve fibers of the autonomic nervous system is thought to underlie the dysfunction. It is incumbent upon the physician to rule out systemic causes of autonomic dysfunction (i.e., pulmonary emboli, sepsis).

The temporal course of the illness is an important diagnostic criterion. Three phases have been distinguished. The initial phase, associated with progression of the illness, is of 2- to 4-week duration and is followed by a plateau phase lasting 2 to 3 weeks. The ensuing recovery phase may last from weeks to months. Most patients follow this course and recover without sequelae. Failure to follow this temporal pattern defines an illness termed *chronic polyradiculoneuropathy*. This entity resembles GBS with regard to symptoms, signs, and laboratory evaluation but has a much poorer prognosis for complete recovery. Chronic polyradiculoneuropathy has an initial, progressive phase of more than 3-month duration and protracted plateau and recovery phases. In the chronic relapsing type, there is an overall deterioration in neurologic status, which follows a waxing and waning pattern.

LABORATORY EVALUATION

With the exception of the cerebrospinal fluid (CSF) analysis, the laboratory evaluation is unrevealing. Serum electrolytes, hepatic and renal function tests, serum and urine electrophoresis, VDRL, monospot, and urinary porphobilinogen and δ aminolevulinic acid levels are normal. Acute and convalescent viral titers may have epidemiologic significance but are rarely helpful in making the diagnosis. The CSF is normal with regard to pressure, cell count, and glucose concentration. Elevation of the protein concentration is the only abnormality, a circumstance described as albuminocytologic dissociation. The protein level increases within the first week of the illness and is usually greater than 100 mg per dl. Peaking within 4 to 6 weeks, it may remain elevated for a few months. The increased protein concentration probably reflects the widespread disruption of the blood–brain barrier occurring at the nerve roots. It may impart a xanthochromic appearance to the CSF and may result in the development of papilledema caused by increased CSF viscosity and the resulting impedance of CSF resorption. A mild monocytic pleocytosis of 10 to 50 cells per cubic ml may be noted in 10 percent of cases. Seldom is the cell count greater than 200. Culture of the CSF is negative.

Electrical studies of the peripheral nerves reveal greater than a 40 percent slowing of motor nerve conduction velocities in 80 to 90 percent of patients some time during their illness. This finding is usually not seen in the early phase. Because of the patchy involvement of the nerves by the inflammatory process, multiple electrical studies are required to reveal the conduction defects. Approximately 30 percent of electrically abnormal patients will have "normal" studies if the electromyographer is not diligent in evaluating multiple nerves. The slowing of conduction velocity is indicative of segmental demyelination. Twenty percent of patients exhibit evidence of spontaneous fibrillations. Although there is no consistent relationship between slowing of conduction velocity and clinical disability, there appears to be some correlation between the presence of abundant spontaneous fibrillations and a more prolonged recovery period and generally poorer prognosis. Such an outcome would be expected, because fibrillations are indicative of axonal derangement, with resultant denervation.

DIFFERENTIAL DIAGNOSIS

The differential diagnosis involves consideration of various entities that affect the anterior horn cell as well as other infectious, inflammatory, and toxic neuropathies. The immediate exclusion of a myelopathy or myelitis (i.e., spinal cord compression or infection) is necessary, because the former is considered a neurosurgical emergency. The presence of spinal cord compression can be reliably determined by showing hyperreflexia and a definite pin level on neurologic examination. Only in spinal shock is an acute onset of areflexic paralysis seen. In this situation, all sensorimotor and autonomic functions below a specific spinal cord level are absent.

Paralytic poliomyelitis is distinguished by a febrile course comprised of meningismus and a motor paralysis that is classically asymmetric and results in muscle atrophy and fasciculations. In addition, poliomyelitis usually presents in an epidemic manner in nonimmunized locations, with a July to September seasonal prevalence.

Primary degenerative disorders of the anterior horn cell may occasionally be considered, especially in infants. Werdnig-Hoffman disease (infantile spinal muscular atrophy) and the later onset, Kugelberg-Welander disease, may be differentiated from GBS by their typical symptom complex, time course, and abnormal muscle biopsy.

A progressive motor neuropathy, essentially similar to GBS, can be concurrent with or subsequent to infectious mononucleosis, viral hepatitis, or diphtheria. That which is concurrent with mononucleosis can be diagnosed by the presence of pharyngitis, cervical lymphadenopathy, hepatosplenomegaly, elevated serum transaminases, and a positive monospot test. Likewise, clinical jaundice and abnormal liver function tests, characteristic of viral hepatitis, suggest the hepatitis motor neuropathy. The diphtheritic neuropathy presents 5 to 8 weeks after the primary infection. A history of pharyngitis associated with diplopia (loss of accommodation), dysphagia, and nasal voice suggests the possibility of this diagnosis. A throat culture positive for *Corynebacterium diphtheriae* would confirm diphtheritic neuropathy. The pathogenesis of the neuropathy is secondary to the elaboration of bacterial exotoxin; therefore, a negative throat culture would not rule out the diagnosis.

Another toxin-mediated illness confused with GBS is botulism. The neurologic signs appear 12 to 36 hours following ingestion of *Clostridium botulinum*-tainted food. Initial bulbar involvement is manifested by symptoms such as diplopia, vertigo, dysarthria, and nasal speech. Physical examination shows ptosis, strabismus, ophthalmoplegia, and dysarthria. In 2 to 3 days, the bulbar phase is followed by generalized weakness of axial and appendicular muscle groups associated with areflexia. The clinical manifestations are secondary to the elaboration of an exotoxin that interferes with the presynaptic release of acetylcholine. The diagnosis is suggested by electrodiagnostic evaluation and the typical clinical presentation.

Acute intermittent porphyria (AIP) is a rare autosomal dominant disorder characterized by recurrent episodes of colicky abdominal pain, encephalopathy, and polyneuropathy. The polyneuropathy is predominantly motor and may be concurrent with the other symptoms or may present independently. The initial paresis is bibrachial, with later involvement of the trunk and lower extremities. In severe cases, a cranioneuropathy may follow. The temporal course is variable and may last from weeks to months. The metabolic defect in this disease is marked by the presence of increased concentrations of the hepatic mitochondrial enzyme, aminolevulinic acid (ALA) synthetase. There is a resulting overproduction of the porphyrin precursors, δ aminolevulinic acid, and porphobilinogen. Elevated urinary concentrations of these substances confirm the diagnosis of AIP. Examination of the CSF reveals a normal protein level.

Other toxic neuropathies, including nitrofurantoin, organophosphate insecticide, and dapsone-induced neuropathies may simulate GBS.

TREATMENT

The therapy of GBS can be divided into general supportive care and specific pharmacologic intervention. The former is the most important, because the illness is self-limited and the objective of treatment is to prevent secondary complications. Close monitoring of pulmonary function is imperative, especially during the progressive phase. The 2 to 5 percent mortality rate of GBS is usually the consequence of pulmonary complications, including pneumonia and pulmonary embolus. Serial arterial blood gas determinations and vital capacity measurements are necessary to assess the adequacy of ventilatory effort and gas exchange. In cooperative patients, vital capacity is easily measured at the bedside by the use of a spirometer. A somewhat crude, but reliable, clinical test is the quantitation of forward serial number counting ability accomplished after a single, maximal inspiration. In practice, this test is especially valuable when a facial diplegia interferes with the tight lip-pursing required for proper use of the spirometer.

Modalities of respiratory support such as vigorous chest physiotherapy, nasotracheal suctioning, and necessary oxygen supplementation must be provided. Endotracheal intubation is indicated if respiratory failure occurs or if improved access for pulmonary toilet is required. If a prolonged intubation is anticipated, a tracheostomy should be performed. Approximately one fourth of all affected patients require tracheostomy. A mechanical ventilator with an intermittent mandatory ventilation (IMV) circuit should be used, because respiratory failure is the result of muscle fatigue, not primary pulmonary pathology. Most often, the inspired gas concentration is room air, unless arterial hypoxemia is shown.

Autonomic instability must first be considered a manifestation of a superimposed process, and a diligent search for sepsis, pulmonary embolus, or other source of hemodynamic compromise must be initiated. The autonomic dysfunction of GBS is short-lived but requires close monitoring. The specific autonomic manifestations (tachycardia, bradycardia, hypertension, or hypotension) are often transient and do not require therapy. Pharmacologic intervention is indicated if cardiac output and tissue perfusion are compromised. Drugs should be selected for their rapid onset and brief duration of action.

Alimentation to ensure positive nitrogen balance must not be neglected. Feeding should be by the enteral route, with a nasogastric (NG) tube used during periods of dysphagia secondary to cranioneuropathy and during endotracheal intubation (see Chapter 8, Enteral Alimentation). Inappropriate secretion of antidiuretic hormone (SIADH) is not an infrequent occurrence and is thought to be the result of dysfunction of peripheral volume sensors secondary to involvement of afferent neurons. The hyponatremia that ensues is managed by fluid restriction (see Chapter 31, Syndrome of Inappropriate ADH). Hypercalcemia is often seen in these patients following prolonged immobilization. Serum calcium determinations should be obtained, and urine should be examined on a regular basis for evidence of nephrolithiasis. Fluid intake may need to be increased, and dietary composition may require alteration if significant hypercalcemia is identified.

Proper bowel and bladder hygiene is essential, especially in quadriplegic patients; this will prevent perineal irritation and decubitus formation. Because urinary retention is not usually present, an external condom catheter is helpful in male patients. Penile excoriation and necrosis must be avoided during prolonged use of condoms. Constipation is a frequent occurrence, and use of stool softeners may be required.

Early involvement of a physiatrist is important for a successful outcome. A daily physical therapy program, initially including passive range-of-motion exercises, will help prevent muscle atrophy and contractures, pressure ulcers, pressure neuropathies, and deep venous thrombosis. The latter predisposes to pulmonary emboli and may be prevented by the administration of low-dose subcutaneous heparin. The physical therapy program should coincide with the course of the illness so that ambulatory training begins as soon as the paralysis resolves. Patient involvement in such a program will help prevent depression. During the initial progressive phase, the patient and family must be reassured repeatedly as to the relatively benign nature of this illness. A mor-

tality rate of 2 to 5 percent and a chronic severe disability rate of 5 to 10 percent are realistic figures of disease outcome. Sixty percent of patients with GBS will recover without residua. Initial avoidance of sedative medication is advisable, but when respiratory stability is ensured, administration of such medication should be liberalized and titrated against the patient's emotional state. Some cases are notable for pain. The pain is not localized and may be of neurogenic origin. Analgesics are usually only partly successful in managing this pain; some reports suggest that quinine may be useful. Most important, a humanistic and compassionate approach toward the patient must be continued throughout the course of the illness. The nature of this disease and its protracted hospital stay can result in emotional regression, and some patients may become overly dependent or demanding.

The effect of specific pharmacologic therapy upon the course and prognosis of GBS is difficult to assess because of the self-limited nature of the disease. Without large scale, randomized, and controlled studies, valid interpretation of drug efficacy is impossible. Although still advocated by some, use of steroids does not seem to have a beneficial effect and is not indicated in GBS. Aside from the potential for the usual complications of steroid therapy, concern has been raised that administration of corticosteroids may result in a higher relapse rate by interfering with the function of suppressor cells, which normally "turn off" the inflammatory process. The fact that steroid therapy is not beneficial is surprising, because the pathogenesis of GBS is thought to be an immunologically mediated attack upon the myelin of the peripheral nervous system. Similarly, other immunosuppressive agents such as azothiaprine and cyclophosphamide have proved ineffective. Plasmapheresis has also not proved efficacious.

CASE PRESENTATION

A 15-year-old white male was in his usual good state of health until 2 weeks prior to admission (PTA) when he developed an illness characterized by rhinorrhea, cough, and sore throat. The symptoms were not severe and resolved within 10 days. Four days PTA, he complained of vague, painful paresthesias that were most pronounced in his lower extremities. This complaint was soon followed by "clumsiness" in the use of his legs. Initially, most apparent during jogging, it progressed to the point that routine ambulation was impeded. In addition, he noted loss of hand dexterity. One day PTA, his family noted that his face appeared "drawn," and he was confined to bed because of weakness. He denied recent fevers, spinal pain, bladder or sexual dysfunction, headaches, dysarthria, dysphagia, and diplopia. The history did not reveal any contact with known neurotoxins.

Examination and Test Results

Initial physical examination was pertinent for a blood pressure of 190/110 mm Hg, a regular pulse rate of 120 beats/min, a respiratory rate of 18 breaths/min, and a temperature of 99°F. Neurologic examination revealed that the patient was alert and fluent, with a facial diplegia and an areflexic quadriparesis, with little sensory dysfunction. No other cranioneuropathy was noted. Coordination was judged to be normal, given the muscular weakness. He was unable to walk, because he could not support his own weight.

Routine laboratory tests, including hemogram, erythrocyte sedimentation rate, serum sodium, potassium, calcium, glucose, creatinine, blood urea nitrogen (BUN), bilirubin, and transaminases, and urinalysis were normal. An electrocardiogram (EKG) was significant for sinus tachycardia. Arterial blood gases were normal.

While in the emergency room, his blood pressure and heart rate fluctuated erratically, returning to normal levels periodically. The hypertension and tachycardia were of predominant concern, and he was admitted for further diagnostic evaluation. No specific diagnosis was considered at this time. During the night, he appeared restless and unable to sleep. A hypnotic was given, and 3 hours later he was noted to be agitated and delirious. Severe bradypnea was apparent. An arterial blood gas revealed marked hypercarbia with moderate hypoxemia, compatible with primary hypoventilation. The patient was intubated and transferred to the ICU. Following correction of his respiratory acidosis, his mental status returned to baseline. The diagnosis of GBS was considered, and a lumbar puncture was performed. The CSF was slightly xanthochromic, acellular, and under normal pressure. The CSF glucose concentration was normal, but the protein was elevated to 200 mg per dl. These results confirmed the clinical impression. The patient remained stable and improved over the course of the next 6 to 8 weeks. Intermittent mandatory ventilation was gradually weaned. Two months after admission, he was discharged in good condition with approximately 90 percent recovery.

SUGGESTED READING

Asburg, A.: Diagnostic consideration in Guillain-Barre syndrome. Ann. Neurol. (Suppl) 9:1, 1981.

Dalakas, M., and Engel, W.: Chronic relapsing polyneuropathy: pathogenesis and treatment. Ann. Neurol. (Suppl) 9:134, 1981.

Hughes, R., and Kadlubowski, M.: Treatment of acute inflammatory polyneuropathy. Ann. Neurol. (Suppl) 9:125, 1981.

McLeod, J.: Electrophysiological studies in the Guillain-Barré syndrome. Ann. Neurol. (Suppl) 9:20, 1981.

Schonberger, L., Hurwitz, E., Katona, P., et al.: Guillain-Barré syndrome: its epidemiology and associations with influenza vaccination. Ann. Neurol. (Suppl) 9:31, 1981.

Nursing Process for Patient Care:

Guillain–Barré Syndrome

The outstanding clinical feature of Guillain-Barré syndrome is a progressive ascending areflexic paralysis. Pulmonary involvement secondary to neuromuscular dysfunction should be anticipated in any patient with Landry-Guillain-Barré-Strohl (LGBS) syndrome during the initial phase.

NEUROMUSCULAR

Frequent assessment of the neuromuscular status of the patient is one of the key elements in the nursing management of Guillain-Barré syndrome.

Assess, Monitor, and Document

Motor response and strength: lower extremities, upper extremities, trunk, face (ability to swallow)

Autonomic dysfunction: cardiovascular, episodic diaphoresis, episodic pallor and/or flush

Anticipate

Alteration in neuromuscular status
  Initial phase (2–4 weeks): progressive symmetrical areflexic paralysis (minimal paraparesis, complete quadriplegia)

Plateau phase (2–3 weeks)
Recovery phase (weeks to months)

PULMONARY

Frequent assessment of pulmonary status is necessary, especially in the initial progressive phase. Neuromuscular dysfunction may result in hypoventilation and subsequent respiratory insufficiency.

Assess, Monitor, and Document

Respiratory rate
Respiratory pattern, including depth
Vital capacity: incentive spirometer
Breath sounds
Color

Arterial blood gases
Response to pulmonary hygiene
  Chest physical therapy: clapping, vibration
  Suctioning: secretions (amount, description)

Anticipate

Alteration in pulmonary function
  Muscle fatigue: hypoventilation
  Respiratory failure

Pneumonia
Pulmonary embolus

CARDIOVASCULAR

In the initial phase of GBS, autonomic dysfunction is a relatively common occurrence. It is episodic in nature, rarely lasting longer than 2 to 3 weeks, and usually requires no specific therapy. The nurse must be alert for signs of decreased cardiac output and tissue perfusion as a result of this dysfunction.

Assess, Monitor, and Document

Heart rate
Rhythm
Blood pressure: arterial
Peripheral pulses

Skin color and condition: pallor, flush
Capillary filling
Response to therapy (if necessary): pharmacologic agents

Anticipate

Alteration in cardiovascular status
    Cardiac dysrhythmias: tachycardia, brady-
      cardia

Hypertension
Hypotension

FLUID AND ELECTROLYTE BALANCE

Fluid and electrolyte balance is important in the overall management of patients with GBS. Associated with GBS is the development of the syndrome of inappropriate secretion of antidiuretic hormone (SIADH). Hypercalcemia may result from prolonged immobilization.

Assess, Monitor, and Document

Weight
Fluid intake
Urine output, including specific gravity
Laboratory data

Serum electrolytes
Serum osmolality
Urine electrolytes
Urine osmolality

Anticipate

SIADH
    Decreased urine output
    Hyponatremia

Altered sensorium
Hypercalcemia

NUTRITIONAL

Assess, Monitor, and Document

Ability to eat: chew, swallow
Daily caloric intake
Daily weight

Anticipate

Alteration in nutritional status
Negative nitrogen balance

INTEGUMENTARY

The prolonged bedrest and immobility associated with GBS predispose the patient to pressure sores and infection.

Assess, Monitor, and Document

Skin condition
    Special attention to bony prominences
Skin care

Turning schedule
Use of adjuncts to care: egg crate foam, gel
    pad, water bolster, Clinitron bed

Anticipate

Alteration in skin condition
Decubiti

RESPONSE OF CHILD

Assess, Monitor, and Document

Developmental level: psychosocial, cognitive, motor, verbal
Behavioral response: fearful, angry, depressed

Level of understanding of condition and limitations
Expected outcome
Response to interventions

Anticipate

Emotional crisis
Inability to cope
Need for referral: social service, psychiatrist

RESPONSE OF FAMILY

Assess, Monitor, and Document

Behavioral response: fearful, verbal, angry, depressed
Level of understanding of child's condition
Expected outcome

Educational needs related to rehabilitative management
Response to nursing interventions

Anticipate

Family crisis
  Disruption in normal family life
Inability to cope

Educational needs regarding rehabilitation and home management
Referral: social service, psychiatrist, rehabilitation

MIND SET

Assess

Neuromuscular status
Pulmonary status
Cardiovascular status
Fluid and electrolyte balance

Nutritional status
Integumentary system
Response of child and family

Anticipate

Alteration in neuromuscular function
  Initial (2–4 weeks): Progressive symmetrical ascending areflexic paralysis
  Plateau phase (2–3 weeks)
  Recovery phase (weeks to months)
Alteration in pulmonary function
  Hypoventilation
  Respiratory insufficiency
  Pneumonia
  Pulmonary embolus

Alteration in cardiovascular function
  Autonomic instability
Alteration in fluid and electrolyte balance
  SIADH
  Hypercalcemia
Alteration in nutritional status
Alteration in skin condition
Emotional crisis
Family crisis

Postoperative Care Following Intracranial Neurosurgery

JEFFREY H. WISOFF, M.D.
FRED J. EPSTEIN, M.D.

Although current neurosurgical and neuro-anesthetic techniques have reduced morbidity and mortality dramatically in pediatric neurosurgical patients, the immediate postoperative period remains a critical time. In this chapter, routine postoperative management and common complications following intracranial surgery are discussed.

Preoperatively, an arterial catheter is placed in every patient; a central venous catheter should be used in operations performed in the sitting position (to aspirate air from the right atrium if an air embolus occurs) or where a large blood loss is anticipated. All patients must be admitted to the intensive care unit (ICU) following surgery. Continuous evaluation and monitoring by ICU nurses who have specialized training in neurosurgery is essential for a smooth postoperative course. Pulse, blood pressure, respiration, and neurological status are checked every 15 minutes for the first 2 hours and then, if the patient remains stable, at hourly intervals for the next 24 to 48 hours. The nursing neurologic examination should include level of consciousness, pupillary size and response to light, and motor function in each limb. Alteration in level of consciousness is the most important parameter to follow.

The head of the bed is kept elevated at 30 degrees for routine craniotomy and at 45 to 60 degrees for operations performed in the sitting position. This elevation promotes venous drainage and helps to reduce postoperative cerebral edema. Additionally, when the sitting position is used, hemostasis is partially accomplished by collapse of small vessels secondary to negative venous pressure; if the patient's head is lowered, these vessels may open and result in postoperative hemorrhage. The patient should be turned in bed from side to side every 2 hours. Patients are permitted out of bed the

day after surgery, and ambulation is allowed as tolerated.

A Foley catheter is placed in all patients. Hourly urine output and specific gravity, with urine fractionals every 4 hours, is recorded for the first 24 to 48 hours. If a drain is used, it should be emptied and recorded at least every 6 hours. Humidified oxygen by mask or face tent is administered for the first day. Coughing, deep breathing, and pulmonary toilet is essential.

Intravenous (IV) fluids consist of D5W $\frac{1}{3}$ normal saline (NS) with 20 mEq of KCl per L in young children and D2.5W $\frac{1}{2}$ NS with 20 mEq of KCl per L in older children and adolescents. Fluid is administered at two thirds normal maintenance. This regimen helps promote a mild dehydration, which decreases cerebral edema. Low-sodium solutions (e.g., D5W) will lower serum osmolality and increase diffusion of water into the brain, with resultant increased edema. Because most patients are on large doses of corticosteroids and have a tendency to hyperglycemia, a solution containing 2.5 percent dextrose is used whenever possible. If fully awake, patients may have ice chips or sips of fluid the evening following surgery. A clear fluid diet is begun the following morning, and the diet is advanced as tolerated.

Routine CBC, serum electrolytes, and arterial blood gases are obtained in the recovery room, 6 hours later, and the following morning. Further laboratory data are obtained when needed.

Medications administered include:

1. Corticosteroids, dexamethasone, 1.5 mg per kg per dose, or methylprednisolone, 4 to 6 mg per kg per dose IV, every 6 hours for 48 to 72 hours and then gradually tapered over 7 to 10 days.

2. Anticonvulsants (for supratentorial tumors only); dilantin, 2 to 3 mg per kg intravenously

every 12 hours; and phenobarbital, 5 mg per kg per day IM, in divided doses, every 8 to 12 hours. These medications are given orally as soon as the patient is tolerating a diet.

3. Antibiotics, oxacillin, 200 mg per kg per day intravenously, in divided doses, is given prophylactically for 48 hours. Vancomycin may be used in patients with penicillin allergies. (The use of prophylactic antibiotics is controversial, although most medical centers use them.)

4. Acetaminophen is given every 4 hours, rectally or orally, for temperature above 99.5°F.

5. Insulin may be needed, in a sliding scale, for hyperglycemia.

6. Antacids are given orally or NG every 2 to 4 hours. Cimetidine is not used.

In patients undergoing surgery in the posterior fossa (e.g., medulloblastoma, cerebellar or brain stem astrocytoma, intravenously ventricle ependymoma), there are several special postoperative considerations. Because these procedures are often performed in the sitting position, the patient must be cared for with the head of the bed elevated 45 to 60 degrees, as previously discussed.

Resection of these tumors usually involves exposure of the fourth ventricle. Disturbances of autonomic function from stimulation of vagal and parasympathetic nuclei in the floor of the fourth ventricle rarely lead to gastric perforations and erosions; frequent administration of antacids is essential. Small amounts of postoperative blood may irritate the floor of the fourth ventricle, leading to hypertension and/or hyperpyrexia. Prompt and aggressive treatment of increased blood pressure with hydralazine is essential to prevent the rare hypertensive hemorrhage in the tumor bed. Body temperature may rapidly rise to 105° to 106° F, with disastrous results.

A hypothermia blanket is mandatory for temperature over 100° F during the first 48 to 72 hours. If lower cranial nerves have been manipulated at surgery or if the tumor was attached to the floor of the fourth ventricle at the calamus, patients must fast until their swallowing and gag reflex are intact. A nasogastric (NG) tube is inserted in these patients. If these deficits persist, tracheostomy and gastrostomy may ultimately be indicated. If patients have a fifth nerve deficit and diminished corneal reflex, the eye is taped closed and artificial tears are given every 4 hours to prevent corneal abrasions and keratitis. The combination of ipsilateral fifth and facial nerve paresis may require a tarsorrhaphy or Arion implant.

Another group of patients deserving special mention are those with suprasellar and parasellar lesions (e.g., craniopharyngioma, pituitary adenoma). Surgery in this region invariably involves manipulation of the hypothalamus and pituitary stalk. Fluid intake and output and urine specific gravity must be measured hourly for early detection of diabetes insipidus (see Chapter 32, Diabetes Insipidus). Serum and urine electrolytes and osmolality are checked at least twice daily. These patients may have wide fluctuations in temperature, requiring alternately vigorous efforts to cool the patient, followed by rewarming for hypothermia. Preoperative and postoperative evaluation of endocrine status is essential; maintenance doses of cortisone acetate should be continued until normal pituitary and adrenal function are documented.

Children undergoing surgery for craniosynostosis and other craniofacial anomalies follow a protocol similar to that for brain tumor patients. Frequent monitoring of vital signs, IV fluids at two-thirds maintenance, and nursing care with the head of the bed elevated is performed as discussed previously. Neonates having sagittal suture resection are not given steroids. All other patients have the steroids tapered over 5 to 7 days. Anticonvulsants are administered only if the dura was opened extensively, or if there is a history of seizures. In many medical centers, prophylactic antibiotics are given routinely until the drains are removed. The major problem encountered in these patients is massive intraoperative blood loss, often 50 to 100 percent of total blood volume, especially with craniofacial repairs. Drains must be emptied and measured hourly, input and output carefully monitored, and serial hematocrits and coagulation studies obtained. Although it is beyond the scope of this chapter to discuss the complete scope of potential coagulation difficulties that may be encountered, it is important to realize that a pediatric hematologist is an essential member of the team caring for these patients.

COMPLICATIONS

Patients usually are reversed from anesthesia and extubated in the operating room (OR) or soon after admission to the recovery room. The patient who does not awaken promptly or who awakens and then deteriorates must be evaluated rapidly. Additional narcotic antagonists are administered when narcotic technique is used. If there is no response, the patient is immediately reintubated. Serum electrolytes, blood glucose, and an arterial blood gas are checked. Recovery room and OR nurses are questioned regarding the possibility of a seizure. If there are new focal deficits or a dilated pupil, an intracranial hematoma must be suspected. The dressing is removed, and the wound and drains are inspected. In infants, the fontanelle is palpated. Unless the patient has herniated acutely, an emergency CT scan is obtained. If a hematoma is present, emergency surgical evacuation is mandatory. In the absence of a hematoma, an intracranial pressure (ICP) monitor (e.g., Richmond screw or ventricular catheter) should be inserted, and any increased ICP should be controlled medically with hyperventilation (Pa_{CO_2}, 25–28), mannitol and furosemide (see Chapter 12, Increased Intracranial Pressure and Chapter 43, Management of Pediatric Head Trauma, for discussion of management of increased ICP).

In patients who have had posterior fossa surgery, who deteriorate suddenly, an epidural hematoma is a strong possibility. The dressing is removed, the decompression is palpated, and if indicated, the wound should be opened at the bedside by the surgeon. If no hematoma is found, the lateral ventricle should be cannulated for decompression, following which, a CT scan is obtained to exclude hemorrhage in the tumor bed or a supratentorial subdural hematoma.

Brain edema occurs to some degree following any intracranial procedure. Severe edema is more likely in patients with subtotally resected malignant tumors in which "wounding" of the tumor causes massive swelling; with tumors that are deep, requiring prolonged retraction of superficial brain for exposure; and following surgery in which venous drainage has been impaired. Postoperative edema may manifest itself with immediate stupor and focal neurologic deficits, mimicking a hematoma, or may present subacutely with deterioration in mental status or progressive deficits 48 to 72 hours following surgery. Only CT scan can differentiate hematoma from edema.

Maximal brain swelling occurs during the first 72 hours following surgery. Medical treatment includes steroids, mild dehydration with restricted fluids, and furosemide or mannitol. Because hypoxia and hypercarbia exacerbate brain edema, Pa_{O_2} greater than 80 mm Hg and Pa_{CO_2} less than 30 should be maintained. If the patient is stuporous or deteriorating, reintubation and hyperventilation are indicated. An ICP monitor is recommended in intubated patients.

Postoperative seizures are another complication in patients undergoing supratentorial surgery. (The cerebellum and brain stem are not epileptogenic; the rare seizure following posterior fossa surgery usually represents subarachnoid air or a supratentorial subdural hematoma.) Patients with a prior history of seizures and those with lesions near the motor cortex are especially prone to postoperative seizures. Postoperative hematoma, infarction, or metabolic derangement may be heralded by seizure. A CT scan and evaluation of blood gases and chemistries are essential.

The primary treatment is rapid control of the seizure activity with maintenance of a good airway and oxygenation. By increasing cerebral metabolic demands, seizures may increase postoperative edema and cause anoxic damage to already edematous brain surrounding the surgical site. This may lead to new transient or permanent neurologic deficits.

Mild hyperglycemia is the most common metabolic derangement seen following intracranial surgery. It is almost always a result of the large doses of corticosteroids used to control edema and corrects itself as steroids are tapered. Blood glucose levels should be obtained at least daily, and urine fractionals should be determined every 4 hours. If hyperglycemia becomes severe, a sliding scale of regular insulin can be used for control after correlation between blood glucose and glycosuria has been established. Patients with diabetes insipidus must be vigorously monitored to prevent dangerous levels of hyperglycemia. Caution must be exercised in treatment; mild hyperglycemia is preferable to hypoglycemia.

The syndrome of inappropriate secretion of antidiuretic hormone (SIADH) occurs as a nonspecific reaction to intracranial surgery and head trauma and is a common cause of electrolyte abnormalities. Mild SIADH usually responds to fluid restriction. More severe SIADH can follow surgery around the hypothalamus (see Chapter 31, Syndrome of Inappropriate ADH).

Neurogenic hypernatremia has been observed following surgery around the hypothalamus (e.g., craniopharyngioma), usually caused by failure of the thirst mechanism. Meticulous fluid balance must be recorded to maintain hydration. Hypernatremia associated with increased osmolality and dehydration results from excessive use of loop and osmotic diuretics. If serum sodium rises above 150 mEq per L or osmolality becomes greater than 310 mOsm per kg, rehydration is necessary.

Diabetes insipidus results from surgery

around the hypothalamus and pituitary stalk (see Chapter 32, Diabetes Insipidus).

In patients with persistent alterations of consciousness beyond 24 to 48 hours, NG feedings should be begun to prevent iatrogenic malnutrition. Rarely is parenteral hyperalimentation required.

Good pulmonary toilet is necessary. Adequate respiratory function is essential for a smooth postoperative course. Aspiration and hypostatic pneumonias are major causes of morbidity in patients with a complicated course and are usually avoidable.

SUGGESTED READING

McLaurin, R. (ed.): Pediatric Neurosurgery. Surgery of the Developing Nervous System. New York, Grune & Stratton, Inc., 1982.

HEMATOLOGIC

Inherited Disorders of Hemostasis

FRANCES FLUG, M.D.
MARGARET KARPATKIN, M.D.

Several hemorrhagic disorders are encountered in the pediatric intensive care setting. These disorders fall under the heading of the coagulopathies, which may be divided into the congenital and acquired disorders of hemostasis. In this chapter, the congenital disorders are discussed. Although congenital deficiencies of each of the factors in the coagulation cascade have been described, attention will be directed to the most common and clinically significant disorders, Factor VIII:C deficiency (hemophilia A), Factor IX deficiency (hemophilia B), and von Willebrand's disease.

ETIOLOGY

The syntheses of Factors VIII:C and IX are controlled by widely separated loci on the X chromosome. Deficiencies are transmitted as X-linked recessive disorders occurring almost always in males. On a statistical basis, carrier mothers transmit the disease to 50 percent of their male offspring and the carrier state to 50 percent of their female offspring. Approximately 25 percent of newly diagnosed patients have no family history of bleeding; these cases are thought to represent new mutations in either mother or son.

Factor VIII:C deficiency is by far the more common of the two hemophilias, accounting for 80 percent of the cases. The incidence is approximately 1 in 10,000 live male births in the United States. Factor VIII:C is a glycoprotein that acts as a cofactor in the reaction in which Factor X becomes activated by activated Factor IX (Fig. 49–1). In plasma, Factor VIII:C circulates complexed via noncovalent bonds to the von Willebrand factor. The site of synthesis of Factor VIII:C is unclear, although the liver appears to play a role. The average half-life is 12 hours.

Factor IX deficiency, also known as hemophilia B, or Christmas disease, has an incidence of 0.25 per 10,000 live male births. Factor IX is synthesized in the liver and is a vitamin K dependent factor. It circulates as a zymogen and is converted to the active form by Factor XIa. In turn, activated Factor IX activates Factor X in the presence of Factor VIII:C, calcium, and platelets. The half-life of Factor IX is approximately 24 hours.

In both hemophilias A and B, the vasculature, platelets, and levels of other factors are normal. The patient's prothrombin time (PT) is normal, but the partial thromboplastin time (PTT) is prolonged.

The degree of severity of hemostasis impairment is classified according to the level of factor found in the patient's plasma. Normal pooled plasma is arbitrarily defined as having 100 percent coagulant activity. Deficiency may be severe (less than 1 percent activity), moderate (1 to 5 percent), or mild (greater than 5 percent). The degree of deficiency usually correlates with the clinical severity and is almost invariably similar in all affected members of a family.

Patients with mild disease often go unrecognized until such time as excessive postop-

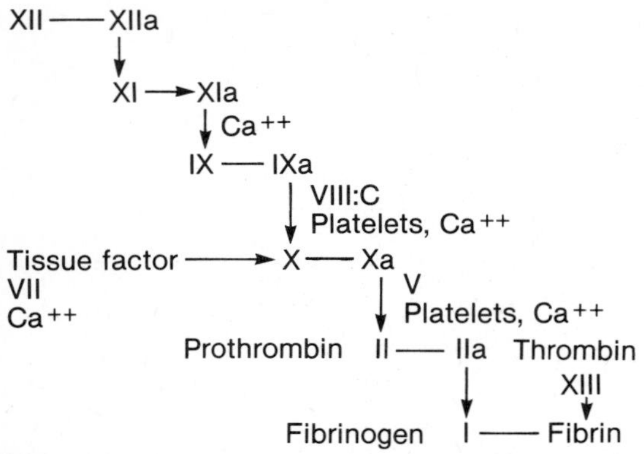

Figure 49–1. The coagulation cascade. Activated factors are designated "a."

erative bleeding occurs. In contrast, patients with moderate or severe hemophilia are subject to recurrent hemorrhage, following mild or moderate trauma in the former, and often spontaneous or following minor trauma in the latter.

The prompt diagnosis and institution of appropriate therapy is essential in all bleeding episodes in hemophiliac patients. In Table 49–1, guidelines are given for management of specific bleeding episodes.

When considering serious bleeding disorders, von Willebrand's disease must be mentioned. This disorder is characterized by a quantitative or qualitative defect in the von Willebrand factor portion of the Factor VIII complex. In most cases, patients experience a mild bleeding diathesis. Type III von Willebrand's disease, how-

ever, is a severe disorder transmitted as an autosomal recessive trait in which life-threatening bleeding episodes may occur.

MANAGEMENT

Treatment of bleeding in hemophilia is based on specific replacement of the deficient factor. Freeze-dried preparations derived from large donor pools of human plasma are commercially available for replacement of Factors VIII:C and IX. Factor IX preparations (prothrombin complex concentrate) also contain Factors II, VII, and X. In addition cryoprecipitate, prepared from individual donor units of fresh plasma, supplies Factor VIII:C and fibrinogen and is the best source of von Willebrand's factor. Fresh frozen plasma supplies variable amounts of all the clotting factors. Blood products used in the treatment of hemophilia are summarized in Table 49–2.

The rules concerning the amount of factor replacement necessary for hemostasis are easy to understand: 1. One unit is the amount of Factor VIII:C or Factor IX in 1 ml of normal pooled plasma, yielding 100 percent factor activity. 2. Infusion of 1 unit per kilogram of body weight will raise the amount of Factor VIII by 2 percent; the half-life of Factor VIII:C is 12 hours. 3. Infusion of 1 unit per kilogram of body weight will raise Factor IX level by 1 percent. This is supposedly because Factor IX is a small molecule that equilibrates rapidly between the intravascular and extravascular

Table 49–1. Management of Specific Bleeding Episodes in Patients with Factor VIII:C or Factor IX Deficiency*

Type of Bleed	Minimal Factor Level for Initial Infusion (percent)	Subsequent Infusion	Other
Early spontaneous joint or muscle	10–15	Usually unnecessary	
Post-traumatic/later joint or muscle	40–50	Daily, 2–3 days	
Soft tissue	25–30	Usually unnecessary	
Oral mucosa laceration/ dental extraction	50–75	May be unnecessary	Epsilon aminocaproic acid (EACA), 200 mg/kg initial, 100 mg/kg every 6 hrs for 7–10 days, maximum single dose 6 gm
Central nervous system	100	Daily for 7–14 days on 12–24-hr basis; 30–50 percent level to be maintained at all times	
Surgery/major laceration	100	Daily for 7–14 days; 30–50 percent level to be maintained at all times	

*Patients with von Willebrand's disease are treated by infusion of cryoprecipitate, 2–4 bags/10 kg depending upon the severity of the bleeding episode.

Table 49–2. Products for Treatment of Bleeding Episodes in Hemophilia

Product	Major Content	Volume (per bag/vial)	Average Amount of Factor VIII:C or IX (per bag/vial)
Fresh frozen plasma	All coagulation factors	200–300 ml	160–240 units
Cryoprecipitate	Factor VIII:C, fibrinogen, von Willebrand's factor	10–30 ml	60–120 units
Factor VIII:C concentrate	Factor VIII:C	10–30 ml	250–1500 units recorded individually on vial label
Factor IX concentrate (pro-thrombin complex)	Factors II, VII, IX, X	20–30 ml	400–600 units as per vial label
Anti-inhibitor coagulation complex	Activated clotting factors	30 ml	180–1050 VIII:C correctional units as per vial label

spaces. The half-life of Factor IX is 24 hours. 4. Von Willebrand's factor is replaced by infusing 2 to 4 bags of cryoprecipitate per 10 kilograms of body weight.

Although hemophiliacs encounter many problems that demand attention, two types of hemorrhagic events, bleeding in the tissues surrounding the airway and bleeding in the central nervous system, can be acutely life threatening.

Airway Compromise

Spontaneous submucosal bleeding in the floor of the mouth, pharynx, or larynx is a rare complication of hemophilia. It can be catastrophic because of obstruction of the airway. Signs of impending obstruction may develop slowly over a period of hours. Patients may complain of dysarthria, dysphagia, or sore throat. Lateral neck films may be useful, especially in cases in which adequate examination of the hypopharynx may be impossible because of swelling of the tongue or floor of the mouth. The patient should be given immediate factor replacement to raise the plasma level to at least 60 percent with follow-up every 12 to 24 hours to maintain a level of 30 to 50 percent until swelling diminishes significantly. If swelling increases in the soft tissues of the neck or the mouth, nasotracheal intubation (under general anesthesia if necessary) may be prudent to ensure the airway. It is best to undertake this electively rather than to wait until severe respiratory distress is evident. With proper replacement therapy, bleeding should stop and swelling should diminish in 2 to 5 days; thus, this approach is superior to tracheotomy, which may result in bleeding from the wound and possible further compromise of the airway.

Traumatic injury to the nasopharynx is treated in a similar manner to spontaneous hemorrhage. With dental manipulation or mucosal laceration, proper management will avoid potential airway compromise. It should be noted that bleeding from the injection site of a local anesthetic may constitute a grave danger to the airway. Thus, the appropriate clotting factor should be infused before local anesthesia is administered. Epsilon aminocaproic acid (EACA)* is an inhibitor of fibrinolysis, which prevents the activation of plasminogen to plasmin. It may be useful in bleeding episodes involving the mouth, because saliva contains potent activators of fibrinolysis. The usual dose is 200 mg per kg P.O. initially, followed by 100 mg per kg every 6 hours (maximum daily dose 24 gm) until healing in evident (7–10 days). This may obviate the need for further replacement therapy; however, each case must be judged individually.

Central Nervous System Bleeding

Central nervous system (CNS) hemorrhage includes bleeding into the intracranial and intravertebral spaces. Intracranial bleeding is considered the leading cause of death in hemophiliacs. Since the increased availability of factor replacement, mortality from this serious condition has declined. Morbidity, as a result of this event, still remains high.

The incidence of CNS bleeding ranges from 2 to 3.5 percent of hemophiliac patients per year. Most reviews show the mean age for intracranial bleeding episodes to be in the mid teens. In one report, one third of the patients

---

* Amicar–Lederle Labs, Wayne, New Jersey.

were 3 years of age or younger, half of the patients were 10 years old or younger, and more than two thirds of the patients were younger than 18 years of age. This probably reflects the increased trauma to which individuals of this age group are subjected in their every day lives. There are remarkably few episodes of intracranial bleeding in the newborn period, given the degree of trauma to the presenting head during passage through the birth canal.

The ratio of patients suffering intracranial bleeding with Factor VIII deficiency to those with Factor IX deficiency is similar to the ratio in the hemophiliac population as a whole. There is a relationship between the severity of the hemostatic defect and the likelihood of developing intracranial hemorrhage. Most cases occur in those with severe disease; however, CNS bleeding has been reported in patients with moderate or mild disease. Bleeding may occur in the subdural or epidural space, intracerebrally or in the intracerebellar space, or in the subarachnoid or intraventricular spaces.

A history of trauma may not be obtained in many patients in whom intracranial bleeding occurs. The proportion of cases preceded by identifiable injury to the head ranges between 26 and 65 percent in various reviews. Thus, any hemophiliac presenting with neurologic signs or symptoms must be suspected of CNS bleeding. One may search for other conditions associated with intracranial bleeding such as hypertension, congenital intracranial anomalies, neoplasms, and CNS infections; however, these will rarely be found.

The evaluation of patients with suspected intracranial bleeding involves a careful history, physical examination, and pertinent diagnostic tests. Most patients present with headache and/or vomiting. Seizures, lethargy, irritability or confusion, obtundation, or coma may also be among the presenting signs and symptoms. Persistent headache as the sole symptom in a hemophiliac should be taken seriously as possible evidence of intracranial bleeding and should be treated with factor replacement therapy and observation. It is a notable fact that hemophiliacs tend to have a long symptom-free interval from the time of trauma; one study showed 4 ± 2.2 days as the average symptom-free interval.

Physical examination should include assessment of the patient's vital signs for evidence of increased intracranial pressure (ICP). A search for scalp lacerations and superficial hematomas may provide evidence of head trauma, the presence of which is an indication for replacement therapy. A careful neurologic examination with serial examinations at frequent intervals may allow early detection of an expanding lesion.

Generally, at the time of suspected intracranial bleeding, the diagnosis of the clotting disorder will already have been made. The plasma should, however, be checked for the presence of an inhibitor. Serial hematocrits should be followed and typed, and cross-matched blood should be made available. Skull x-rays should be taken, because the finding of a fracture may also be evidence of trauma and is an indication for replacement therapy, even without neurologic signs. CT scan, of course, has become the diagnostic procedure of choice in patients with presumed or suspected intracranial bleeding. It is invaluable for its noninvasive nature and ability to localize a lesion. Occasionally, lumbar puncture after factor replacement may be considered necessary to rule out CNS infection or to document subarachnoid or intraventricular bleeding.

It cannot be overemphasized that with proper replacement therapy, management should proceed according to basic medical and neurosurgical principles, with no indicated diagnostic or therapeutic maneuver withheld from the hemophiliac patient. This includes surgical procedures such as emergency relief of ICP via burr holes and craniotomy with evacuation of the hematoma. During surgery, attention should be paid to local hemostasis.

Postoperatively, corticosteroids may be used to reduce edema; special care should, however, be taken to prevent gastric bleeding, which may be related to steroids, stress, or intracranial injury. Attempt should be made to maintain gastric pH greater than 5.0 by frequent use of antacids and/or H_2 blockers (cimetidine). The use of prophylactic antibiotics is controversial. It should be recognized, however, that wound hematomas may promote infection and, conversely, infection may make bleeding more likely. Anticonvulsant therapy is an important supplement to management. A hematoma or the site of surgical manipulation may act as a seizure focus. In fact, seizures are one of the major sequelae in hemophiliac survivors of intracranial bleeding. Seizure control should be tight to avoid additional injury secondary to the convulsion, such as possible airway obstruction from hemorrhage in the mouth or further head injury. Finally, it should be remembered that aspirin, aspirin-containing products, and the nonsteroidal anti-inflammatory agents have no place in the management of pain in hemophiliacs because of their actions in inhibiting platelet aggregation.

Until now, we have alluded to proper replacement therapy. Certain guidelines can be outlined in the management of intracranial bleeding, with prompt, aggressive, prolonged therapy being the basis for treatment. All hemophiliacs with head injury should be treated immediately. If the injury is minor and unaccompanied by neurologic deficit, a single dose of factor replacement can be infused to raise the plasma level to 40 to 50 percent, followed by a period of observation. If, however, trauma is major or accompanied by neurologic findings, the initial infusion should raise the plasma level to 100 percent. It is of the utmost importance that the initial treatment be given before any diagnostic steps are undertaken. If intracranial bleeding is documented, replacement therapy should continue on a 12-hour basis to maintain a minimum level of 30 to 50 percent for a minimum of 10 to 14 days. It may be necessary to keep the level closer to 100 percent during the first few days following injury or during the first few postoperative days. The clinical situation may also require a prolonged course of factor replacement up to 20 to 30 days. If bleeding is not documented but symptoms persist, treatment should probably be continued during an observation period of several days, maintaining a factor level of 30 to 50 percent. Persistent headache, nausea, vomiting, or other neurologic signs are indications for replacement therapy to 30 to 50 percent, followed by appropriate diagnostic studies. This is true even in the absence of a history of trauma. Because of the long symptom-free interval in many hemophiliacs, the patient seen initially within 5 days of head trauma should be treated according to the previous guidelines.

With prompt, aggressive therapy, the outcome of intracranial bleeding in hemophiliacs has improved greatly, from a mortality rate of 70 percent prior to 1960 to approximately 35 percent in patients followed after 1960, with intracerebral bleeds carrying the poorest prognosis. Nevertheless, persistent neurologic deficits run as high as 50 percent in patients with documented CNS hemorrhage. These include seizure disorders (in 20–25 percent), motor impairment, mental retardation, and hydrocephalus. In addition, the incidence of rebleeding is significant, ranging from 13 to 25 percent in recent studies. The recurrence is often without intervening trauma, may occur more than 1 year following the initial injury, and may be located at a different site than the original. Thus, those who have had an intracranial hemorrhage appear to be at significant risk for recurrence. A patient who has had two apparently spontaneous intracranial hemorrhages should be placed on maintenance replacement therapy indefinitely. This usually consists of infusion of 20 U per kg three times a week that will maintain a low level of the defective clotting factor and will hopefully protect against further intracranial hemorrhage. The concentrate can be administered at home by a family member or by the patient himself after appropriate training.

Intravertebral bleeding occurs in hemophiliacs much less frequently than intracranial bleeding. The presentation may be with back pain or paralysis. A history is often unobtainable and, as with intracranial bleeds, a symptom-free interval following trauma may be seen. Rapidly progressive symptoms may occur with flaccid paralysis, decreased deep tendon reflexes, and a sensory level obtained on physical examination. Bleeding may occur anywhere along the vertebral column, with that in the cervical region being immediately life threatening because of paralysis of the respiratory muscles. Hemorrhage may be extramedullary or intramedullary. The latter has the poorer prognosis. The principles of management are the same as those for intracranial bleeding. Immediate factor replacement should be administered, followed by any indicated diagnostic procedure. Lumbar puncture and myelogram may be performed, and laminectomy is often necessary.

The care of hemophiliacs with spinal injuries demands special attention to areas considered routine in other patients with spinal cord trauma (see Chapter 44, Pediatric Spinal Cord Trauma). For example, physical therapy with range-of-motion exercises must be done with great care to avoid hemarthroses and soft-tissue bleeding. Skin care must be rigorous, because hemophiliacs are at risk to bleed from the open wound of a decubitus, as well as at sites exposed to prolonged pressure. Finally, urinary retention may necessitate bladder catherization, which can be associated with significant bleeding.

Patients With Inhibitors

The treatment of hemophiliac patients who have developed inhibitors presents a special problem. Approximately 10 percent of patients with hemophilia A and 2 to 3 percent of those with hemophilia B develop an antibody to the transfused factor. These inhibitors occur unpredictably, often in childhood, and are not related to the number of infusions the patient has had. The possibility of an inhibitor should be considered when a patient does not respond as expected to replacement therapy; also, screening at regular intervals and prior to elective surgery should be routine in the care of hemophiliacs.

Inhibitors to Factor VIII are IgG antibodies, which specifically neutralize Factor VIII coagulant activity. Patients with inhibitors do not bleed more frequently than hemophiliacs without inhibitors, but their bleeding episodes are often difficult to control.

Patients with inhibitors may have low or high titers. Those with low titers may show an anamnestic response to factor replacement. Low titer inhibitors may be treated with one to two times the usual dose of Factor VIII:C concentrate. High doses appear to "saturate" the antibody. Patients with low titers and anamnestic reponses (low titers because they have not recently received treatment) may generally be treated with large amounts of Factor VIII:C (sometimes necessitating as much as 20,000 units per day) for several days until the anamnestic response occurs. In some cases, the few days of treatment may be sufficient. This type of management can be undertaken with the understanding that these patients will then be resistant to Factor VIII therapy until the inhibitor activity drops to a low level (which may take many months).

Patients with high titer activity present the most difficult management problem. A variety of approaches have been attempted, including immunosuppressive drugs, exchange transfusion, plasmapheresis, and animal Factor VIII preparations, all with little success. Over the past 10 years, it has been recognized that concentrates used in the treatment of Factor IX deficiency (prothrombin complex concentrates) may be useful in treating patients with Factor VIII deficiency with inhibitors. These concentrates,* known to contain Factors II, VII, IX, and X, also contain activated coagulation factors that theoretically trigger clotting beyond the position of Factor VIII:C in the cascade. The mechanism for this "bypass" is unknown. The dose is 50 to 100 U per kg.

Caution is indicated, because prothombin complex concentrates have been known to be thrombogenic and/or to induce disseminated intravascular coagulation in nonhemophiliacs with liver disease, as well as in Factor IX deficient patients postsurgically. Because of this,

manufacturers have attempted to produce a product containing less activated clotting factors. It is not known whether the agents responsible for bypassing Factor VIII:C activity are the same as those that cause thrombotic events; however, since the changes in production have occurred, these agents seem less useful in treating bleeding episodes in patients with inhibitors. Despite this finding, there have been several reports of young men with inhibitors who have developed myocardial infarcts after repeatedly receiving prothrombin complex concentrates in large doses (post-production changes). Thus, caution is indicated in the use of these agents. They should not be used repeatedly in patients with inhibitors unless life-threatening bleeding persists and alternative therapy is not feasible. The concomitant use of inhibitors of fibrinolysis (i.e., Amicar) should be avoided. Special attention must be given to patients with liver disease who receive these substances, because the liver plays an important role in clearing activated clotting factors.

Two preparations that contain greater levels of activated factors are currently available. These are known as Autoplex* and FEIBA.† There have been reports of good to excellent results in the presence of high titer inhibitors using doses of 50 to 100 Factor VIII:C correctional U per kg at 6- to 24-hour intervals. Transient hypofibrinogenemia has been observed in children receiving these substances. In addition, there have been reports of serious thrombotic events, including death from myocardial infarction in adults receiving these concentrates. Thus, these agents should be used with extreme caution.

In summary, when faced with a major hemorrhagic event, patients with low titer inhibitors may be treated with large doses of Factor VIII:C infusion until an anamnestic response occurs. At this point, as with those who start out with high inhibitor levels, nonactivated prothrombin complex concentrates may be cautiously used, followed by activated prothrombin complex concentrates if hemostasis is not achieved.

COMPLICATIONS OF THERAPY

Many complications of replacement therapy result from the fact that the plasma of thou-

---

* Proplex–Hyland Therapeutics, Glendale, California, and Konyne–Cutter Biological, Emoryville, California.

* Hyland Therapeutics, Glendale, California.
† Immuno, A.G. Vienna, Austria.

sands of donors is pooled for each lot of concentrate. From this pooling, several problems arise. First, anti-A and anti-B isoagglutinins present in the concentrates place recipients with blood types A, B, and AB at risk for development of a hemolytic process, manifested by anemia, reticulocytosis, and jaundice. One must be aware of the possibility of this syndrome in patients receiving intensive therapy.

Second, the transmission of hepatitis is a major complication of treatment of hemophiliacs. Although potential donors are routinely screened for hepatitis B antigen, it is non-A, non-B hepatitis that currently constitutes the major risk for these patients. Acute clinical disease does not occur with great frequency; however, many hemophiliacs have transient or persistent abnormalities in liver function values and most are positive for antibody to hepatitis B. The clinical significance of transfusion–associated liver disease is not completely understood at this time.

A life-threatening complication of therapy has recently developed. Since 1981, a total of 59 cases of acquired immune deficiency syndrome (AIDS) have been reported in hemophiliacs in the United States; 30 have died. The causative virus is presumably transmitted in concentrate. The Centers for Disease Control has recommended that patients with hemophilia A should receive cryoprecipitate, or heat-treated, freeze-dried concentrates (commercially available). Patients with hemophilia B should receive fresh frozen plasma whenever possible.

CASE PRESENTATION

W.K., a 2-year-old, 18 kg (39 lb), Oriental male with known severe Factor VIII:C deficiency (less than 1 percent VIII:C) was admitted to the hospital. During the 2 days prior to admission, he complained of headache and vomiting. A history of trauma was not elicited. Factor VIII:C concentrate was immediately administered at 50 U/kg (900 U). A CT scan revealed a left subdural hematoma and a mild left-to-right midline shift. Past medical history was remarkable for a left subdural hematoma, which had presented with headache and seizures, 2 months prior to admission. There was no history of trauma at that time. The child had been successfully treated with factor replacement and discharged on phenobarbital, with no obvious sequelae. CT scan at the time of discharge was normal.

Physical Examination

Physical examination revealed an irritable child who was able to follow commands. Vital signs were normal for his age. Examination of the skull showed no palpable fracture or abrasion. Cranial nerves and motor and sensory examinations were normal. Deep tendon reflexes were symmetrical, and a positive Babinsky sign was elicited on the right.

Laboratory Data

WBC = 12,300/mm^3, hgb = 11.5 gm/dl, hct = 34 percent, and PLT = 234,000/mm^3. PT: patient = 12 sec, control = 11.5 sec and PTT = 160 sec, control = 40.5 sec. Factor VIII:C < 1 percent. There was no evidence of a Factor VIII:C inhibitor. Skull x-ray series was normal.

Problem List

Hematologic

Hemophilia with evidence of CNS hemorrhage requires administration of Factor VIII:C concentrate at 50 U/kg to raise the level to 100 percent. 50 U/kg infusion is to be administered q12h until neurologic status is improved. Thereafter, a level of 30–50 percent is to be maintained for 10–14 days. Peak and trough levels of Factor VIII:C are to be obtained to ensure adequacy of levels and to guide dosage. Following discharge, this patient will require prophylactic administration of concentrate because of his previous history of CNS hemorrhage. An infusion of 20 U/kg will be given at home at 2- to 3-day intervals.

Neurologic

Subdural hematoma with evidence of midline shift: Lasix 1 mg/kg IV was administered to effect a diuresis, to decrease ICP; Solu-Medrol was administered to decrease cerebral edema. Phenobarbital was continued.

Intake and Output

Because of vomiting and possible progressive deterioration in mental status, the patient was made NPO. IV fluids were administered at two thirds maintenance rate so as not to contribute to intracranial hypertension.

Gastrointestinal

Antacids and cimetidine were administered to decrease the possibility of upper gastrointestinal hemorrhage.

SUGGESTED READING

Abildgaard, C.F.: Management of inhibitors in hemophilia. *In* Hilgartner, M.W. (ed.): Hemophilia in the Child and Adult. New York, Masson Publishing USA, Inc., 1982.

Aledort, L.M.: Current concepts in diagnosis and management of hemophilia. Hosp. Pract. October, 1982, pp. 77–92.

CDC: Update: Acquired Immune Deficiency Syndrome (AIDS) in Persons with Hemophilia. MMWR. 33:589, 1984.

Corrigan, J.J.: Oral bleeding in hemophilia: treatment with epsilon aminocaproic acid and replacement therapy. J. Pediatr. 80:124, 1972.

Eyster, M.E., et al.: Central nervous system bleeding in hemophiliacs. Blood 51:1179, 1978.

Gilchrist, G.S., Piepgras, D.G., and Roskos, R.R.: Neurologic complications in hemophilia. *In* Hilgartner, M.W. (ed.): Hemophilia in the Child and Adult. New York, Masson Publishing USA, Inc., 1982.

Sjamsoedin-Liesbeth, J.M., et al.: The effect of activated prothrombin-complex concentrate (FEIBA) on joint and muscle bleeding in patients with hemophilia A and antibodies to factor VIII. N. Engl. J. Med. 305:717, 1981.

Stanievich, J.F., Marshak, G., and Stool, S.: Airway obstruction in a hemophiliac child. Ann. Otol. 89:572, 1980.

Nursing Process for Patient Care:
Inherited Disorders of Hemostasis

Children with inherited disorders of hemostasis require admission to the critical care unit based not only on severity but also on anatomic site of hemorrhage. Bleeding in the CNS or in the tissues surrounding the airway, although not of large magnitude, is potentially life threatening. Children with moderate or severe hemophilia may bleed in response to mild or moderate trauma. Children with severe hemophilia may bleed spontaneously. Anticipating a spontaneous bleed in the common sites is of prime importance in the nursing management of these children.

HEMATOLOGIC

Assess, Monitor, and Document

Signs of bleeding: gastrointestinal, joints, muscle, soft tissue, CNS
Status of factor deficiency
   Laboratory results
   Discussion with physician
Status of factor replacement

Accurate administration of clotting factors
Fresh frozen plasma
Cryoprecipitate
Factor VIII: C concentrate
Factor IX concentrate

Anticipate:

Alteration in hematologic status
   Hemorrhage
   Shock

Complications of therapy: hemolytic process (anemia, jaundice, reticulocytosis)

NEUROLOGIC

CNS hemorrhage, particularly intracranial bleeding, is considered the leading cause of death in children with hemophilia. Although the mortality rate has declined since the availability of factor replacement, morbidity remains high.

Assess, Monitor, and Document

Headache
Vomiting
Irritability
Level of consciousness: lethargy, confusion, stupor
Pupillary response
Reflexes
Posturing

Blood pressure
Pulse
Respiratory rate and pattern
Seizures: type, duration
Back pain
Paralysis
Altered sensory level

Anticipate

Increased ICP
   Headache
   Alteration in level of consciousness
   Alteration in pupillary response
   Alteration in reflexes
   Increased blood pressure
   Decreased pulse
   Decreased respiratory rate
   Altered respiratory pattern

Seizures
Intravertebral hemorrhage
   Back pain
   Flaccid paralysis
   Decreased deep tendon reflexes
   Altered sensory level

FLUID AND ELECTROLYTE BALANCE

Assess, Monitor, and Anticipate

Weight
Urine output, including specific gravity
Fluid intake: accurate administration of par-

enteral fluids (use infusion pump if available)
Serum electrolytes

Anticipate

Alteration in fluid and electrolyte balance
status
Increased ICP

RESPONSE OF CHILD

Assess, Monitor, and Document

Developmental level: verbal, psychosocial,
cognitive, normal fears (separation)
Behavioral response: anxious, fearful, non-
threatened, compliant, friendly

Ability to relate to staff
Ability to cope
Response to nursing interventions

Anticipate

Emotional distress
Inability to cope
Disruption in normal growth and development

RESPONSE OF FAMILY

Assess, Monitor, and Document

Behavioral response: anxious, fearful
Level of knowledge of disease and child's
condition
Expected outcome
Ability to cope

Learning needs related to discharge
Medication administration
Special techniques
Signs and symptoms of bleeding (CNS)

Anticipate

Family crisis
Inability to cope

Learning needs related to discharge planning
Referral: social service

MIND SET

Assess

Hematologic status
Neurologic status

Fluid and electrolyte balance
Response of child and family

Anticipate

Alteration in hemostasis
  Hemorrhage: CNS (intracranial, intravertebral), soft tissue, joints, gastrointestinal, submucosal, floor of mouth, pharynx, larynx (airway obstruction)

Shock
Emotional distress of child
Family crisis

50

Acquired Disorders of Hemostasis

FRANCES FLUG, M.D.
MARGARET KARPATKIN, M.D.

Hemostasis depends upon the interaction of blood vessels, platelets, and blood coagulation factors. The most common acquired defect seen in the pediatric age group is immune thrombocytopenic purpura. However, this disorder is rarely seen in the intensive care setting and will not be discussed here. We shall limit our remarks to four of the more common causes of hemostatic failure seen in the pediatric intensive care unit (ICU), namely disseminated intravascular coagulation (DIC), vitamin K deficiency, liver disease, and the coagulopathy of the massively transfused patient.

DISSEMINATED INTRAVASCULAR COAGULATION

Disseminated intravascular coagulation (DIC) refers to an acquired coagulopathy whereby the coagulation cascade is activated and leads to the generation of thrombin within the circulation. This, in turn, promotes further activation of the clotting mechanism, formation and deposition of fibrin, depletion of some of the coagulation factors, and secondary activation of the fibrinolytic system.

The clinical syndrome of DIC results from activation of the coagulation mechanism, leading to fibrin formation and thrombosis, and activation of the fibrinolytic pathway, causing dissolution of the clot and hemorrhage. Thus, DIC manifests itself along a spectrum. If the intravascular clotting process is dominant compared with the fibrinolytic process, thrombosis will be the major clinical expression. If fibrinolysis is more prominent, the patient will exhibit signs of impaired hemostasis.

In addition, DIC can exist in a compensated form, whereby the production of clotting factors keeps up with their consumption. In this state, the coagulopathy may be clinically insignificant. It is only when production cannot keep up with consumption (leading to bleeding) or when tissue damage occurs from fibrin thrombi that the situation becomes decompensated and clinically apparent. Most cases occurring in the pediatric age group present as an acutely decompensated bleeding diathesis.

Pathogenesis

To understand the pathogenesis of DIC, it is useful to refer to an experimental animal model known as the generalized Shwartzman reaction. This reaction is induced by two intravenous (IV) injections of endotoxin, 8 to 24 hours apart, and results in formation of fibrin in the glomerular capillaries, bilateral renal cortical necrosis, and activation of the coagulation mechanism. The first dose of endotoxin triggers intravascular coagulation, and the reticuloendothelial system (RES) removes the resulting fibrin. The second injection of endotoxin, in the presence of a blocked RES, leads to a more exaggerated burst of intravascular coagulation, resulting in fibrin deposition in the glomerular capillaries and other small vessels throughout the body. Prior blockade of the RES will cause a single injection of endotoxin to produce this reaction. IV injection of antigen–antibody complexes can trigger the reaction in rabbits prepared with 1 dose of endotoxin. Administration of heparin and depletion of neutrophils protect rabbits from the endotoxin-triggered reaction.

Among the events thought to trigger DIC in human beings in vivo are the presence in the circulation of endotoxin; antigen–antibody complexes or other particulate matter; tissue injury with liberation of tissue thromboplastic activity; damage to red blood cells, platelets, or endothelial cells; blood stasis; and disorders of the reticuloendothelial system, leading to decreased clearance of activated coagulation factors. The coagulation system is apparently activated by each of these events, via either the intrinsic and/or extrinsic pathways. The result of this is generation of thrombin. Thrombin has several direct effects (Fig. 50–1). It enzymatically degrades fibrinogen to the fibrin monomer, which, in turn, polymerizes and is stabilized by activated Factor XIII. Factor XIII is activated by thrombin. Thrombin also increases the potencies of Factors V and VIII:C many fold, thus facilitating both the intrinsic and extrinsic pathways. In addition, thrombin induces platelet aggregation, with attendant thrombocytopenia and release of platelet contents, which may further stimulate coagulation. Some of the excess fibrin polymer formed via these mechanisms becomes deposited in the microvasculature, leading to poor perfusion, ischemia, possible necrosis of end organs, entrapment of platelets, and further thrombocytopenia. Damage to red blood cells may occur as they pass through these small vessels (microangiopathic hemolytic anemia). These damaged red cells may, upon release of their contents, trigger additional intravascular coagulation, thus perpetuating the cycle. Lastly, thrombin is known to activate the fibrinolytic system, that is, it facilitates the formation of plasmin from plasminogen. Plasmin acts to degrade fibrinogen, fibrin monomer, and fibrin polymer (fibrin clot) to form the fibrinolytic degradation products (FDP), which are among the hallmarks of DIC.

Clinical Syndromes

DIC is not a primary disease entity. It is a secondary phenomenon that is triggered by a variety of underlying disorders. In many cases, the ability to make the diagnosis of DIC demands a high index of suspicion and a knowledge of the clinical disorders associated with the coagulopathy. In Table 50–1, an extensive listing of such conditions is provided.

Among pediatric patients, DIC is most commonly seen in sick newborns. After the neonatal period, the most common cause of DIC is bacterial sepsis. It has been reported in association with various gram-negative as well as gram-positive organisms. Hypotension (i.e., a shock state) appears to be necessary for development of DIC associated with bacterial sepsis. Other infectious states, including disseminated viral infections (varicella being a notable type), rickettsial diseases, and fungal and protozoal infections, may also precipitate DIC.

Purpura fulminans, also known as post–in-

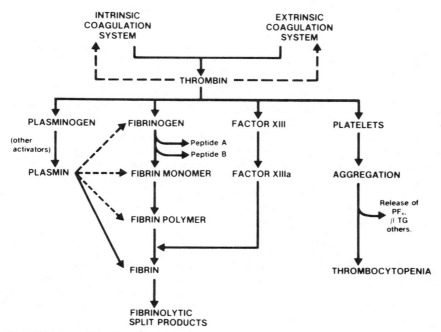

Figure 50-1. Effects of thrombin upon coagulation and fibrinolysis. (From Corrigan, J.J.: Disseminated intravascular coagulation. Pediatrics in Review 2:39, 1979. Used by permission.)

Table 50-1. Etiologic Factors for Disseminated Intravascular Coagulation (DIC)

I. Injury to endothelial cells and/or activation of intrinsic system:
    Gram-negative sepsis
      Escherichia coli
      Hemophilus influenzae
      Klebsiella sp.
      Neisseria meningococcus and gonococcus
      Proteus mirabilis
      Pseudomonas aeruginosa
      Salmonella sp.
      Serratia sp.
    Gram-positive sepsis
      Staphylococcus aureus and *albus*
      Streptococcus spp.
      Pneumococcus pneumoniae
    Rocky mountain spotted fever
    Fungal infections
      Aspergillus sepsis
      Disseminated *Candida albicans*
      Toxoplasmosis
    Protozoa
    Viruses
      Cytomegalovirus
      Disseminated herpes simplex
      Hemorrhagic fever (Korean, Thai)
      Influenza
      Rubella
      Varicella
    Prolonged hypotension from any cause
    Severe acidosis
    Hypoxemia or asphyxia
    Systemic vasculitis
    Hypothermia
    Polycythemia and stasis
    Intrauterine growth retardation
    Cavernous hemangioma
    Lymphangioma
II. Tissue injury with liberation of tissue thromboplastic activity and activation of extrinsic system:
    Obstetric complications
      Abruptio placentae
      Amniotic fluid embolism

II. (*continued*)
      Dead twins
      Eclampsia and pre-eclampsia
    Brain injury
    Surgical procedures and cardiopulmonary bypass
    Trauma
    Extensive burns
    Heat stroke
    Rhabdomyolysis due to various causes
    Necrotizing enterocolitis
    Neoplasm
      Acute promyelocytic leukemia
      Rarely, acute and chronic granulocytic leukemia, acute lymphatic leukemia, or lymphoma
      Pediatric solid tumors (Ewing's sarcoma, neuroblastoma, rhabdomyosarcoma, Wilms' tumor)
III. Direct activation of fibrinogen, Factor II, or Factor X:
    Snake bite (procoagulant venoms)
    Mucin-secreting adenocarcinomas of adults
IV. Red blood cell, platelet, or immunologic injury:
    Intravascular hemolysis
      Incompatible red blood cell transfusions
      Severe erythroblastosis fetalis
      Drowning
    Antigen–antibody reactions
      Renal transplant rejection
      Graft-versus-host disease
V. Reticuloendothelial system injury, with decreased clearance of activated coagulation factors:
    Reticuloendothelial hypofunction
    Hepatic diseases
VI. Miscellaneous:
    Types II and IV hyperlipidemias
    Nonbacterial thrombotic endocarditis
    Exposure to 100 percent oxygen in experimental animals

From Stuart, M., and McKenna, R.: Diseases of coagulation: the platelet and vasculature. *In* Nathan, D., and Oski, F. (eds.): Hematology of Infancy and Childhood, 2nd ed. Philadelphia, W.B. Saunders Company, 1981, p. 1272.

fectious gangrene is a rare disorder that occurs following a viral or bacterial infection. It is associated with striking purpuric skin lesions on the extremities that progress rapidly to gangrene. The laboratory findings of DIC accompany this acute syndrome.

DIC can also occur as a result of a localized event. Such is the case with giant hemangiomas (Kasabach-Merritt syndrome) or arterial aneurysms. In these disorders, trapping of platelets or circulatory stasis may be the initiating event leading to activation of coagulation, fibrin deposition, and, ultimately, DIC.

Malignancies may be associated with DIC. In these cases, DIC may present as local or diffuse thromboses or as minor or diffuse hemorrhage. In childhood, the acute leukemias are the most common malignancies with this as-

sociation, and, of these, acute promyelocytic leukemia is best known for this complication. The coagulation cascade is apparently directly activated as promyelocytes lyse and release specific tissue factors from their granules. Sometimes DIC becomes overt or aggravated during initial chemotherapy with its rapid cell lysis. Generally, it is an additional hemostatic problem to an already present thrombocytopenia caused by bone marrow replacement by the malignancy.

Any shock state, including septic, hypovolemic, cardiogenic, and anaphylactic states, can precipitate DIC. Hypotension, hypoxia, and acidosis lead to poor perfusion and increased venous stasis, which may promote coagulation. Head injuries and crush injuries release large amounts of tissue factors that can activate the coagulation cascade. A similar etiology is involved in DIC related to acute intravascular hemolysis as may occur in transfusion of mismatched blood or hemolysis of other etiologies such as in malaria or drowning. Here, release of red cell contents into the circulation stimulates the coagulation system and induces a consumptive coagulopathy.

A somewhat different mechanism is involved when a snake bite precipitates DIC. The venom of certain poisonous snakes (rattlesnakes, copperheads, and water moccasins) contains proteases, which convert fibrinogen to fibrin. Bites from these snakes provoke acute DIC through direct action on fibrinogen. Other venoms bring about DIC by activation of other clotting factors (e.g., *Echis carinatus carinatus* and the Russell's viper).

Diagnosis

How does one recognize the clinical syndrome of DIC among this vast array of underlying disorders? Clinical presentations may vary, and a key factor is a high degree of suspicion based upon knowledge of the disorders that accompany the coagulopathy. Sometimes DIC adds no additional symptoms to the underlying disorder and is suspected only because of its known association with the disease.

Pediatric patients with DIC usually present with bleeding at one or more sites. It may be in the form of petechiae or ecchymoses of the skin or mucous membranes. Epistaxis or hemoptysis may be present, there may be oozing from mucous membranes or from sites of venipuncture, or there may be bleeding from the gastrointestinal or genitourinary tracts. When thrombosis is part of the clinical picture, one may observe diffuse phlebitides as well as acral cyanosis or further manifestations of ischemia. Several other manifestations of fibrin deposition leading to organ dysfunction have been suggested as being secondary to DIC, including acute renal failure and adult respiratory distress syndrome (ARDS). There is, however, little conclusive evidence that these dysfunctions result from the fibrin deposition of DIC.

When DIC is suspected, various laboratory tests can help in confirming the diagnosis. Generally, in fulminant DIC, the diagnosis is not a difficult one to make. In most cases, a blood count will reveal thrombocytopenia (platelet count less than 150,000/mm^3) and may indicate anemia. Examination of the peripheral smear may show a microangiopathic hemolytic process (i.e., red cell fragments or schistocytes) in approximately 50 percent of patients with acute

DIC. It should be noted that this sign can be present in other disorders, such as renal diseases and various vasculitides and in the presence of artificial heart valves and that DIC can be present in the absence of this sign. Next, a "coagulation profile" must be obtained. The prothrombin time (PT), which measures the intactness of the extrinsic pathway; the partial thromboplastin time (PTT), which measures the intrinsic pathway; and the thrombin time (TT), which measures the conversion of fibrinogen to fibrin, will all be prolonged in most cases of DIC because of depletion of multiple coagulation factors. Caution is indicated in analyzing these tests, because in selected cases, one or more may be in the normal range. This may be because the production of clotting factors is keeping pace with their consumption, leaving levels in the normal range, or because early on, the high biologic activity of certain activated clotting factors may actually shorten the PT or PTT, even while levels of other factors are low.

The fibrinogen level will be low (less than 150 mg/dl) in most cases of DIC. One must keep in mind, however, that fibrinogen is an acute phase reactant and may therefore be elevated in instances of inflammation or malignancy, despite the simultaneous presence of DIC. In addition, fibrinogen, as most of the coagulation factors, is produced in the liver. Thus, in liver disease where DIC may not be present, the level of fibrinogen will be decreased.

The presence of fibrinolytic degradation products (FDP) is usually considered a hallmark of DIC. However, the absence of FDP does not rule out the diagnosis, because they may be rapidly cleared by the reticuloendothelial system.

Finally, measurement of the levels of some of the clotting factors may be helpful in establishing the presence of DIC. Generally, Factors II, V, and VIII:C are measured in this context and are frequently found to be low. The finding of a low level of Factor VIII:C can be particularly helpful in distinguishing DIC from liver disease as in the latter disorder elevated Factor VIII:C levels are almost invariable. However, a normal or elevated level of Factor VIII:C may also be seen in DIC, so this does not rule out the diagnosis. Demonstration of the presence of soluble fibrin monomer in the plasma (3P Test*) may also be helpful in making the diagnosis of DIC.

---

* 3P Test refers to plasma protamine paracoagulation and depends upon the ability of protamine sulfate to precipitate fibrin monomer from plasma.

In rare cases, additional investigations, including demonstration of shortened in vivo platelet and fibrinogen survival and biopsy proven evidence of fibrin deposition in the microvasculature, may be necessary to confirm the diagnosis of DIC.

Management

In the same way that the presentation of DIC and the underlying associated disorders are varied, so too is the approach to management of this entity, with each case requiring consideration by an experienced physician. Not all cases require specific treatment. When clinical bleeding or thrombosis is not present and surgery is not contemplated, compensated DIC may be left untreated. However, in most pediatric cases, when a bleeding diathesis is involved, an attempt to modify the process becomes mandatory.

The most important therapeutic modality is to remove or treat the underlying disorder. Supportive measures such as institution of proper antimicrobial therapy, infusion of fluids, correction of acid base and electrolyte disturbances, and stabilization of cardiac status may be the only measures necessary to abolish the consumptive coagulopathy. In the case of malignancy or giant hemangioma, surgical removal, radiotherapy, or chemotherapy may be of significant benefit in diminishing or stopping the clotting process. In many instances, however, the triggering disorder cannot be corrected immediately and other approaches are necessary.

The first approach to be considered is replacement of depleted coagulation factors and platelets to hemostatic levels. This may be accomplished in the form of fresh frozen plasma (FFP, 10–15 ml/kg); platelet concentrates (1 U/ 5 kg), or cryoprecipitate (3–4 bags/10 kg) to replace fibrinogen. The idea of "feeding the fire" and enhancing intravascular coagulation by providing a fresh supply of clotting factors is a theoretical consideration only and, in practice, does not appear to have validity. In fact, many patients seem to stabilize through this method of treatment, particularly in conjunction with treatment of the underlying disorder. Factor IX concentrates, which contain activated Factors II, VII, IX, and X, should not be used, because these materials may be thrombogenic, thereby aggravating the situation.

Much debate has occurred regarding the use of heparin as therapy for DIC. The apparent paradox of giving an anticoagulant to a bleeding patient is clear. However, it is easier to understand if one remembers that by its inactivation of thrombin and other clotting factors, heparin can interrupt the coagulation process and diminish fibrinolysis. When this occurs, hemorrhage and/or thrombosis will also be decreased.

Current information suggests that heparin in conjunction with replacement therapy is effective only in very specific cases of DIC and has no effect on outcome or may be harmful in many other cases. When patients with DIC manifest evidence of fibrin deposition as in venous thrombosis, pulmonary embolism, or dermal necrosis, the use of heparin is probably indicated. Specifically, heparin has been shown to reduce morbidity and mortality associated with purpura fulminans. A treatment course of 2 to 3 weeks may be required to treat this entity. Efficacy has also been shown in several other disorders. In acute promyelocytic leukemia, heparin is successfully used in the prevention or treatment of DIC during the initial induction therapy. In this disorder, because of impaired platelet production by the bone marrow, it is important to supplement heparin therapy with platelet transfusions in order to keep the platelet count greater than 50,000 per mm^3. There is evidence to suggest that heparin may be helpful in cases of incompatible blood transfusions. Here, early institution of heparin therapy may be of value, whereas delay may allow time for irreversible damage to occur. Finally, heparin is thought to be of value in cases of giant hemangioma involving hemorrhage. It is generally palliative in this situation, and the coagulopathy may resume when heparin is discontinued unless measures have been taken to reduce the hemangioma.

When heparin is used, it may be administered as a continuous IV infusion. A loading dose of 50 to 100 U per kg, followed by a maintenance dose of 10 to 25 U per kg per hour is an appropriate dose; however, the dose must be titrated between clinical response and toxicity. Caution should be taken so that the heparin therapy does not escalate bleeding. When heparin is used, the PTT and TT cannot be used to follow the progress of the coagulopathy, because heparin interferes with these tests. Instead, response should be based on the clinical status as well as the platelet count, fibrinogen level, and the levels of specific clotting factors. All these levels should rise if the therapy is successful. A response may be seen within hours but should definitely be evident within 24 to 48 hours in most cases.

Heparin has been shown not to affect the

outcome of children with DIC secondary to septic shock. Heparin therapy has also been useless for snake bites, because proteases in the various venoms are not inactivated by heparin. For this situation, anti-venom should be used, and coagulation factors should be replaced by plasma infusion.

Other therapeutic modalities, including fibrinolytic activators and inhibitors and platelet aggregation inhibitors, have been explored as treatments for DIC, both in experimental models and in patient trials, without conclusive results. It is generally agreed that the use of fibrinolytic inhibitors, for example, epsilon aminocaproic acid (EACA),* can be dangerous, because by stopping the fibrinolytic process, there is an excessive risk of promoting thrombosis. In rare, selected cases, however, in which bleeding persists despite attempts at supportive care, replacement therapy and heparin administration, EACA may be used as a last resort, but only with simultaneous heparin infusion. The loading dose is 50 to 100 mg per kg, followed by a maintenance dose of 15 to 25 mg per kg per hour. This substance may be administered orally or intravenously. When given intravenously, it should be given slowly and should be well diluted, because rapid administration may be associated with hypotension, ventricular dysrhythmias, hypokalemia, and intravascular thromboses. In most cases, if a favorable response is not apparent within 12 to 24 hours, this therapy should be stopped.

VITAMIN K DEFICIENCY

Etiology

Vitamin K is a fat-soluble vitamin upon which the production of functional molecules of prothrombin (Factor II) as well as Factors VII, IX, and X are dependent. After one of these vitamin K dependent proteins is synthesized by the liver, certain glutamic acid residues near the N-terminal portion of the factor are carboxylated, producing γ-carboxyglutamic acid. This confers a strong negative charge, which serves to tightly bind calcium, which, in turn, promotes interaction of the clotting factor with the phospholipid surface of the platelets. Deficiency of vitamin K prevents this carboxylation and results in production of abnormal coagulation factors with impaired clotting activity.

Vitamin K is acquired via dietary sources, particularly leafy, green vegetables. The daily requirement is probably less than 1 mcg per kg of body weight, an amount that is easily obtained in most normal diets. In addition, vitamin K is synthesized by bacterial flora and absorbed from the colon.

Deficiency of Vitamin K can occur because of a generalized malabsorption syndrome. Celiac disease, cystic fibrosis, sprue, chronic gastroenteritis, excessive intestinal resections, or protracted diarrhea of any cause can result in vitamin K deficiency.

Biliary obstruction, either intrahepatic or extrahepatic, may also cause vitamin K deficiency because of the absence of bile salts to aid in absorption of this fat-soluble vitamin. Disorders of this nature may include biliary atresia and chronic hemolytic anemias, with secondary gallstone formation and obstructive jaundice. In these disorders, vitamin K malabsorption may coexist with malabsorption of the other fat-soluble vitamins, namely vitamins D, A, and E.

In the absence of a malabsorption syndrome, vitamin K deficiency occurs in patients who have inadequate oral intake and who are concomitantly on broad-spectrum antibiotics that may alter the intestinal flora. Postoperative patients or patients receiving IV hyperalimentation to which vitamin K has not been added are examples of cases in which hemostatic defects due to vitamin K deficiency may occur.

The symptoms of vitamin K deficiency may range from easy bruisability to large ecchymoses, mucous membrane bleeding, or oozing from venipuncture or surgical sites.

Special mention must be made of hemorrhagic disease of the newborn. This category of vitamin K deficiency occurs because of low vitamin K stores and hepatic immaturity, leading to marked deficiencies of Factors II, VII, IX, and X. Several circumstances may predispose to hemorrhagic disease of the newborn. Prematurity accentuates hepatic immaturity. Breast-feeding promotes vitamin K deficiency, because human breast milk supplies much less vitamin K than does either cow's milk or proprietary formulas. Breast-feeding may also delay the colonization of the gastrointestinal tract by bacteria. The infant in whom feeding is delayed or in whom vomiting or diarrhea may occur or to whom broad-spectrum antibiotics may be administered is a likely victim of this hemorrhagic tendency. In addition, infants whose mothers have taken coumarin or anticonvulsants (particularly diphenylhydantoin) are at high risk for hemorrhagic disease of the

---

* Amicar–Lederle Labs, Wayne, New Jersey.

newborn. When possible, these mothers should have vitamin K supplements administered to them during late pregnancy.

Today, because of the wide acceptance of prophylactic administration of vitamin K to neonates, the incidence of hemorrhagic disease of the newborn is quite low. It may still occur, however, because vitamin K administration may occasionally be overlooked. Usually, one or more of the predisposing factors just mentioned are present. In such cases, bleeding, which may be severe, occurs most commonly on the second or third day of life. Vitamin K deficiency is one of the major causes of bleeding in otherwise healthy infants. It may manifest as large cephalohematomas, bleeding from the umbilical stump or after circumcision, large ecchymoses, or intramuscular hemorrhages. Intracranial bleeding may also occur.

A delayed form of this condition has occurred occasionally in infants in whom the combination of gastroenteritis, prolonged antibiotic therapy, and breast-feeding has been present. These infants have had hemorrhagic manifestations secondary to vitamin K deficiency, which has responded to administration of the vitamin.

The final cause of vitamin K deficiency to be considered is coumarin-induced deficiency. Coumarin is a vitamin K antagonist that prevents γ-carboxylation. Rarely in the pediatric age group, patients are treated with coumarin for pulmonary embolus or deep vein thrombosis. In these cases, difficulties may arise in the therapeutic dosage regulation. More commonly, accidental ingestions of the medication of an adult household member or of warfarin-containing rat poison may occur. Hemorrhagic symptoms may be delayed for up to 2 to 3 days. Symptoms may be prevented by early administration of vitamin K.

Laboratory Diagnosis

The laboratory diagnosis of vitamin K deficiency is relatively straightforward. Generally, the PT is most prolonged, because, of the four vitamin K dependent clotting factors, Factor VII has the shortest half-life. As the vitamin K deficient situation persists, the PTT will also become prolonged. Specific factor assays can be helpful, because vitamin K dependent factors such as Factor VII will be low, whereas others such as Factor V will be in the normal range, as will the fibrinogen level and the platelet count.

Treatment

The treatment of vitamin K deficiency depends upon the severity of the symptoms. When bleeding is not immediately life threatening, vitamin K, in a dose of 1 to 10 mg (depending upon the patient's size), may be administered parenterally. It is administered in the water soluble form either by intramuscular (IM) or IV injection.

In cases in which severe hemostatic impairment prohibits intramuscular injections or when severity of hemorrhagic symptoms demands more immediate availability, slow IV administration is indicated. Rare anaphylactic reactions have occurred with this form of therapy; epinephrine should be available when vitamin K is given by this route. Hemostasis should improve within hours, and coagulation assays will usually return to normal within 24 hours if vitamin K deficiency is indeed the only problem. It should be noted that in cases in which coumarin overdose is the cause of vitamin K deficiency and when the overdose occurs in a patient receiving coumarin for therapeutic reasons, administration of vitamin K may cause the patient to be refractory to further coumarin for days to weeks. In such cases or when more rapid reversal of the hemostatic defect is necessary than will be afforded by vitamin K administration, fresh frozen plasma (FFP), in a dose of 10 to 15 ml per kg of body weight should raise the concentrations of the deficient clotting factors to hemostatic levels. The dose may have to be repeated at 4- to 6-hour intervals. Vitamin K can be administered immediately, along with the first infusion of FFP, when therapeutic coumarin is not involved.

The prothrombin complex concentrates, which supply the vitamin K dependent clotting factors, should not be used unless there is serious hemorrhage that is uncontrolled by FFP and vitamin K. This is because of the greater risk of viral hepatitis with these materials and the possibility of thromboembolic complications.

LIVER DISEASE

Liver disease, an uncommon occurrence in the pediatric age group, has long been associated with defects in coagulation. Although most patients with severe liver disease have abnormalities in their hemostatic functions, only a few actually undergo bleeding. The diseased liver participates in hemostatic abnormalities by impaired synthesis of coagulation factors, defective clearance of products of clotting and fibrinolysis, quantitative or qualitative changes in platelets, and induction of disseminated intravascular coagulation or fibrinolysis.

Pathophysiology

Impaired synthesis of clotting factors plays a major role in the coagulopathy associated with liver disease. The levels of the vitamin K dependent Factors (II, VII, IX, and X) are often prominently reduced because of this, with Factor VII showing the earliest and greatest reduction because of its short half-life (approximately 2 hours). Occasionally, vitamin K deficiency is simultaneously present as in obstructive jaundice or when other clinical situations predispose to this. Administration of vitamin K in these cases may partially and transiently improve the coagulopathy; however, failure of complete response is a good indication of hepatocellular disease causing defective synthesis.

The non–vitamin K dependent Factors V, IX, XI, XII, and XIII are also synthesized by the hepatocytes, and these factors are generally low in patients with liver disease.

Fibrinogen represents a special situation. Although it is synthesized by the liver, it is an acute phase reactant and tends to increase in situations of infection and inflammation. Therefore, in some instances of liver disease, the fibrinogen level may be increased, whereas in others, it may be normal or decreased. In either case, fibrinogen produced by the diseased liver is often abnormal. This is most commonly recognized by a prolonged TT, which measures the time required for fibrinogen to form a fibrin clot after adding thrombin to plasma. The abnormal fibrinogen resembles fetal fibrinogen, because it has an increased number of sialic acid residues, having the effect of delaying polymerization of fibrin monomers.

Factor VIII:C also represents a special situation, because it is found in the plasma of patients with liver disease in levels as high as 20 times normal. The explanation for this is not entirely clear. Apparently, Factor VIII:C also acts as an acute phase reactant and is elevated in states of infection or inflammation. Although there is evidence for its synthesis by the hepatocytes, these high levels of Factor VIII:C are taken to imply synthesis in organs other than the liver.

In addition to the clotting factors, hemostasis is controlled partially by naturally occurring inhibitors of coagulation and fibrinolysis. These are also produced by the liver and are decreased in quantity by liver disease. Thus, antithrombin III and antiplasmin deficiencies may be severe in hepatocellular disease and may also contribute to defects in hemostasis.

In addition to decreased and aberrant synthesis of clotting factors, evidence suggests that catabolism of the clotting factors may be increased in liver disease and that a further decrease in the plasma levels of these factors may occur through losses into ascitic fluid or via bleeding.

Another aspect of the hemostatic derangement associated with liver disease involves platelet number and function. Thrombocytopenia is often associated with liver disorders. Splenomegaly and sequestering of platelets are responsible for perhaps half of these cases. In other cases, a viral agent may directly suppress bone marrow formation of platelets. Though rarely applicable to pediatric patients, it should be noted that chronic alcohol consumption seems to directly suppress marrow thrombopoiesis. In other cases of liver disease, the cause of thrombocytopenia is not known. Finally, there is evidence to suggest that platelets may be functionally defective in many cases of liver disease.

The liver plays an important role in removing from the circulation activated clotting factors, plasminogen activators, and products of the fibrinolytic system. Thus, damage to the liver may aggravate clotting and lysis, lead to large amounts of fibrinolytic degradation products in the circulation, and predispose to disseminated intravascular coagulation. Whether the coagulopathy of liver disease is related to or caused by DIC is a controversial issue. Certainly, the picture of hypofibrinogenemia, thrombocytopenia, prolonged PT, PTT, and TT, and the presence of FDP may be common to both. Often, it is not possible to separate the two syndromes.

Clinical Manifestations

As mentioned previously, although there are many hemostatic abnormalities associated with liver disease, only a small percentage of patients with these disorders manifest clinical bleeding. The gastrointestinal tract is the most common site of bleeding. Usually the source is a local lesion such as gastritis, varices, or a peptic ulcer.

In addition, patients may manifest petechiae and ecchymoses, gingival bleeding, epistaxis, and menorrhagia. When hemostasis is challenged by surgery or trauma, severe bleeding may ensue.

Laboratory Diagnosis

The laboratory findings in liver disease vary with the cause and severity of the underlying disorder. Patients with obstructive jaundice generally develop a state of vitamin K deficiency with prolonged PT and PTT and deficiencies in Factors II, VII, IX, and X. Patients with acute or chronic hepatocellular disease may show a more widespread deficiency of the clotting factors, depending upon the severity of the disease. In severe decompensated disease, one may see prolonged PT, PTT, and TT, decreased levels of all the clotting factors except Factor VIII:C and, rarely, the presence of FDP.

At times, the clinical picture and initial laboratory results found in DIC, vitamin K deficiency, and liver disease may look similar. Here, analysis of the plasma levels of certain individual coagulation factors can greatly aid in distinguishing between the various coagulopathies (Table 50–2). Factor V will generally be decreased in liver disease and DIC but should be normal in vitamin K deficiency. Factor VIII:C will usually be elevated in liver disease, may be decreased in DIC, and is approximately normal in vitamin K deficiency. However, Factor VIII:C is occasionally normal or elevated in DIC. It is sometimes impossible to be certain whether a patient with known hepatic dysfunction has superadded DIC.

Treatment

Treatment of the coagulation abnormalities in liver disease should include the administra-tion of parenteral vitamin K (IM or IV), in a dose of 1 to 10 mg, depending upon the patient's weight. This may produce a partial or temporary improvement in hemostatic factors. Patients with chronic liver disease may receive maintenance therapy, with vitamin K administered at regular intervals. Other prophylactic measures may be beneficial, such as the reduction of gastric acidity with H_2 receptor antagonists in patients who are prone to upper gastrointestinal hemorrhage.

Further therapy is indicated only if the patient must have a surgical procedure or shows serious bleeding. In the former case, the patient can be prepared by infusion of FFP, in a dose of 10 to 20 ml per kg of body weight at 4- to 6-hour intervals, depending upon the necessity and the limitation of the patient's fluid tolerance. For the latter case, replacement therapy may be effected with packed red blood cells and FFP. Platelet transfusions may be helpful in cases in which platelets are qualitatively or quantitatively deficient. Local measures to control bleeding may be indicated. For upper gastrointestinal hemorrhage, iced saline lavage, balloon compression, or local arterial infusions of vasopressin may be lifesaving maneuvers.

Prothrombin complex concentrates have been used in the replacement therapy of bleeding patients with liver disease. They are extremely hazardous in this situation, because they contain activated clotting factors that cannot be cleared by the malfunctioning liver. Thus, they have been known to cause severe DIC and should not be given to patients with liver disease.

Despite the possibility of DIC contributing to the coagulopathy of liver disease, there is no evidence that the use of heparin improves the clinical situation in these cases. Similarly, antifibrinolytic agents have been advocated for use in liver disease when fibrinolysis is believed to be a factor contributing to bleeding. Again, there is no good evidence for clinical efficacy,

Table 50–2. Comparison of Laboratory Values in Acquired Coagulopathies

	DIC	Vitamin K Deficiency	Liver Disease	"Washout"
Prothrombin time (PT)	↑	↑	↑	↑
Partial thromboplastin time (PTT)	↑	N,↑	↑	↑
Thrombin time (TT)	↑	N	↑	N,↑
Fibrinogen	↓	N	↓,N,↑	N,↓
Fibrin degradation products (FDP)	↑	N	N,↑	N
Factor V	↓,N	N	↓	↓
Factor VII	↓	↓	↓	N,↓
Factor VIII:C	↓,N,↑	N	↑	↓
Platelet count	↓	N	N,↓	↓

↑ = increased, ↓ = decreased, and N = normal.

and there is the danger of thrombotic complications when these agents are used.

THE MASSIVELY TRANSFUSED PATIENT

Transfusion of large quantities of stored blood into an actively bleeding patient can lead to further alteration of hemostasis in the already bleeding patient. These alterations result from loss and inadequate replacement of platelets and certain factors, the so called "washout phenomenon." A large degree of blood loss and replacement, approximately 1 to 2 times the individual's blood volume, is necessary before these changes become apparent.

If patients with excessive bleeding are transfused with packed red blood cells and FFP, the levels of most of the clotting factors will be reasonably maintained. Stored whole blood is not appropriate for replacement, because Factors V and VIII:C, as well as platelets, are labile under the conditions in which blood products are stored (4°C). Factor V may fall to low levels (approximately 15 percent of normal) after 21 days of storage. Factor VIII:C may fall to levels as low as 20 percent within 48 hours of storage at 4°C. This level may not be sufficient for hemostasis; however, it should be remembered that because Factor VIII:C is an acute phase reactant, it is generally elevated in stressed patients in whom DIC is not a concomitant factor. Thus, the overall level of Factor VIII:C usually remains hemostatic, but it can fall lower than the 25 to 30 percent required.

Blood stored at 4°C is almost devoid of normal platelet function by 48 hours, because platelet function is markedly altered by refrigeration and storage. Thus, massively transfused patients are at risk for dilutional thrombocytopenia. When the platelet count falls below 75,000 per mm³, bleeding may be aggravated. Factors other than dilutional, such as hypotension, hypoxia, and tissue necrosis, leading to DIC, can exacerbate thrombocytopenia in the briskly bleeding patient.

Another consideration in the massively transfused patient is citrate toxicity. Donor blood is anticoagulated with citrate, which acts by chelating the ionized calcium necessary for coagulation. Very rapid transfusions can theoretically cause marked hypocalcemia in the recipient. In practice, this is rarely a problem except in newborns and patients with liver disease in whom toxic levels are more easily achieved (citrate being metabolized in the liver).

Diagnosis

In terms of diagnosis of this disorder, the setting of a patient with excessive bleeding requiring massive transfusion to maintain blood volume is necessary. The PT, PTT, and TT may be prolonged. The platelet count should be decreased and may continue to fall for 1 or 2 days after blood replacement. Factors V and VIII:C may be found in the ranges previously mentioned. Other factors such as Factor VII and fibrinogen should be in the normal range if FFP has been given unless DIC is also present. In the latter situation, FDP may be present.

Treatment

Treatment of the massively transfused patient includes local measures to stop the bleeding. It must be understood that loss of blood must not be replaced by packed red blood cells alone. If this is done, the coagulopathy will be exaggerated, because deficiency of all clotting factors will occur. Along with proper replacement of red cells and FFP, platelet transfusions should be given to keep the platelet count above 100,000 per mm³. Cryoprecipitate, with its concentrated Factor VIII:C and fibrinogen, is useful when massive transfusion results in a Factor VIII:C level of less than 30 percent. The latter two therapeutic modalities must be considered when blood loss and replacement approach the patient's total blood volume. Because a person's blood volume is approximately 80 ml per kg, it is prudent to remember that in a small child, the "washout phenomenon" may occur with the loss of a relatively small volume of blood.

In summary, the four most commonly acquired coagulopathies have been discussed. By appropriate laboratory testing it may be determined which of these four conditions is causing bleeding in a specific patient. Accurate diagnosis is essential, because treatment of each disorder is specific.

CASE PRESENTATION

M.F., a 10-year-old black female with biliary atresia was admitted to the hospital complaining of tarry stools for 3 days and having vomited bright red blood on the day of admission. Past medical history was significant for progressive jaundice, first noted at 3 weeks of age. At 14 months of age, an exploratory laparotomy revealed extrahepatic biliary atresia. Corrective surgery was not attempted. Between the ages of 1 and 10 years, the child was hospitalized many times for episodes of epistaxis and infection. One year prior to admission, the child had presented with melena and hematemesis. An upper gastrointestinal series at that time revealed esophageal varices. Past history was also remarkable for rickets, treated with vitamin D and calcium. The patient's medications at the time of the present admission included:

Vitamin D, 500,000 U daily by mouth
Aldactone, 25 mg t.i.d. by mouth
Multivitamin tablet daily
Vitamin K, 2 mg IM every 2 weeks

Physical Examination

Physical examination revealed an alert, oriented, well-developed child. Her temperature was 38°C, heart rate was 98 beats/min and respiration rate was 18 breaths/min. Blood pressure was 100/60 mm Hg. She weighed 33 kg (72 1b).

The skin was jaundiced, the sclera were icteric, and the lungs were clear. Examination of the heart revealed a grade 2–3 systolic murmur at the left lower sternal border. The abdomen was distended. The liver, palpable 11 cm below the right costal margin was firm and not tender. The spleen was palpable 8.5 cm below the left costal margin. Examination for shifting dullness was suspicious for ascites. The lower extremities showed 2+ edema, and the neurologic examination was normal.

Laboratory Data

Hemoglobin = 7.1 gm/dl, hematocrit = 22.5 percent, platelet count = 200,000/mm³,
White blood count = 6,400/mm³, 75 percent neutrophils, 5 percent band forms, and 20 percent lymphocytes
Urinalysis—trace protein, 3+ bilirubin, 2+ blood
Serum glutamic–oxaloacetic transaminase (SGOT) = 200 IU
Serum glutamic–pyruvic transaminase (SGPT) = 66 IU
Akaline phosphatase = 450 IU
Total bilirubin = 14.4 mg/dl, direct bilirubin = 10.3 mg/dl
Total protein = 4.7 gm/dl, albumin = 1.5 gm/dl
Prothrombin time (PT) = 15.5 sec, control = 12.7 sec
Partial thromboplastin time (PTT) = 78 sec, control = 45 sec
Thrombin time (TT) = 20 sec, control = 18 sec
Fibrinogen = 170 mg/dl
Fibrinolytic degradation products (FDP) = 1.69 μg/ml (normal < 8 μg/ml
Factor V = 37 percent, Factor VII = 30 percent, Factor VIII = 515 percent

Problem List

The patient's management was directed toward the following aspects:

Upper Gastrointestinal Bleed

Iced saline lavage, performed through a nasogastric (NG) tube, continued to show bloody return. Endoscopy revealed large, actively bleeding esophageal varices as well as gastric varices, which were not actively bleeding. Balloon tamponade was attempted with a pediatric Sengstaken-Blakemore tube. Bleeding was temporarily diminished but resumed soon after. The child underwent a superior mesenteric arteriogram, which revealed massive varices in the esophagus and stomach. A catheter was left in place for selective vasopressin (Pitressin) administration at 12 U/hr. Following this, bleeding subsided and the Pitressin infusion was tapered over 36 hours, without recurrence of gross hemorrhage. The hematocrit stabilized at 30 percent.

Coagulopathy

The initial coagulation profile was characteristic of liver disease, with possible superimposed vitamin K deficiency. Five mg of vitamin K were immediately given IM. Six hours after admission, the platelet count was noted to have dropped to 29,000/mm³. Coagulation profile at the time revealed:

PT = 18 sec, control = 11.5 sec
PTT = 114.5 sec, control = 45 sec
TT = 29.5 sec, control = 15.2 sec
Fibrinogen = 117 mg/dl
FDP = 108.16 μg/ml

These results were indicative of DIC. The child was transfused with a total of 12 U of red blood cells, 10 U of platelets, and 6 U of FFP until the bleeding subsided. Six hours post-arteriography, studies showed:

PT = 17.7 sec, control = 11.7 sec
PTT = 69.5 sec, control = 45.5 sec
TT = 23 sec, control = 16.8 sec
Fibrinogen = 210 mg/dl
FDP = 13.52 μg/dl
Hematocrit = 30 percent, platelet count = 106,000

Upon discharge from the hospital 1 week later, the platelet count was 220,000/mm³, and the coagulation profile was similar to that on admission. The child was scheduled to return to the clinic every 2 weeks for IM injection of 2 mg vitamin K.

Fluid and Electrolytes

A bladder catheter and central venous line were placed early in the course to accurately monitor the patient's fluid status. Care was taken to avoid both overexpansion of the vascular space and hypovolemia.

SUGGESTED READING

Bick, R.L.: Disseminated intravascular coagulation and related syndromes: etiology, pathophysiology, diagnosis, and management. Am. J. Hematol. 5:265, 1978.
Corrigan, J.J.: Disseminated intravascular coagulopathy. Pediatr. Rev. 1:37, 1979.

Feinstein, D.I.: Diagnosis and management of disseminated intravascular coagulation: the role of heparin therapy. Blood. 60:284, 1982.

Flute, P.T.: Clotting abnormalities in liver disease. *In* Popper, H., and Schaffner, F. (eds.): Progress in Liver Disease, Vol. VI. New York, Grune & Stratton, Inc. 1979, pp. 301–312.

Karpatkin, M.: Screening tests in hemostasis. Pediatr. Clin. North Am. 27:831, 1980.

Lechner, K., Niessner, H., and Thaler, E.: Coagulation abnormalities in liver disease. Semin. Thromb. Hemostas. 4:40, 1977.

Merskey, C.: DIC identification and management. Hosp. Pract. December 1982, pp. 83–94.

Owens, C.A.: Coagulation disorders associated with hepatocellular disease. *In* Lusher, J.M., and Barnhart, M.I. (eds.): Acquired Bleeding Disorders in Children. Abnormalities of Hemostasis. New York, Masson Publishing USA, Inc., 1981, pp. 41–59.

Wintrobe, M., et al.: Clinical Hematology, 8th ed. Philadelphia, Lea & Febiger, 1981, pp. 1206–1246.

Nursing Process for Patient Care:

Acquired Disorders of Hemostasis

Disorders of hemostasis are not uncommon occurrences in the intensive care unit (ICU). Shock, hypoxia, sepsis, and acidosis may trigger disseminated intravascular coagulation (DIC). Inadequate nutrition as the consequence of either poor intake or malabsorption, particularly if associated with the use of broad-spectrum antibiotics, may result in a bleeding diathesis secondary to vitamin K deficiency. Patients requiring massive transfusions may develop a coagulopathy as a result of the "washout phenomenon." Children with liver disease may have insufficient synthesis of coagulation factors and may present with bleeding.

HEMATOLOGIC

Assess, Monitor, and Document

Bleeding: oozing from puncture sites, petechiae, ecchymoses, epistaxis, hemoptysis, gastrointestinal, genitourinary
Thrombosis: purpura fulminans, phlebitis, acrocyanosis

Laboratory data: platelet count, coagulation profile (PT, PTT, TT, FDP)

Anticipate

Alteration in hematologic status
  Bleeding
  Shock
  Thrombus formation

Embolic phenomenon
Organ dysfunction related to ischemia: pulmonary, renal

CARDIOVASCULAR

Assess, Monitor, and Document

Heart rate
Rhythm
Blood pressure: arterial, central venous
Peripheral perfusion: capillary filling, skin condition

Color
Level of consciousness
Urine output, including specific gravity
Fluid intake

Anticipate

Shock
  Tachycardia
  Hypotension
  Poor peripheral perfusion

Restlessness, agitation
Decreased urine output
Cyanosis
Cardiac arrest

RESPIRATORY

Assess, Monitor, and Document

Respiratory rate and pattern: work of breathing
Breath sounds

Color
Secretions: amount, description
Arterial blood gases

Anticipate

Respiratory insufficiency
   Tachypnea
   Tachycardia
   Decreased breath sounds
   Rhonchi and/or rales, rub

Increased secretions
Cyanosis
Arterial blood gases: hypoxemia, hypercarbia, acidemia

RENAL

Assess, Monitor, and Document

Weight
Urine output, including specific gravity
Blood pressure
Fluid intake

Serum: electrolytes, BUN, creatinine, osmolality
Urine: electrolytes, osmolality

Anticipate

Acute renal failure
   Decreased urine output
   Increased weight
   Increased blood pressure

Alteration in laboratory data: hyponatremia, hyperkalemia, increased BUN, creatinine, and osmolality

RESPONSE OF CHILD

Assess, Monitor, and Document

Developmental level: cognitive, motor, verbal, fears, tasks
Behavioral response: anxious, fearful, aggressive, compliant

Response to nursing interventions

Anticipate

Emotional distress
Inability to cope
Disruption in normal growth and development

RESPONSE OF FAMILY

Assess, Monitor, and Document

Behavioral response: anxious, fearful, angry
Level of understanding of child's condition

Expected outcome
Response to nursing interventions

Anticipate

Inability to cope
Family crisis

MIND SET

Assess

Hematologic status
Cardiovascular status
Respiratory status

Renal status
Response of child and family

Anticipate

Alteration in hematologic status
   Bleeding
   Thrombotic/embolic phenomenon
Alteration in cardiovascular status
   Shock
Alteration in respiratory status

Pulmonary embolism
Adult respiratory distress syndrome (ARDS)
Alteration in renal status
   Acute renal failure
Emotional distress
Family crisis

INFECTIOUS

Encephalitis

ANNE A. GERSHON, M.D.

Infectious encephalitis is an acute inflammatory reaction of the brain, caused by a viral infection. The disease may be the direct result of viral replication in the central nervous system (CNS) (e.g., due to herpes simplex virus, HSV) or a complication following a viral infection (as after measles), presumably secondary to an abnormal immune response.

Epidemic forms of encephalitis are unusual in the United States. When they occur, they are most often caused by arthropod-borne or arboviruses, including Eastern, Western, and Venezuelan equine encephalitis viruses, St. Louis encephalitis virus, and California virus. Mumps virus, once a major cause of encephalitis and meningoencephalitis in the United States, has virtually disappeared with the widespread use of mumps vaccine.

The clinical features of arbovirus encephalitides are similar, although Eastern equine tends to be more devastating than the others. Typically, the patient presents with the abrupt onset of high fever, headache, nuchal rigidity, and vomiting, soon followed by drowsiness or coma and focal or generalized seizures. Focal neurologic signs may also be present. The cerebrospinal fluid (CSF) is under increased pressure and exhibits pleocytosis, at first with a predominance of polymorphonuclear cells, and later with increased lymphocytes. The protein is usually elevated, and the glucose is normal.

There is no specific treatment for these forms of encephalitis. Eastern equine encephalitis is associated with a 75 percent mortality rate; the others carry a 5 to 20 percent mortality rate.

The most common nonepidemic form of encephalitis in the United States is that caused by HSV type I. This is a disease that may be gradual or fulminant in onset and, if untreated,

carries a mortality rate of 80 percent. Survivors are often severely neurologically impaired. HSV encephalitis occurs most often in people older than 15 years of age, but it may also occur in children and, occasionally, in infants. In the latter case, it must be distinguished from neonatal HSV infection (caused by HSV type II) with encephalitis.

HSV type I has a predilection for involvement of the temporal or parietal lobes of the brain, and the illness often presents with personality change, focal seizures, and fever. The spinal fluid may be normal or may show an increase in pressure, cells, and/or protein. Laboratory tests such as electroencephalogram (EEG) and CAT scan will usually indicate a unilateral mass effect, involving the temporal and/or parietal lobe. Patients with HSV encephalitis usually progress from lethargy to semicoma to coma within hours to days. Early treatment with the anti-viral drug adenine arabinoside (ARA-A) is associated with a decrease in mortality and morbidity. Successful therapy is most often achieved in patients treated during the lethargic state and in those younger than 30 years of age.

Several other forms of acute infectious encephalitis deserve mention. Mumps virus causes both an acute encephalitis, probably related to direct invasion of the CNS, and a less common post–infectious encephalitis, similar to that which may follow measles and chickenpox. Mumps encephalitis is usually self-limited. When not associated with parotitis, it may present a diagnostic problem and resemble acute bacterial meningitis. Post–infectious viral encephalitides, such as those following measles, rubella, and chickenpox, tend to be severe and are usually associated with high morbidity and mortality rates. Characteristically, they occur 5 to 10 days after the onset of the original viral illness. Infectious mononucleosis, caused by the Epstein-Barr (EB) virus, is rarely associated with an encephalitis that is part of the illness itself. Encephalitis due to rabies virus is rare in the United States; it usually can be related to prior contact with a rabid animal (e.g., a bat or skunk). Toxoplasmosis may occasionally be associated with an encephalitic syndrome, particularly in immunosuppressed patients.

Chronic viral encephalitides include those caused by the so-called slow viruses (e.g., kuru, seen in New Guinea: Creutzfeld-Jakob disease, a rare dementia that occurs in adults; and progressive multifocal leukoencephalopathy (PML), which presents in immunocompromised patients). Measles virus has also been associated with subacute sclerosing panencephalitis (SSPE), observed most often in children who experienced measles before the age of 2 years. With the widespread use of measles vaccine, SSPE has become rare. Patients with SSPE undergo gradual intellectual and motor deterioration, progressing to dementia and death. A similar illness attributed to rubella virus has been described in long-term survivors of the congenital rubella syndrome. In both cases, it appears that the disease is due to abnormal persistence of the virus in the CNS.

PATHOPHYSIOLOGY

Arbovirus infections, which are mosquito-borne, tend to occur in epidemic form during warm months of the year, when mosquitos are prevalent. The infection in man is initiated following the bite of a mosquito when the virus invades first the blood, followed by lymphoid, and then neural tissue. HSV encephalitis may be due to primary or recurrent HSV infection, the latter being due to reactivation of latent HSV. HSV type I remains latent in cervical sensory ganglia following primary infection. Mechanisms concerning how and why latent HSV reactivates and why, in some cases, the CNS is invaded are poorly understood. There seems to be no relationship between a history or previous facial HSV (e.g., fever blisters) and the development of HSV encephalitis.

In all types of acute viral encephalitis, the brain pathology is similar, showing edema, petechial hemorrhages, necrosis, inclusion bodies, cellular infiltration, and neuronal degeneration. In SSPE and post–infectious encephalitides, demyelination is the rule.

DIAGNOSIS AND DIFFERENTIAL DIAGNOSIS

The diagnosis of acute viral encephalitis can usually be made on clinical grounds. The patient characteristically manifests fever, a change in the state of consciousness, nuchal rigidity, headache, cranial nerve palsies, seizures, and abnormal CSF. The presence of mucosal HSV infection is not a diagnostic sign of HSV encephalitis. Differentiation between arboviral and HSV encephalitis first requires investigation to determine whether there is focal involvement of the brain. This is best accomplished by EEG and a CAT scan. Despite the availability and sensitivity of CAT scanning, however, the diagnosis of HSV encephalitis cannot be made securely, even if focal involvement is found. Biopsy of the focal area of the involved brain is required. In one study involving more than 100 patients who presented with characteristic signs of HSV encephalitis, the brain biopsy was positive for HSV in only approximately 50 percent. Other illnesses with which it was confused included vascular disease, brain abscess, cryptococcal infection, tumor, toxic encephalopathy, toxoplasmosis, Reye's syndrome, tuberculosis, and other viral encephalitides (Coxsackie, mumps, SSPE, St. Louis, post-influenza, infectious mononucleosis, and lymphocytic choriomeningitis). In more than half the patients who underwent brain biopsy and did not have HSV encephalitis, the biopsy was important in identifying the actual diagnosis. The rate of false-negative results of brain biopsy and morbidity from the biopsy itself were minimal (2–4 percent). Until a better test for HSV encephalitis becomes available (e.g., demonstration of HSV antigen in CSF), brain biopsy remains crucial for diagnosis. In addition to the recognition of HSV encephalitis so that anti-viral treatment may be given, it is also important to determine or rule out other potentially treatable conditions (e.g., brain abscess). Clinical response (or lack thereof) to ARA-A cannot be used as a diagnostic criterion for the presence or absence of HSV encephalitis.

To document arboviral encephalitis, culture of the CSF (or brain if a biopsy is done or the illness is fatal) should be performed to try to isolate a virus. Acute and convalescent serum specimens should be studied for an antibody response to the arboviruses that might presumably be involved. These tests may be performed through state health departments. Prior to collecting specimens, it is important to discuss the patient with the laboratory staff so that the specimens are collected and transported properly.

A variety of tests may implicate other agents as causative of encephalitis. For example, SSPE is associated with high measles antibody titers in serum and CSF; mumps, even without parotitis, is often accompanied by an increase in serum amylase. Infectious mononucleosis may often be diagnosed quickly by a monospot test; if this is negative and the diagnosis is still considered, specific antibody responses to EB virus may be looked for in serum. Reye's syndrome, which may be confused with viral encephalitis, is associated with elevated serum transaminase levels, but a liver biopsy may be necessary to make an accurate diagnosis. Skin tests for tuberculosis (as well as chest x-rays) are often negative in tuberculous meningitis; thus, treatment with isoniazid and rifampin may have to be instituted on a presumptive basis in certain patients when a specific diagnosis has not yet been made. CSF culture should yield mycobacteria within 4 to 6 weeks in such cases, and a repeat tuberculin test is usually positive. In cases of suspected brain abscess, bacterial culture, both aerobic and anaerobic, should be performed on the brain biopsy specimen. Blood cultures may also be helpful in identifying a causative organism. Cryptococcal infection is best diagnosed by examining CSF for presence of the fungal antigen.

A blood lead level is helpful in assessing whether lead encephalopathy is present. Rabies is diagnosed by history of an animal bite or scratch, serum antibody titers, and pathologic examination of brain tissue. Toxoplasmosis is diagnosed by studying antibody in paired serum samples and also by microscopic analysis of brain biopsy material.

TREATMENT

Nonspecific

Supportive therapy such as fluid and electrolyte balance, monitoring of intracranial pressure (ICP), maintenance of respiratory function, if indicated, and prevention of decubiti all play an important part in the eventual outcome of the patient.

Specific

There is no specific treatment for arboviral or postinfectious encephalitides. Specific therapy is available for HSV encephalitis. ARA-A,

an inhibitor of viral and host DNA, should be started after performance of the brain biopsy. It is preferable *not* to withhold the drug until results of the viral culture are available, because this may take 2 to 3 days and the outcome of HSV encephalitis is improved with early therapy. Patients who are younger than 30 years of age and who are treated prior to development of semicoma or coma have the best response to ARA-A. Toxicity to ARA-A includes nausea, vomiting, rash, tremors, and depression of the bone marrow. ARA-A should not be administered in conjunction with interferon because of an increased potential for toxicity when both drugs are given together. Long-term effects of ARA-A are unknown. The new antiviral, acyclovir, is under study for treatment of HSV encephalitis. Until data are available concerning acyclovir for treatment of this disease, ARA-A should be used, although theoretically acyclovir may be the less toxic drug.

ARA-A is administered intravenously (IV), at a dose of 15 mg per kg per day, given over a 12-hour period. The concentration of drug should not exceed 0.7 mg per ml of standard IV solution. Frequent mixing is required, because ARA-A is poorly soluble in aqueous solutions. Some patients respond quickly to ARA-A, whereas others may experience more gradual improvement. It is not uncommon for recovery to take as long as 1 year. Even with early institution of ARA-A, the total mortality of HSV encephalitis is decreased only from 80 percent to 30 percent, and, even in treated survivors, some residua are not uncommon.

CASE PRESENTATION

A healthy 16-year-old boy had the sudden onset of behavioral changes characterized by inability to study and failure to recognize his family. He also had fever, sore throat, and visual hallucinations, and he spoke incoherently.

Examination and Test Results

Physical examination was pertinent for a temperature of 104°F and nuchal rigidity. His weight was 60 kg (132 lb). Soon after presentation to the hospital emergency room, he became semicomatose and experienced a grand mal seizure. The peripheral white blood count and urinalysis were within normal limits. A lumbar puncture revealed cloudy CSF with a pressure of 200 mm H_2O. There were 300 WBC/cu mm³ (90 percent lymphocytes); the glucose was 80 mg/dl, and the protein was 100 mg/dl. An EEG showed right focal temporal slowing and spikes. A CAT scan revealed focal attenuation in the right temporal lobe. The patient was taken to the operating room, where a brain biopsy was performed under general anesthesia. At surgery, congestion and brain swelling were noted, with an area of necrosis in the right temporal area. There was no sign of tumor or brain abscess. The biopsy specimen was sent to pathology and prepared for routine light microscopy, electron microscopy, and viral culture. Spinal fluid was tested for cryptococcal antigen and cultured for viruses. Blood cultures were obtained. Acute (and later convalescent) serum samples were obtained for titers of antibody to viral agents.

Problem List

Neurologic

Increased Intracranial Pressure: A subarachnoid bolt was placed to monitor intracranial pressure (ICP) because of the patient's deteriorating mental status and evidence of cerebral edema. The initial pressure determination was 19 cm H_2O. Fluid restriction, lasix, and a hypothermia blanket were ordered. Repeat ICP measurement was 14 cm H_2O.

Seizures: Phenobarbital therapy was instituted in the emergency room and continued in the ICU. Following another seizure, dilantin was begun. Serum levels of both anticonvulsants should be routinely monitored.

Infectious

The history of fever, personality change, seizure, and altered state of consciousness in a previously healthy boy suggests the possibility of HSV encephalitis. The presence of a predominant lymphocytosis and a normal glucose in the spinal fluid support a viral process. The EEG and CAT scan indicate unilateral temporal lobe involvement, strongly suggestive of HSV encephalitis. ARA-A 15 mg/kg/day, was ordered. The dose is administered by continuous IV infusion over a 12-hour period.

Intake and Output

Because of the increase in ICP, fluid intake was restricted to two thirds maintenance. (maintenance = 2300 ml, therefore 1550 ml). The use of ARA-A often complicates fluid therapy because of the large volumes required for its infusion; the concentration of ARA-A should not exceed 0.7 mg/ml of infusate. In this child, 900 mg/day will require that approximately 1300 ml of the daily fluid total be given over 12 hours.

On Day 3 of hospitalization, the virology lab reported the growth of HSV from the brain biopsy specimen but not from the CSF. The ARA-A was continued for a 10-day course. Clinical improvement was noted on Day 7 of treatment, when the patient began to regain consciousness. Within 3 weeks of the initiation of ARA-A therapy, he was walking and beginning to speak coherently.

SUGGESTED READING

Carey, R.M. et al.: Toxoplasmosis. Am. J. Med. 54:30, 1973.

Frenkel, J.K. et al.: Immunosuppression and toxoplasmic encephalitis. Human Pathol. 6:97, 1975.

Miller, J.R. et al.: Acute viral encephalitis. Med. Clin. North Am. 56:1393, 1972.

Whitley, R.J. et al.: Adenine arabinoside: therapy of biopsy-proved herpes simplex encephalitis. N. Engl. J. Med. 297:289, 1977.

Whitley, R.J. et al.: Herpes simplex encephalitis. N. Engl. J. Med. 304:313, 1981.

Nursing Process for Patient Care:

Encephalitis

Infectious encephalitis is caused by a viral infection that produces inflammation of the brain paren-chyma. This inflammatory response alters neurologic function, and evaluation of the status of the CNS is essential to patient management. Fluid balance is important because of the potential effect of overload on intracranial pressure (ICP).

The child with encephalitis is usually impaired neurologically. Dealing with the child and the parents requires careful assessment and creative nursing strategies.

NEUROLOGIC

Assess, Monitor, and Document

Headache
Nuchal rigidity
Personality
Level of consciousness

Blood pressure
Pulse
Respiratory rate and pattern
ICP (if available)

Anticipate

Increased ICP
  Headache
  Altered level of consciousness: lethargy, stupor, coma
  Altered pupillary response
  Increased blood pressure (widening pulse pressure)

Bradycardia
Decreased respiratory rate
Altered respiratory pattern
Seizures
Focal
Generalized

INFECTIOUS PROCESS

Assess, Monitor, and Document

Temperature
The nurse should be aware of the CSF lab-oratory determinations.

Anticipate

Fever
It is important to note that a hypo-thermia blanket may be used in the man-agement of increased ICP, and fever would then be lost as a parameter.

FLUID BALANCE

Careful attention must be given to the child's intake and output. Children with encephalitis often have a fluid restriction of two-thirds maintenance. The use of ARA-A requires a large volume of fluid, which can complicate fluid therapy.

Assess, Monitor, and Document

Weight
Fluid intake: accurate administration of par-enteral fluids (use infusion pump if avail-able), accurate recording of oral fluids (if level of consciousness permits oral intake)
Urine output, including specific gravity

Anticipate

Fluid overload

RESPONSE OF CHILD

Assess, Monitor, and Document

Developmental level: tasks, fears
Behavioral response: sociable, quiet
Degree of distress

Ability to cope
Strategies to reduce stress

Anticipate

Emotional distress

RESPONSE OF FAMILY

Assess, Monitor, and Document

Behavioral response: anxious, fearful
Level of understanding of disease and child's
   condition

Expected outcome
Ability to cope

Anticipate

Fear
Distress

Inability to cope
Family crisis

MIND SET

Assess

Neurologic status
Infectious disease status

Fluid balance
Emotional response of child and family

Anticipate

Increased ICP
Seizures
Altered level of consciousness

Emotional distress
Family crisis

Bacterial Meningitis Beyond the Neonatal Period

KEITH KRASINSKI, M.D.
PHILIP LaRUSSA, M.D.

Bacterial meningitis in infants and children is most commonly due to *Hemophilus influenzae, Streptococcus pneumoniae* (pneumococcus), or *Neisseria meningitidis,* which together account for 90 to 95 percent of infections. *H. influenzae* is the most common organism in toddlers. Unusual organisms such as *Pseudomonas aeruginosa, Staphylococcus aureus* or *epidermidis,* and virtually any other bacterium may cause meningeal infection when there are host defense deficits or penetrating trauma. In the abnormal host, the pathogens isolated tend to be those organisms with which the patient has been previously colonized.

The most common pathophysiologic mechanism for the development of meningitis is probably primary respiratory colonization with bacteria, with subsequent bloodstream invasion and hematogenous spread to distant foci, including the cerebral ventricles and meninges. This mechanism explains the frequent occurrence of multiple anatomic sites of infection at the time of presentation of meninigitis. Another major pathway for bacterial invasion of the central nervous system (CNS) is by contiguous spread from an adjacent focus of infection such as otitis media, mastoiditis, or paranasal sinusitis. This may occur by direct extension secondary to destruction of intervening tissue or via blood vessels that drain nasal sinuses to dural venous sinuses. Bacterial infection also occurs by direct inoculation as a result of trauma or through a pre-existing defect such as dural sinus or myelomeningocele.

Specific alterations of host defense mechanisms have been associated with increased risk of infection. Humoral deficiencies of immunoglobulins, complement, and properdin have been associated with infections caused by encapsulated organisms such as *Streptococcus pneumoniae.* Congenital and traumatic absence of the spleen as well as splenic infarction or hypofunction are similarly associated with sepsis. Defects of cellular immunity, particularly defective polymorphonuclear leukocyte chemotaxis, phagocytosis and killing, also increase susceptibility to infection. Cardiovascular malformations with venous to arterial circulatory shunts allow blood to bypass the lung, subverting its filtering and phagocytic capabilities. Thus, potentially contaminated venous blood has direct access to the cerebral arterial circulation.

Approximately 50 percent of children with meningitis have a history of a preceding or concurrent upper respiratory infection. There is experimental evidence that viral infection may alter host defense mechanisms, including the structure and function of respiratory epithelium and the function of polymorphonuclear leukocytes. Viral infections may also interfere with a normal humoral antibody response. Despite this information, no virus or group of viruses is known to be routinely associated with bacterial meningitis.

Bacterial infection of the CNS involves a broad-spectrum of disease, from primary encephalitis, including irritability, headache, stupor, or seizures to frank meningitis, which manifests as nuchal rigidity. Patients commonly present with fever, but they may be hypothermic. Evidence of elevated intracranial pressure (ICP) is common and can be subtle (headache) or dramatic (bulging fontanelle or sutural diastasis). Young infants commonly do not have focal signs of infection. These children frequently present with a history of fever and irritability, and the parents may complain of a general feeling of unease about the health of the child. Older patients with meningitis frequently have cranial nerve involvement demonstrable on the physical examination. Cranial nerves III, VI, and VIII are most frequently involved in bacterial meningitis. Other neurologic findings include reflex changes and alterations of muscle tone. Other physical findings associated with meningitis in children include cutaneous petechiae or ecchymoses and tache cérébrale, a red streak with pale margins produced by stroking the skin. A careful search for infections at other sites (otitis media, purulent pneumonia, septic arthritis, buccal cellulitis, and purulent pericarditis) will aid in establishing the diagnosis and directing therapy.

DIAGNOSIS

No single symptom or sign of bacterial meningitis is consistently present. Consequently, the diagnosis must be based on review of cerebrospinal fluid (CSF) findings. CSF culture should be taken. The physician's immediate review of the CSF gram stain for the presence of organisms and an inflammatory response is mandatory. The CSF white blood cell (WBC) total and differential counts, as well as CSF protein and glucose, should be obtained. Alterations of the CSF/serum glucose ratio is a particularly helpful sign. There is typically an increase in WBCs, predominately polymorphonuclear leukocytes, elevated protein levels, and depressed glucose. Although oral antibiotic pretreatment occurs commonly and may decrease the recovery of bacterial pathogens (particularly meningococcus), the CSF cell count and glucose are not dramatically altered, thus permitting a diagnosis of bacterial meningitis.

Ancillary laboratory tests that provide additional evidence of bacterial infection or a specific bacterial etiology or uncover a primary focus of infection include complete blood count (CBC) with differential WBC, chest roentgenogram, and blood cultures. Cultures should also be obtained from other accessible sites of infection, such as the middle ear. Although not widely available or of established reliability, CSF lactic (acid) dehydrogenase (LDH) activity, CSF lactate, and Limulus lysate test for endotoxin have been used to diagnose bacterial infection. None of these is more useful than careful interpretation of standard information. Furthermore, these tests do not establish the specific bacterial etiology. CSF and urine counterimmunoelectrophoresis (CIE) and latex agglutination to detect bacterial antigen are useful diagnostic aids for *H. influenzae* type B streptococcus, meningococcus, and pneumococcus.

Urine CIE is particularly useful because bacterial antigen is excreted and large volumes of urine can be collected and concentrated. Urine CIE may be positive when CSF CIE has become negative. A negative test does not exclude the diagnosis of bacterial meningitis.

TREATMENT

Early intravenous (IV) therapy for meningitis should be empiric, based on likely pathogens for the age of the patient, and instituted rapidly. Ampicillin, 200 mg per kg per day, and chloramphenicol, 75 to 100 mg per kg per day, provide antibiotic coverage for *H. influenzae, Streptococcus pneumoniae,* and *Neisseria meningitides,* penetrate the CSF, and do not demonstrate antagonism against these organisms. Combination therapy is recommended up to 6 years of age to provide activity against beta-lactamase–producing *H. influenzae* and insensitive or relatively resistant pneumococci. Antibiotics administered should be adjusted on the basis of culture and sensitivity reporting. *H. influenzae* should be routinely tested for beta-lactamase production and chloramphenicol susceptibility. *S. pneumoniae* isolated from significant sites should also be tested for penicillin susceptibility using a 1 μg oxacillin disc. To investigate the possibility of antimicrobial resistance among organisms and to assess the therapeutic response, repeat CSF examination at 24 to 48 hours after institution of therapy is of value, particularly in patients who are not doing well. Repeat CSF examination is useful in establishing the efficacy of therapy and for investigating the presence or emergence of resistant organisms while on therapy. In special circumstances, it may be helpful to document therapeutic concentrations of antibiotic in the CSF.

There is evidence that oral chloramphenicol palmitate results in serum levels of antibiotic comparable to those achieved after IV administration of chloramphenicol succinate. Oral chloramphenicol palmitate, 75 mg per kg per day, may be indicated for in-hospital therapy of a patient who is stable and mechanically and physiologically able to tolerate and absorb oral medication. Outpatient oral therapy for meningitis should never be considered. The anticonvulsants phenytoin and phenobarbital interact with chloramphenicol to produce elevated or depressed serum chloramphenicol concentrations, respectively. When given concurrently with anticonvulsants, the dosage of chloramphenicol should be adjusted to provide therapeutic concentrations. Monitoring serum levels of antimicrobial agents is desirable.

Several factors have converged to stimulate interest into other antibiotic regimens. First, some *H-influenzae* are resistant to chloramphenicol due to the presence of acetyl transferase and some are ampicillin-resistant even though they do not produce beta-lactamase. Second, it is desirable to avoid both the predictable and the idiosyncratic reactions to chloramphenicol. Third, it is necessary to alter chloramphenicol dosage and monitor levels in patients with liver disease and in those receiving interacting drugs. Fourth, the causes of meningitis vary among neonates and those beyond the neonatal period.

Many new drugs with broad-spectrum coverage, enhanced CSF penetration, or increased activity against specific pathogens are or will become available. Cephalosporin-related drugs, including cefuroxime, cefotaxime, ceftizoxime, moxalactam, ceftriaxone, cefoperazone, and ceftazidime, seem to be useful for meningitis due to *H. influenzae* and meningococcus. At the time of publication cefuroxime 200 mg per kg per day and cefotaxime 200 mg per kg per day are available and acceptable empiric monotherapy for bacterial meningitis beyond the neonatal period. The role of these drugs in replacing traditional therapy will be determined as experience with their use develops. Moxalactam, cefuroxime, and cefotaxime also appear to be useful for infections due to Enterobacteriaceae. Ceftazidime has improved activity against Pseudomonas species. These drugs should not be used as sole agents for empiric therapy of meningitis in newborns, because most are inactive against enterococci and *Listeria monocytogenes*. Moxalactam is also inactive against group B streptococci and *S. pneumoniae*. Another group of drugs, including the beta-lactam agents azlocillin and mezlocillin and the piperazine piperacillin, are primarily indicated for serious infections due to Pseudomonas, though they also have increased activity against many other organisms.

Patients with bacteremic diseases, including meningitis, require careful initial evaluation for other co-primary or secondary sites of infection such as septic arthritis and pericarditis. The physical examination should be reviewed completely during the hospital stay and repeated for new or persistent fever or other untoward clinical events. Treatment for specific complications such as elevated ICP, subdural effusion, or empyema must be instituted as these complications arise. The syndrome of inappropriate antidiuretic hormone (SIADH) secretion occurs with such frequency that routine management of meningitis should include initial fluid restriction (except for patients in shock) and fre-

quent measurement of serum and urine electrolytes and osmolality.

The common practice of maintaining a patient in the hospital for 24 to 48 hours after completion of antibiotic therapy and repeating the CSF examination is not informative. Patients commonly have abnormal CSF WBC counts after successful therapy. Furthermore, relapse or recurrence of meningitis tends to occur after the 48-hour period of observation. It is more useful to carefully review the physical examination of a patient to uncover a sequestered site of infection that could be responsible for relapse. CSF examination, at the conclusion of therapy, should be reserved for patients with complicated hospital courses.

SUMMARY

The mortality rate due to meningitis beyond the neonatal period is approximately 7 to 10 percent. Fifteen to 20 percent of survivors will have CNS sequelae, including seizures, gross mental and/or motor retardation, and hearing loss at the time of discharge. A much larger proportion of patients will have psychomotor retardation demonstrable by careful testing as well as other subtle abnormalities such as learning disabilities or behavioral problems.

CASE PRESENTATION

An 18-month-old male was brought to the emergency room with fever and a history of a generalized seizure of 5-minute duration. The patient had developed an upper respiratory infection 4 days previously. Two days later, the child developed fever to 102.8°F, and a diagnosis of left otitis media was made. There were no known allergies to medicine, and the patient was treated with amoxicillin; however, the fever persisted.

A second generalized seizure of short duration was observed in the emergency room.

Examination and Test Results

The physical examination on admission showed a weight of 11 kg (24 lb), temperature = 104°F, heart rate = 120 beats/min, respiratory rate = 40 breaths/min, and blood pressure = 98/64 mm Hg. The child was lethargic but arousable and was irritable when aroused. The tympanic membranes were erythematous, and mobility was decreased on tympanometry. Kernig's and Brudzinski's signs were present. The neurologic examination was abnormal for paresis of the left VI cranial nerve and weakness of the right leg. The hemoglobin was 11.4 gm/dl and the WBC count was 24,000/cu mm³, with 64 percent neutrophils, 18 percent band forms, and 18 percent lymphocytes. The platelet count was 210,000/cu mm³. A chest roentgenogram was normal. The CSF WBC count was 342/cu mm³, with a differential count of 80 percent neutrophils, 8 percent band forms, and 12 percent lymphocytes. The CSF glucose and protein were 24 mg/dl and 68 mg/dl, respectively. The concurrent serum glucose was 85 mg/dl. Many neutrophils and a few pleomorphic gram-negative bacilli were observed on a gram-stained specimen of CSF. The serum sodium was 128 mEq/L, potassium = 4.6 mEq/L, and chloride = 101 mEq/L.

Problem List

Infectious: Meningitis

Blood and CSF cultures were sent to the laboratory. No other focus of infection was apparent at the time of admission. An IV line was placed, and the patient was treated with ampicillin, 50 mg/kg, and chloramphenicol, 25 mg/kg IV, to be immediately followed by ampicillin, 200 mg/kg/day, and chloramphenicol, 75 mg/kg/day, each in four divided doses.

Respiratory isolation was ordered for the first 24 hours of hospitalization.

Neurologic

The patient was treated with phenobarbital for seizures. Focal neurologic findings occur frequently in children with meningitis and commonly involve cranial nerves with long intracranial pathways. The weakness of the right side was diagnosed as Todd's paresis, and CT was deferred.

Intake and Output

Intake and output were monitored because of the relatively frequent occurrence of SIADH. Children with meningitis, in the absence of shock, should have fluid intake restricted to one half to two thirds of normal maintenance requirements. This patient received two thirds of maintenance requirements, and simultaneous serum and urine sodium, potassium, and osmolalities were measured routinely.

Hospital Course

CSF and urine CIE were both positive for *H. influenzae* type b. On Day 2 of hospitalization, the child remained febrile. There was no recurrence of seizure activity. The first CSF culture was positive for *H. influenzae* type B, which did not produce beta-lactamase, and was susceptible to chloramphenicol by disc testing. Chloramphenicol was subsequently discontinued.

Meningitis

Repeat CSF examination was performed. The CSF WBC count was 400/cu mm³, with a differential count of 80 percent neutrophils, 5 percent band forms, and 15 percent lymphocytes. The CSF glucose and protein were 30 mg/dl and 70 mg/dl, respectively. The concurrent serum glucose was 120 mg/dl. No microorganisms were demonstrable on gram stain of the CSF.

Intake and Output

Simultaneous serum and urine sodium, potassium, chloride, and osmolalities indicated a continued problem with SIADH; consequently, fluid restriction was continued.

Epidemiology/Prophylaxis

Antimicrobial prophylaxis for contacts of meningococcal disease is routinely recommended. Rifampin (or sulfa for susceptible organisms) is frequently used for this purpose. Rifampin prophylaxis for contact of *H. influenzae* disease is controversial at present. The American Academy of Pediatrics Committee on Infectious Diseases currently recommends oral rifampin prophylaxis (20 mg/kg/dose as a single daily dose for 4 days) for all household members and day care center contacts where there are children younger than 4 years of age. Rifampin is contraindicated in pregnancy. If prophylaxis is administered to contacts, the index case should also receive prophylaxis prior to discharge.

Hospital Course

The patient continued to be febrile to 102°F through Day 7. Careful review of the physical examination revealed mild swelling, warmth, and limitation of the range of motion of the right knee. Cerebral CAT scan established the presence of bilateral sudural effusions.

Infectious

Roentgenograms of the right knee suggested the presence of effusion, and subsequent needle aspiration confirmed the diagnosis of septic arthritis. Repeated needle aspiration and continued antibiotic therapy were prescribed. Fever typically lasts 4 to 5 days in patients with bacterial meningitis. Persistent fever should precipitate a search for intercurrent illness such as aspiration pneumonia, urinary tract infection, phlebitis, and gastroenteritis. Emphasis should be placed on discovering occult sites of infection with the primary organism such as sinusitis, otitis media, subdural empyema, septic arthritis, and pericarditis.

Neurologic

Subdural paracentesis was deferred due to the absence of new focal neurologic signs or signs of elevated ICP.

Intake and Output

Normal serum sodium and osmolality determinations allowed the fluid intake of this patient to be liberalized to maintenance levels.

After completion of antibiotic therapy for meningitis and septic arthritis, the patient was discharged on anticonvulsant medication. Physical examination at the time of discharge was normal. The patient was referred for brain stem evoked responses to test auditory function, as well as for continued routine care.

SUGGESTED READING

Bolagtas, R.C., Levin, S., Nelson, K.E., et al.: Secondary and prolonged fevers in bacterial meningitis. J. Pediatr. 77:957, 1970.

Carpenter, R.R., and Petersdorf, R.G.: The clinical spectrum of bacterial meningitis. Am. J. Med. 33:262, 1962.

Chartrand, S.A., and Cho, C.T.: Persistent pleocytosis in bacterial meningitis. J. Pediatr. 88:424, 1976.

Colding, H., and Lind, I.: Counterimmunoelectrophoresis in the diagnosis of bacterial meningitis. J. Clin. Microbiol. 5:405, 1977.

Dodge, P.R., and Swartz, M.R.: Bacterial meningitis. N. Engl. J. Med. 272:725–731, 779–787, 842–848, 898–902, 954–960, 1003–1010, 1975.

Feldman, W.E.: Concentrations of bacteria in cerebrospinal fluid of patients with bacterial meningitis. J. Pediatr. 88:549, 1976.

Johnson, D.: Some important pitfalls in the diagnosis and treatment of bacterial meningitis in children. Clin. Pediatr. 14:191, 1975.

Kraskinski, K., Kusmiez, H., and Nelson, J.D.: Pharmacologic interactions among chloramphenicol, phenytoin, and phenobarbital. Pediatr. Infec. Dis. 1:232, 1982.

McCracken, G.H., and Nelson, J.D.: The third generation cephalosporins and the pediatic practitioner. Pediatr. Infec. Dis. 1:123, 1982.

Nelson, J.D., and McCracken, G.H.: Mezlocillin and related antibiotics. Pediatr. Infec. Dis. 1:42, 1982.

Nyhan, W.L., and Richardson, F.: Complications of meningitis. Ann. Rev. Med. 14:243, 1963.

Schaad U.B., Krucko, J., and Pfenninger, J.: Cefuroxime therapy in childhood bacterial meningitis. Ped. Infect. Dis. 3:410, 1984.

Schaad, U.B., Nelson, J.D., and McCracken, G.H., Jr.: Recrudescence and relapse in bacterial meningitis of childhood. Pediatrics 67:188, 1981.

Sell, S.H., Merril, R.E., Doyne, E.O., et al.: Long-term sequelae of Haemophilus influenzae meningitis. Pediatrics 49:206, 1972.

Sell, S.H., Webb, W.W., Pate, J.E., et al.: Psychological sequelae to bacterial meningitis: two controlled studies. Pediatrics 49:212, 1972.

Spitz, E.B., Wagner, S., Sataloff, J., et al.: Cerebrospinal fluid otorrhea and recurrent meningitis. J. Pediatr. 59:397, 1961.

Bacterial Meningitis Beyond the Neonatal Period

Bacterial meningitis is a potentially life-threatening infection of the central nervous system (CNS), making assessment of neurologic function a priority. The infectious process is not necessarily limited to the CNS. The nurse must be alert to signs and symptoms of sepsis.

Fluid and electrolyte balance is always a concern in children. This is especially important in children with meningitis because of the frequency of inappropriate antidiuretic hormone secretion (SIADH).

Assessment parameters in terms of growth and development and emotional response are difficult to measure and interpret. The impact of the illness and hospitalization on the family must be anticipated and appropriate nursing interventions must be implemented.

NEUROLOGIC

Assess, Monitor, and Document

Headache
Nuchal rigidity
Level of consciousness
Reflexes
Muscle tone

Cranial nerve function (especially III, VI, and VIII)
Blood pressure
Pulse
Respiratory rate and pattern

Anticipate

Increased intracranial pressure (ICP)
  Headache
  Altered level of consciousness
  Altered pupillary response
  Increased blood pressure (widening pulse pressure)

Bradycardia
Decreased respiratory rate
Altered respiratory pattern
Seizures

INFECTIOUS PROCESS

Children with bacteremic disease require periodic evaluation for other sites of infection or intercurrent illness.

Assess, Monitor, and Document

Temperature
Changes in physical assessment parameters
  Vital signs
  Respiratory status: breath sounds

Inflammation of joints: pain, redness, edema
Renal: pain (flank, dysuria), appearance of urine

Anticipate

Persistent fever
  Secondary sites: sinuses, ears, joints
  Intercurrent illness: aspiration pneumonia, urinary tract infection

Septic shock

FLUID AND ELECTROLYTE BALANCE

Careful attention must be given to the child's fluid and electrolyte status. The effect of fever is well known and anticipated. In children with meningitis, there is a relatively frequent occurrence of SIADH.

Assess, Monitor, and Document

Weight
State of hydration: thirst, mucous membranes, skin turgor, blood pressure
Urine output, including specific gravity

Fluid intake, both oral and parenteral
Laboratory data
   Serum electrolytes and osmolality
   Urine electrolytes and osmolality

Anticipate

SIADH
   Weight gain
   Decreased urine output: specific gravity
     > 1.015

Altered serum and urine values: serum, (Sodium, potassium, osmolality), urine (sodium, potassium, osmolality)

RESPONSE OF CHILD

Assess, Monitor, and Document

Developmental level: fears, tasks
Degree of distress
Ability to cope

Strategies to reduce trauma and normalize experience

Anticipate

Emotional crisis

RESPONSE OF FAMILY

Assess, Monitor, and Document

Behavioral response: shock, fearful
Level of understanding of disease and child's condition

Expected outcome
Communicability
Ability to cope

Anticipate

Fear
Distress

Inability to cope
Family crisis

MIND SET

Assess

Neurologic status
Infectious disease status

Fluid and electrolyte balance
Emotional response of child and family

Anticipate

Increased ICP
Seizures
Infection
  Persistent fever
  Other infection sites
SIADH
  Urine output

Specific gravity
Serum and urine electrolytes and osmolality
Communicability among family members and
  close contacts
Emotional trauma
Family crisis

53

Sepsis

PHILIP La RUSSA, M.D.
KEITH KRASINSKI, M.D.

The concept of bacterial sepsis encompasses a spectrum of disease from asymptomatic bacteremia to septic shock. The clinical presentations and responsible etiologic agents vary with the ages of the patients. Whereas older children may present with more easily identifiable signs and symptoms, young infants are likely to present with fever and/or a general impression of lack of well being on the part of the caretaker. The most common pathogens in infants beyond the neonatal period and young children are *Streptococcus pneumoniae, Hemophilius influenzae* type b, *Neisseria meningitidis, Escherichia coli,* and Salmonella. The major causes of sepsis in older children are *S. pneumoniae* and *N. meningitidis.* Bacterial sepsis in immunocompromised children is likely to be due to gram-negative enteric organisms, *Pseudomonas aeruginosa,* or Staphylococci.

PREDISPOSING FACTORS

Predisposing factors are those that violate physical defense barriers, alter the natural flora of the host, or alter the ability of the host to respond to infection.

Physical Defense Barriers

Conditions that disrupt the integrity of the skin increase the risk of invasion with saprophytic organisms normally present at the site. Severe atopic dermatitis, burns, and trauma all predispose to early infection with skin colonizers and to later systemic infection. Dental work is a recognized cause of bacteremia, with organisms normally inhabiting the mouth and nasopharynx. Iatrogenic violation of natural barriers with insertion of urinary and intravenous (IV) catheters, cerebral spinal fluid (CSF) shunts, diagnostic instrumentation, and surgery can also disrupt the integrity of the gastrointestinal tract, skin, or urinary bladder, causing spillage of saprophytic organisms into sterile spaces or the vascular system.

Children with indwelling foreign bodies or damaged endothelial surfaces are at additional risk for disposition of organisms at these sites during bacteremia of any etiology.

Normal Flora

The normal flora results from a dynamic interaction of host and environment. Conditions that upset this equilibrium favor the proliferation and invasion of organisms that are normally not pathogens. Prolonged hospitalization and the use of antibiotics favor the gradual replacement of a patient's normal flora with organisms that tend to display multiple drug resistance.

Immune Response

Conditions that alter the host's immune response to infection also increase the risk of invasive disease.

Cellular Immunity

Granulocytopenia due to primary illness (cyclic neutropenia, leukemia, lymphoma) or therapeutic measures (immunosuppressive agents, radiation) is associated with invasive disease caused by endogenous organisms, especially those residing in the gastrointestinal tract and on the skin. The risk increases when granulocyte counts fall below 500 per mm^3 and is particularly severe with counts below 100 per mm^3.

Impaired granulocyte function also predisposes to invasive disease. In chronic granulomatous disease, the neutrophil is unable to generate the hydrogen peroxide necessary to kill ingested bacteria and fungi. Bacteria that make hydrogen peroxide but not the catalase that normally degrades it, autodigest within the neutrophil. Organisms capable of generating catalase (*Staphylococcus aureus*, gram-negative enterics) are not killed when ingested. Disseminated disease sometimes results from the chronic cutaneous and hepatic granulomata or osteomyelitis that characterize this condition. Defective chemotaxis may play a role in the pathogenesis of infection in patients with diabetes mellitus. Pyelonephritis and perinephric abscess due to *S. aureus*, *E. coli*, proteus species, and actinomycetes, and secondary bacteremia occur more commonly in diabetics than in the general population.

Humoral Immunity

Patients with agammaglobulinemia lack opsonizing antibodies necessary to kill encapsulated organisms (*S. pneumoniae*, *H. influenzae* type b, *N. meningitidis*), increasing the risk of invasive disease with these pathogens. Selective IgA deficiency predisposes to recurrent pulmonary infection and meningitis. Although primary defects of the classic complement system are rare, they are associated with recurrent pneumonia and meningitis caused by *S. pneumoniae*, *N. meningitidis*, and klebsiella species. Defective activation of the C3 component of the alternate complement pathway also impairs opsonization of these organisms.

The spleen is active in the production of opsonizing antibodies and functions as part of the reticuloendothelial system in removing organisms and particulate matter from the circulation. Patients who are functionally asplenic due to hematologic disease (sickle cell disease, hereditary spherocytosis, β-thalassemia) or who have been splenectomized for any of a variety of reasons (e.g., trauma, Hodgkin's disease) have an increased risk of invasive disease as a result of encapsulated organisms.

Combined Immunodeficiency

Both cellular and humoral immunity are impaired in patients with adenosine deaminase (ADA) deficiency, ataxia telangectasia, and Wiskott-Aldrich syndrome. These patients are in danger of invasive disease due to saprophytic bacteria, viruses, fungi (candida species), and protozoans (e.g., *Pneumocystis carinii*, *Toxoplasma gondii*).

PATHOPHYSIOLOGY

Septicemia due to gram-positive or gram-negative organisms can evolve into the state of septic shock. Although differences in the degree of expression of individual clinical and laboratory parameters occur, these are not reliable indicators of a specific bacterial pathogen.

Experimental work with the lipid A component of endotoxin and with similar components of the cell wall of gram-positive organisms demonstrates their widespread effect. Endotoxin provokes the initiation of the clotting cascade by damaging endothelial surfaces with subsequent activation of the complement pathway and release of vasoactive agents. The resulting tissue damage, peripheral vasodilatation, and decreased peripheral vascular resistance cause peripheral pooling of blood and diminish venous return to the heart. Cardiac output decreases, compounding cellular hypoxia and acidosis and provoking relaxation of precapillary sphincters. The resulting congestion of the capillary bed and leakage of fluid into interstitial spaces further decrease central intravascular pressure. Although a compensatory release of catecholamines acts to maintain central intravascular pressure by increasing heart rate and stroke volume, it also causes constriction of both pre- and post-capillary sphincters. Cellular hypoxia becomes irreversible and results in terminal vascular collapse.

CLINICAL PRESENTATION

Focal infections can progress, leading to bacteremia and clinical sepsis. Bacteremia, without an obvious focus of infection, in a febrile child is usually discovered when concern of high fever prompts the drawing of blood cultures. Although bacteremia is often cleared without specific therapy, some infections progress within days, with patients manifesting signs of focal infection or septic shock.

The earliest signs of septic shock are tachypnea and tachycardia, representing an attempt to compensate for hypoxia at the cellular level. The patient's temperature may be elevated. Systolic blood pressure is slightly elevated with a widened pulse pressure. The child may be agitated and have warm flushed skin and bounding pulses. Urine output is adequate or slightly increased. As compensatory mechanisms begin to fail, the child becomes dyspneic. The skin is cold and clammy, with increasing peripheral cyanosis and poor capillary filling. The pulse becomes rapid and faint, urine output falls, and hypothermia develops. The child lapses into coma, and hypotension becomes refractory to resuscitative efforts.

LABORATORY EVALUATION

The CBC typically shows an initial leukocytosis, and a predominance of segmented and juvenile neutrophils. As sepsis progresses, the WBC count may fall as a result of developing neutropenia. Neutropenia may be the cause of infection, or it may be due to peripheral use and destruction of WBCs. Erythrocyte sedimentation rates and C-reactive protein levels may be normal or increased.

Laboratory parameters reflect the evolving picture of shock. Serum electrolyte determinations are characterized by decreased sodium and bicarbonate ions and increased blood urea nitrogen (BUN) and creatinine. Serum glucose may be increased early in the course of septic shock, but soon falls to levels of absolute hypoglycemia. Arterial blood gases initially reflect a compensated metabolic acidosis with respiratory alkalosis (normal or slightly decreased pH, depressed Pa_{O_2} and Pa_{CO_2}). Later, they reflect the progression from decompensated metabolic acidosis (decreased pH, Pa_{O_2} and Pa_{CO_2}) to combined metabolic and respiratory acidosis (depressed pH and Pa_{O_2} and increased Pa_{CO_2}).

Coagulation profiles reflect the consumptive coagulopathy initiated by endotoxin (prolonged prothrombin time, PT, partial thromboplastin time, PTT, decreased fibrinogen, and increased fibrin split products).

DIAGNOSIS

A presumptive diagnosis of sepsis should be considered on the basis of early clinical signs and symptoms. Every effort should be made to identify the source and specific etiology of septicemia, allowing selection of the most appropriate therapy. Careful history and physical examination will help determine the direction of the diagnostic work-up. Although examination and cultures of indicated clinical specimens (blood, sputum, urine, stool, and CSF) and appropriate roentgenograms will localize most sources of infection, additional measures are necessary in certain situations. For example, in patients with pulmonary infiltrates who are not responding to appropriate empiric antibiotic therapy, a lung biopsy can often make a specific diagnosis.

Rapidly obtainable microbiologic information such as gram-stain characteristics, morphology, and metabolic markers of organisms will help identify likely pathogens and guide initial therapy (Fig. 53–1).

Counterimmunoelectrophoresis and latex agglutination use antisera to identify organism specific antigens in a variety of clinical specimens (CSF, serum, urine, and pus).

MANAGEMENT

Successful management of patients with sepsis requires early recognition and eradication of primary sites of infection, appropriate antibiotic therapy, and aggressive supportive care. After the site of infection has been identified, any areas of loculated infection should be drained. In patients with nosocomial infection, special attention should be paid to operative sites, indwelling catheters, and areas of skin breakdown. Foreign bodies should be removed and cultured. Careful chest physical therapy can minimize postoperative pulmonary atelectasis and prevent infection due to stasis of secretions.

Persistently positive blood cultures or continued fever when appropriate antibiotic therapy is being administered suggests a sequestered site of infection. A new murmur or signs of septic emboli suggest an echocardiogram to identify vegetations responsible for destruction of a valve. Similarly, in patients with abdominal findings, ultrasound, CT, and laparotomy may be indicated. In patients with focal neurologic signs, transillumination, brain scan, CT, and electroencephalogram (EEG) can help identify a focus of infection.

Antibiotic Therapy

Identification of a probable primary focus of infection will help direct initial antibiotic therapy (Table 53–1). Initial therapy of nosocomial infections should take into account the antibiotic susceptibility patterns of hospital organisms. When a focus is not obvious, initial therapy should be directed against the most common pathogens for that age group, considering the immune status of the patient (Table 53–2). When *H. influenzae* type b is a likely path-

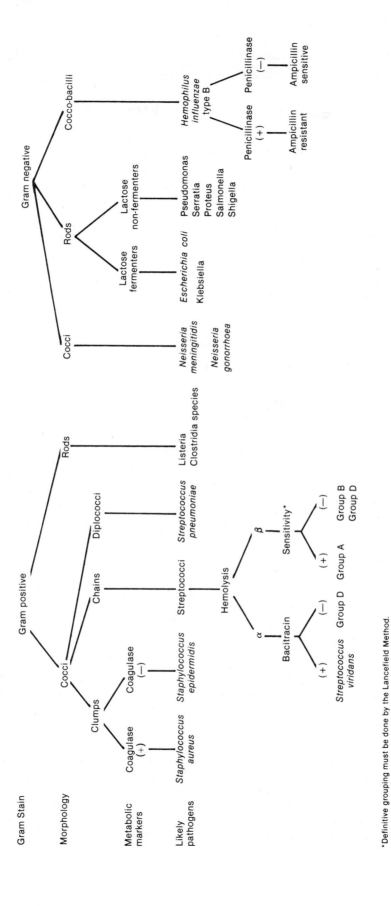

Figure 53-1. Initial microbiologic findings.

*Definitive grouping must be done by the Lancefield Method.

Table 53–1. Guidelines for Initial Therapy When a Probable Primary Focus Has Been Identified

Focus	Most Common Organisms	Initial Therapy
Skin		
With a history of trauma	Staphylococci	Nafcillin
Without a history of trauma		
Periorbital and buccal cellulitis	*H. influenzae* type b	Ampicillin and chloramphenicol
Below the waist-line or hands	Staphylococci, Streptococci, enterics, *H. influenzae* type b	Nafcillin and aminoglycoside
Other Sites	Staphylococci, Streptococci	Nafcillin
Burns		
Early onset of infection	Streptococci	Penicillin
Late onset of infection	Pseudomonas	Carbenicillin and aminoglycoside
Gastrointestinal Tract		
Above the level of the diaphragm	Mouth flora*	Penicillin
Below the level of the diaphragm	Enterobacteriaceae	Cefoxitin and aminoglycoside
	Pseudomonas	or
	S. faecalis	Clindamycin and aminoglycoside
	B. fragilis, other anaerobes	
Genitourinary Tract	Anaerobes (gram-positive and gram-negative)	Cefoxitin and aminoglycoside
	Enterobacteriaceae	
	Neisseria species	
Respiratory Tract		
Upper respiratory tract and sinuses	Mouth flora	Penicillin
	S. pneumoniae, H. influenzae	
Lower respiratory tract		
Mild to moderately ill	*S. pneumoniae*	Penicillin
Severely ill, rapid onset	Staphylococci, *H. influenzae* type b	Nafcillin and chloramphenicol
Probable aspiration	Mouth flora	Penicillin and steroids
Musculoskeletal System		
Bone	Staphylococci	Nafcillin
Joints		
Younger than 6 years of age	Staphylococci, *H. influenzae* type b	Nafcillin and chloramphenicol
Older than 6 years of age	Staphylococci	Nafcillin
Muscle		
Without gas formation	Staphylococci	Nafcillin
With gas formation	Clostridia species, Streptococci	Penicillin
Cardiovascular System	*Streptococcus viridans*	Penicillin and aminoglycoside
	Staphylococci	
Central Nervous System		
Focal infection (brain abscess)	Staphylococci	Nafcillin and chloramphenicol
	Streptococci	
	Anaerobes	Metronidazole†
Meningitis	(see Chapter 52)	

*Mouth flora: Aerobic and anaerobic streptococci, gram-negative anaerobes, Fusobacterium, and Veillonella
†Not approved for use in children

ogen, combination therapy should be used until the susceptibility pattern of the organisms is known. When an organism has been isolated, the most appropriate antibiotic therapy can be selected based on susceptibility data (Table 53–3). The recommendations in Tables 53–1 through 53–3 are guidelines that may need to be modified to obtain the most favorable balance of efficacy and toxicity for each patient.

When an organism is difficult to eradicate, antibiotic therapy can be optimized by special studies. The ability to monitor serum antibiotic concentration permits dosage adjustments, maintaining peak serum concentrations within the therapeutic range. Identification of tolerant organisms, that is, those showing a 16- or 32-fold difference between the concentration of antibiotic required to inhibit its growth in vitro (minimum inhibitory concentration) and that necessary to kill the organism (minimum bactericidal concentration) indicates the need for more aggressive antibiotic therapy. Synergy and antagonism studies evaluate the ability of combination therapy to enhance or impede in vitro killing of a organism compared with single drug therapy. Combinations that are synergistic in vitro can enhance survival, especially in compromised patients.

Table 53–2. Guidelines for Initial Antibacterial Therapy When a Source is Not Obvious

	Most Common Organisms	Initial Therapy
Immunologically Normal		
Younger than 6 years of age	*S. pneumoniae, H. influenzae* type b *N. meningitidis*, Salmonella species	Ampicillin and chloramphenicol
Older than 6 years of age	*S. pneumoniae* *N. meningitidis*	Penicillin
Immunologically Compromised		
Granulocytopenic patients	Skin and enteric organisms	Carbenicillin or ticarcillin and cephalothin and aminoglycoside or Mezlocillin and nafcillin and aminoglycoside
Defective granulocyte function	*S. aureus*	Nafcillin
Agammaglobulinemia and asplenia	*S. pneumoniae* *H. influenzae* *N. meningitidis*	Penicillin

Supportive Therapy

Volume Expansion

Volume expansion should be carefully guided by measurement of central venous and pulmonary wedge pressures. In patients with septic shock, volume expansion can result in decreased stroke volume and cardiac output as left ventricular filling pressure is increased, precipitating pulmonary edema at relatively low pulmonary wedge pressures.

Pressors

Agents with both inotropic and chronotropic effects (dobutamine, dopamine, epinephrine) increase tissue perfusion if intravascular volume has been reconstituted.

Digitalizaton

There is some evidence that rapid digitalization can be helpful in septic shock when central venous pressure is elevated.

Metabolic Acidosis

Sodium bicarbonate should be used to partially correct severe acidosis after adequate ventilation is ensured. Some patients who do not respond to fluids and pressors may respond to glucose-insulin-potassium infusions.

Steroids

The use of steroids in septic shock is still controversial. Their ability to suppress activation of complement, aggregation of leukocytes, and destabilization of lysosomal membranes decreases pulmonary leukoembolization, release of toxic superoxide radicals, and resulting damage to endothelial surfaces. Studies showing increased survival with steroids use high-dose glucocorticoids (methylprednisolone, 10–30 mg/kg, or dexamethasone, 2–6 mg/kg) as an IV bolus early in the course of septic shock, with repeated doses at 4- to 6-hour intervals. A disadvantage of steroids is their ability to inhibit migration and function of neutrophils and monocytes. Prolonged use of steroids can be complicated by gastric erosions, nonketotic hyperglycemia, dysrhythmias, and psychosis, as well as secondary infection.

Control of Coagulopathy

Although vitamin K, fresh frozen plasma (FFP), and whole blood can help control the consumptive coagulopathy associated with sepsis, heparin therapy has little or no effect on survival.

New Modes of Therapy

Although animal studies clearly show the benefit of granulocyte transfusions in the treatment of septicemia in neutropenic hosts, their efficacy has not been established in human infection. Patients with documented septicemia who continue to remain granulocytopenic and febrile in spite of optimal antibiotic therapy are those most likely to benefit. The peripheral circulating granulocyte pool can be temporarily reconstituted with approximately 10^9 granulocytes per kg IV. Because transfused granu-

Table 53–3. Therapy of Choice

Pathogens	Therapeutic Agent	Dose
Gram-Positive Organisms		
Staphylococci		
Methicillin-sensitive	Methicillin, nafcillin	100 mg/kg/d ÷ q6h
Methicillin-resistant	Vancomycin	40 mg/kg/d ÷ q6h
Streptococci		
Penicillin-sensitive	Penicillin	100,000–200,000 U/kg/d ÷ q4–6h
Penicillin-resistant	Chloramphenicol	50–100 mg/kg/d ÷ q6h
S. viridans		
In endocarditis	Penicillin	50,000–100,000 U/kg/d ÷ q4–6h
	and	
	Gentamicin	5 mg/kg/d ÷ q8h
Other sites	Pencillin	50,000–100,000 U/kg/d ÷ q4–6h
S. faecalis	Ampicillin	100–200/mg/kg/d ÷ q6h
	or	
	Vancomycin	40 mg/kg/d ÷ q6h
	and	
	Gentamicin	5 mg/kg/d ÷ q8h
Gram-Negative Organisms		
N. meningitidis	Penicillin	50,000–100,000 U/kg/d ÷ q4–6h
H. influenzae type b		
β-lactamase ⊖	Ampicillin	100–200 mg/kg/d ÷ q6h
β-lactamase ⊕		
Chloramphenicol-sensitive	Chloramphenicol	50–100 mg/kg/d ÷ 6h
Chloramphenicol-resistant	3rd generation cephalosporin (moxalactam, cefotaxime)	50–150 mg/k/d ÷ q6h
E. coli		
Ampicillin-sensitive	Ampicillin	100–200 mg/kg/d ÷ q6h
Ampicillin-resistant	Aminoglycoside*	
	3rd generation cephalosporin	50–150 mg/kg/d ÷ q6h
Klebsiella-Enterobacter-Serratia	Aminoglycoside	
(KES)	±3rd generation cephalosporin	50–150 mg/kg/d ÷ q6h
Salmonella	Ampicillin	100–200 mg/kg/d ÷ q6h
	or	
	Chloramphenicol	50–100 mg/kg/d ÷ q6h
Shigella species	Trimethoprim-sulfamethoxazole	8 mg trimethoprim/40 mg sulfamethoxazole/kg/d ÷ q12h
Pseudomonas species	Mezlocillin	300 mg/kg/d ÷ q4h
	and aminoglycoside	
Anaerobes		
S. fragilis	Clindamycin	25–40 mg/kg/d ÷ q6h
	Chloramphenicol	50–100 mg/kg/d ÷ q6h
	Cefoxitin	50–150 mg/kg/d ÷ q6h
	Metronidazole†	15 mg/kg/d ÷ q6h
Others	Penicillin	50,000–200,000 U/kg/d ÷ q4–6h

*Aminoglycosides: Tobramicin 5 mg/kg/day ÷ q8h
                 Gentamicin 5–7.5 mg/kg/day ÷ q8h
                 Amikacin 15–22 mg/kg/day ÷ q8h
†Not approved for use in children.

locytes remain in the peripheral circulation for only 4 to 6 hours, recommendations for the number of transfusions vary from at least one to as many as four per day. These transfusions should be continued until the peripheral granulocyte count is greater than 500 per mm³ or until the patient is afebrile and blood cultures are consistently sterile. Granulocytes should be irradiated (1500–2500 rads) to prevent potentially fatal graft versus host disease and should be red cell–type compatible. There is no evidence that prophylactic transfusions are helpful in preventing sepsis. Potentially serious respiratory distress can develop during the

infusion if transfused granulocytes aggregate in the pulmonary vascular bed.

Other modes of therapy currently under study include antiserum to endotoxin, calcium channel blockers and prostaglandin inhibitors, and naloxone and thyrotropin releasing hormone (TRH). Antiserum prepared against the core lipopolysaccaride common to most gram-negative organisms increases survival when given as an IV bolus early in the course of sepsis. It may act by binding to endotoxin, inhibiting its ability to initiate shock. In animal models of endotoxin shock, naloxone and TRH significantly increase mean arterial pressure

(MAP) for prolonged intervals. Naloxone may function by competing for central nervous system (CNS) binding sites of endorphins released during septic shock. The mechanism of action of TRH and calcium and prostaglandin inhibitors is uncertain.

Special Situations

The neutropenic patient without a bacterial etiology of infection who continues to be febrile in spite of appropriate empiric antibiotic therapy should be evaluated for unusual pathogens (Table 53–4). Pneumonia and septicemia due to fungi (candida species, aspergillus) and *Pneumocystis carinii* are likely in this situation. Although diagnosis is usually made on biopsy of involved organs, techniques for detection of specific antigen in serum are being studied for candida and pneumocystis.

DiGeorge syndrome, malignancies (Hodgkin's disease, acute lymphocytic leukemia), and the therapeutic regimens used to treat malignancies are examples of conditions that depress the cellular immune response and thus increase the risk of disseminated infection with intracellular pathogens (see Table 53–4).

Because therapy is now available for treatment of many of these pathogens, it is important to make a specific diagnosis. Biopsy of involved organs will show the pathogens on histology, electron microscopy, immunofluorescence, or culture.

Preventive measures for nonbacterial pathogens are limited. Although long-term prophylaxis with trimethoprim-sulfamethoxazole is effective in preventing *P. carinii* infection in high-risk patients, it is associated with an increased incidence of fungal infections. Until recently, postexposure use of varicella-zoster immune globulin was the only prophylactic measure available to decrease the severity of varicella-zoster infections in immunocompromised patients. A live attenuated vaccine is currently being studied.

Table 53–4. Unusual Pathogens Associated With The Clinical Picture of Sepsis

Predisposing Conditions	Pathogens	Therapy
Neutropenia	Fungi	
	Aspergillus	Amphotericin B
	Candida	Amphotericin B
	Protozoa	
	P. carinii	Trimethoprim-sulfamethoxazole or Pentamidine
Defects in Cellular Immunity	Herpes Viruses	
	Herpes simplex	Antivirals (adenine-arabinoside [ARA-A], acyclovir)
	Varicella-Zoster	
	Cytomegalovirus	
	Epstein-Barr virus	
	Fungi	
	Candida	Amphotericin B
	Aspergillus	Amphotericin B
	Cryptococcus	Amphotericin B
	Protozoa	
	Toxoplasma gondii	Pyrimethamine and sulfadiazine and spirmycin
	Pneumocystis carinii	Trimethoprim-sulfamethoxazole or Pentamidine
	Bacteria	
	Atypical Mycobacteria	Isonicotinic hydrazide (INH), rifampin
	Listeria monocytogenes	Penicillin and gentamicin

PREVENTION

Attempts to reduce invasive disease due to endogenous organisms in neutropenic patients include prophylactic use of antibiotics, vaccines, and isolation precautions. Oral colistin, polymyxin, gentamicin, and nystatin have been used to suppress the gastrointestinal flora. Killed vaccines, made from mutant *E. coli,* are currently under study. Their specific colony morphology exposes the lipid A component of endotoxin common to most gram-negative organisms, provoking the production of antibodies, which hopefully will provide protection against a wide variety of gram-negative organisms. Protective isolation, as ordinarily practiced, is probably the most commonly used, but least successful, preventive measure.

Children with agammaglobulinemia are at lower risk for infection with encapsulated organisms if they receive monthly immune serum globulin intramuscularly (IM).

A multivalent pneumococcal vaccine has been shown to be effective for the prevention of pneumococcal disease in asplenic adults and children older than 2 years of age. Because the vaccine does not contain all pneumococcal serotypes and because some of the serotypes included are poor immunogens, lifelong oral penicillin prophylaxis is also recommended.

Children who are close contacts of patients with invasive disease due to *N. meningitidis* or *H. influenzae* type b are also at increased risk for invasive disease. Prophylaxis with rifampin or sulfadiazine is effective in reducing the secondary attack rate of meningococcal disease. Unless the organism is known to be sensitive to sulfonamides, contacts should receive rifampin. The effectiveness of prophylaxis in contacts of children with invasive disease caused by *H. influenzae* type b has not been proved. The Committee on Infectious Diseases of the American Academy of Pediatrics recommends prophylactic rifampin for household and day-care center contacts.

SEQUELAE

Sequelae of sepsis are a function of the primary infectious process and the vascular instability that can result.

Septic emboli seed new sites, extending the range and gravity of the primary infection. This is exemplified by the development of a brain abscess in a patient with bacterial endocarditis or septic arthritis in a patient with invasive disease due to *N. meningitidis* or *H. influenzae* type b.

Vascular collapse causes ischemic damage in poorly perfused areas. Necrosis of distal extremities and acute renal failure following septicemia are examples. "Shock lung" or adult respiratory distress syndrome (ARDS) typically occurs 1 to 3 days following septic shock. The pathogenesis of ARDS is uncertain but probably involves hypoxic damage to the endothelial surface of the pulmonary capillary bed, local aggregation of leukocytes, and decreased production of surfactant. As compliance decreases, tachypnea progresses to dyspnea and respiratory failure (see Chapter 23, Adult Respiratory Distress Syndrome).

PROGNOSIS

Mortality rates vary with the age and underlying condition of the patient, the specific pathogen involved, and the rapidity with which appropriate therapy is initiated. In Table 53–5, the mortality rates in large series of children and adults are provided.

CASE PRESENTATION

A 7-month-old female was admitted to the hospital for elective surgical repair of a rectovaginal fistula and imperforate anus. Past medical history was remarkable for urinary tract infections due to *E. coli* at 3 and 5 months of age, both treated successfully with amoxicillin.

Examination and Test Results

Vital signs on admission were temperature = 99° F, heart rate = 150 beats/min, respiratory rate = 24 breaths/min, and blood pressure = 90/60 mm Hg. Physical examination revealed a small-for-age infant with an excoriated erythematous perineum. Stool was discharged through the vaginal orifice. Laboratory examination showed a WBC count of 20,000/mm³ (20 percent mature neutrophils, 12 percent band forms, 68 percent lymphocytes), platelet count of 150,000/mm³, and hematocrit of 33 percent; urinalysis was unremarkable. A pull through ano-

Table 53–5. Mortality in Children and Adults With Septicemia

Pathogen	Mortality Rate (%)
Pseudomonas species	70
E. coli	40
Klebsiella species	32
N. meningitidis	30
Staphylococci	10
H. influenzae type b	7
S. pneumoniae	6

plasty with division of the rectovaginal fistula was accomplished without complications.

Six hours after surgery, she became febrile to 102° F. Vital signs were heart rate = 170 beats/min, respiratory rate = 48 breaths/min, and blood pressure = 100/50 mm Hg. Physical examination was reported as unremarkable. Therapy was limited to antipyretics (acetaminophen, 10 mg/kg P.O.) Ten hours after surgery, perioral and peripheral cyanosis was noted. Twelve hours after surgery, she suffered a generalized tonoclonic seizure followed by cardiorespiratory arrest. She was orotracheally intubated and mechanically ventilated. Sinus tachycardia was restored with IV sodium bicarbonate, epinephrine, and calcium gluconate. Blood pressure post-resuscitation, was 60/40 mm Hg. Physical examination showed a flaccid, cyanotic child, with areas of ecchymosis forming over the buttocks and perineum. Blood pressure and urine output responded to IV administration of lactated Ringer's solution (20 ml/kg). IV antibiotics were started (ampicillin, 100 mg/kg/day; oxacillin, 100 mg/kg/day; gentamicin, 5 mg/kg/d).

Laboratory Data

Laboratory values at the time of the arrest were serum sodium = 127 mg/dl, serum, CO_2 = 14 mEq/L, WBC count = 16,500/mm³ (15 percent mature neutrophils, 2 percent bands, 83 percent lymphocytes), platelet count = 159,000/mm³, hematocrit = 30 percent. Arterial blood gases prior to intubation were pH = 6.9, PO_2 = 56 mm Hg, and PCO_2 = 86 mm Hg. After intubation pH = 7.39, PO_2 = 123 mm Hg, and PCO_2 = 23 mm Hg. No infiltrate or atelectasis was seen on roentgenogram of the chest.

Focal seizures of the right arm began 18 hours after surgery and recurred intermittently over the next 48 hours. They were controlled with IV diazepam and phenobarbital.

Twenty hours after surgery, the child became mottled. Vital signs were: heart rate = 190 beats/min, respiratory rate = 25 breaths/min (ventilator driven), and blood pressure = 70/50 mm Hg. Arterial blood gases showed pH = 7.3, PO_2 = 90 mm Hg, and PCO_2 = 20 mm Hg; urine output was 0.5 ml/kg/hr. WBC count was 1800/mm³ (4 percent mature neutrophils, 10 percent band forms, 86 percent lymphocytes); platelet count was 27,000/mm³ and hematocrit was 32 percent. Lumbar puncture revealed no cells, protein = 18 mg/dl, and glucose = 60 mg/dl (serum glucose = 90 mg/dl). A pressor (dopamine, 5 mcg/kg/min) was begun. Dexamethasone, 6 mg/kg, was given as an IV bolus and repeated at 6-hour intervals for 48 hours. A granulocyte transfusion (10⁹ granulocytes/kg irradiated with 1500 rads) was given over 4 hours, and repeated 16 hours later.

Twenty-four hours after surgery, the patient's vital signs had stabilized, but the ecchymotic areas on the buttocks and perineum became necrotic, without evidence of crepitus. The abdomen was tense, without bowel sounds. Blood cultures taken at the time of the cardiopulmonary arrest were reported to be growing a gram-negative lactose-fermenting bacillus

sensitive to gentamicin and cephalosporins, but resistant to ampicillin. Oxacillin and ampicillin were replaced with cefoxitin, 150 mg/kg/d, and gentamicin was continued.

Two days after surgery, the necrotic tissue was débrided, and a colostomy was established. After 24 hours of therapy, peak and trough serum gentamicin concentrations were 2 mcg/ml and 0 mcg/ml, respectively. The gentamicin dose was increased to 7.5 mg/kg/d. Repeat peak and trough serum concentrations were 8 mcg/ml and 0.9 mcg/ml, respectively.

Three and one half days after surgery, the child was afebrile, with stable vital signs off the respirator. The WBC count was 19,800/mm³ (9 percent mature neutrophils, 46 percent band forms, 45 percent lymphocytes). *E. coli* was isolated from blood, necrotic perineal tissue, and peritoneal fluid. Group B streptococcus was isolated from perineal tissue and peritoneal fluid. Ten days after surgery, the débrided areas of perineum and buttocks were covered with a split thickness skin graft.

The patient's subsequent hospital course was unremarkable. Repeat blood cultures were sterile, and antibiotic therapy was discontinued after a 14-day regimen of cefoxitin and gentamicin. The child was discharged on phenobarbital and scheduled for cosmetic repair of the perineum and buttocks.

Problem List

Preoperative

A history of two urinary tract infections with an enteric organism is suggestive of an anomaly involving the gastrointestinal and urinary systems. Although the rectovaginal fistula may be the source of contamination of the urinary tract, renal anomalies are associated with enterourinary malformations. During a subsequent hospitalization, elective abdominal ultrasound and IV pyelograms demonstrated absence of the right kidney and an abnormal left kidney and collecting system.

Because the rectovaginal fistula was to be divided, it would have been appropriate to suppress the bowel flora with oral colistin, gentamicin, and nystatin prior to surgery, decreasing the risk of bacteremia. Second generation cephalosporins given IV at the time of colon surgery and for 72 hours after surgery have been shown to decrease the risk of infection with enteric organisms.

Although WBC counts are not sensitive indicators of infection, a preoperative count of 20,000/mm³ in a patient with an excoriated inflamed perineum and an anatomic anomaly suggests infection. It would have been appropriate to delay surgery until the situation was clarified.

Postoperative

Tachycardia, tachypnea, and cyanosis 6 to 10 hours after surgery indicate compensatory efforts to increase cardiac output and are suggestive of impending shock.

Fever of unknown cause should prompt further investigation. It would have been appropriate to look for signs of postoperative wound infection, phlebitis, and atelectasis at the time of the initial postoperative fever. CBC and blood cultures should be done at this time.

Infectious

Initial antibiotic coverage (ampicillin, oxacillin, and gentamicin) was appropriate, considering the likely sources of infection. Surgical incision in the perineum predisposes to invasive disease with skin and enteric organisms. Enteric organisms are also likely pathogens following manipulation of the colon. Preliminary laboratory findings (gram-negative, lactose-fermenting bacillus) suggested *E. coli* as a likely pathogen and the possibility that other enteric organisms were involved. Cefoxitin was substituted for ampicillin and oxacillin to cover enteric anaerobes, specifically *B. fragilis,* which can be resistant to ampicillin and penicillin. Isolation of group B streptococcus and *E. coli* from peritoneal fluid and necrotic perineal tissue suggests a gastrointestinal source of infection resulting from manipulation of the colon during surgery or hypoxic damage to the colon during the cardiopulmonary arrest and seizure. A lumbar puncture was appropriately performed. It is necessary to rule out infection of the CNS in patients with possible sepsis, especially when CNS involvement (e.g., seizure activity) is present.

Granulocyte transfusions were appropriate, considering the absolute neutropenia (252 neutrophils/mm^3) at 24 hours after surgery. Because granulocyte transfusions do not increase the peripheral WBC count appreciably, the rapid increase to 19,000 WBC/mm^3 was a good prognostic sign, indicating the patient's own bone marrow response to infection. The use of steroids in septic shock is controversial; if used, they should be administered early in the course of treatment.

Sequelae of Infection

The extensive necrosis of tissue in the perineum and buttocks will require cosmetic repair. Although the child exhibited no further seizure activity, long-term follow-up will be necessary to determine the extent of CNS damage.

SUGGESTED READING

Blaisdell, W.F.: Controversy in shock research, con: the role of steroids in septic shock. Circ. Shock 8:673, 1981.

Kaplan, S.L.: Endotoxin shock, *In* Feigin, R., and Cherry, J. (eds.): Textbook of Pediatric Infectious Diseases. Philadelphia, W.B. Saunders Company, 1981, p. 507.

Kaye, W.: Catheter and infusion related sepsis. Heart Lung 11:221, 1982.

Perkin, R.M., and Levin, D.L.: Shock in the pediatric patient. Part I. J. Pediatr. 101:163, 1982.

Perkin, R.M., and Levin, D.L.: Shock in the pediatric patient. Part II. J. Pediatr. 101:319, 1982.

Pfenninger, J., Gerber, A., Tschappelar, H., and Zimmerman, A.: Adult respiratory distress syndrome in children. J. Pediatr. 101:352, 1982.

Schumer, W.: Controversy in shock research, pro: the role of steroids in septic shock. Circ. Shock 8:667, 1981.

Washington, J.A.: The clinician and the microbiology laboratory. *In* Mandell, G., Douglas, R., and Bennett, J. (eds.): Principles and Practice of Infectious Diseases. New York, John Wiley & Sons, 1981, p. 145.

Winston, D., Ho, W., and Gale, R.: Therapeutic granulocyte transfusions for documented infections. Ann. Intern. Med. 97:509, 1982.

Young, L.S.: Gram-negative sepsis. *In* Mandell, G., Douglas, R., and Bennett, J. (eds.): Principles and Practice of Infectious Diseases. New York, John Wiley & Sons, 1981, p. 571.

Zieglar, E., McCutchan, J., Fierer, J., et al.: Treatment of gram-negative bacteremia and shock with human antiserum to a mutant *Escherichia coli.* N. Engl. J. Med. 307:1225, 1982.

Nursing Process for Patient Care:

Sepsis

Although most infections that are encountered are localized, sepsis is not an uncommon occurrence, especially in the intensive care unit (ICU). The use of IV and urinary drainage catheters, endotracheal tubes, and respiratory apparatus predisposes the already acutely ill child to bacteremia and systemic infection. The critical care nurse must be aware of the clinical presentation of sepsis and septic shock and anticipate its occurrence.

INFECTIOUS PROCESS

Assess, Monitor, and Document

Temperature
Localizing signs of pain or discomfort
Changes in physical assessment parameters:
  Vital signs— pulse, respiratory rate, blood pressure
  Potential sites of infection— IV catheter,

Foley catheter, drains, wounds, secretions (color, odor)
Laboratory data— CBC with differential and platelet count, cultures and sensitivities
Response to antibiotics

Anticipate

Persistent fever
Localized signs of infection: pain, redness, swelling, drainage

Septic shock

CARDIOVASCULAR

Endotoxin and other vasoactive substances released from infected tissue cause decreased peripheral vascular resistance. Cardiac output drops as a consequence of diminished venous return, and the metabolic needs of the body can no longer be met. A cycle of tissue hypoxia and acidosis ensues.

Assess, Monitor, and Document

Heart rate
Rhythm
Perfusion
Blood pressure
Color

Skin condition
Respiratory rate
Level of consciousness
Urine output
Arterial blood gases

Anticipate

Septic Shock
  Initial hyperdynamic state
    Tachypnea
    Tachycardia
    Bounding pulses
    Mild hypertension
    Widened pulse pressure
    Elevated temperature
    Warm, flushed skin
    Adequate urine output
  Subsequent hypodynamic state
    Dyspnea
    Tachycardia
    Faint pulses

Decreased blood pressure
Decreased temperature
Cold, clammy skin
Peripheral cyanosis
Poor capillary filling
Decreased urine output
Altered level of consciousness
Complications of shock
  Cerebral edema
  Seizures
  Adult respiratory distress syndrome (ARDS)
  Acute renal failure
  Disseminated intravascular coagulation

FLUID AND ELECTROLYTE BALANCE

Assess, Monitor, and Document

Systemic arterial blood pressure
Central venous pressure
Urine output, including specific gravity
Urine electrolytes and osmolality
Serum electrolytes, BUN, creatinine, and os-
   molality

Fluid intake: accurate administration of parenteral fluids (use infusion pump if available)
Weight
Thirst

Anticipate

Relative hypovolemia
Acute renal failure

Decreased urine output
Increased serum BUN, creatinine

RESPONSE OF CHILD

Assess, Monitor, and Document

Developmental level: verbal, psychosocial,
   cognitive, fears
Behavioral response: anxious, fearful, withdrawn, passive

Response to nursing interventions

Anticipate

Emotional distress
Disruption in normal growth and development

RESPONSE OF FAMILY

Assess, Monitor, and Document

Behavioral response: anxious, fearful
Level of knowledge of disease process and
   child's condition

Expected outcome
Ability to cope
Response to nursing interventions

MIND SET

Assess

Infectious disease status
Cardiovascular status

Fluid and electrolyte balance
Response of child and family

Anticipate

Septic shock
   Hyperdynamic state
   Hypodynamic state
ARDS
Neurologic sequelae
   Cerebral edema

Seizures
   Altered level of consciousness
Acute renal failure
Disseminated intravascular coagulation
Emotional distress
Family crisis

Toxic Shock Syndrome

SOL S. ZIMMERMAN, M.D.

Although toxic shock syndrome (TSS), associated with *Staphylococcus aureus,* has received considerable attention in the adult medical and lay literature because of its predominant occurrence in menstruating females and its relation to tampon usage, it was initially described in the pediatric population and occurs in a variety of clinical settings. TSS has significant associated morbidity and mortality, and only enhanced awareness of its possible presentation in children and adolescents will lead to timely and appropriate medical intervention.

CLINICAL PRESENTATION

Toxic shock syndrome is a multisystem disorder characterized by fever, hypotension, syncope, headache, vomiting, diarrhea, myalgias, arthralgias, inflammation of mucous membranes, and an erythematous rash that progresses to desquamation. Renal, hepatic, hematologic, and central nervous system (CNS) dysfunction are also often evident. The revised Center for Disease Control (CDC) criteria for diagnosis are outlined in Table 54–1. Because this entity remains a syndrome with no specific diagnostic test, strict adherence to all the listed criteria is required for a definitive diagnosis. Table 54–1 includes the 1981 modifications, which recognize orthostatic dizziness as evidence of hypotension and allow the inclusion of cases with positive blood cultures for *S. aureus,* to the original criteria.

The syndrome typically has an acute onset, with fever to levels of 38.9°C or higher, vomiting, and pronounced diarrhea. Complaints of lightheadedness, headache, sore throat, and joint and muscle pain are common. Physical examination reveals absolute or postural hypotension and is pertinent for nonpurulent conjunctivitis, a "strawberry" tongue, pharyngitis, and a diffuse blanching, erythematous,

macular rash that is scarlatiniform in character. Discomfort elicited upon joint examination is more often due to muscle tenderness than to synovitis. Periorbital and nonpitting pedal edema are frequent findings. The patient's state of consciousness ranges from lethargic to confused or agitated, but detailed neurologic examination generally reveals no focal deficits. In the presence of vaginitis, there is edema of the vulva, hyperemia of the vaginal mucosa, and adnexal tenderness.

Laboratory evaluation reveals no specific or uniformly present diagnostic signs, but there are several abnormalities commonly seen in patients with TSS. These abnormalities represent multiorgan system involvement and include leukocytosis with left shift, thrombocytopenia, sterile pyuria, hypocalcemia, hypoalbuminemia, hypoproteinemia, elevations of blood urea nitrogen (BUN), creatinine, bilirubin, creatine phosphokinase (CPK), serum aspartate transaminase (SGOT), and serum alanine transaminase (SGPT) and prolongation of prothrombin (PT) and partial thromboplastin (PTT) times. Laboratory data should be interpreted as to which abnormalities are more likely the consequence of shock-induced hypoperfusion than the direct result of the underlying disease process.

Cultures of infected sites and mucous membranes reveal *S. aureus.* Most of these organisms belong to phage group I. The exact incidence of positive blood cultures is uncertain. In one series, 4 percent of blood cultures were positive for *S. aureus.* The original definition of TSS, however, prohibited the inclusion of patients with positive blood cultures; thus, the low incidence must be interpreted in that context.

Chest x-ray examination upon admission is generally normal. Following volume expansion, a pulmonary edema pattern may be evident. If the hypotension is severe, the radiographic picture of adult respiratory distress syndrome (ARDS) may evolve. In the absence of myo-

Table 54–1. Revised Case Definition of Toxic Shock Syndrome

Fever: temperature ≥ 38.9°C (102°F)

Rash: diffuse macular erythroderma

Desquamation 1 to 2 weeks after onset of illness, particularly of palms and soles

Hypotension: systolic blood pressure ≤ 90 mm Hg for adults or below 5th percentile by age for children younger than 16 years of age, orthostatic drop in diastolic blood pressure ≥ 15 mm Hg from lying to sitting, orthostatic syncope, or orthostatic dizziness

Multisystem involvement—three or more of the following:

Gastrointestinal: vomiting or diarrhea at onset of illness

Muscular: severe myalgia or creatine phosphokinase level at least twice the upper limit of normal for laboratory

Mucous membrane: vaginal, oropharyngeal, or conjunctival hyperemia

Renal: blood urea nitrogen (BUN) or creatinine at least twice the upper limit of normal for laboratory or urinary sediment with pyuria (≥ 5 leukocytes per high-power field) in the absence of urinary tract infection

Hepatic: total bilirubin, SGOT*, SGPT† at least twice the upper limit of normal for laboratory

Hematologic: platelets ≤ 100,000/mm³

Central nervous system: disorientation or alterations in consciousness without focal neurologic signs when fever and hypotension are absent

Negative results on the following tests, if obtained:

Blood, throat, or cerebrospinal fluid cultures (blood culture may be positive for *Staphylococcus aureus*)

Rise in titer to Rocky Mountain spotted fever, leptospirosis, or rubeola

---

*SGOT denotes serum aspartate transaminase.
†SGPT denotes serum alanine transaminase.

From Reingold, A.L., Hargrett, N.T., Shands, K.N., et al.: Toxic shock syndrome surveillance in the United States, 1980–1981. Ann. Intern. Med. 96:875, 1982.

---

carditis and electrolyte abnormalities, the electrocardiogram (EKG) is normal.

Diseases that must be differentiated from toxic shock syndrome include scarlet fever, staphylococcal scalded skin syndrome, Kawasaki syndrome, Rocky Mountain spotted fever, leptospirosis, Stevens-Johnson syndrome, and rubeola.

EPIDEMIOLOGY

More than 90 percent of reported cases occur in association with menstruation; only 2 to 3 percent of the total reported cases are in males. In the menstruation-related group, 99 percent of the women used vaginal tampons compared with 85 percent in control groups. *S. aureus* was isolated from cervical or vaginal cultures in 96 percent of these women compared with 10 per-

cent of control subjects. Ninety-eight percent of the menstrual TSS cases occurred in white females.

TSS does occur, however, in numerous other clinical situations and can occur at any age. It is associated with pyoderma, abscesses, cellulitis, postoperative wound infections, adenitis, burns, empyema, osteomyelitis, septic abortion, and colonization of mucous membranes with *S. aureus*. The focus of staphylococcal infection may be trivial or very significant. The clinical findings in the menstrual and nonmenstrual cases are the same. Only 87 percent of nonmenstrual cases, however, were in white patients.

One or more recurrences of TSS occurred in approximately 25 percent of menstrual-related cases. Often, the severity of these recurrences was less than that of the original episodes. The incidence of such recurrences was markedly reduced if the first episode had been treated with a beta-lactamase–resistant antibiotic.

PATHOGENESIS

The association of TSS with *S. aureus* is clear. The general absence of bacteremia, the multiorgan system involvement, and the cutaneous manifestations suggest the action of a toxin. Two toxins have been isolated from strains of *S. aureus* obtained from patients with TSS. Bergdoll and associates identified enterotoxin F, which was present in 94 percent of isolates from TSS patients and in only 6 percent of controls. Staphylococcal pyrogenic exotoxin C was identified by Schlievert and colleagues in 100 percent of TSS strains as opposed to 16 percent of controls. These toxins have similar physical and chemical properties and may, in fact, be the same. A specific etiologic role for this toxin, however, has not yet been identified.

Additional support for the role of *S. aureus* is provided by the reduced incidence of recurrences after beta-lactamase–resistant antibiotic treatment.

The association of tampon use with TSS is statistically significant. In most of the tampon-related cases, tampon use was continuous throughout menstruation. The role of the tampon may be as a local irritant causing microulcerations of the cervix and vagina, which allow systemic entry of toxin produced at these sites.

TREATMENT

Specific therapy is directed at treatment of the staphylococcal infection and removal of toxin from the site. Abscesses should be drained, and foreign bodies such as sutures and tampons should be removed. Infected sites should be irrigated with normal saline (NS). Most of the TSS-related *S. aureus* is resistant to pencillin and ampicillin but sensitive to nafcillin, vancomycin, cephalosporins, and aminoglycosides. The use of antibiotics does not appear to affect the acute course, but it decreases the frequency of recurrences and treats those few patients who are bacteremic. The use of gamma globulin or antitoxin in the acute management and toxoid in the prophylaxis of TSS awaits identification and confirmation of the role of toxin as the causative agent. Prevention, at present, rests upon discontinuation of tampon use in menstruation-related cases and use of beta-lactamase–resistant antibiotics to prevent recurrences.

The remainder of therapy is supportive and directed at ensurance of adequate oxygenation, reversal of hypovolemic shock, and correction of acid-base and electrolyte disturbances. Central venous and arterial catheters should be placed to assess adequacy of circulation. A urinary drainage catheter should be passed to permit continuous monitoring of urine output. Crystalloid or colloid infusions should be administered as in any circumstance of hypovolemic shock (see Chapter 10, Shock). It has been suggested that colloid, especially albumin, infusion is associated with an increased incidence of radiographically demonstrated pulmonary vascular congestion. There is, however, no proven statistical correlation, and the patients receiving albumin tended to be those most ill. Pressors may be required as an adjunct to volume replacement.

Hypoproteinemia and hypocalcemia are common, but hypocalcemic tetany is rare. Supplementary calcium, however, appears to have a beneficial effect in the management of hypotension, but its specific role in the treatment of TSS has not been clarified.

Patients developing acute renal failure (Chapter 38), ARDS (Chapter 23), dysrhythmias (Chapter 18), and disseminated intravascular coagulation (Chapter 50, Acquired Disorders of Hemostasis) as a consequence of TSS should be managed according to the respective protocols for these complications.

PROGNOSIS AND SEQUELAE

Toxic shock syndrome carries with it a case fatality rate of 5 to 9 percent. Irreversible shock, acute renal failure, and ARDS are the primary causes of death. The remaining patients tend to recover within 5 to 6 days and exhibit desquamation 1 to 2 weeks after onset of the disease.

As previously noted, one or more recurrences can occur in the menstrual-related group. Subsequent episodes, however, tend to be less severe, and the likelihood of occurrence can be reduced by initial use of beta-lactamase–resistant antibiotics.

One of the sequelae of TSS is a pruritic, erythematous, maculopapular rash that develops in the second week after onset of the syndrome. The rash occurred in one third of the patients in one series. Other sequelae are less frequent and include decreased renal function, reversible loss of nails and hair, muscle weakness, and paresthesias.

CASE PRESENTATION

An 8-year old male was brought to the emergency room because of fever, headache, sore throat, vomiting, and a rash. Physical examination revealed an ill-appearing but well-hydrated child with diffuse erythroderma involving the face and the trunk.

History and Physical Examination

Vital signs were: heart rate = 120 beats/min, respiratory rate = 28 breaths/min, and temperature = 102.4°F. The examination was pertinent for marked erythema of the pharynx and a "strawberry" tongue. A throat culture was taken; and a diagnosis of scarlet fever was made. Penicillin was prescribed, and the child was taken home.

Over the subsequent 12 hours, he began to complain of severe pain in his extremities and he passed several watery bowel movements. While returning from the bathroom, he became dizzy and fell.

He was brought back to the hospital by ambulance and upon arrival appeared ashen. Vital signs were: BP = 60/35 mm Hg, heart rate = 160 beats/min, respiratory rate = 30 breaths/min, and temperature = 104°F. Repeat physical examination revealed a pharyngitis, a scarlatiniform rash, thready peripheral pulses, and slow capillary filling of the nailbeds. The abdomen was slightly distended but soft, nontender, and without organomegaly. Over the lateral aspect of the right mid-thigh, there was a 1 cm round carbuncle, with a surrounding zone of erythema. The patient subsequently recalled an insect bite at that location a few days earlier.

A central venous catheter was placed, and the central venous pressure (CVP) was determined to be 1 cm H_2O. A Foley catheter was passed, and 25 ml of concentrated urine was obtained.

Laboratory Data

Initial laboratory results were: ABG: pH = 7.12, Pa_{O_2} = 81 mm Hg, Pa_{CO_2} = 34 mm Hg, HCO_3 =

11 mEq/L, hematocrit = 39 percent, WBC = 21,400, with 56 percent segmented neutrophils, 25 percent bands, 15 percent lymphocytes, 3 percent monocytes, and 1 percent eosinophils; platelets = 130,000. Urine specific gravity was 1.029, with 15–20 WBC/hpf, and 0–1 RBC/hpf. Urine dipstick was positive for 2+ proteinuria. BUN = 26 mg/dl, creatinine = 1.4 mg/dl, sodium = 142 mEq/L, potassium = 4.3 mEq/L, chloride = 106 mEq/L, HCO_3 = 12 mEq/L, calcium = 6.2 mg/dl, total protein = 4.7 gm/dl, albumin = 2.4 gm/dl, bilirubin = 1.4 mg/dl, SGOT = 194 mU/ml (N: 7–40 mU/ml), SGPT = 176 mU/ml (N: 0–50 mU/ml), CPK = 515 mU/ml (N: 25–225 mU/ml), PT = 17/13 sec, PTT = 40/32 sec. EKG and chest x-ray were negative.

Cultures of blood, urine, and the thigh lesion were obtained. Gram stain of pus aspirated from the thigh carbuncle revealed gram-positive cocci in clusters. Blood was drawn for serologic determinations for Rocky Mountain spotted fever, leptospirosis, rubeola, and streptococcal infection.

The child was admitted to the pediatric ICU.

Problem List

Hypotension/Intake and Output

Three "pushes" of 20 ml/kg of NS were infused over the first 1½ hours to raise the CVP to 5 cm H_2O. Blood pressure rose to 105/70 mm Hg. Urine output increased to greater than 1 ml/kg/hr. No pressors were required.

Acid–Base Balance

Sodium bicarbonate was given to partially correct the acidosis. Administration of bicarbonate is a temporizing measure, because restoration and maintenance of a normal pH is dependent upon fluid resuscitation and return of adequate perfusion.

Hypocalcemia

Both hypocalcemia and hypoproteinemia are present. The ionized calcium fraction, however, is low and calcium chloride, 20 mg/kg, was administered IV.

Infectious

The fever, hypotension, scarlatiniform rash, pharyngitis, vomiting, myalgias, pyuria, hypoproteinemia, prolongation of PT and PTT, and elevation of the serum transaminases and CPK are all compatible with the diagnosis of TSS. The carbuncle on the right thigh probably represents the site of *S. aureus* infection. Nafcillin, 200 mg/kg/day, was ordered to be given IV in four divided doses.

Hematologic

The platelet count, although depressed, was not at thrombocytopenic levels. Prolongation of PT and PTT were mild. There was no clinical evidence of a bleeding diathesis.

The child showed dramatic improvement over the next 36 to 48 hours. The fever subsided, and the rash began to fade. Blood, urine, and throat cultures were negative. The thigh lesion grew *S. aureus*. All acute and convalescent serologic data were subsequently negative. Eight days after onset of his illness, the child had desquamation of the skin on his back, fingers, and toes.

SUGGESTED READING

Bergdoll, M.S., Crass, B.A., Reiser, R.F., et al.: A new staphylococcal enterotoxin, enterotoxin F, associated with toxic shock syndrome *Staphylococcus aureus* isolates. Lancet 1:1017, 1981.

Chesney, P.J., Crass, B.A., Polyak, M.B., et al.: Toxic shock syndrome: management and long-term sequelae. Ann. Intern. Med. 96:847, 1982.

Davis, J.P., Chesney, P.J., Wand, P.J., et al.: Toxic shock syndrome: epidemiologic features, recurrence, risk factors, and prevention. N. Engl. J. Med. 303:1436, 1980.

Nusser, R., Rowe, P., Frierson, J.G., and Murphy, C.: Hypotension in the toxic shock syndrome [letter]. Ann. Intern. Med. 95:124, 1981.

Reingold, A.L., Hargrett, N.T., Dan, B.B., et al.: Nonmenstrual toxic shock syndrome: a review of 130 cases. Ann. Intern. Med. 96:871, 1982.

Reingold, A.L., Hargrett, N.T., Sands, K.N., et al.: Toxic shock syndrome surveillance in the United States, 1980–1981. Ann. Intern. Med. 96:875, 1982.

Schlievert, P.M., Shands, K.N., Dan, B.B., et al.: Identification and characterization of an exotoxin from *Staphylococcus aureus* associated with toxic shock syndrome. J. Infect. Dis. 143:509, 1981.

Shands, K.N., Schmid, G.P., Dan, B.B., et al.: Toxic shock syndrome in menstruating women: its association with tampon use and *Staphylococcus aureus* and the clinical features in 52 cases. N. Engl. J. Med. 303:1429, 1980.

Todd, J., Fishaut, M., Kaprai, F., and Welch, T.: Toxic shock syndrome associated with phage group I staphylococci. Lancet 2:116, 1978.

Tofte, B.W., and Williams, D.N.: Clinical and laboratory manifestations of toxic shock syndrome. Ann. Intern. Med. 96:843, 1982.

Nursing Process for Patient Care:

Toxic Shock Syndrome

Toxic shock syndrome (TSS) is a multisystem disorder characterized by fever, hypotension, vomiting, diarrhea, inflammation of mucous membranes and rash. Although most often thought of as a disease associated with menstruation, it was first reported in children and occurs in other clinical settings.

CARDIOVASCULAR

Irreversible shock is one of the primary causes of death associated with TSS.

Assess, Monitor, and Document

Pulse
Blood pressure: arterial, central venous
Perfusion: peripheral pulses, capillary filling, skin color, skin condition
Respiratory rate
Urine output hourly, including specific gravity
Thirst
Altered level of consciousness

Response to:
 Crystalloid replacement
 Colloid infusion
 Pressors (if indicated)
 Accurate administration of parenteral fluids (use infusion pump if available)
Laboratory data: arterial blood gases, serum electrolytes

Anticipate

Shock
 Hypotension
 Tachycardia
 Tachypnea
 Poor capillary filling
 Cold, clammy skin
 Cyanosis
 Decreased urinary output
 Altered level of consciousness
Complications of shock
 Adult respiratory distress syndrome (ARDS)
  Tachypnea
  Retractions

 Rales
 Rhonchi
 Increased secretions (may be blood tinged)
Acute renal failure
 Decreased urine output
 Increased BUN, creatinine
Disseminated intravascular coagulation
 Petechiae
 Bruises
 Oozing from wound or puncture sites
 Frank bleeding
 Altered laboratory data: thrombocytopenia, prolonged PT, PTT levels

INFECTIOUS PROCESS

Assess, Monitor, and Document

Temperature
Site of infection
Response to management

Antibiotic administration
Local wound care (if appropriate)
Subsequent cultures

Anticipate

Fever
Persistent positive cultures

INTEGUMENTARY

The appearance of a diffuse, erythematous maculopapular rash is associated with TSS. Desquamation usually occurs 1 to 2 weeks after onset of illness, particularly on the palms of the hands and soles of the feet.

Assess, Monitor, and Document

Status of rash: description, location

Anticipate

Desquamation

GASTROINTESTINAL

The gastrointestinal system is involved early in the course of TSS. The initial clinical presentation is associated with vomiting and diarrhea. Fluid loss related to alteration in gastrointestinal function can have a significant effect on fluid balance and the total hemodynamic status of the child.

Assess, Monitor, and Document

Alteration in gastrointestinal function
  Vomiting: amount, description

Diarrhea: amount, description
Total body output

Anticipate

Fluid loss
Electrolyte loss and imbalance

CENTRAL NERVOUS SYSTEM

Assess, Monitor, and Document

Level of consciousness
Blood pressure
Pulse

Respiratory rate and pattern
Headache

Anticipate

Alteration in level of consciousness

Cerebral edema
Seizures

RESPONSE OF CHILD

Assess, Monitor, and Document

Developmental level: verbal, psychosocial, cognitive, fears
Behavioral response: anxious, fearful, compliant, quiet, aggressive

Response to nursing interventions

RESPONSE OF FAMILY

Assess, Monitor, and Document

Behavioral response: anxious, fearful, verbal, angry
Level of understanding of disorder and child's condition
Expected outcome

Educational needs
  TSS
    Possibility of recurrence
    Clinical manifestations
Response to nursing interventions

Anticipate

Inability to cope
Family crisis
Educational needs related to discharge

MIND SET

Assess

Temperature
Cardiovascular status
Integumentary system
Gastrointestinal system
Muscular system
Mucous membranes
Central nervous system

Laboratory data that reflect status of other
    systems
    Renal
    Hepatic
    Hematologic
Emotional response of child and family

Anticipate

Fever
Shock
    Complications of shock: ARDS, acute renal
        failure, disseminated intravascular coag-
        ulation DIC)
Rash
    Diffuse macular erythroderma
    Desquamation 1 to 2 weeks after onset of
        illness
Vomiting

Diarrhea
Myalgia
Arthralgia
Inflammation of mucous membranes: vagi-
    nal, oropharyngeal, conjunctival
Alteration in level of consciousness
Alteration in laboratory data reflecting multi-
    organ system involvement
Emotional crisis
Family crisis

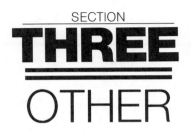

SECTION

THREE

OTHER

CHAPTER

55

Burns

JOHN M. STEIN, M.D.

Burns are among the severest injuries suffered by humans. Management of children with major thermal trauma taxes the personnel of the most sophisticated critical care unit. As with all trauma, initial care focuses on airway, breathing, and circulation, but even during this earliest phase, attention should be given to clean or preferably sterile technique to avoid early contamination of the burn wound with the virulent and antibiotic-resistant organisms hospital personnel carry on their hands.

Because cutaneous burns are such an obvious physical finding, and because the child is often struggling and in pain, the usual careful physical examination is sometimes abbreviated; this is a mistake that one will later regret when wondering if the heart murmur or the neurologic deficit was there on admission. If the burn is associated with other trauma (e.g., a jump from a burning building, car crash, child abuse), a diligent search for associated injuries must be made. Associated injuries should be cared for as soon as possible and almost always should take precedence over the burn. Craniotomy, thoracotomy, laparotomy, and fracture fixation carry the least risk of infection and complications when carried out during the first 24 hours after burn while resuscitation is continued.

Severely burn-injured children face a multitude of problems during initial hospitalization, including: 1) upper airway compromise due to edema; 2) lower airway damage due to smoke inhalation; 3) respiratory distress syndrome; 4) restriction of chest wall movement due to constriction by an unyielding burn eschar and subcutaneous edema; 5) impaired limb

perfusion by similar eschar constriction and edema; 6) fluid and electrolyte management; 7) multiple operative procedures with the difficult anesthetic management problems of fluid control, blood replacement, and regulation of body temperature; 8) recognition of sepsis and use of potentially toxic antibiotics in an immunocompromised host; 9) overgrowth by opportunistic organisms, particularly fungi and viruses; 10) nutrition; 11) pain control; 12) psychological problems involving patient, parents, siblings, and medical staff; and 13) rehabilitation for both function and cosmesis. This chapter focuses on the critical care of burned children and only *touches* on many of the important problems just enumerated.

ETIOLOGY

The etiology of burns is presented in Table 55–1. Although the depth of the burn (see Pathophysiology) is often determined by its cause, this relationship is not constant. Child abuse must always be considered, but it is difficult to prove from the appearance of most burns except for the obvious cigarette burn, contact with the pattern of the stove top burner or flatiron branded on the skin. Some scald burns, particularly those with a sharp level of demarcation and no splash marks, are typical of inflicted burns. Child neglect and improper supervision are more common than actual willful abuse.

If the history of thermal injury is vague, a differential diagnosis of other problems with

Table 55–1. Etiology of Burns With Clinical Correlation

Etiology	Usual Depth*	Common Clinical Findings*	Comments
Sun	1° 2° 3°	Erythema with blanching Erythema and blisters Erthema w/o blanching	Uncommon Rare; may occur in infants
Scald	2° 1° 3°	Erythema with blisters Erythema Erythema w/o blanching	Most common Depth depends upon water temperature, duration of exposure, and skin thickness
Flame	3°	Dry, firm, parchment-like	
Flash flame	2°	Dry or blistered	Illuminating gas explosion w/o sustained fire Look for perforated TMs
Chemical	Any depth	Early erythema. Takes days to determine actual depth Multiple splash marks often present	Depends upon strength of chemical and concentration Rapidity of washing it off Commonly strong acid or base
Contact	Usually 3°, but can be any depth	Sharply demarcated injury Recognizable pattern, e.g., stove top, common	Duration of contact, skin thickness, and temperature determine depth
Electrical low voltage (household)	3°	Sharply demarcated	Hairpin in socket and electric cord bites common May cause ventricular fibrillation
Electrical high voltage	3°	Depressed hard entry wound. Blast-like exit wound.	Tissue damage extends far beyond visible skin burn.
Radiation	Any depth	Early erythema. Late skin necrosis	Systemic effects of radiation
Microwave	Skin usually spared	Deep pain of ischemia and neural damage	

*Depth and clinical findings vary by case. See sections of text entitled Etiology and Pathophysiology.

similar appearance should be considered. The scalded skin syndrome is aptly named, and diagnosis is made by culturing *Staphylococcus aureus* from the patient. Drug reaction with epidermolysis or epidermal necrosis (Stevens-Johnson syndrome), as well as pemphigus, may be considered.

PATHOPHYSIOLOGY

Major burn injury is more than a dermatologic problem; multiple organ systems respond to the trauma and show varying degrees of derangement during the course of treatment.

Superficial or first-degree burns are erythematous without blistering, painful, and sensitive to pinprick. Partial-thickness or second-degree burns are characterized by blister formation or erythema, with a wet, exudative wound. Sensation to pinprick is variable; in burns that penetrate deep into but not through the dermis, the cutaneous nerve endings may be damaged and insensitive. Areas of full-thickness or third-degree burns extend beyond the depths of the hair follicles and into the subcutaneous tissue. These areas are generally blanched and appear depressed; they swell less rapidly than the surrounding second-degree burn, and destruction of nerve endings causes local anesthesia. (Fig. 55–1).

Infants younger than 2 years of age have particularly thin skin and are prone to full-thickness burns, which, by the usual criteria, at first appear to be second-degree burns. There is a general tendency to underestimate depth and to overestimate size of burns.

The burn is less deep at its perimeter than at its center. There are also variations in depth as a result of differences in intensity of exposure to thermal trauma, in body positions, and in skin thickness. The etiology of the thermal injury usually provides some indication of the depth of the burn.

Within moments of injury the skin is laminated into three zones that have a three-dimensional bowl-like configuration, with the deepest burn usually at the center of the lesion (Fig. 55–2). The central area (zone of coagulation) contains cells that have been heated to a temperature sufficient to coagulate their proteins; they are dead without hope of salvage. Surrounding the zone of coagulation is a layer of tissue that has sustained thermal damage but not to the point of instant death. This injured layer or zone of stasis is so named because bloodflow in its capillaries is markedly slowed. The zone of stasis may be salvaged by immediate (within minutes) cooling of the burned area, use of prostaglandin inhibitors aimed at reducing local thromboxane elaboration, and

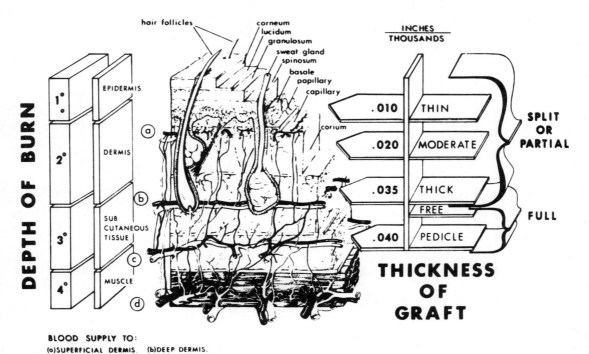

Figure 55–1. Cross section of skin depicting blood supply, depth of burn, and relative thickness of skin grafts. (From Artz, C.P., Moncrief, J.A., and Pruitt, B.A.: Burns: A Team Approach. Philadelphia, W.B. Saunders Company, 1979, p. 434. Used by permission.)

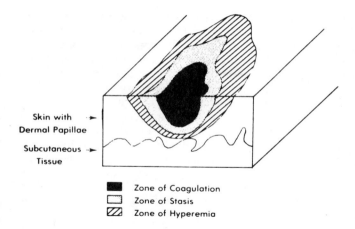

Skin with → Dermal Papillae

Subcutaneous → Tissue

■ Zone of Coagulation
▢ Zone of Stasis
▨ Zone of Hyperemia

Figure 55–2. The burn wound is characteristically made up of several zones of tissue death, with confluent wounds of equal depth being unusual except in very deep burns. The zone of coagulation is the site of irreversible skin death. The zone of hyperemia is the site of minimal cell involvement and early spontaneous recovery. In the zone of stasis, infection or drying of the wound results in conversion of this potentially salvageable area to full-thickness skin destruction with irreversible cell death. (From Artz, C.P., Moncrief, J.A., and Pruitt, B.A.: Burns: A Team Approach. Philadelphia, W.B. Saunders Company, 1979, p. 171. Used by permission.)

prevention of burn wound desiccation with artificial membranes, amnion or porcine, or human cadaveric skin. Failure to resuscitate the zone of stasis will lead to an apparent deepening of the burn wound several days after the injury, because the cells in this layer die from lack of circulation. Surrounding the zone of stasis is a layer of minimally injured and uninjured cells, which react to the adjacent tissue injury by vasodilatation (zone of hyperemia). This less than 1-mm-wide red line of hyperemia can be seen surrounding most burns within an hour and represents one of the earliest events in wound healing.

Two factors make the zone of coagulation important. First, being an avascular and unprotected tissue in contact with the outside environment, it is susceptible to colonization and invasion by all microbes, usually bacteria. As the bacterial burden of this avascular burn *eschar* increases, a critical mass of bacteria may occur, which then allows invasion of deeper, viable tissue, heralding the start of burn wound sepsis. Second, in the earliest phase of the burn (during the first several days), myocardial depressant polypeptides and lipoproteins may be leached from the eschar into the circulation, reducing cardiac output to subnormal levels even when there is apparently sufficient intravascular volume, as judged by measurements of right and left heart filling pressures. Four to 5 days after the burn when the myocardial depressant factors from the eschar have been exhausted and the hypermetabolism of burn injury supervenes, supranormal cardiac output is noted. (Fig. 55–3).

It is in the zone of stasis and in its junction with the zone of hyperemia that the massive *edema* associated with burns develops. The injured capillaries in the region develop large pores, allowing egress of plasma with all its protein fractions. In contact with tissue thromboplastin, a gel-like clotted protein-rich edema

forms. Subsequent clot lysis with resorption of fibrin split products may account in part for the pulmonary infiltrates sometimes seen 2 to 5 days after burn injury, even in the absence of smoke inhalation or pneumonia. The edema fluid lost from the intravascular space accounts for much of the volume required for *resuscitation,* but uninjured tissues also become edematous due to decreased serum oncotic pressure secondary to protein loss in the burn. Because the amount of edema formation has been related to the volume of fluid used for resuscitation, some burn centers use hypertonic sodium solutions (containing 200 to 250 mEq Na/L) to draw water from the intracellular into the intravascular space, thereby reducing the amount of exogenous fluid volume required for resuscitation. Because large quantities of protein are lost into the burn wound during the first 24 hours following the burn, other centers have used colloid (albumin) during early resuscita-

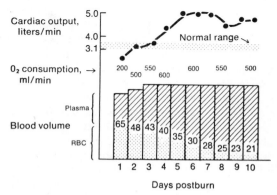

Figure 55–3. Typical response of cardiac output, O_2 consumption, and blood volume in burns of more than 50 percent full-thickness injury. Emphasis is placed on the low cardiac output during the first 3 days, followed by elevated output as hypermetabolism occurs. (From Practical Approaches to Burn Management. Deerfield, Illinois, Flint Laboratories, Division of Travenol Laboratories, Inc., 1977. Used by permission.)

tion. Albumin-containing resuscitative solutions were successfully used in the past in the old Brooke and Evans formulae, but few centers now use colloid during the first 12- to 24-postburn hours because of the increased leak of colloid into the burn wound and an increase in pulmonary complications. Today, most centers use Ringer's lactate solution alone during the first 12 to 24 hours and start albumin administration after that time, because the massive capillary leaks in the zone of stasis seem to seal in that time period, allowing the administered albumin to stay in the circulation.

Another feature found in the zones of stasis and hyperemia is margination and diapedesis of polymorphonuclear leukocytes. A child seen within 1 to 4 hours of burn will have a peripheral white blood cell (WBC) count of 15,000 to 25,000 per mm³, with a marked shift to the left. Within 2 to 4 days, a precipitous drop to 3,000 to 6,000 is seen, with even more of a left shift and the appearance of a high percentage of bands and even more juvenile forms in the WBC series. This is a consumptive leukopenia. The use of topical silversulfadiazine on the burn wound may further depress the nadir of the leukopenia. Over the next several days, the WBC count slowly rises, usually settling in the range of 8,000 to 18,000, with a continued left shift. Failure of the WBC count to return to these levels should alert the clinician to the possibility of early sepsis.

Several *respiratory* problems will complicate burn care considerably. *Glottic* and *subglottic* edema are associated with burns of the face and neck and are treated by orotracheal or nasotracheal intubation. Early intubation is particularly important in the very young, because minimal amounts of edema will severely compromise their small airways. The volume of resuscitative fluid should be kept as sparse as possible to minimize edema and, unless other pulmonary problems develop, extubation can be expected within 3 to 5 days.

Inhalation injury is also associated with burns of the face and neck, particularly in closed space fires. Vaporized aldehydes, ketones, acrolein, and other toxins produced by burning fabrics, plastics, and wood combine with the moist endotracheal and endobroncheal epithelium, causing a chemical burn. Early bronchoscopy will aid in making the diagnosis, which may not become obvious on chest x-rays for several days. The extent and depth of the damage to the respiratory epithelium is determined by the nature and concentration of the toxins in the inhaled smoke as well as the duration of exposure. Hydrocarbon soot, although highly visible, does not cause severe damage to the ciliated respiratory epithelium and is cleared within hours or days, with little residual damage. The presence of soot, however, should alert the clinician that other more toxic chemicals may have been inhaled.

True toxic inhalation injury may be classified as mild, moderate, or severe. In mild injury, there is temporary paralysis of the cilia, with resultant pooling of secretions and possibly the development of pneumonia. In moderate injury, portions of the respiratory epithelium are destroyed, leading to pneumonia, which will be difficult to eradicate. Healing takes place with squamous metaplasia, which lacks a ciliated surface and leads to recurrent pulmonary infections. Patients who survive this injury are apt to have permanent reduction in pulmonary function and recurrent infection and may develop bronchiectasis. In severe inhalation injury, large portions of the respiratory epithelium and the underlying tissues are involved. There is a profuse and uncontrollable bronchorrhea, followed in several days by sloughing of the necrotic tissue. Entire casts of the bronchial tree are sometimes recovered from the endotracheal tube or tracheostomy in such cases, and survival is uncommon (Fig. 55–4).

Carbon monoxide poisoning should be suspected with any flame burn, but it is more common with closed space injuries. The diagnosis is made by measurement of blood carboxyhemoglobin levels. Carbon monoxide is not toxic to the lungs, but rather, it combines 200 times more firmly with the hemoglobin molecule than does oxygen, thereby interfering with O_2 transport. The half-life of carboxyhemoglobin is 4 hours with 100 percent O_2 treatment at atmospheric pressure. Although the presence of

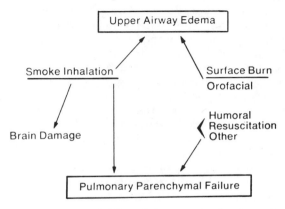

Figure 55–4. Factors in respiratory failure in burn patients. (From Stein, J.M.: Burns in childhood. *In* Rudolph, A.M. (ed.): Pediatrics, 17th ed. Norwalk, Appleton-Century-Crofts, 1982. Used by permission.)

carboxyhemoglobinemia should alert the clinician to the possibility of toxic smoke inhalation, it is not diagnostic.

Although some facts about the *hemic* system, such as the initial leukocytosis and the subsequent consumptive leukopenia, have already been stated, other matters deserve mention. Burned children will generally maintain some degree of leukocytosis throughout the course of treatment until the burn wound is completely healed or grafted. The WBC with differential should be monitored frequently, looking for abrupt changes. Sepsis, which is often difficult to diagnose early in burned children, may be heralded either by a rise in WBC or by a fall to leukopenic levels. In either case, the differential WBC count will be shifted more markedly to the left, showing not only bands but also myelocytes, metamyelocytes, and occasionally promyelocytes in a leukemoid-like reaction. Red cell production is decreased, and the marrow seems less responsive to erythropoietin than normal. Examination of the marrow reveals a dearth in the erythroid series. Frequent blood sampling accentuates the anemia.

The *hypermetabolism* of burns is generally related to the size of the burn. Little increase is seen until the burn size reaches about 10 percent of the total body surface area. From 10 to 50 or 60 percent, there is an almost linear increase in metabolic rate, which peaks at 2 to 2.5 times normal. There is little or no further increase in metabolic rate as burn size increases from 60 to 100 percent.

Accompanying the hypermetabolism, there is constant hyperthermia to levels of about 38.5°C. The hyperthermia follows a reset of the brain's thermoregulatory center, caused in part by leukocyte pyrogens and in part by endocrine responses. No attempt should be made to reduce the fever unless it reaches levels that may cause convulsions or brain damage, arbitrarily 39.5° to 40°C. Use of cooling blankets or a cool environment will only cause the child to shiver to maintain the preset temperature and to waste valuable calories in the attempt. Most burn victims are comfortable and have a neutral thermal environment at an ambient temperature of about 33°C. Focal external heating devices should be used to maintain this environmental temperature without causing excessive discomfort to the personnel who are treating the victim. Maintenance of sufficient environmental temperature is particularly important during the prolonged operative procedures that the child is likely to require.

Almost every *endocrine system* is affected by burn injury. Hypermetabolism immediately raises the possibility of excessive thyroid function. Indeed, T_3 and T_4 levels are usually normal, but there is significant elevation of the metabolically inactive reverse T_3. Marked catecholamine elevation is consistently found and is probably a major cause of the hypermetabolism.

Adrenal cortical hormones are also elevated, as are estrogens and progesterone, but testosterone is low in the adults who have been studied. Antidiuretic hormone (ADH) is also elevated, making the syndrome of inappropriate ADH (SIADH) a common occurrence.

Abnormally elevated *liver* function tests (SGOT, SGPT, alkaline phosphatase) are also seen often; these abnormal findings were noted even before the use of aggressive intravenous (IV) nutritional support.

Although acute *renal* failure (ARF) following underresuscitation in the acute phase of the burn is often cited as the reason for giving generous volumes of fluids early, acute tubular necrosis (ATN) caused by insufficient volume of resuscitative fluids is rarely seen in the United States today. The opposite is usually seen, with overly generous fluid administration causing massive edema, weight gain, and even pulmonary edema. During resuscitation, IV fluids should be administered at a rate to produce low normal urinary output, approximately 0.20 to 0.25 ml per minute for infants younger than 1 year of age, 0.4 to 0.5 ml per minute for children 1 to 5 years of age, and 0.5 to 0.8 ml per minute for older children. Somewhat higher urinary outputs should be sought in those patients who have free hemoglobin or myoglobin (not just red cells) in the urine in order to prevent precipitation of these hemochromogens in the collecting tubules. Free hemochromogens in serum and urine are often seen following high-voltage electrical injury and after very deep flame burns.

Today, renal failure is seen more commonly as a consequence of aminoglycoside antibiotic administration than as a result of inadequate resuscitation. Creatinine and aminoglycoside clearance are considerably increased following major burn injury; hence, antibiotic levels in the serum must be carefully monitored, and unusually large doses with increased frequency are often required to attain adequate serum and tissue levels.

The *gastrointestinal system* is also a participant in burn injury. Children with burns exceeding 20 to 30 percent of the total body surface tend to get an adynamic ileus, which seems to affect the stomach and colon more than the small intestine; it usually lasts 1 to 3 days. Acute gastric dilatation with vomiting and aspiration is dangerous. Although a few burn centers start intestinal feedings with liquid elemental diets during the period of ileus, most await resolution of the ileus before starting enteral alimentation.

Gastroduodenal ulceration of clinical importance has almost disappeared with aggressive use of antacids and cimetidine. Monitoring gastric pH while the nasogastric (NG) tube is in place is recommended, and the dose of antacid is appropriately modified. Although massive hemorrhage from and perforation of acute peptic ulcers is rare, some slow blood loss through the stool may still be detected. Indeed, those victims who die of massive burns continue to show superficial erosions of stomach and duodenum at autopsy. Duodenal obstruction due to superior mesenteric artery syndrome may be seen.

Acute pancreatitis and calculous, as well as acalculous cholecystitis continue to be seen, albeit infrequently.

Both the circulating and cellular arms of the *immune system* are impaired following severe burns. There is accelerated turnover of all plasma proteins, including immunoglobulins of all types and nonspecific opsonic factors (e.g., fibronectin). Synthesis can rarely keep pace with destruction; thus, plasma levels of all these proteins are generally low. During septic episodes, the already low levels are depressed even further.

Despite the usually elevated total WBC count, the absolute lymphocyte count is often low. Furthermore, there may be an imbalance between helper and suppressor T lymphocytes.

Although the total number of WBCs in the polymorphonuclear neutrophil (PMN) series is generally increased, the function of the WBCs is depressed, as measured by chemotactic, phagocytic, and bacterial killing indices. Thus, it is evident that the body's entire defense system against invading microbes, from the intact mechanical skin barrier to the internal circulating and cellular mechanisms, is weakened.

Adequate *nutritional* support strengthens all these weakened defense systems, but it fails to return them to normal. Administration of exogenous immune factors such as globulin may be helpful. Fibronectin (cold insoluble globulin) can be supplied by undepleted fresh frozen plasma (FFP) and, in a more concentrated form, by cryoprecipitate and may be beneficial. Studies are currently being done using various immunostimulants, such as thymosin, to determine whether lymphocyte function can be improved. The use of transfused WBCs has not been found to be helpful.

TREATMENT

Fluid Resuscitation

Most clinicians who treat burn victims agree that the volume of resuscitative fluids should be kept to the minimum required to sustain vital functions in order to avoid excessive edema formation in the burn wound and lungs. The total volume that will be required during the first 24 hours can be estimated as follows: 3 ml $\times$ percentage of total body surface burn $\times$ preburn body weight (kg; Fig. 55–5). One half of the calculated volume should be given during the first eight postburn hours, because edema formation is most rapid during that time. Remember to take into account the fluids that were given before you took over the care of the child. The operative word in the formula is "estimate." The estimated rate of administration must be altered in response to close monitoring of the patient, just as one would do with any hypovolemic child. Adequate information can usually be obtained by monitoring urinary output (which should be kept at low normal for the child's age and size), pulse and blood pressure (which can be obtained from noninvasive electronic blood pressure cuff systems), and physical examination (mental status, capillary refill in unburned areas, venous filling, chest auscultation). Arterial blood gases help to determine sufficiency of oxygenation, and metabolic acidosis is a measure of insufficient tissue perfusion. Again, noninvasive means such as transcutaneous O_2 electrodes and capillary blood gases from an unburned extremity or earlobe should be used whenever feasible, because invasive lines are likely to become infected in burned children. Invasive central venous, pulmonary arterial, and systemic arterial lines are, of course, indicated if noninvasive measurements are insufficient. Body weight should be measured. **Danger Sign**: Severely burned children are more likely to be overhydrated than to develop hypovolemic shock or ATN.

Changes in the rate of fluid administration in response to monitored findings should be made gradually; usually not more than a 20 percent increase or decrease in rate is made at any one time unless the child is in obvious hypovolemic shock or pulmonary edema. If changes are made too rapidly, one will oscillate between overhydration and underhydration, never attaining that particular child's ideal requirement. It should be remembered that as the rate of edema formation slows, fluid requirements will diminish.

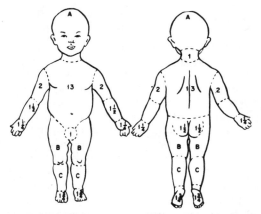
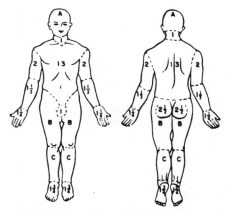
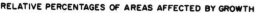

RELATIVE PERCENTAGES OF AREAS AFFECTED BY GROWTH

AREA	AGE 0	1	5
A = ½ of Head	$9\frac{1}{2}$	$8\frac{1}{2}$	$6\frac{1}{2}$
B = ½ of One Thigh	$2\frac{3}{4}$	$3\frac{1}{4}$	4
C = ½ of One Leg	$2\frac{1}{2}$	$2\frac{1}{2}$	$2\frac{3}{4}$

% BURN BY AREAS

RELATIVE PERCENTAGES OF AREAS AFFECTED BY GROWTH

AREA	AGE 10	15	ADULT
A = ½ of Head	$5\frac{1}{2}$	$4\frac{1}{2}$	$3\frac{1}{2}$
B = ½ of One Thigh	$4\frac{1}{2}$	$4\frac{1}{2}$	$4\frac{3}{4}$
C = ½ of One Leg	3	$3\frac{1}{4}$	$3\frac{1}{2}$

% BURN BY AREAS

Figure 55–5. The percent of body surface area (BSA) burned can be calculated from this drawing and the accompanying chart. Knowing the percent of the burn is helpful in estimating fluid requirements, nutritional requirements, and likelihood of survival. (From Practical Approaches to Burn Management. Deerfield, Illinois, Flint Laboratories, Division of Travenol Laboratories, Inc., 1977. Used by permission.)

Although there is consensus about the quantity of resuscitative fluid required, there is less agreement as to its quality. Most commonly, lactated Ringer's solution without dextrose is used initially. Some clinicians use hypertonic sodium solutions and others add albumin to the initial solution; the rationale for each was discussed in the section entitled Pathophysiology.

There is agreement that the capillary leaks in the zone of stasis begin to seal around 24 hours after injury and that albumin administration should be started at this time to replenish serum oncotic pressure.

Surgical intervention directed at either excision of portions of the burn wound with grafting or correction of associated traumatic injuries may be undertaken during the first 24 to 48 hours during the resuscitative phase. Blood lost should be replaced with red cells, albumin, or FFP and platelets. Resuscitation must continue under anesthesia, again guided by the appropriate methods that are least invasive.

Respiratory and Airway

Endotracheal intubation is necessary to bypass upper airway edema. The orotracheal or nasotracheal route is preferred. Fiberoptic endoscopes may be required to accomplish this if considerable edema has occurred before the decision was made to intubate. The endotracheal tube must be securely fastened using strings passed around the head and neck or sutures or even wiring it to the teeth, because adhesive tape will not stick firmly to the burned face. Because replacement of a dislodged endotracheal tube in the presence of massive facial and cervical edema is a very difficult task, some clinicians prefer tracheostomy (despite its complications when there are contiguous neck burns) except in very young patients in whom tracheomalacia will develop, making decannulation impossible.

In cases of inhalation injury with damage to the tracheal and bronchial mucosa, intubation and early use of positive pressure ventilation are advised. Humidified, warmed gas with the lowest possible O_2 tension consistent with adequate arterial blood gases is used. Steroids are withheld. The endotracheal tube must be large enough to allow suction of the profuse bronchorrhea. N-acetylcysteine (Mucomyst) may help loosen secretions and débride necrotic mucosa, but it causes bronchospasm and should be used with a bronchodilator such as isoproterenol or terbutaline.

Infection and Antibiotics

The most common cause of death among burned patients is infection. No matter what type of isolation procedure is used, ranging from the strictest procedures with caps, masks, gowns, gloves, shoe covers, and laminar flow to minimal isolation, using gloves only to change the dressings, all burn wounds will eventually become colonized, at first with the patient's own endogenous bacteria and later with hospital strains. Protecting the rest of the hospital from the bacteria in the burn treatment area is another consideration for isolation.

Because the coagulated zone of the burn wound is avascular, neither the body's own defense mechanisms nor systemic antibiotics are effective in combating bacteria in that area. Therefore, topical antimicrobial agents are applied to the burn wound. Although these topical agents can reduce the number of bacteria in the eschar, they do not render the wound sterile. Several topical agents are available, each with its own advantages, disadvantages, indications, contraindications, and complications. The most commonly used topical agent today is silver sulfadiazine. Its popularity stems from its moderate effectiveness against the most common bacteria found in the burn wound, namely, staphylococci and pseudomonas, and its relative lack of complications. More detailed information about this drug and the other commonly used topical agents, such as mafenide, povidone-iodine, and silver nitrate, is available in other sources.

Deciding when a burned child is septic and in need of antibiotic treatment is not always a straightforward procedure, because elevation of body temperature and leukocytosis with left shift are physiologic reactions to uninfected burn injury. One must look to other findings such as a change in mental status, commonly lethargy, recurrence or persistence of ileus after the third postburn day, sudden rise or fall of WBC with an even more accentuated left shift, and glucose intolerance. Any of these findings should make the clinician suspicious that sepsis is occurring.

The five most common sites of sepsis are 1) burn wound, 2) lungs, 3) urine, 4) any presently or previously used IV sites, and 5) abdomen. Meningitis is uncommon but should be considered if no other focus is found. Diagnostic cisternal puncture may be required if the back is burned. Burn–unrelated intercurrent processes such as otitis, appendicitis, and viral diseases such as chickenpox should not be forgotten.

The entire burn wound must be thoroughly and closely inspected daily. In uninfected burn wounds, there is an absolutely sharp demarcation between the burned skin and the adjacent normal skin. The slightest erythema around the burn perimeter is often the earliest sign of burn wound infection and should be treated with antibiotics. Focal color changes within the burn, changes in the type of wound exudate, ulceration of the burn wound below the general level of the surrounding skin, and deteriorating or pale waxy granulation tissue are also among the gross findings of burn wound infection. In order that appropriate antibiotics can be started as soon as the gross findings become evident, it should be routine procedure to culture the burn wound periodically (usually once or twice weekly). Quantitative biopsy cultures are the most accurate, but surface cultures (after the topical antimicrobial has been removed) and wound scrapings generally allow identification of the bacteria. The results of these routine cultures and antibiotic sensitivities are stored so that if gross findings of wound infection occur, appropriate antimicrobial therapy can be started immediately. In addition to systemic antibiotic therapy, débridement of the wound and occasionally subeschar injection of antibiotics may be helpful.

Aggressive early excision of the dead burn wound with skin grafting is now considered the best way to prevent burn wound sepsis.

Diagnosis and treatment of lung infections are the same as in unburned patients. In intubated patients, it is good practice to obtain routine tracheal aspirates for gram stain, culture, and sensitivity.

Recurrent urinary tract infections are common, because essentially all severely burned patients will have indwelling urinary catheters for varying lengths of time. These catheters should, of course, be removed at the earliest possible time to minimize this source of infection.

Venous and arterial access sites are in constant danger of infection. In general, no line should be left in place for more than 48 hours; 72 hours is an absolute maximum. Suppurative thrombophlebitis in a currently or previously used site may be an insidious and hard-to-find septic focus, causing bacteremia. Surgical drainage or excision may be required if the process fails to respond to antibiotic therapy.

Abdominal sepsis from antibiotic-related enterocolitis, perforated viscus, cholecystitis, and pancreatitis should be considered and treated if found. Fungal overgrowth, commonly Candida, in the gastrointestinal tract is common during prolonged and repeated courses of antibiotics and may become the source of bloodstream invasion and systemic candidiasis; oral mycostatin reduces this risk.

Nutrition

The nutritional support of the burned child is extremely important because of the high metabolic rate and the deleterious effect of undernutrition and malnutrition on the immune system and wound healing. The aim of nutritional support is stable weight, using preburn weight or admission weight as a baseline. The weight should stabilize 3 to 5 days after the day of burn, when the excess fluid given during resuscitation has been eliminated through the urine and by insensible routes. Evaporative water losses are increased through the burn wound and can be estimated at about 1 to 2 ml per kg per percentage of burn. Burn tissue excised at surgery should be weighed and subtracted from baseline weight, because it may account for a considerable proportion of total body weight, particularly in the very young.

There are several formulas that can be used to estimate nutritional requirements. A simple method used to estimate the daily caloric requirement is

maintenance requirement
plus
calories for the burned area

$$= 1800 \text{ Kcal/m}^2 \text{ of BSA/day}$$
plus
$$= 2000 \text{ Kcal/m}^2 \text{ of burn wound/day}$$

The area of the burn wound is found by multiplying the body surface area (BSA) by the percentage of burn.

A calorie: nitrogen ratio of 150:1 is a usual starting point. Many patients, however, will require more nitrogen, and ratios as low as 80:1 or 90:1 may be required and tolerated. The importance of adequate amounts of high-quality protein to maintain the immune system has been stressed. In general, 15 to 20 percent of calories will come from protein, about 48 percent from carbohydrates, and the balance from fats.

Because of the dangers of IV lines, enteral nutrition is preferred, even if gavage feeding is necessary. Minerals, particularly zinc, magnesium, and phosphate, must be supplied along with multivitamin supplements, stressing A and C.

Nutritional monitoring by body weight and measurement of plasma proteins, particularly albumin, globulin, and transferrin, should be carried out. All enteral and parenteral intake should be recorded. Nitrogen balance studies are usually inaccurate, because much protein is lost through the burn wound itself.

Team Approach

From the foregoing discussions, it is evident that modern therapy for severely burned children requires a multidisciplinary team that communicates well and frequently. In recognition of the need for teamwork, the American Burn Association includes in its membership not only physicians from all specialties but also nurses, Ph.D. researchers, occupational and physical therapists, administrators, social workers, dietitians, and some former patients who have recovered from burn injury.

SUGGESTED READING

Artz, C.P., Moncrief, J.A., and Pruitt, B.A.: Burns: A Team Approach. Philadelphia, W.B. Saunders Company, 1979.

Burke, J.F., Bondoc, C.C., and Quinby, W.C.: Primary burn excision and immediate grafting: a method shortening illness. J. Trauma 14:389, 1974.

Caldwell, F.R., and Bowser, B.A.: Critical evaluation of hypertonic and hypotonic solution to resuscitate severely burned children: a prospective study. Ann. Surg. 189:546, 1979.

Durtschi, M.B., Kohler, T.R., Finley, A., and Heimbach, D.M.: Burn injury in infants and young children. Surg. Gynecol. Obstet. 150:651, 1980.

Hildreth, M., and Carvajal, H.F.: Caloric requirements in burned children: a simple formula to estimate daily caloric requirements. J. Burn Care Rehab. 2:78, 1982.

Lemoski, E.F., and Hunter, K.A.: Specific patterns of inflicted burn injuries. J. Trauma 17:842, 1977.

Lewis, P.J., and Zucker, R.M.: Childhood scald burns: an inquiry into severity. J. Burn Care Rehab. 3:95, 1982.

Moylan, J.A., and Chan, C.K.: Inhalation injury—an increasing problem. Ann. Surg. 188:34, 1978.

Myers, R.A., Linberg, S.E., Cowley, R.A., et al.: Carbon monoxide poisoning: the injury and its treatment. J. Am. Coll. Emer. Phys. 8:479, 1979.

Neal, G.D., Lindholm, G.R., Lee, M.J., et al.: Burn wound histologic culture—a new technique for predicting burn wound sepsis. J. Burn Care Rehab. 2:35, 1981.

Robbins, A.B., Doran, J.E., Reese, A.C., et al.: Clinical response to cold insoluble globulin replacement in a patient with sepsis and thermal injury. Am. J. Surg. 142:636, 1981.

Robson, M.C., Del Beccaro, E.J., Heggers, J.P., et al.: Increasing dermal perfusion after burning by decreasing thromboxane production. J. Trauma 20:722, 1980.

Shires, T.G., and Black, E.A., (eds.): Second conference on supportive therapy in burn care. J. Trauma (Suppl) 21:665, 1981.

Stein, J.M.: Burns in childhood. In Rudolph, A.M. (ed.): Pediatrics, 17th ed. Norwalk, Connecticut, Appleton-Century-Crofts, 1982.

Wallner, S.F., Vautrin, R.M., Buerk, C., et al.: The anemia of thermal injury: studies of erythropoiesis in vitro. J. Trauma 22:774, 1982.

Wilmore, D.W., and Aulick, L.H.: Metabolic changes in burned patients. Surg. Clin. North Am. 58:1173, 1978.

56

Multiple Trauma

KAREN W. WEST, M.D.

JAY L. GROSFELD, M.D.

THOMAS R. WEBER, M.D.

Accidents are the most frequent cause of death in children. Automobile–pedestrian and passenger-related injuries are the cause of most childhood injuries. Eighty percent of multiple injuries is due to blunt trauma. In 1978, the National Safety Council reported 12,448 deaths of children due to accidents; 5,796 were due to automobile-related injuries. For each child recorded as an accidental death, four additional children are permanently disabled from this type of traumatic episode. Children with multiple injuries should be stabilized at the community hospital and immediately transported to a trauma center in an attempt to decrease morbidity and increase survival rates. On admission, a multidisciplinary approach to the injuries is taken, with the child admitted to the pediatric surgery service.

ASSESSMENT

A thorough physical examination is undertaken while the airway is being secured, breathing is established, and adequate circulation is ensured. Because cardiopulmonary resuscitation may complicate a cervical spine fracture, modified procedures to maintain the airway, using continuous longitudinal traction, should be undertaken. Evidence of external trauma is recorded graphically or is photographed. Pictures are especially important to document injuries in cases of suspected child abuse.

The highest priorities are those injuries that lead to death if not immediately corrected: cardiorespiratory compromise by neck, chest, or maxillofacial injuries and severe external hemorrhage. Next, possible retroperitoneal, intraperitoneal, cranial and spinal, and extensive soft-tissue injuries may be assessed.

The potential for hypovolemia related to un-

diagnosed retroperitoneal and intraperitoneal injuries requires prompt evaluation. Abdominal paracentesis (peritoneal lavage) provides a 95 to 97 percent accuracy in the detection of intra-abdominal injuries and is an extremely useful diagnostic test in selected cases. When the airway has been secured, cardiac status has been ensured, and placement of a large bore IV has been achieved, a nasogastric (NG) tube and a Foley catheter are placed. Abdominal and chest x-rays are obtained. Peritoneal lavage is performed under local anesthesia, using an infraumbilical incision carried down through muscle fascia and peritoneum. A short dialysis catheter, or No. 10 feeding tube with multiple side ports, is directed toward the pelvis. An isotonic solution (Ringer's lactate or normal saline, NS) at 20 ml per kg is infused. The bottle is placed on the floor, and the color of the return is noted. The fluid is sent for cell count, hematocrit, amylase, and bilirubin. Criteria for a positive tap include the presence of bilirubin, greater than 75,000 RBC per mm^3, gross blood, and a hematocrit greater than 1 percent. In children, the greater accuracy of abdominal paracentesis (compared with adults) is related to a decreased amount of omentum, less likelihood of previous abdominal procedures and adhesions, and the shallowness of the peritoneal recesses.

Liver-spleen scan and computerized axial tomography (CAT) with intravenous (IV) and gastrointestinal contrast are important adjunctive methods for evaluating intra-abdominal injuries. If the patient has stable vital signs and hematocrits, CAT evaluation may be performed prior to or instead of the paracentesis. The mortality rate is often related to a delay in diagnosis following pediatric trauma. Unsuspected retroperitoneal injuries accounted for 40 percent of initial deaths in children with combined blunt abdominal trauma and head injuries. These are also frequently documented on CAT scan, which is performed with both oral and IV contrast.

Cranial CAT scans are performed on comotose patients to evaluate the severity of the closed injury and to exclude epidural, subdural, or intraventricular hemorrhage and cerebral contusion. Insertion of intracranial pressure (ICP) monitors may be required to best maintain appropriate fluid and sedation management. This procedure is performed under the direction of the neurosurgery team and may be placed even under local anesthesia in the intensive care unit (ICU). The cerebral perfusion pressure (CPP—the difference between the mean systemic pressure and the ICP) is maintained at 40 to 50 mm Hg. High ICP may be indicative of cerebral edema and brain herniation (see Chapter 43, Management of Pediatric Head Trauma, and Chapter 12, Increased Intracranial Pressure).

Lower priorities (not life threatening) include lower urinary tract injuries, peripheral nerve and minor vascular injuries, and moderate soft-tissue damage. Blood at the urinary meatus must be evaluated with a retrograde urethrogram prior to the insertion of a Foley catheter. Soft-tissue injuries must be débrided and closed, even if an underlying nerve injury is to be repaired secondarily. Contaminated wounds are débrided and left open for delayed wound closure. Vascular injuries may require evaluation by arteriography. Extremities should be immobilized temporarily as the overall evaluation of the patient continues. Extremity pulses, capillary refilling, and movement must be carefully documented distal to the injury to ensure adequate arterial inflow.

Decisions must then be made concerning disposition: immediate operative therapy, further diagnostic evaluation (CAT scans, arteriograms, isotope studies), or admission to the ICU for further observation and close monitoring (Table 56–1).

MANAGEMENT

Thoracic Injuries

Thoracic trauma accounts for one fourth of early pediatric trauma deaths, most of which occur after reaching the hospital. Resuscitative measures, including endotracheal intubation and tube thoracostomy, adequately treat 85 percent of these patients. The overall treatment of these injuries in children is identical to that of adults. A child's thorax is elastic, and severe

Table 56–1. Emergency Management

Unresponsive Patients	Responsive, Unstable Patients
Cervical collar protection	Vital signs
Ensure airway patency	History and physical examination
Cardiac resuscitation	Blood work
Effective monitoring (EKG and BP)	IV access
Thorough physical examination (control external hemorrhage)	NG tube (prevent air swallowing)
IV access	Monitoring
Blood work (CBC, liver function tests, amylase, electrolytes, type and crossmatch)	Further evaluation
Fluid resuscitation	
Further evaluation	

Stable Patients
History and physical examination, monitoring
IV access
Laboratory tests
Appropriate tubes
Further evaluation

injuries may be present even in the absence of rib or sternal fractures. The mediastinum is also mobile and may be displaced to the side opposite a tension pneumothorax. This interferes with the volume of the functional lung and cardiac filling.

Evaluation for airway patency is mandatory. The airway should be cleared, and intubation should be performed in the apneic patient by direct vision using a laryngoscope. Portable chest x-ray examination will reveal pneumohemothorax, widened mediastinum, pneumomediastinum, or subcutaneous emphysema. The diaphragm must be inspected to exclude a rupture.

Pulmonary lacerations leading to pneumohemothorax are the most common cause of bleeding into the chest. In children, this may be indicative of great vessel injury if present on the left or pulmonary hilar injuries if on the right, especially with associated first, second, and third rib fractures. Blood must be evacuated by a tube thoracostomy placed in the anterior midaxilliary line at the nipple level. Forty percent of the blood volume may be lost in one hemothorax, and rapid replacement via a heparinized collection system (a form of closed autotransfusion) may be needed.

Hyperresonance to percussion, absent breath sounds, and deviation of the trachea may be evident when there is a tension pneumothorax. The child will be tachypneic and anxious due to hypoxemia and may have central cyanosis. When this has been confirmed by chest x-ray, a tube thoracostomy is placed under local anesthesia. A French catheter can be tunneled in the subcutaneous tissue over the chosen rib to avoid disruption or injury to the neurovascular bundle (which runs along the under surface of the rib). The tube is then sutured, placed, and added to an underwater seal with continuous negative pressure.

Flail chest (necessitates 6–8 rib fractures) is uncommon in children, but if present, it should be treated with intubation and positive pressure ventilation. Children with traumatic wet lung (shock lung) or pulmonary contusion may be hypovolemic and cyanotic upon presentation and may initially have a normal chest x-ray. Over the ensuing hours, fluffy infiltrates develop. Bronchospasm and pulmonary edema develop; lactic acidosis and hypoxia worsen. The treatment remains controversial but includes ventilatory support, oxygen supplementation, fluid restriction, diuretics, and the administration of salt-poor albumin (to increase intravascular colloid oncotic pressure). In instances of bilateral involvement, extracorporeal membrane oxygenation (ECMO) has occasionally been used. Bilateral cases can be lethal, regardless of associated injuries.

Rapidly developing shock, pneumomediastinum, and left pneumothorax are the hallmarks of esophageal injuries. These tears occur at the level of the carina and may be diagnosed by esophagoscopy and barium studies. If diagnosed within 12 hours, the injuries may be repaired primarily via a right thoracotomy approach. If diagnosis is delayed, diversion of the saliva (nasopharyngeal continuous drainage or esophagostomy), chest tube drainage, high-dose broad-spectrum antibiotics, and total parenteral nutrition are used in the treatment. Repeat contrast evaluation is performed in 1 week or earlier if the condition deteriorates. Complications include mediastinal abscess, persistent esophageal leak, and traumatic tracheoesophageal fistula.

Approximately 10 percent of blunt traumatic injuries in children involve the thorax. Among these cases, traumatic diaphragmatic hernia is a relatively uncommon injury because of the increased elasticity of the rib cage. The initial chest x-ray film is diagnostic in 25 to 50 percent of the cases and is highly suggestive in the remainder of the cases. These findings include elevated diaphragm; discoid atelectasis, shift of the mediastinum and heart, extraneous gas bubbles, and abdominal shadows above the diaphragm. An NG tube passed into the stomach and then appearing in the thoracic cavity may confirm the diagnosis. Acute respiratory distress and chest and abdominal pain are present. The incidence of associated injuries is significant, and 50 to 60 percent of the cases will have associated long-bone, pelvic, or spinal injuries. Only 20 percent of the injuries involve the right side because of the buffering capacity of the liver and the increased bursting pressure of the right hemidiaphragm. A transabdominal operative approach is used for the repair. This approach provides adequate exposure for reduction of herniated viscera, treatment of accompanying intra-abdominal injuries, and access for diagnosis of possible bilateral diaphragmatic injury.

Rupture of the tracheobronchial tree is diagnosed in patients with hemoptysis and initial subcutaneous emphysema. Children with tracheobronchial injuries who die at the scene of an accident often have an associated injury to the heart and great vessels. Prompt surgical repair is required in those patients who reach the emergency room alive. Resuscitative measures include tube thoracostomy and placement of a cuffed entotracheal tube via emergency tracheostomy. If adequate ventilation cannot be achieved, partial or complete cardiopulmonary bypass may be required for the repair. Emergency open thoracotomy with aortic cross-clamping in the emergency room may be required.

Seventy-five percent of thoracic injuries are due to blunt trauma. One half of these patients will have injuries to multiple systems. The mortality rate increases from 5 to 15 percent when additional organs are involved, necessitating prompt recognition of associated injuries if the mortality rates are to be decreased.

Abdominal Injuries

The evaluation of patients with abdominal trauma is critical. Efforts must be made to be thorough and to expedite both the diagnosis and the course of treatment. Acute conditions requiring emergency surgery include uncontrollable external hemorrhage, refractory hypotension, free intraperitoneal air, and extruding abdominal viscera. Most patients, however, do not require an emergency operation; thus, further diagnostic evaluation can be undertaken. All patients with penetrating or blunt abdominal trauma should have chest and abdominal x-rays taken and urinalysis, complete blood count (CBC), liver function tests, and serum amylase drawn. Of primary importance during this evaluation is repeated physical examination by an experienced examiner.

The spleen is the most commonly injured organ in children. Tachycardia, hypotension, left upper quadrant tenderness, and Kehr's sign (referred pain to the left shoulder) may be present. Leukocytosis is common, and hematuria may be present, because associated renal trauma may occur in as many as 40 percent of the cases. The abdominal films may reveal colon or stomach displacement, loss of psoas and renal shadows, and a serrated appearance of the greater curvature of the stomach. Liver-spleen scintiscans are the mainstay of splenic injury diagnosis. CAT is also accurate in establishing the diagnosis and for post-injury follow-up. These injuries may be successfully managed nonoperatively if uncontrolled hemorrhage does not occur. Patients must be managed in an ICU setting, with frequent monitoring of vital signs and serial hematocrits. An acceptable blood loss is less than 30 ml per/kg. Blood loss that is greater than this associated with unstable vital signs dictates a surgical exploration. Observation continues in the hospital for 7 to 10 days; physical activity is limited for 4 weeks. A repeat scintiscan is performed at that time to assess splenic healing.

Prompt operative management of persistent splenic bleeding should be undertaken. However, total splenectomy is avoided if possible to decrease the 1.5 percent incidence of pediatric post-splenectomy sepsis. Splenorrhaphy (primary splenic repair) is performed when possible, with simple suturing techniques using chromic catgut, omental patches, and stimulation of platelet aggregation, using topical thrombin or microfibrillar collagen for surface oozing. Partial splenectomy, splenic artery ligation, and autoimplants of fragmented splenic tissue (preferably thin slices placed in the omentum) are alternative modes of therapy that may preserve immune competence and reduce the risk of pneumococcal sepsis.

Hepatic injuries are associated with rapid loss of large blood volumes. Forty percent of children with major liver injuries die before reaching the hospital. Eighty percent of these injuries involve the right lobe. Children who present in profound shock with evidence of right upper quadrant trauma require rapid evaluation, fluid resuscitation, and, in cases of major liver injury, surgical exploration. In cases of blunt trauma, 20 percent will involve the major hepatic vein or vena cava. If this form of injury is suspected, upper extremity large-bore IV catheters should be inserted. When major vascular damage is encountered, it may be necessary to extend the midline abdominal incision to allow access to the right atrium and supradiaphragmatic vena cava. Vessels in the porta hepatis may require intermittent 15- to 20-minute periods of clamping to control life-threatening hemorrhage (Pringle maneuver). Simple linear fractures may be observed if not actively bleeding or oversewn with chromic catgut if bleeding is noted. Subhepatic and subdiaphragmatic drainage may be used in selected cases. T-tube insertion is not advised. The placement of an intracaval shunt may be necessary in the treatment of complex injuries involving the hepatic veins. In cases of extensive hemorrhage, hepatic artery ligation is an alternative to major hepatic resection. Postoperative complications of liver injury include bile leak, subhepatic and subdiaphragmatic abscess, hemobilia, and infection related to retained devitalized hepatic tissue. Subcapsular hematomas (diagnosed on liver spleen or CAT scan) can often be managed conservatively. Sophisticated radiologic and nuclear technology, (abdominal sonography, scintiscan, CAT scan) have provided a sensitive means for evaluating the extent of hepatic injuries and, in selective cases, have allowed for conservative, nonoperative management.

The pancreas is susceptible to injury, because the midportion of the gland crosses the vertebral column. Elevated serum and urinary amylase, duodenal atony, and associated duodenal and splenic injuries are commonly associated with pancreatic contusions or lacerations. Commonly, the cause is a bicycle handlebar. Treatment is variable according to the extent of injury and may involve simple observation in some instances, drainage, or conservative resection of the involved gland. For persistent pancreatitis, prolonged total parenteral nutrition and NG decompression may be required. Ultrasonography is an excellent method to use to follow the course of pancreatic injury, including the development of pancreatic pseudocysts (see Chapter 42, Pancreatitis).

Isolated gastrointestinal injuries are rare. Most commonly, these injuries involve the small bowel, with perforation of the antimesenteric border. Gastrointestinal injuries may result from relatively mild blunt abdominal trauma in postprandial children, with relative distention of the small bowel. The proximal jejunum (ligament of Treitz) and ileocecal region are most commonly involved. Other injuries result from direct contact over the vertebral column. Abdominal x-rays may reveal an ileus pattern or free air. Surgical repair is required.

Duodenal hematomas result from contusion of this fixed retroperitoneal structure. Mild tenderness, edema of the second and third portions of the duodenum, obstruction, and a history of epigastric trauma are noted. Bilious vomiting may be present. On barium study, the "stack of coins sign" may be seen. These injuries may be managed nonoperatively with NG decompression and parenteral nutrition. The bleeding occurs in the bridging vessels between the submucosa and muscularis layers; the submucosa remains intact. Surgery is required if symptoms do not improve in 7 to 10 days of conservative therapy.

Gastric perforations are handled operatively and usually involve simple débridement and closure. The rib cage protects this organ from blunt trauma unless it is distended following a meal.

Renal

Most renal injuries in children follow blunt trauma. These organs are less protected because of decreased perirenal fat and their abdominal location. Pre-existing congenital renal abnormalities (found in 10 percent of patients with renal trauma) such as renal cyst, Wilms' tumor, ectopic location, and horseshoe kidney render this organ more susceptible to even minimal trauma. Hematuria, abdominal pain, or flank hematomas may be associated with renal injuries. Renal injuries may be classified as 1) contusion, 2) superficial lacerations, 3) deep lacerations, 4) hilar disruption, and 5) shattered kidney. Forty percent of the cases are associated with liver or splenic injuries.

The psoas shadow may be obliterated with urinary extravasation or retroperitoneal bleeding. After the possibility of urethral trauma has been eliminated, a cystogram is obtained. Sites of extravasation are looked for on anteroposterior (AP) and lateral exposures. An IV pyelogram should be obtained to assess bilateral function and possible delayed extravasation. The CAT scan, with IV contrast, assesses renal artery continuity. Selective aortography may be required in patients with nonvisualizing collecting systems. The management of blunt renal trauma is outlined in Figure 56–1.

In patients with minimal extravasation, antibiotic therapy is initiated and nonoperative management is used. Eighty percent of such cases may be observed safely. Hematuria is serially evaluated, and repeat physical examinations are performed for evidence of expanding flank masses (urinoma or hematoma). If renal salvage is to be possible, prompt surgical intervention must be undertaken in selected cases of renal arterial or venous disruption. Expanding hematomas of Gerota's fascia noted on abdominal exploration for other injuries must be evaluated. This increases the renal salvage rate. Complications include infected urinomas, ureterocutaneous fistulas, and hypertension.

Bladder injuries may result in urine extravasation extraperitoneally (bladder neck injury) or intraperitoneally (bladder dome). The child may not be able to void and clinically presents with increasing abdominal distention. Catheterization may yield large volumes of urine. The cystogram will reveal the disruption. Rectal examinations may reveal bogginess of the bladder neck. Minor extraperitoneal injuries may be treated with catheter drainage and antibiotic prophylaxis. Closure of the defect and suprapubic cystostomy drainage may be required for large intraperitoneal bladder injuries.

Posterior urethral injuries are associated with

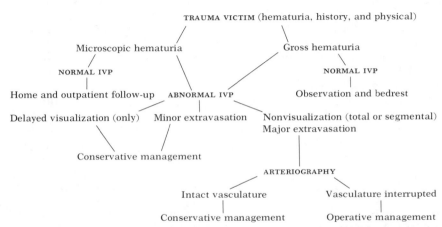

Figure 56–1. Proposed management of blunt renal trauma. (From Peters, P.C., and Bright, T.C.: Blunt renal injuries. Urol. Clin. North Am. 4:122, 1977. Used by permission.)

pelvic fractures. Children with pelvic fractures, blood at the urinary meatus, and urinary retention should be evaluated for this type of injury. Rectal examination reveals anterior displacement of the prostate in boys and a soft mass in girls. Blood may also be seen in the scrotum or labia. A retrograde urethrogram is obtained, and attempts are made to pass the urethral catheter. If the catheter is passed easily, drainage is maintained for 21 days. Most children are treated with immediate cystostomy and passage of a splinting urethral catheter. These children must be followed for the development of a urethral stricture.

CASE PRESENTATION

A 14-year-old pedestrian was struck by an automobile, thrown 10 feet and was found by the side of the road. He was arousable. On arrival at the emergency room, vital signs showed BP = 80/50 mm Hg; HR = 130 beats/min, and RR = 35 breaths/min. He remained arousable but not coherent. Hematomas were present over the left parietal region and the left flank. The chest was clear to percussion and auscultation. Abdominal examination revealed moderate tenderness in the left upper quadrant and pelvic instability. Rectal examination revealed a non-displaced prostate, with hematest negative stools. A right central venous catheter was inserted in the subclavian vein, and 500 ml Ringer's lactate was rapidly infused. BP rose to 100/80 mm Hg and HR decreased to 100 beats/min. Initial laboratory values were: hgb = 10.0 gm/dl, hct = 30 percent, WBC = 15,000 mm³, UA = 5–10 RBC/hpf on spontaneous voiding, amylase = 601 U, and alkaline phosphatase = 250 IU. Chest x-ray revealed no rib or vertebral fractures, and haziness of the left lower lobe. KUB (kidney, ureter, and bladder) revealed bilateral pubic fractures. Arterial blood gas results on room air: pH = 7.35, PO_2 = 60 mm Hg, and PCO_2 = 40 mm Hg.

Problem List

1. **Respiratory**—tachypnea and hypoxemia. Oxygen supplementation in a concentration of 40 percent was administered by face mask. Repeat chest x-ray revealed increased fluffiness of the left lower lobe, consistent with pulmonary contusion. Arterial blood gas results revealed pH = 7.38, PO_2 = 80 mm Hg, and PCO_2 = 35 mm Hg.

2. **Cardiac**—EKG with no dysrhythmias. Cardiac CPK isoenzymes were sent to the laboratory evaluate for possible cardiac contusion.

3. **Anemia**—The repeat hemaglobin was 8.5 gm/dl. The patient was transfused with 250 ml of whole blood. Blood pressure remained stable at 100/80 mm Hg, with maintenance fluids.

4. **Neurologic compromise**—no localizing signs.

5. **Hematuria**—The catheter was placed without difficulty, and 200 ml of blood tinged urine were obtained.

6. **Leukocytosis** with elevated liver function tests suggested splenic and liver injuries.

The patient was transported with continuous EKG and BP monitoring to the x-ray department where CAT scans of the head and abdomen were done. IV and gastrointestinal contrast were used. The cranial evaluation was normal. A subcapsular splenic hematoma and liver laceration were noted. Both kidneys functioned promptly. A retroperitoneal hematoma was noted but there was no extravasation of dye.

The patient was transported to the ICU. Continuous EKG and arterial BP, hourly neurochecks, and vital signs were monitored. Blood counts were obtained every 4 hours. Fluids were restricted to two thirds maintenance for treatment of the cerebral concussion and pulmonary contusion. BP remained 100/80 mm Hg. Over the next 12 hours, blood transfusion requirements were 1000 ml (< 20 ml/kg). Pulmonary status remained static. Urinalysis for pH and presence of myoglobin (muscle trauma) were monitored serially and remained normal.

Within 36 hours, the neurologic status returned to normal and the abdominal examination was benign. Pelvic tenderness persisted. A repeat CAT scan of the abdomen at 1 week revealed improvement in the subcapsular splenic hematoma. Urinary drainage was discontinued after 14 days, and spontaneous voiding was achieved. The hematoma was no longer present. The patient was discharged on Day 20, with continued bedrest as treatment for the pelvic fractures. Progressive weight bearing was instituted at 10 days and was continued on an outpatient basis. A repeat liver-splenic scintiscan was obtained 1 month following injury and showed healing of both the hepatic and splenic injury.

SUGGESTED READING

Accident Facts: Chicago, National Safety Council, 1971.

Bevine, B.A., and Jona, J.Z.: Diagnostic peritoneal lavage. Pediatr. Trauma. 16:739, 1976.

Chapman, N.D., and Braun, R.A.: The management of traumatic tracheoesophageal fistula caused by blunt chest trauma. Arch. Surg. 100:681, 1970.

Cooney, D.R.: Splenic and hepatic trauma in children. Surg. Clin. North Am. 61:1165, 1981.

Drew, R., Perry, J.F., and Fisher, R.P.: The expediency of peritoneal lavage for blunt trauma in children. Surg. Gynecol. Obstet. 145:885, 1977.

DuPriest, R.W., Rodriquez, A., and Shataey, C.H.: Peritoneal lavage in children and adolescents with blunt abdominal trauma. Am. Surg. 48:460, 1982.

Epstein, L.I., and Lempke, R.C.: Rupture of right diaphragm due to blunt trauma. J. Trauma 7:19, 1968.

Lewis, F.R.: Thoracic trauma. Surg. Clin. North Am. 62:97, 1982.

Meyer, A.A., and Cross, R.A.: Abdominal trauma. Surg. Clin. North Am. 62:105, 1982.

Olsen, W.R., Redman, H.C., and Hildieth, D.H.: Quantitative peritoneal lavage in blunt abdominal trauma. Arch. Surg. 104:536, 1972.

Peters, P.C., and Bright, T.C.: Blunt renal injuries. Urol. Clin. North Am. 4:17, 1977.

Pontes, J.E.: Urologic injuries. Surg. Clin. North Am. 57:77, 1977.

Powell, R.W., Smith, D.E., Zorins, C.Z., and Parvin, S.: Peritoneal lavage in children with blunt abdominal trauma. J. Pediatr. Surg. 11:973, 1976.

Randolph, J.: Children and accidents. *In* Randolph J.G., Ravitch, M.M., Welch, K.J., et al. (eds.): The Injured Child: Surgical Management. Chicago, Year Book Medical Publishers, Inc., 1979, pp. 1–5.

Steichen, F.M.: Emergency management of the severely injured child. *In* Randolph, J.G., Ravitch, M.M., Welch, K.J., et al. (eds.): The Injured Child: Surgical Management. Chicago, Year Book Medical Publishers, Inc., 1979, pp. 7–24.

Welch, K.J.: Thoracic injuries. *In* Randolph, J.G., Ravitch, M.M., Welch, R.J. (eds.): The Injured Child: Surgical Management. Chicago, Year Book Medical Publishers, Inc., 1979, pp. 215–229.

West, K.W., Weber, T.R., and Grosfeld, J.L.: Traumatic diaphragmatic hernias in childhood. J. Pediatr. Surg. 16:392, 1981.

Nursing Process for Patient Care:

Multiple Trauma

Children who have been victims of accidents and present with multiple injuries are true medical emergencies. Such crises require knowledge and skill in physical assessment and resuscitation techniques. A multidisciplinary approach must be taken by an organized team of practitioners.

The first priority is to secure an airway, establish breathing, and ensure adequate circulation. When these measures have been accomplished, a systematic evaluation of major body systems should take place.

RESPIRATORY

Assess, Monitor, and Document

Patency of airway
Secretions
Respiratory rate
Pattern of respiration, including depth
Symmetrical chest expansion
Bilateral breath sounds
Color
Restlessness

Agitation
Arterial blood gases
Response to therapy
  Chest Tube: underwater seal maintained,
    continuous negative pressure maintained
  Drainage: description, amount
  Insertion site: clean, dry, dressing

Anticipate

Airway obstruction
Pneumohemothorax
Tension pneumothorax: absent breath sounds, deviation of the trachea
Flail chest
Adult respiratory distress syndrome (ARDS, shock lung): pulmonary edema, bronchospasm

Esophageal injuries: pneumomediastinum, left pneumothorax
Traumatic diaphragmatic hernia
Rupture of the tracheobronchial tree: hemoptysis, subcutaneous emphysema

CARDIOVASCULAR

Assess, Monitor, and Document

Heart rate
Respiratory rate
Blood pressure: arterial, central venous
Perfusion: peripheral pulses, capillary filling

Color
Condition of skin
Urine output

Anticipate

Shock
  Decreased urine output
  Altered level of consciousness
  Decreased blood pressure

  Increased pulse rate
  Increased respiratory rate
  Poor perfusion: decreased capillary filling
  Cardiac arrest

NEUROLOGIC

Head injury is a common occurrence in multiple trauma. The child's neurologic status may be altered by insults such as concussion, contusion, fracture and epidural, subdural, and intraventricular hemorrhage.

Assess, Monitor, and Document

Headache
Vomiting
Blood pressure
Pulse
Respiratory rate and pattern
Intracranial pressure (if available)
Level of consciousness: lethargy, stupor, coma

Pupillary response
Reflexes
Motor response
Posture
Seizures (if applicable)

Anticipate

Increased intracranial pressure (ICP)
  Headache
  Vomiting
  Increased blood pressure
  Decreased heart rate
  Decreased respiratory rate
  Altered respiratory pattern: Cheyne-Stokes
  Altered level of consciousness

Altered reflex responses: pupillary, oculo-vestibular, oculocephalic
  Posturing: decorticate, decerebrate
Seizures
Coma
Respiratory arrest
Cardiac arrest
Posthypoxic encephalopathy

GASTROINTESTINAL

Assess, Monitor, and Document

Pain: location, description
Abdominal girth

Anticipate

Injury to spleen
  Tachycardia
  Hypotension
  Left upper quadrant tenderness
  Kehr's sign: referred pain to left shoulder
Injury to liver
  Profound shock

Injury to pancreas
  Elevated serum amylase
  Pain
Injury to bowel
  Vomiting
  Tenderness
  Obstruction

RENAL

Assess, Monitor, and Document

Pain: location, description
Urine output: color, amount, abdominal girth

Anticipate

Hematuria
Flank pain
Abdominal pain

Inability to void
Abdominal distention
Acute renal failure

MUSCULOSKELETAL

Assess, Monitor, and Document

Pulse distal to injury
Temperature of extremity
Color of extremity

Movement of extremity
Condition of cast (if applicable)
Diameter of thighs

Anticipate

Neurovascular compromise
  Decreased or absent pulse: distal to injury
  Inability to move extremity

Thrombophlebitis: swelling, redness, pain
Pulmonary embolism: chest pain, dyspnea,
  respiratory insufficiency

RESPONSE OF CHILD

Assess, Monitor, and Document

Developmental level: verbal, motor, psychosocial, cognitive, perception of accident
Behavioral response: fearful, anxious, tearful,
  angry

Response to nursing interventions

Anticipate

Emotional crisis
Inability to cope

RESPONSE OF FAMILY

Assess, Monitor, and Document

Behavioral response: anxious, fearful, verbal,
  angry
Perception of accident
Feelings of guilt

Level of understanding of child's condition
Expected outcome
Response to nursing interventions

Anticipate

Inability to cope
Family crisis
Need for referral: social service, psychiatry

MIND SET

Assess

Status of airway
Respiratory status
Cardiovascular status
Neurologic status

Gastrointestinal system
Renal system
Musculoskeletal system
Response of child and family

Anticipate

Alteration in respiratory status
  Airway obstruction
  Respiratory failure
Alteration in cardiovascular status
  Hemorrhage
  Shock
  Cardiac arrest
Alteration in neurologic status
  Increased ICP

Seizures
Coma
Alteration in gastrointestinal function
Alteration in renal function
Alteration in musculoskeletal system
  Fractures
  Soft-tissue injury
Emotional crisis
Family crisis

Kawasaki Syndrome

SOL S. ZIMMERMAN, M.D.

Kawasaki syndrome is an acute febrile illness associated with nonpurulent conjunctivitis, inflammation of mucous membranes, hand and foot changes, lymphadenopathy, and an erythematous rash that progresses to desquamation. These features overlap with those of several well-recognized diseases, including scarlet fever, leptospirosis, meningococcemia, toxic shock syndrome, measles, atypical measles, Rocky Mountain spotted fever, acute rheumatic fever, juvenile rheumatoid arthritis, Reiter's syndrome, Stevens-Johnson syndrome, and acrodynia, but the occurrence of coronary arteritis, aneurysm formation, and thrombosis make Kawasaki syndrome a distinct entity that must be diagnosed accurately. Also known as mucocutaneous lymph node syndrome, this illness has a 1 to 2 percent mortality rate.

EPIDEMIOLOGY

Kawasaki syndrome occurs in a worldwide distribution, and all ethnic groups are represented, but it is most prevalent in children of Japanese ancestry. Caucasian children appear to have the lowest incidence. Although the association with specific human leukocyte antigen (HLA) has been investigated and some links have been suggested, no definite relationship has been established.

Cases occur both in a sporadic and an epidemic manner. No environmental or dietary factors have been incriminated, and there is no evidence of person-to-person transmission. A seasonal pattern, with an increased incidence between February and May, has recently been reported in the United States by the Centers for Disease Control.

The syndrome affects primarily younger children with most cases occurring in patients younger than 5 years of age. Cases reported in

adolescents and adults most often are not Kawasaki syndrome but rather toxic shock syndrome (TSS, see Chapter 54, Toxic Shock Syndrome). The incidence in males exceeds that in females in a ratio of 1.5:1.

ETIOLOGY

The cause of Kawasaki syndrome is unknown. The fever, rash, mucosal inflammation, aseptic meningitis, and epidemiology suggest an infectious process, but no specific bacterial or viral agent has been isolated. Particles resembling rickettsia were reported in electron micrographs of skin and lymph node tissue from patients with Kawasaki syndrome, but attempts at confirmation have been unsuccessful.

The presence of vasculitis, arthralgias, arthritis, and elevated IgE point to immune involvement, but no etiologic role has been demonstrated. Toxins and heavy metals have been proposed as possible explanations because of the resemblance of the mucous membrane involvement, rash, and desquamation to acrodynia. Finally, the higher incidence in males and in Japanese people and the possible relation to HLA type suggest at least some genetic influence.

CLINICAL PRESENTATION

Because this entity is a syndrome, diagnosis is dependent upon strict adherence to the clinical criteria listed in Table 57–1. At least five of the six principal criteria must be present to ensure accuracy of the diagnosis. Because the syndrome has a protracted course, all the manifestations may not be present at the time of the initial examination. As new findings occur,

Table 57–1. Principal Diagnostic Criteria

Fever, persisting for more than 5 days
Conjunctival injection
Changes in the mouth, including
   Erythema, fissuring, and crusting of the lips
   Diffuse oropharyngeal erythema
   Strawberry tongue
Changes in the peripheral extremities, including
   Induration of hands and feet
   Erythema of palms and soles
   Desquamation of finger and toetips approximately 2
     weeks from onset
   Transverse grooves across fingernails 2–3 months after
     onset
Erythematous rash
Enlarged lymph node mass measuring greater than 1.5
   cm in diameter

From Melish, M.E.: Kawasaki syndrome (The mucocutaneous lymph node syndrome). Pediatr. Ann. 11:2, 255–268, 1982.

the entire clinical picture and time course will have to be reassessed if the syndrome is to be recognized. Associated manifestations are listed in Table 57–2.

Kawasaki syndrome has a relatively predictable triphasic course. The acute phase is characterized by the evolution of the principal clinical manifestations: fever, conjunctivitis, mucosal inflammation, edema of the extremities, rash, and lymphadenopathy. Aseptic meningitis and gastrointestinal symptoms occur during this phase. Defervescence and resolution of rash and adenopathy (7–14 days) mark the end of the acute and the beginning of the subacute phase. Cardiac involvement, desquamation, and joint manifestations characterize this period. Thrombocytosis occurs, and the risk of sudden death is greatest. The subacute phase ends as all clinical symptoms and signs subside (approximately 4 weeks after onset of fever), and the convalescent phase extends from this point until return of the erythrocyte

Table 57–2. Associated Features (in order of frequency)

Pyuria and urethritis
Arthralgia and arthritis
Aseptic meningitis
Diarrhea
Abdominal pain
Myocardiopathy
Pericardial effusion
Obstructive jaundice
Hydrops of gallbladder
Acute mitral insufficiency
Myocardial infarction

From Melish, M.E.: Kawasaki syndrome (The mucocutaneous lymph node syndrome). Pediatr. Ann. 11:2, 255–268, 1982.

sedimentation rate to normal (6–8 weeks past onset).

The abrupt onset of fever is usually the first sign of disease and is present in all cases. Most often, there are multiple daily temperatures of 40°C or greater without return to a normal baseline in the intervals. The fevers are relatively refractory to standard antipyretic therapy and persist for a minimum of 5 days, with an average duration of 10 to 11 days.

Bilateral conjunctivitis is present in 96 percent of cases and consists of bulbar conjuctival vascular engorgement. There is neither generalized erythema nor discharge. The onset of conjunctivitis is usually 2 days following the fever and may be of 3- to 5-week duration.

Inflammation of mucous membranes occurs in 99 percent of cases and is characterized by erythema and fissuring of the lips, injection of the oropharynx, and hypertrophy of the tongue papillae ("strawberry tongue"). Onset of these findings is generally within 3 days of onset of the fever.

Extremity changes that include erythema of the palms and soles and firm, "wooden" edema of the hands and feet occur in 99 percent of patients. The skin overlying the hands and feet is so tense that it resembles scleroderma. Appearance of these changes follows the onset of fever by 3 days, and duration is approximately 1 week. Two to 3 weeks after onset of fever, desquamation begins in a periungual distribution that extends to involve the entire palm and sole.

An erythematous rash is found in 99 percent of patients, but there is no pathognomonic appearance or distribution. The rash is most often maculopapular (morbilliform) or urticarial. A small percentage of patients may have an erythroderma that is scarlatiniform in character.

Lymph node enlargement is the least constant finding, occurring in 80 percent of cases. The adenopathy is generally unilateral in the form of a single, large cervical node that is nonsuppurative. The node rapidly decreases in size as the patient defervesces.

Other clinical manifestations include urethritis and sterile pyuria, which is present in 70 percent of cases. Arthritis and arthralgias occur in 35 to 40 percent of patients toward the end of the acute febrile course. Weight-bearing joints are affected predominantly, but both large and small joints are involved. Duration of symptoms is 1 to 2 weeks.

Central nervous system (CNS) manifestations are common and range from irritability and emotional lability to lethargy and stupor.

Aseptic meningitis is found in 25 percent of patients.

Abdominal pain and diarrhea are indicative of the gastrointestinal involvement seen in 25 percent of the cases. Less frequently found are hepatitis (10 percent) and hydrops of the gallbladder (5 percent).

Cardiac Manifestations

Cardiac involvement occurs in 20 percent of patients with Kawasaki syndrome but is often asymptomatic. In the acute phase, the only findings suggestive of myocarditis may be tachycardia disproportionate to the magnitude of fever and gallop rhythm. The EKG may reveal prolonged PR and QT intervals, decreased R wave amplitude, and flattened T waves.

In the subacute phase, cardiac manifestations escalate in severity and include dysrhythmias, pericardial effusion, and congestive heart failure (CHF). Papillary muscle dysfunction may result in mitral insufficiency. Coronary artery aneurysms develop in approximately 20 percent of patients. The aneurysms generally affect both coronary arteries and arise proximally but tend to spare the first 10 mm. The combination of coronary arteritis, aneurysmal dilatation, and thrombotic occlusion is responsible for sudden death in 1 to 2 percent of cases, the majority of which are males younger than 2 years of age. The EKG may reveal deep Q waves characteristic of a myocardial infarction, but absence of these Q waves does not rule out significant myocardial damage. Even in the presence of coronary aneurysms, the EKG may be interpreted as normal. Chest x-ray examination is most often normal, but it may show an enlarged cardiac silhouette that represents either true cardiomegaly or pericardial effusion. Decreased ventricular contractility, mitral insufficiency, and pericardial effusion may be evident on echocardiogram. Two-dimensional echocardiography accurately detects aneurysms of the left coronary artery and is a valuable tool for both screening and serial evaluation of patients with aneurysms. An initial echocardiogram should be performed during the acute phase and repeated 3 weeks later. Coronary angiography is the most sensitive diagnostic modality for complete evaluation of both coronary arteries. Its invasive nature, however, makes it unacceptable for routine screening; it is reserved for evaluation of children with significant cardiac symptoms or persistent echocardiographic evidence of aneurysm.

Angiographic data demonstrate resolution of aneurysms in over half the affected patients within 1 year. The remainder of the patients have persistent aneurysms or other coronary pathology such as tortuosity or narrowing. Whether all the children with coronary arteritis are at risk for accelerated atherosclerosis is unknown; the answer awaits the passage of time. Death from acute myocardial infarction in young adults conceivably could be the consequence of unrecognized Kawasaki syndrome in early childhood.

Cardiac pathology has been correlated with duration of illness, as shown in Table 57–3. Most deaths occur in stages 2 and 3, between 11 and 50 days.

Arteritis is not confined to involvement of the coronaries; other arteries, including cerebral, renal, mesenteric, hepatic, splenic, pancreatic, testicular, and axillary, may also be affected, although less commonly. The resulting symptoms vary and are dependent upon the location of the affected vessel and its pattern of distribution.

LABORATORY FINDINGS

The laboratory findings in Kawasaki syndrome are not diagnostic. They include leukocytosis with left shift, elevated erythrocyte sedimentation rate (ESR), positive C-reactive protein (CRP), and sterile pyuria. Total immunoglobulin levels are within normal limits, but IgE levels are frequently elevated. Total

Table 57–3. Pathology of Kawasaki Syndrome

Stage 1—Disease Duration Less Than 10 Days
Acute perivasculitis of coronary arteries
Microvascular angiitis of coronary arteries and aorta
Pancarditis with pericardial, myocardial, endocardial inflammation
Inflammation of AV conduction system
Stage 2—Disease Duration 12–28 Days
Acute panvasculitis of coronary arteries
Coronary artery aneurysms
Coronary obstruction and thrombosis
Myocardial and endocardial inflammation less intense
Stage 3—Disease Duration 28–45 Days
Subacute inflammation in coronary arteries
Coronary artery aneurysms
Myocardial and endocardial inflammation much depressed
Stage 4—Disease Duration More Than 50 Days
Scar formation and calcification in coronary arteries
Stenosis and recanalization of coronary vessel lumen
Myocardial fibrosis without acute inflammation

From Melish, M.E.: Kawasaki syndrome (The mucocutaneous lymph node syndrome). Pediatr. Ann. 11:2, 255–268, 1982.

hemolytic complement is normal or increased. Antinuclear antibodies (ANA), lupus erythmatosis (LE) preparation, and rheumatoid factor are negative. Elevation of serum bilirubin and transaminases occurs in the presence of hepatitis. The myocardial fraction of creatine phosphokinase (CPK–MB) is increased in those patients who survive an acute myocardial infarction. Patients with aseptic meningitis will have cerebrospinal fluid (CSF) that shows pleocytosis with lymphocytic predominance and normal glucose and protein.

Thrombocytosis is the most characteristic laboratory finding. Platelet counts are initially normal and begin to increase during the second week of the illness. Peak values may be well in excess of 1 million per cu mm. Platelet counts return to normal toward the end of the first month. This period of thrombocytosis correlates with the time frame in which coronary thrombosis occurs.

TREATMENT

In addition to general supportive measures, aspirin is given because of its anti-inflammatory and anti-platelet aggregation effects. Aspirin, in a dose of 80 to 100 mg per kg per day, has a beneficial effect upon the length of the febrile course, shortening it by a few days. The high-dose salicylates are continued until the fever resolves or the thrombocytosis becomes evident, at which time the dose is decreased to 10 mg per kg per day. Reduction in dosage with increasing platelet count is necessary to avoid the stimulation of vascular thrombogenic factors associated with higher aspirin doses. The low dose is effective in inhibiting platelet aggregation. Duration of therapy will vary with the complexity of the course, but aspirin should be continued at least until the ESR returns to normal.

Although steroids have classically been used in the treatment of vasculitis, the only controlled study of steroid efficacy in Kawasaki syndrome showed their association with an increased incidence of aneurysm formation. Aneurysms were identified in 20 percent of those patients given no medication, 11 percent of those taking salicylates, and 65 percent of those taking steroids. Based on these data, steroids are contraindicated in Kawasaki syndrome.

CHF is treated in the conventional manner, with fluid restriction, diuretics, and digitalization (see Chapter 19, Congestive Heart Failure). Dysrhythmias and myocardial infarction are managed according to routine protocols (see Chapter 18, Dysrhythmias in Children).

CASE PRESENTATION

A 6-year-old Oriental male presented to his physician with a 4-day history of fever, sore throat, and a "swollen gland." A throat culture was obtained and was subsequently negative. Fever to 104° F persisted for the next 3 days, despite antipyretic therapy. Because of a toxic appearance, he was admitted to a local hospital.

Physical Examination

Physical examination was pertinent for marked pharyngeal injection, hypertrophy of the tongue papillae, bulbar conjunctivitis, and right posterior cervical adenopathy.

Laboratory Evaluation

Laboratory evaluation revealed an elevated white blood cell (WBC) count with left shift, normal platelet count, elevated ESR, positive CRP, negative ANA, latex fixation, and monospot tests, and normal hepatic and renal function tests. A urinalysis was unremarkable. CSF was acellular, with normal protein and glucose. Cultures of blood, CSF, and urine were ultimately negative. Chest x-ray examination upon admission revealed a normal cardiac silhouette and no pulmonary infiltrates.

On hospital Day 2, a generalized erythematous maculopapular rash and edema of the hands and feet were noted. Tachypnea to 60 breaths/min and tachycardia to 170 beats/min occurred the following day, and the child was transferred to the pediatric ICU of a tertiary medical center. Physical examination was remarkable for a gallop rhythm, bibasilar rales, and hepatomegaly, with the liver edge palpable 3 cm below the right costal margin. Chest x-ray examination revealed bilateral perihilar engorgement and an increase in size of the cardiac silhouette. An echocardiogram showed a pericardial effusion. Diuretics and salicylates at anti-inflammatory doses were administered.

The early hospital course was marked by persistence of fever, the appearance of jaundice, progressive hepatomegaly, and increasing complaints of painful hands and feet. Laboratory evaluation demonstrated hyperbilirubinemia, elevated transaminases, prolongation of the prothrombin (PT) and partial thromboplastin (PTT) times, and hypoalbuminemia. Thrombocytosis became evident on Day 8, with the count ultimately increasing to 1.5 million/cu mm. The picture of hepatic involvement resolved clinically and biochemically by Day 7. The hands and feet were remarkable for a firm, painful edema that prevented use of the extremities. Periungual desquamation was noted at the end of the second week of the illness.

Although symptoms and changes in vital signs that were attributed to the cardiac status improved early in the hospital course, pericardial effusion remained evident on ultrasound examination for 4 weeks. Dilatation of the coronary arteries was shown on echocardiogram at the end of the first hospital week and remained unchanged throughout the hospital course. The child was discharged 1 month following admission. "Low-dose" salicylate therapy, originally instituted when the thrombocytosis became evident, was continued as an outpatient. The ESR at the time of discharge remained moderately elevated.

At home, the child did well. He was maintained on salicylates and was restricted in terms of vigorous physical activity. Echocardiograms performed on an outpatient basis revealed persistence of the coronary artery aneurysms. EKGs were unremarkable. Approximately 4 months after discharge, the child began to complain of episodic epigastric pain. His mother discontinued the salicylates because she thought that they were related to the abdominal discomfort. On the day of readmission, he had an episode of abdominal pain associated with left shoulder pain, nausea, and diaphoresis. An EKG revealed Q waves in leads II, III, and aVF and ST elevation in all the precordial leads; occasional PVCs were present. CPK was markedly elevated.

Problem List

Cardiac

Morphine was administered for pain. Lidocaine was infused as a continuous IV drip in a dose of 0.3 mg/kg/hr to protect against dysrhythmias. It was continued for the first 72 hours of hospitalization. Salicylate therapy was reinstituted.

Respiratory

Although the patient was comfortable in room air mild hypoxia was evident on blood gas analysis, and oxygen was administered by face mask in a concentration of 35 percent.

Intake and Output

Initially the patient was made NPO, and maintenance fluids were administered intravenously.

Gastrointestinal

Stool softeners were administered in an attempt to avoid the need for a Valsalva maneuver.

The patient underwent further diagnostic evaluation. A gated pool study revealed markedly impaired ventricular function. Coronary angiography showed total obstruction of the right coronary artery and aneurysmic involvement of the left anterior descending and left circumflex arteries, with good patency peripherally. A decision was made to perform a coronary artery bypass, and this was accomplished uneventfully.

SUGGESTED READING

Bell, D.M., Morens, D.M., Holman, M.S., et al.: Kawasaki syndrome in the United States. Am. J. Dis. Child. 137:211, 1983.

Fujiwara, H., and Hamashima, Y.: Pathology of the heart in Kawasaki disease. Pediatrics 61:100, 1978.

Kato, H., Koike, S., and Yokoyama, T.: Kawasaki disease: effect of treatment in coronary artery involvement. Pediatrics 63:175, 1979.

Melish, M.E., Hicks, R.V., and Reddy, V.: Kawasaki syndrome: an update. Hosp. Pract. March 1982, pp. 99–106.

Melish, M.E.: Kawasaki syndrome (The mucocutaneous lymph node syndrome). Pediatr. Ann. 11:2 255, 1982.

Morens, D.M., Anderson, L.J., and Hurwitz, E.S.: National surveillance of Kawasaki disease. Pediatrics 65:21, 1980.

Nursing Process for Patient Care:
Kawasaki Syndrome

PRINCIPAL CHARACTERISTICS

Assess, Monitor, and Document

Temperature
Conjunctiva
Mucosal involvement: lips, tongue, throat

Extremities: hands/feet, palms/soles
Skin: erythematous rash
Lymph node mass

Anticipate

Fever persisting for more than 5 days
Conjunctival injection without exudate or discharge
Mouth changes
    Erythema, fissuring, and crusting of the lips
    Erythema of oropharynx
    "Strawberry" tongue
Changes in extremities

Induration of hands and feet
Erythema of palms and soles
Desquamation of fingers and toes
Erythematous rash
Enlarged lymph node mass
    Cervical
    Unilateral

ASSOCIATED FEATURES

Assess, Monitor, and Document

Cardiovascular status
    Heart rate
    Rhythm
    Blood pressure
    Perfusion
    Respiratory rate
    Breath sounds
Renal status
    Urine output: amount, description
    Dysuria

Joints
    Swelling
    Erythema
    Warmth
Central nervous system (CNS)
    Level of consciousness
    Mood
Gastrointestinal status
    Bowel movements
    Presence of pain

Anticipate

Cardiovascular system
    Is affected in approximately 20 percent of children
    Tachycardia
    Gallop rhythm
    Congestive heart failure (CHF): tachypnea, rales
    Pericardial effusion
    Mitral insufficiency
    Dysrhythmias: first and second degree AV block, premature ventricular contractions, paroxysmal atrial tachycardia
    Coronary artery aneurysms
    Myocardial infarction
    Sudden death
Renal system

    Urethritis
    Pyuria
Joints
    Arthritis
    Arthralgia
CNS
    Irritability
    Labile mood
    Lethargy
    Aseptic meningitis
Gastrointestinal system
    Diarrhea
    Abdominal pain

RESPONSE OF CHILD

Assess, Monitor, and Document

Developmental level: verbal, motor, cognitive, psychosocial, fears
Behavioral response: fearful, passive, aggressive, degree of distress

Ability to cope
Strategies to reduce stress and facilitate coping
Response to nursing interventions

Anticipate

Emotional distress
Disruption of normal growth and development

RESPONSE OF FAMILY

Assess, Monitor, and Document

Behavioral response: anxiety, fear, anger, depression
Level of understanding of child's condition
Expected outcome

Ability to cope
Educational needs related to home care management and follow-up
Response to nursing interventions

Anticipate

Family crisis
Inability to cope

Educational needs related to discharge and home management

MIND SET

Assess

Principal characteristics
  Temperature
  Conjunctiva
  Mucosal involvement
  Extremities
  Skin
  Lymph node mass

Associated features
  Cardiovascular status
  Renal status
  Joints
  CNS
  Gastrointestinal system
Response of child and family

Anticipate

Acute phase
  Fever
  Conjunctivitis
  Mucosal inflammation
  Edema of extremities
  Rash
  Lymphadenopathy
  Aseptic meningitis
  Gastrointestinal symptoms
Subacute phase
  Defervescence

  Resolution of skin rash
  Desquamation
  Resolution of adenopathy
  Joint manifestations
  Cardiac involvement
Convalescent phase
  Clinical signs and symptoms subside
  Return of erythrocyte sedimentation rate to normal
  Continued observation for cardiac complications

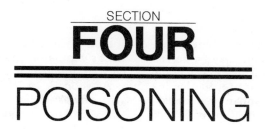

CHAPTER

58

Poisoning: General Principles of Management

LORRAINE HARTNETT, M.D.
ALAN G. KULBERG, M.D.

Childhood poisoning accounts for a substantial number of emergency room visits and hospital admissions each year. The number is increasing as children and adolescents are exposed to a wider variety of chemical or pharmaceutical substances accidentally and intentionally. Physicians in the pediatric emergency service and intensive care unit (ICU) must be prepared to care for a wide range of patients; for instance, the 4-year-old child who drank turpentine and is now coughing, the vomiting 3-year-old child who has eaten his mother's prenatal vitamin and iron tablets, and the comatose 17-year-old adolescent who has taken some pills to "get high."

The therapeutic maneuvers necessary to adequately treat these patients are often technically difficult and frustrating. These patients are frequently physically, emotionally, and intellectually demanding. The best long-term prognosis often requires coordination of medical, social, and psychiatric services.

The proper approach to poisoned or overdosed patients depends upon rigorous attention to stabilization of vital signs, followed by a therapeutic strategy based upon the patient's age, mental status, presence or absence of the gag reflex, and presence of other clinical signs of systemic toxicity.

INITIAL ASSESSMENT

As with any patient presenting to the emergency service, the initial assessment must ensure adequacy of the airway and stability of the cervical spine. If the patient is not breathing adequately, the airway must be controlled and adequate oxygenation and ventilation ensured. Because trauma is a frequent complication of drug usage in older patients, the cervical spine must be properly immobilized if there is *any* suspicion of injury, and cervical spine radiographs must be obtained. The circulatory status must then be assessed and appropriate measures taken to ensure cardiovascular stability. It is at this point that specific poison management may proceed. It is useful to separate poisoned or overdosed patients into three basic categories because of the distinct management principles of each group: 1) the comatose or convulsing patient, 2) the agitated or uncooperative patient, and 3) the patient with a normal mental status. This approach applies to all patients, regardless of age.

While the initial assessment is being made, as much history as possible must be obtained from the family or friends accompanying the child or adolescent. Sensitivity is paramount, because often the parents have feelings of guilt, thinking that they were careless or neglectful. On the other hand, the parents may be defensive about having had illicit drugs in the home and therefore may be reluctant to divulge information. The friends accompanying the adolescent may withhold information for fear of parental or legal punishment. All parties must be assured that any information obtained is vital to the patient's welfare and is privileged. The interviewer must be rigorous in his questioning about any drugs or chemicals present in the home. Poisoning as a form of child abuse should be considered whenever the history given does not seem to adequately explain the clinical picture.

The patient's belongings must be searched for clues to the ingestion such as empty containers, residual pills, or characteristic odors. Any clothing that is saturated with chemicals should be removed from the patient and taken from the area, and the skin should be washed. Continued absorption of a toxin, such as an organophosphate insecticide, may occur if this step is neglected.

PATIENTS WITH ALTERED MENTAL STATUS OR IN COMA

Evaluation and Management

The initial assessment should proceed as previously outlined, with proper resuscitative measures and cervical spine evaluation. All comatose patients should be given 100 percent oxygen (O_2) by either face mask or endotracheal tube, depending upon respiratory effort, pending determination of arterial blood gases, and exclusion of carbon monoxide poisoning as the possible diagnosis. Cardiac monitoring should be instituted, and a full 12-lead EKG should be obtained; all intervals should be measured in addition to the routine evaluation of wave amplitude and duration and baseline position.

Intravenous (IV) access must be established. If the patient is hypotensive or has poor peripheral perfusion, a large-bore catheter should be inserted either percutaneously or, if necessary, by surgical cutdown and a fluid challenge (20 ml/kg of normal saline (NS) or Ringer's lactate infused rapidly) should be administered. Volume must be restored before consideration of pressor therapy. At the time of IV placement, blood for electrolytes, BUN, glucose, calcium, complete blood count (CBC), and appropriate toxicologic studies should be sent for laboratory determination. An arterial blood gas should always be obtained to assess the patient's ventilatory status and to detect the presence of any acid-base abnormalities.

As soon as an IV line is started in patients with any alteration in mental status (coma, seizures, agitation) and *regardless* of the presence or absence of focal neurologic findings or pupil size, the following should be given IV: dextrose, 0.5 to 1.0 gm per kg, and naloxone, 0.01 to 0.1 mg per kg *or more.*

If the coma or altered mental status is due to hypoglycemia, patients will usually respond to the previous dose of dextrose within minutes unless the hypoglycemia has been of prolonged duration. When a patient responds to dextrose, further monitoring of blood glucose is necessary and the etiology of the hypoglycemia should be sought. Reagent strips (Dextrostix and Chem-BG) may be useful in establishing the diagnosis but also may be erroneous or misread; therefore, they should not be the only method relied upon in the emergency setting. A large initial dose of naloxone may be necessary to reverse the effects of some opiate poisonings because of the intrinsic properties of the opiate (e.g., methadone, codeine, and propoxyphene) or the amount ingested. Repeat doses of naloxone and/or initiation of a continuous naloxone infusion may be necessary if the patient responds to the initial dose. A starting dose for a continuous infusion should be calculated to deliver 0.4 to 0.8 mg of naloxone per hour, more if the clinical situation mandates it.

If the patient is an adolescent or has a history of chronic ethanol abuse, 100 mg of thiamine hydrochloride should be given intramuscularly (IM) or IV to prevent development of Wernicke's encephalopathy.

After respiration and circulation have been stabilized, a rectal temperature must be obtained. Severe hypothermia or hyperthermia must be recognized and treated appropriately, because the presence of either may hamper further efforts to stabilize the patient. The presence of fever may indicate an infectious etiology for the altered mental state.

A complete physical examination must be performed. It is essential that signs of trauma be noted and investigated. Serious trauma may be the sole cause of the coma or may be the result of the toxic derangement, and may raise the suspicion of child abuse or neglect.

Correct management of a toxicologic emergency may still result in the patient's demise if occult trauma such as ruptured spleen or liver or a cervical spine injury remains undiagnosed. A neurologic examination, with special attention to level of consciousness, pupil size and reactivity, and presence or absence of nystagmus and reflexes, should be recorded in a reproducible manner. Any focal neurologic abnormalities should be noted and, if present, a structural intracranial lesion should be suspected. A cerebral CAT scan is useful in the evaluation of such a patient. The physician should keep in mind that the Glasgow Coma Scale is prognostic in patients with head trauma (see Chapter 43, Management of Pediatric Head Trauma) but has no prognostic value in poisoned or overdosed patients.

At this point, the vital signs should be reassessed. The patient who remains hypotensive may need another fluid challenge, with 10 to 20 ml per kg of NS or Ringer's lactate. If hypotension persists, one must consider several possibilities: 1) ingestion of a direct myocardial depressant, 2) ingestion of a potent vasodilator, and 3) concomitant trauma (usually abdominal) with hypovolemia. Invasive monitoring with a central venous catheter or, less commonly, a Swan-Ganz catheter may be indicated for assessment of intravascular volume and guidance in the use of pressors.

Prevention of absorption of the ingested toxin is the next priority. In patients in coma or with altered mental status, gastric lavage is the only acceptable mode of removal. The airway should be protected with an endotracheal tube (with an outer cuff in patients older than 8 years of age) to prevent aspiration of gastric contents. Ideally, the size of the tube used to lavage should be large enough to accommodate whole pills or capsules. This is possible in adolescents using a 30–40-French orogastric tube.

The size of orogastric tubes available for use in children range from 16–28-French tubes; the largest that the child can accommodate is the one to be used. Most 2- or 3-year-old children can comfortably allow passage of a 28-gauge tube. The Ewald-type may be used, but it has only one end hole and is easily clogged, whereas the orogastric tube has multiple sideholes in addition to the distal hole. Nasogastric (NG) tubes are inadequate for the purpose of lavage when particulate substances have been ingested. When it is certain that only a liquid has been swallowed, an NG tube is sufficient.

After checking for proper tube placement, the lavage should be performed with the patient in the left lateral decubitus, head-down position to prevent aspiration. A funnel attached to the end of the tube can be used to deliver 50 to 100 ml aliquots of NS in children, 150 to 200 ml in adolescents. The empty tube with funnel attached is then lowered below the patient to facilitate easy emptying into a pail or basin. The process should be continued until the lavage return is clear of particulate matter for at least 1 L. The first return of lavage fluid may be saved for toxicologic testing. In Table 58–1, the proper technique and contraindications to lavage are explained.

The tube should then be used to administer activated charcoal and a cathartic. The powdered form of activated charcoal (not tablets) is an efficacious adsorbent for most organic and inorganic substances (except small ions such as magnesium, iron, and lithium). The dose is 1 gm per kg, which is mixed in a slurry with water in a ratio of 1:4 (charcoal:water). Guide-

---

Table 58–1. Lavage

Tube
Adolescents
   30–40 French orogastric-type tube
Children
   16–28-French orogastric-type tube
Lavage Procedure
  1. Endotracheal or nasotracheal intubation should precede gastric lavage in unconscious or seizing patients, or patients with absent gag reflexes.
  2. *If patients can tolerate intubation without trauma, they should be intubated.* In any case, the airway must be meticulously protected.
  3. When the tube is introduced, confirmation of position of the tube in the stomach is essential.
  4. The patient should be kept in the left lateral decubitus position.
  5. A saline-lavage solution initiated with 200 ml aliquots should be instilled in adolescents (or 50–100 ml aliquots in children).
  6. This procedure should be continued for at least several liters of lavage or until no particulate matter is seen and the lavage is clear.
  7. The tube should then be used for instillation of activated charcoal and a cathartic.
Contraindications
Strong acid or alkali ingestion
Significant hemorrhagic diathesis (relative contraindication)

Modified from Goldfrank, L.R.: Toxicologic Emergencies, 2nd ed. Norwalk, Connecticut, Appleton-Century-Crofts, 1982.

Table 58–2. Activated Charcoal (Powder Form Only)

Dose
 Adults and Children
  1 gm/kg body weight
Procedure
  1. Add chosen quantity of activated charcoal to four parts of water.
  2. This mixture will form a transiently stable slurry that the patient can drink or have placed down an orogastric hose.
  3. The activated charcoal can be given in a mixture with the chosen cathartic.
  4. If the patient vomits the dose, it may be repeated.
  5. Multiple doses can be used if the drug ingested (tricyclic antidepressants, PCP) is suspected of having an entero-gastric recirculation or an entero-enteral recirculation (phenobarbital, theophylline).
Contraindications
  Do not use the universal antidote.
  Do not give until the syrup of ipecac has evoked emesis.

Modified from Goldfrank, L.R.: Toxicologic Emergencies, 2nd ed. Norwalk, Connecticut, Appleton-Century-Crofts, 1982.

lines for administration, dosage, and contraindications are listed in Table 58–2. Multiple doses of activated charcoal have been shown to be efficacious in increasing clearance of certain drugs. An ionic cathartic may be placed down the tube with the charcoal slurry. Ionic cathartics (magnesium sulfate, sodium sulfate, and Fleet's Phospho-Soda) will not be absorbed by the charcoal. Dosage guidelines and contraindications to the use of cathartics are listed in Table 58–3. Fleet's Phospho-Soda should not be used in children because of the potential for severe electrolyte imbalances (hypocalcemia, hypernatremia, and hyperphosphatemia).

Deterioration of the patient after a charcoal stool is produced may signify that 1) the toxin has an enterohepatic circulation, 2) an occult injury (subdural hematoma, ruptured spleen) is present, 3) additional toxin has been ingested

during hospitalization, or 4) a bolus of pills allows continuing absorption.

The lavage/charcoal/cathartic regimen should be performed in all eligible patients *regardless* of the time elapsed since ingestion. Whole pills or fragments can be recovered from the gastrointestinal tract a day or more after the presumed ingestion, especially under conditions that produce slowing of gastrointestinal motility and delayed absorption (food, anticholinergics, opiates, drugs with sustained release absorption characteristics, acute abdomen, trauma, ileus).

Etiology and Differential Diagnosis

The major drugs or toxins that may cause an altered mental status or coma are listed in Table

Table 58–3. Cathartics (Tonic)

Dose
 Adults
  Magnesium sulfate   30 gm
  Sodium sulfate   30 gm
  Phospho-Soda   30 ml (diluted 1:4)
 Children
  Magnesium sulfate   250 mg/kg body weight
  Sodium sulfate   250 mg/kg body weight
  Magnesium   4 ml/kg body weight
Administration
  1. Laxatives and nonionic cathartics should not be used in overdosed patients because of the likelihood that they will adsorb to activated charcoal and become inactivated.
  2. Oil cathartics should not be used for overdosed patients because of the risks of enhanced absorption of hydrocarbons and pesticide substances and the increased danger if aspirated.
Contraindications
  Adynamic ileus
  Severe diarrhea
  Abdominal trauma
  Intestinal obstruction
  Renal failure (magnesium sulfate)
  Congestive heart failure (sodium sulfate)
  Ethylene glycol (Phospho-Soda)

Modified from Goldfrank, L.R.: Toxicologic Emergencies, 2nd. ed. Norwalk, Connecticut, Appleton-Century-Crofts, 1982.

Table 58–4. Common Drugs or Toxins Causing Alterations in Mental Status

CNS Depressants	CNS Stimulants
Barbiturates	Amphetamines
Ethanol	Caffeine
Ethylene glycol	Cocaine
Isopropyl alcohol	Lithium
Lithium	Phencyclidine
Methanol	Salicylates
Opiates	Strychnine
Phencyclidine	Tricyclic antidepressants
Tricyclic antidepressants	Phenylpropanolamine
Benzodiazepines	Phenytoin
Phenothiazines	Camphor
Glutethimide	LSD
Meprobamate	Marijuana
Ethchlorvynol	Theophylline
Methaqualone	Menthol
Carbamazepine	
Chloral hydrate	

58–4. Differential considerations should routinely include hypoglycemia, endocrinopathies (hypothyroidism, hypoadrenalism), hypothermia, central nervous system (CNS) infections (meningitis, cerebritis, abscess, encephalitis), Reye's syndrome, and CNS trauma (epidural/subdural hematoma, subarachnoid hemorrhage, contusion, concussion).

AGITATED PATIENTS

Agitated, delirious, or hallucinating patients are found with increasing frequency in the pediatric population because of the availability of and use of illicit drugs. These patients require prompt attention and treatment. Merely placing them in a quiet room to "calm down" is unacceptable and may result in *nontreatment* of life-threatening conditions such as hypoglycemia and hypothermia.

Many drugs, including hallucinogens (LSD, mescaline, peyote, psilocybin mushrooms), phencyclidine (PCP, angel dust), marijuana, amphetamines, cocaine, anticholinergics, alcohol, sedative hypnotics, and barbiturates, cause severe agitation or symptoms of psychosis.

The differential diagnosis includes hypoglycemia and other metabolic abnormalities, hypoxia from any cause, drug withdrawal states, drug-induced psychosis, meningitis or encephalitis, and functional psychoses such as schizophrenia. It is apparent that several of the aforementioned states require immediate treatment.

The first step in treating severely agitated patients is to gain IV access. Depending upon the age of the child or adolescent, several staff members may be needed for this task. Blood should be drawn and sent for CBC, electrolytes, BUN, glucose, calcium, and toxicologic "screen" for drugs that may cause agitation or CNS stimulation. The patient should be given IV glucose in the aforementioned doses, and 100 percent oxygen should be administered pending arterial blood gas determination. If the blood gases are normal and carbon monoxide intoxication is excluded, oxygen therapy may be discontinued.

Attempts should be made to calm that patient with verbal reassurance if he or she is awake. If necessary, padded extremity restraints can be used with safety. "Straight jackets" or camisole restraints should *never* be used, because they may lead to severe, life-threatening hyperthermia. In severely agitated patients, the rectal temperature should be monitored and hyperthermia should be treated rapidly by using a cooling blanket and ice water soaks. Cooling to the point of violent shivering should be avoided.

If physical restraint is unsuccessful, pharmacologic restraint may be required. The drug of choice is IV diazepam, in small doses (starting dose 0.3 mg/kg). The use of haloperiodol or phenothiazines for sedation is relatively contraindicated, because they may lower the seizure threshold, cause hyperthermia on an anticholinergic basis, and lead to acute dystonic reactions.

Attempts to remove the ingested material and decrease absorption may now proceed in the same manner as for comatose patient, with the following recommendations:

1. Agitated patients who are alert and responsive can be given syrup of ipecac.

2. An NG tube may be used to instill the syrup of ipecac if the patient is alert yet agitated and uncooperative.

3. When the ingestion is potentially life threatening, no effort should be spared in attempting to remove the poison.

After completion of all procedures and full evaluation, the patient should be placed in a quiet environment in which the patient can be observed.

Physostigmine (0.5 mg in children up to maximum dose of 2.0 mg IV *slowly*) may be used in adolescents to control the hallucinations resulting from anticholinergic toxicity. Following an effective first dose, it may be repeated in 20 to 30 minutes if needed, but multiple doses without a clear response or too-rapid administration will precipitate a cholinergic crisis.

ALERT PATIENTS

Alert poisoned patients should have a complete set of vital signs taken. A complete history may be obtained from the patient, depending upon his or her age and the reliability of the parents or friends. The suspected suicidal patient should be interviewed alone to get as accurate a history as possible.

If all vital signs are stable, basic poison management should then proceed. In older patients, all procedures and their significance should be explained fully in order to achieve cooperation. Constant reassurance should be given to the patient and the parents that all procedures are for the patient's benefit. A complete physical examination should be performed.

The first priority is to remove the ingested toxin. The decision to use emesis or lavage is determined by age, presence or absence of the gag reflex, and the presence of a contraindication to either procedure.

Emesis

Alert patients older than 6 months of age who have a gag reflex and are cooperative may receive syrup of ipecac as an emetic. The appropriate dosage according to age is listed in Table 58–5. Ipecac is not recommended for infants younger than 6 months of age. Other contraindications to its use are listed in Table 58–5. If no contraindications are present, vomiting should be induced by administration of ipecac, regardless of the suspected time elapsed since ingestion.

Syrup of ipecac is a mixture of several natural alkaloids that will induce emesis in 80 percent of children within 20 minutes and 95 percent of children within 30 minutes. It is a safe preparation, without intrinsic systemic toxicity. In contrast to the safety of the syrup, the formerly used *fluid extract* of ipecac was 14 times more potent and was reported to result in serious toxicity in the form of gastrointestinal irritation, CNS depression, and cardiac dysrhythmias.

The patient who does not vomit after 30 minutes may require mechanical stimulation to induce emesis. A second dose of syrup of ipecac may be given if no emesis has occurred by this time. If emesis has not ocurred 15 to 30 minutes after the second dose, lavage should be performed for removal of the toxin.

Lavage

Lavage may be an extremely difficult procedure in alert patients. Technically, the procedure is identical to that in unconscious patients (see Table 58–1) except that, in alert patients, the airway does not need to be protected with endotracheal intubation. The physician must be patient and persistent. Most patients will eventually cooperate, but, at times, restraint may be necessary. Lavage should be

Table 58–5. Emesis With Syrup of Ipecac

Dose
   6–12 months, 10 ml (2 tsp)
   1–5 years, 15 ml (1 tbsp)
   Over 5 years, 30 ml (2 tbsp)
Administration
   1. Emesis should be induced regardless of the number of hours that have passed since ingestion provided there are no contraindications present.
   2. Give the appropriate dose of syrup of ipecac.
   3. Give the patient several glasses of water (150–250 ml each).
   4. Position the patient upright or in the sitting position to prevent aspiration of vomitus.
   5. Carefully supervise all vomiting patients.
   6. One additional dose (a second dose) may be given if the patient has not vomited within 30 min.
Contraindications
   Child younger than 6 months
   Comatose patient
   Patient experiencing seizures
   Patient withoug a gag reflex
   Ingestion of a strong acid or alkali
   Patients with hemorrhagic diatheses (cirrhosis, thrombocytopenia)
   Concomitant ingestion of sharp, solid materials (thermometer, glass, nails, razor blades)
   Evidence of significant vomiting prior to ipecac utilization
   An ingested substance due to its quantity (visualized ingestion of opioid or tricyclic antidepressant) or character, such as chloroquine, camphor or strychnine, where the urgency of *removal* mandates against any potential delay Lavage instead.

From Goldfrank, L.R.: Toxicologic Emergencies, 2nd ed. Norwalk, Connecticut, Appleton-Century-Crofts, 1982.

attempted in infants younger than 6 months of age, in patients who have had massive ingestion of pills (in which case emesis may not effectively remove all pills or concretions of pills), and in patients who have had ingestions of particularly dangerous substances (strychnine, camphor). NG lavage is also an acceptable first method for gastric evacuation if the only ingested substance reported is liquid. After lavage, the appropriate dose of activated charcoal and cathartic (see Tables 58–2 and 58–3) should be placed down the tube prior to its removal.

UNCOOPERATIVE PATIENTS

Uncooperative patients present a difficult problem for physicians. They may refuse to drink ipecac and may not cooperate with the passage of a tube. If this happens, the options available are as follows:

1. Pass an NG tube, and after confirming its presence in the stomach, instill ipecac and water in the amounts used for oral therapy and then remove the tube, allowing the patient to vomit. This does not constitute lavage, but is merely an alternate method of administering ipecac.

2. After restraining the patient, pass the largest size tube that the nasal passages will comfortably permit, with adequate lubrication, and then lavage the stomach.

3. Reassess the situation and decide whether gastric evacuation is necessary. For instance, some substances may be relatively nontoxic or may be used in such a manner that gastric emptying would not be useful.

PSYCHIATRIC CONSULTATION

Every suspected suicide attempt or gesture must be taken seriously. Questions to elicit information about suicidal ideation should be asked of older children as well as adolescents. If the question of suicide arises at any time during interviews with the patient, family, or friends, appropriate psychiatric intervention must be sought before the patient leaves the hospital setting. It is essential that one-to-one observation be maintained at all times with all seriously suicidal patients.

SOCIAL SERVICE EVALUATION

Many cases of poisoning in childhood are the result of some degree of parental negligence

or abuse. Any suspicion of such abuse requires that the physician report the case to appropriate agencies for evaluation of the home setting and protection of the affected child and other children in the home. This is an essential aspect of the total management of the poisoned patient and must not be neglected by the physician.

ADVANCED MANAGEMENT PRINCIPLES

In addition to the basic management principles outlined in the previous sections, certain overdoses require the utilization of other techniques to enhance excretion of the toxin. These techniques include forced diuresis (acid, alkaline, osmotic), dialysis (peritoneal or hemodilysis), and hemoperfusion (charcoal or resin).

Diuresis

The efficacy of any type of diuresis requires that a significant amount of the toxin or active metabolite be excreted by the kidney. Diuresis will not be effective if a drug has a large volume of distribution or a nonrenal excretory mechanism. Contraindications to forced water or osmotic-induced diuresis include renal failure, cardiovascular compromise, and the inability to monitor fluid, electrolyte, or hemodynamic status. Conditions that are relative contraindications include pulmonary edema, cerebral edema, and the syndrome of inappropriate secretion of antidiuretic hormone (SIADH). In such cases, additional monitoring of pulmonary wedge pressure or intracranial pressure (ICP) may facilitate management, or hemodialysis may be a more effective alternative.

Acid diuresis increases the renal clearance of amphetamine, phencyclidine, and strychnine intoxications. Ammonium chloride, 75 mg per kg per day IV or PO in four divided doses, is used to achieve urinary acidification to a pH of 5.5. Appropriate fluids must be given to achieve a urine output of 3 ml per kg per hr. Ascorbic acid is not effective as a urinary acidifier. In phencyclidine overdose, only about 10 percent of the drug is excreted in the urine, so even adequate acidification may not significantly alter drug excretion. Furthermore, intoxication with these substances may be associated with a metabolic acidosis and rhabdomyolysis resulting from extreme muscle activity, and acidification may complicate such a circumstance.

Alkaline diuresis is useful in enhancing excretion of two drugs commonly encountered in overdose patients, salicylates and phenobarbital. It may also be helpful in isoniazid intoxications. Effective alkaline diuresis is defined as a urine output of 3 to 5 ml per kg per hr, with a urine pH greater than 7.5. Alkalinization is achieved by administering sodium bicarbonate IV in an initial bolus of 2 mEq per kg, followed by a constant infusion of 1.0 mEq per kg per hr, as a starting dose. Adequate fluids must also be administered; composition of the fluids is dependent upon the patient's electrolyte status. Alkalinization lowers the serum potassium 1 ml, yet a normal serum potassium must be maintained in order to achieve an alkaline urine. Acetazolamide (Diamox) has no place as a urinary alkalinizing agent, because it alkalinizes the urine at the expense of creating a systemic acidosis. This may have dire consequences in patients with severe salicylism, because the acidosis may favor an intracellular accumulation of salicylate, most significantly in the CNS.

Diuresis with hypertonic agents such as mannitol may decrease proximal tubular reabsorption of solute and, secondarily, water; the result is a decreased tubular concentration of the toxin. Forced water or loop diuretic–induced diuresis has little effect on the proximal tubule and therefore is not efficacious. Forced water diuresis should be avoided because of the possible complications of fluid overload in an already compromised patient.

Dialysis

Dialysis is useful in the management of intoxication in which the toxin has a low volume of distribution and diffuses rapidly across the dialysis membrane. Peritoneal dialysis is less effective than hemodialysis, especially if hypotension is present. In many pediatric patients, however, hemodialysis or hemoperfusion may not be technically possible. If the patient's size and age permit, hemodialysis or hemoperfusion are the procedures of choice when dialysis is indicated.

Certain intoxications, including serious methanol and ethylene glycol ingestions, are clear-cut indications for dialysis. Depending upon the serum concentration of the drug, overdoses with salicylates, lithium, barbiturates, or heavy metals may require dialysis. Clinical criteria for dialysis in the presence of a dialyzable toxin include unstable vital signs; deteriorating fluid, electrolyte, or acid-base status despite corrective measures; and hepatic or renal failure

when the ingested toxin is either metabolized or excreted by the nonfunctional organ.

The use of dialysis in children requires the presence of a medical team that is knowledgeable and experienced in handling this method in children; the intensive care setting is necessary for proper monitoring, both during and after the procedure.

Hemoperfusion

Charcoal or resin hemoperfusion is becoming increasingly popular in the management of certain overdoses. In general, substantially more toxin is removed during hemoperfusion than during peritoneal dialysis or hemodialysis; this is especially true in the case of drugs that are lipid soluble or protein bound. Charcoal hemoperfusion is efficacious in the management of serious intoxications with theophylline and may also be useful in serious poisonings with barbiturates and salicylates. Potential complications of hemoperfusion include thrombocytopenia and infection. As with hemodialysis, a consulting renal service with pediatric experience and an ICU setting for proper monitoring of the patient are prerequisites for the use of charcoal or resin hemoperfusion.

LABORATORY USAGE

The laboratory is an important adjunct in the management of pediatric intoxications. If possible, blood, urine, and gastric contents should be obtained for future analysis in all cases in which the patient is suspected of having an overdose because of the history or the clinical setting; of the three, urine is the most sensitive for qualitative drug detection. Table 58–6 provides guidelines for selection of drug determinations, including those that should be ordered stat. The "toxicologic screen" should be discouraged, because it is expensive and usually delays the identification of the responsible toxin. Ideally, the toxicology laboratory should be provided with clinical information that may suggest specific analyses and facilitate rapid results.

COMMON CARDIOVASCULAR COMPLICATIONS

Hypotension

Hypotension should be managed, as outlined previously, by Trendelenberg positioning and adequate volume administration before the use

Table 58–6. Studies That Should Be Available From a Problem-Oriented Toxicology Laboratory

Stat Studies	**CNS Stimulants**
Acetaminophen	Immediate studies
Carbon monoxide	Amphetamines
Digoxin	Caffeine
Ethanol	Cocaine
Ethylene glycol	Lithium
Iron/TIBC	Phencyclidine
Isopropyl alcohol	Salicylates
Lithium	Strychnine
Methanol	Secondary studies
Methemoglobin	Tricyclic antidepressants
Phenobarbital	Phenytoin
Phenytoin	Camphor
Salicylates	LSD
Theophylline	**Anion Gap Metabolic Acidosis**
CNS Depressants	Ethanol
Immediate studies	Ethylene glycol
Barbiturates—short-acting, long-acting	Iron
Ethanol	Isoniazid
Ethylene glycol	Methanol
Isopropyl alcohol	Paraldehyde
Lithium	Salicylates
Methanol	Toluene
Opiates (if positive, screen for acetamino-	**Heavy Metals**
phen and salicylates)	Arsenic
Phencyclidine	Cadmium
Note: If all negative, assay for CNS stimu-	Copper
lants	Iron
Secondary studies	Lead
Tricyclic antidepressants	Mercury
Benzodiazepines	**Nonstat Studies**
Phenothiazines	Borates
Glutethimide	Bromide
Meprobamate	Iodides
Ethchlorvynol	Organophosphates/carbamates
Methaqualone	Thallium
Carbamazepine	
Chloral hydrate	

Modified from Goldfrank, L.R.: Toxicologic Emergencies, 2nd ed. Norwalk, Connecticut, Appleton-Century-Crofts, 1982.

of pressors. Invasive monitoring may be required to assess fluid status. Usually, fluid management is sufficient to maintain an adequate blood pressure.

If pressors are necessary, dopamine is a good choice. Some clinicians have suggested using norepinephrine for tricyclic antidepressant overdose because of the norepinephrine depletion that may occur as a result of inhibited synaptic reuptake; in many of these cases, even dopamine can be used with success. Epinephrine and isoproterenol should be avoided in cases of overdoses with cardiotoxic drugs, because they may increase the potential for dysrhythmias.

Supraventricular Tachydysrhythmias

Supraventricular tachydysrhythmias may be encountered in overdosed patients. In the absence of associated hypotension, ventricular ectopy, or mental status changes, cardiac monitoring should be continued, but no active intervention is necessary.

Patients with suspected ingestion of a tricyclic antidepressant, phenothiazine, or other anticholinergic substance and a supraventricular tachydysrhythmia must have a 12-lead EKG with measurement of all intervals (PR, QRS, and QTc). If all the intervals are within normal limits, the patient requires monitoring for at least 24 hours after the tachycardia has resolved. If there is prolongation of QRS interval, the patient should receive IV sodium bicarbonate, 2 mEq per kg initially, followed by a bicarbonate drip. The objective of therapy is the maintenance of serum pH between 7.45 and 7.5. The mechanism of action of the sodium bicarbonate in this type of overdose is unknown. The patient should also receive a standard antidysrhythmic loading dose of phenytoin (10 mg/kg, at a rate no greater than 50 mg/min). These maneuvers will most likely bring about normalization of the intervals and prevent the onset of serious ventricular dysrhythmias in the aforementioned overdoses.

Ventricular Tachydysrhythmias

The potentially life-threatening dysrhythmias that must be recognized and treated immediately include ventricular premature contractions, ventricular tachycardia, and ventricular fibrillation. The common overdoses associated with these dysrhythmias include anticholinergics (antihistamines, antiparkinsonians, antipsychotics, tricyclic antidepressants, belladonna alkaloids, scopolamine, and atropine), digitalis preparations, and hydrocarbons. Other diagnoses to consider include hypoxia from any cause (especially associated with carbon monoxide or cyanide poisonings) and electrolyte abnormalities (hypokalemia or hypercalcemia). The presence of even minute quantities of "digoxin" in a patient who is not supposed to be taking any digitalis preparation may indicate the ingestion of digoxin, digitoxin, digitalis leaf, foxglove, or oleander.

The management of patients with ventricular tachydysrhythmia begins with administration of 100 percent oxygen. Lidocaine, 1 mg per kg as a bolus, followed by a drip of 0.1 to 0.4 mg per kg per minute should then be given. The bolus may be repeated, if necessary. If the dysrhythmia is unresponsive to lidocaine, bretylium (3–5 mg/kg IV) may be useful. Phenytoin may also be beneficial in the management of ventricular tachydysrhythmias secondary to anticholinergics or digitalis. The use of quinidine or procainamide is contraindicated, because these agents may exacerbate digitalis or anticholinergic-associated dysrhythmias. Cardioversion is contraindicated in suspected digoxin overdose because of the high association with increased ventricular ectopy.

Bradydysrhythmias

Second or third degree heart block associated with slow ventricular rates, ventricular ectopy, altered mental status, or hypotension requires immediate treatment. Common overdoses associated with such dysrhythmias include digitalis, clonidine, and cholinergic poisoning due to organophosphate or carbamate insecticides. Other nontoxic causes include increased ICP and electrolyte abnormalities. Treatment begins with atropine, 0.01 mg per kg, repeated every 5 minutes, as necessary. If the bradydysrhythmia is unresponsive to atropine, temporary cardiac pacing is indicated.

SEIZURES IN OVERDOSED PATIENTS

Seizures in poisoned or overdosed patients should be managed with administration of oxygen, glucose, naloxone, and anticonvulsants (see Chapter 46, Status Epilepticus). Overdoses of certain opiates, including meperidine, propoxyphene, and codeine, may present with seizures on the basis of intrinsic toxicity, whereas other opiate overdoses present with seizures on a hypoxic basis. Naloxone, therefore, is indicated in all convulsing patients. Seizures should be initially managed with IV diazepam (0.3 mg/kg or starting dose up to 0.5 mg/kg), with careful attention paid to respiratory status. Because diazepam is short-acting, long-term anticonvulsant control should be instituted. This should be achieved by administration of phenytoin rather than phenobarbital, because phenytoin is less sedating.

THE REGIONAL POISON CONTROL CENTER

All physicians caring for overdosed children and adolescents should be familiar with the services available from their regional poison control center. Most such centers provide important information as to differential diagnosis, management guidelines, and advanced management techniques. Any serious overdose should be discussed with a toxicologist associated with a poison control center who will be familiar with the current literature and indications for the various antidotes and advanced management techniques.

CASE PRESENTATION

A 2-year-old female was found lying unresponsive in the bathroom with an open bottle of pills next to her on the floor. She was immediately taken to the emergency room by the baby sitter. Upon arrival, she was responsive only to painful stimuli. Her vital signs were: BP = 140/90 mm Hg, HR = 180 beats/min, RR = 24/min, and T = 102°F. Her weight was 12 kg (26 lb).

Physical Examination

Physical examination was pertinent for pupils dilated to 6 mm and nonreactive; dry mucous membranes; warm, dry skin; absent bowel sounds; and a distended bladder. The fundi were benign in appearance. The patient was unresponsive to pain and there were no focal neurologic deficits or abnormal reflexes. No signs of trauma were evident.

Laboratory Evaluation

An IV line was established, and blood was drawn for CBC, electrolytes, BUN, creatinine, glucose, and calcium. Additional blood was saved for toxicologic determinations. The infusate was D5W 1/3 NS initially, at a rate to keep the vein open. She received 100 percent oxygen by face mask and was given 6 gm of glucose and 1 mg of naloxone IV with no response. An arterial blood gas obtained prior to oxygen therapy revealed pH = 7.39, PO_2 = 93 mm Hg, and PCO_2 = 41 mm Hg. The CBC and electrolytes were within normal limits.

The patient was intubated and lavaged via an orogastric tube with NS until the gastric contents returned clear. Activated charcoal and magnesium sulfate were then administered, after which the lavage tube was removed. A Foley catheter was passed, and 200 ml of urine was obtained. Specimens of both gastric aspirate and urine were saved for toxicologic analysis. The child was transferred to the pediatric ICU.

The parents arrived, and a complete history was obtained. The child was otherwise healthy and receiving no medication. An 8-year-old brother is enuretic, and the only pills in the house were his 25-mg imipramine tablets.

Problem List

Intake and Output

Because of the alteration in mental status, the patient was kept NPO. IV fluids were restricted to two thirds maintenance because of the presence of hypertension. The infusate was changed to D2 1/2W/ 1/2 NS. The initial electrolytes and BUN were normal but were monitored regularly as long as the child was NPO. The urine output was monitored via an indwelling urinary drainage catheter.

Respiratory

Supplementary oxygen was discontinued when the blood gas obtained in room air returned with a normal arterial oxygen tension. The patient received routine pulmonary care, as in any case of decreased level of consciousness. Arterial blood gases were obtained p.r.n.

Cardiovascular

A 12-lead EKG was obtained because of the tachycardia, history of possible tricyclic antidepressant ingestion, and physical findings suggestive of anticholinergic poisoning. All intervals were measured and were found to be normal for rate. Cardiac monitoring was initiated and continued for 24 hours after the child's heart rate returned to normal. The hypertension observed in this case was consistent with the early phase of an anticholinergic overdose and was managed by fluid restriction.

The child was much improved by 18 hours. A urine specimen for toxicologic analysis revealed imipramine. The blood specimen was negative.

SUGGESTED READING

Andersen, R.J., and Hart, G.R.: Clonidine overdose. Ann. Emerg. Med. 10:107, 1981.

Done, A.K.: Aspirin overdosage; incidence, diagnosis, and management. Pediatrics (Part II Suppl) 62:890, 1978.

Goldfrank, L.R.: Toxicologic Emergencies, 2nd ed. Norwalk, Connecticut, Appleton-Century-Crofts, 1982.

Goldfrank, L., Cohen, L., Flomenbaum, et al.: New antidotes and controversies in antidotal therapy. In Wolcott, B.W., and Rund, D.A. (eds.): Emergency Medicine Annual, 1984, 3:223–266, 1984.

Greenblatt, D.J., and Koch-Wieser, J.: Clinical pharmacokinetics. N. Engl. J. Med. 293:702–705 and 964–970, 1975.

Haddad, L.M., and Winchester, J.F.: Clinical Management of Poisoning and Drug Overdose. Philadelphia, W.B. Saunders Company, 1983.

Marshall, J.B., and Forker, A.D.: Cardiovascular effects of tricyclic antidepressant drugs. Am. Heart J. 103:401, 1982.

McCarron, M.M., Schultze, B.W., Thompson, G.A., et al.: Acute phencyclidine intoxication: incidence of clinical findings in 1000 cases. Ann. Emerg. Med. 10:237, 1981.

Milby, T.H.: Prevention and management of organophosphate poisoning. JAMA 216:2131, 1971.

Mitchell, A.A., Lovejoy, F.H., and Goldman, P.: Drug ingestions associated with miosis in comatose children. J. Pediatr., 89:303, 1976.

Moore, R.A., Rumack, B.H., and Conner, C.S.: Naloxone-underdosage after narcotic poisoning, Am. J. Dis. Child. 134:156, 1980.

Rumack, B.H., and Temple, A.R.: Lomotil poisoning. Pediatrics 53:495, 1974.

Rumack, B.H., and Petersen, R.: Acetaminophen overdose: incidence, diagnosis, and management in 416 patients. Pediatrics 62:898, 1978.

Salzberg, M., and Gallagher, E.J.: Propranolol overdose. Ann. Emerg. Med. 9:26, 1980.

Smith, T.W., Butler, V.P., Haber, E., et al.: Treatment of life-threatening digitalis intoxication with digoxin-specific Fab antibody fragments. Experience in 26 cases. N. Engl. J. Med. 307:1357, 1982.

Winchester, J.F., Gelfand, M.C., Knepshield, J.M., and Schreiner, J.F.: Dialysis and hemoperfusion of poisons and drugs—update. Trans. Am. Soc. Artif. Intern. Organs 23:762, 1977.

Nursing Process for Patient Care:

Poisoning: General Principles of Management

Patients who have ingested toxic substances require immediate evaluation and stabilization of vital signs. After this has been accomplished, attention is then directed toward the substance itself and attempts are made to decrease its absorption and increase its elimination. In a few circumstances, specific antidotes may exist. Care is generally supportive, with close monitoring of specific "target" organs.

RESPIRATORY

Initial assessment priorities include ensuring a patent airway and adequate oxygenation and ventilation. Respiratory compromise can occur as a result of CNS depression and pulmonary and systemic toxicity.

Assess, Monitor, and Document

Patency of airway
Respiratory rate
Respiratory pattern, including depth
Breath sounds
Color

Arterial blood gases
Response to oxygen administration
Response to intubation and assisted mechanical ventilation (if applicable)

Anticipate

Alteration in respiratory status
  Hypoventilation
  Hypoxia

Respiratory failure
Respiratory arrest

CARDIOVASCULAR

Assess, Monitor, and Document

Heart rate
Rhythm
Blood pressure: arterial, central venous, and, if indicated, pulmonary artery and capillary wedge
Peripheral perfusion: pulse, skin color, skin condition

Urine output hourly, including specific gravity
Fluid intake
Weight
Serum: electrolytes, glucose, BUN, creatinine
Response to medical management: volume administration, pharmacologic agents

Anticipate

Alteration in cardiovascular status
  Hypotension
  Dysrhythmias: supraventricular tachydys-

rhythmias, ventricular tachydysrhythmias, bradydysrhythmias
Cardiac arrest

NEUROLOGIC

Assess, Monitor, and Document

Level of consciousness: lethargy, stupor, coma
  Behavioral state: agitated, uncooperative
Blood pressure
Pulse

Respiratory rate and pattern
Pupillary response
Reflexes
Motor response
Seizure activity

512

Anticipate

Altered level of consciousness
 Lethargy
 Coma
Altered behavior

Agitated
Uncooperative
Focal signs
Seizures

POISON MANAGEMENT PROTOCOLS

There are essentially three major management protocols based upon the clinical presentation of the patient. They all share common goals in terms of emptying the stomach, decreasing the absorption, and increasing the elimination of the toxic substance. The nurse must be knowledgeable about the principles and practices in order to assess and anticipate the patient's response.

Assess, Monitor, and Document

Response to
 Pharmacologic agents
 Methods to empty stomach and decrease absorption: induce vomiting (syrup of ipecac), lavage, administration of activated charcoal

Methods to increase elimination: cathartic, forced diuresis, dialysis (hemodialysis, peritoneal dialysis), hemoperfusion

Anticipate

Favorable or unfavorable response to specific management modalities

RESPONSE OF CHILD

Assess, Monitor, and Document

Development level: psychosocial, cognitive, motor, verbal
Behavioral response: fearful, tearful, angry
Level of understanding of condition
Perception of events surrounding accident or incident

Expected outcome
Educational needs related to environmental safety and drugs
Response to interventions

Anticipate

Profound emotional crisis
Need for referral: social service agency, psychiatrist

RESPONSE OF FAMILY

Assess, Monitor, and Document

Behavioral response: angry, distressed, verbal
Level of understanding of child's condition
Expected outcome
Educational needs related to environmental safety and substance abuse

Need for referral: social service agency, psychiatrist
Response to nursing interventions

Anticipate

Inability to cope
Family crisis
Educational needs related to environmental
  safety and substance abuse

Need for referral: social service agency, psychiatrist

MIND SET

Assess

Respiratory status
Cardiovascular status
Fluid and electrolyte balance
Neurologic status
Temperature
Response to specific poison management
  protocols

Empty stomach
Decrease absorption
Increase elimination
Response of child and family

Anticipate

Alteration in respiratory status
  Hypoxia
  Respiratory failure
  Respiratory arrest
Alteration in cardiovascular status
  Hypotension
  Dysrthythmias
  Cardiac arrest
Alteration in neurologic status
  Agitated
  Uncooperative
  Comatose
  Seizures

Alteration in body temperature
  Hyperthermia
Favorable or unfavorable response to specific
  poison management protocols
Emotional trauma
Family crisis
Educational needs related to environmental
  safety and substance abuse
Referral to social service agency and/or psy-
  chiatrist

Salicylate Ingestions

HARRIS E. BURSTIN, M.D.

Salicylate ingestions are the most common childhood poisonings. Although the incidence of acute poisonings has decreased as a result of the newer safety-capped bottles and the decreased number of tablets per bottle, chronic poisonings have slightly increased. Though acute poisonings are still more common and have higher salicylate levels, chronic poisonings tend to be more severe, even with lower salicylate levels, and constitute a larger percentage of hospitalized patients.

PATHOPHYSIOLOGY

Excessive ingestion of salicylates has multiple effects on the body's homeostatic mechanisms, leading to profound physiologic disturbances.

Tachypnea and hyperpnea are seen secondary to direct stimulation of the central nervous system (CNS) respiratory center and result in a decreased Pa_{CO_2}. Although causing an initial respiratory alkalosis, this hyperventilation contributes later to a severe metabolic acidosis by decreasing bicarbonate and buffering capacity.

An increase in the metabolic rate caused by uncoupling of oxidative phosphorylation increases heat production (fever), oxygen consumption, and gluconeogenesis.

Inhibition of the Kreb's cycle results in ketone formation. Alterations in amino acid and lipid metabolism are present. The resultant accumulation of metabolic acids is responsible for the severe acidemia that develops.

Fluid and electrolyte loss occur as a consequence of the described metabolic derangements. Increased metabolic rate and heat production lead to increased sweating, resulting in water and sodium loss. Tachypnea increases insensible respiratory water loss. Aciduria causes an osmotic water and electrolyte diuresis. The degree of dehydration can be quite pronounced.

Salicylate intoxication can decrease prothrombin formation, Factor VII production, and platelet aggregation and adhesiveness and increase capillary fragility. Although acute bleeding is rarely a clinical problem, elevation in the prothrombin (PT) time can be seen.

The direct irritant effects of salicylates on gastric mucosa can cause nausea and vomiting. The degree of symptoms depends upon quantity and duration of ingestion. Significant upper gastrointestinal bleeding can be seen in severe chronic ingestions.

DIAGNOSIS AND ASSESSMENT

Vomiting, hyperpnea, and hyperthermia are hallmarks of salicylate intoxication. The symptoms of an acute salicylate ingestion, however, vary depending upon the quantity of poison ingested and the duration of exposure. Mild lethargy, tachypnea, vomiting, and disorientation can progress to severe hyperpnea, hyperthermia, coma, convulsions, oliguria, and shock. The maximum effects of severe acidosis may not be seen for 12 to 24 hours after ingestion.

Although a respiratory alkalosis is said to predominate early in the course, followed by a combined respiratory alkalosis and metabolic acidosis, children are rarely alkalotic. The metabolic derangements are quite severe and acidosis prevails. Hypoglycemia, hypokalemia, and either hyponatremia or hypernatremia are present. Alterations in renal function are consistent with severe dehydration.

A salicylate level is, of course, diagnostic and should be obtained. While awaiting results of a level, a ferric chloride test should be performed. A deep purple color is indicative of the presence of salicylates. Absence of a positive ferric chloride test should alert the physician to the possibility of another drug ingestion. Patients often confuse acetaminophen with aspirin (see Chapter 60). A toxicology screen for other drugs should always be obtained.

Assessment of severity can be gauged by estimating the mg per kg of salicylate ingested acutely. Ingestions of less than 150 mg per kg are associated with no toxicity, 150 to 300 mg per kg with mild to moderate toxicity, 300 to 500 mg per kg with severe toxicity, and greater than 500 mg per kg with potential fatality.

The Done nomogram (Fig. 59–1) gauges severity based upon salicylate level and time elapsed since ingestion. This is only relevant for an acute ingestion at one point in time. Salicylate level is not as indicative of severity in chronic ingestions, because prolonged exposure to the metabolic derangements of salicylates can cause severe symptoms, even at lower levels.

Certainly the most important means of assessment is clinical. The physical condition of the patient, including vital signs, hydrational status, and state of consciousness require frequent monitoring.

THERAPY

As with most drug ingestions, emergency management of acute salicylate ingestion begins with efforts to empty the stomach. This is of limited use after 3 hours postingestion, because peak gastric absorption occurs by 2 hours. Emesis induced by ipecac syrup is used in conscious patients. Gastric lavage via a large-bore nasogastric (NG) or orogastric tube is an alternative, especially in patients with altered mental status. Activated charcoal is given to decrease salicylate absorption. A cathartic such as magnesium sulfate or citrate can be given together in a thick slurry or following the charcoal to induce emptying of the gastrointestinal tract (see Chapter 58).

Fluid and electrolyte therapy is directed at correcting dehydration, electrolyte disturbances, and acidosis, as well as promoting an increased elimination of salicylates.

Emergent fluid resuscitation with a crystalloid such as normal saline (NS, 20 ml/kg pushes) is used to establish a stable blood pressure and urine output if the patient presents in shock. Bicarbonate, in 1 to 2 mEq per kg aliquots, can be given if arterial pH is below 7.2. Glucose should be given in a bolus if the dextrostick reading is critically low.

If the patient presents with dehydration but shows no evidence of cardiovascular collapse, the initial infusate should consist of a solution containing 10 percent dextrose, 75 mEq Na+,

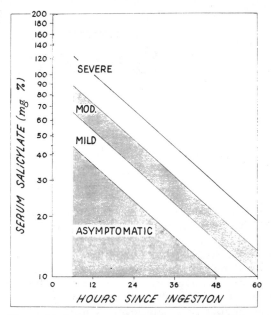

Figure 59–1. Nomogram relating serum salicylate concentration and expected severity of intoxication at varying intervals following the ingestion of a single dose of salicylate. (From Done, A.K.: Salicylate intoxication: significance of measurements of salicylate in blood in cases of acute ingestion. Pediatrics, 26:800–807, 1960, with permission. Copyright American Academy of Pediatrics, 1960.)

25 mEq HCO_3^-, and 50 mEq Cl^- per L (or D10 1/3 NS plus 25 mEq HCO_3^- per L). This solution should be infused at a rate of 10 to 15 ml per kg per hour for 1 to 2 hours. Additional boluses of bicarbonate can be given depending upon the degree of acidosis. Potassium is added after urine output is evident. Because correction of acidosis lowers the serum potassium concentrations, 35 to 40 mEq of potassium per L of fluid may be required.

Subsequent fluid management is based upon individual hydration and electrolyte needs. An attempt is made to maintain urine output between 5 and 6 ml per kg per hour and urine pH above 7.5. An alkaline urine promotes renal salicylate excretion. This goal can be achieved by infusing a solution of 5 to 10 percent dextrose with 0.2 or 0.33 NS, plus 20 to 30 mEq HCO_3^- per L, infused at a rate of 4 to 8 ml per kg per hour. This fluid therapy is continued until the salicylate level decreases to the therapeutic range. The infusion rate then decreases to maintenance, and the solution is changed to D5 1/5 NS, plus 20 mEq HCO_3^- per L. Potassium is added to these solutions in the concentrations necessary to maintain normal serum levels.

Serum calcium, as well as degree of ionization, is affected by alkalinization, and tetany is a possibility during this form of fluid therapy. Calcium levels should be followed, and any deficits should be corrected.

Peritoneal dialysis is required in the presence of cardiac or renal failure, severe CNS manifestations, or progressive deterioration in spite of standard medical therapy that prohibits the use of large fluid volumes. Hemodialysis or exchange transfusions are other alternatives.

CASE PRESENTATION

An 8-year-old male was transferred from a community hospital because of coma, fever and seizures. Two weeks prior, the child had rhinorrhea, cough, and a sore throat. He was treated for a documented streptococcal throat infection with oral penicillin. Over the following 2 weeks, the patient was given multiple over-the-counter salicylate-containing products, including Bayer, Bufferin, Dristan, and Anacin, as well as Tylenol.

Two days prior to transfer the patient began to complain of tinnitus, nausea, and vomiting. The following day, he was taken to a local community hospital because of auditory and visual hallucinations and increasing lethargy.

Examination and Test Results

On initial presentation, the patient was described as comatose and hyperpneic with a temperature of 107°F. The patient's admission salicylate level was 76 mg/dl. He was extremely hypokalemic and hypocalcemic and had an admission glucose of 40 mg/dl. He had a grossly bloody NG aspirate. Platelet count was normal, and a PTT was greater than 2 minutes. His admission arterial pH was 7.27, with a serum bicarbonate of 6.6 mEq/L.

He was treated aggressively with fluids, bicarbonate (over 200 mEq IV), vitamin K, and calcium. Seizures began 2 hours postadmission and were stopped with IV Valium. He was loaded with phenobarbital. Just prior to transfer, he was started on a dopamine drip to maintain blood pressure.

On arrival following transfer, the child was hyperpneic with no signs of seizures and was responsive only to deep pain. He had a central venous pressure line, a peripheral IV, a Foley catheter, and an NG tube with nonbloody aspirate. Physical examination findings included the following vital signs: T = 104.6°F; HR = 120 beats/min; RR = 46 breaths/min; and BP = 130/60 mm Hg. HEENT: benign, discs sharp. Lungs: clear. Heart: regular rhythm with a I–II/VI systolic murmur at left sternal border. Abdomen: distended, with no organomegaly. Skin: numerous ecchymotic areas. Neurologic: no doll's eye movements, positive gag reflex; no deep tendon reflexes could be appreciated and plantar reflexes were equivocal bilaterally.

Laboratory Data

Laboratory values were hematocrit = 36 percent; WBC = 34,800, with 70 percent polys, 9 bands, and 17 lymphs; platelets = 314,000. Coagulation studies showed PT was control and PTT was 1½ times control. UA: pH = 6, positive for blood. Electrolytes: Na = 149, K = 2.5, Cl = 103, CO_2 = 30, BUN = 42, creatine = 1.9, and Ca = 3.8 mEq/L. Glucose: 152 mg/dl. Toxicology: salicylate = 53 mg/dl, acetaminophen = 1.3 mg/dl, and phenobarbital = 0.4 mg/dl. Liver function test (LFT): bilirubin < 1 mg/dl, ammonia = 40 μmol/L, SGOT = 214 mμ/ml, and SGPT = 96 mμ/ml.

Problem List

Intake and Output

D10W/1/3NS, with 25 mEq $NaCO_3$/500 ml and 15 mEq KCl/500 ml, was infused at just under $2\times$ maintenance rate to keep CVP at 6–8 mm H_2O, urine output at 4–5 ml/kg/hr, and urine pH at 7.5. Owing to his neurologic status, fluid volumes were kept to the minimal amount necessary to achieve the above parameters. KCl pushes of 0.5 mEq/kg were given three times. Electrolytes were followed frequently.

Salicylate Intoxication

Level fell to 30 mg/dl by 18 hours and to less than 10 mg/dl by 36 hours postadmission. Social service was contacted about counseling for the family.

Respiratory

The patient maintained blood gases with a pH in the 7.5 range and Pa_{CO_2} between 28 and 32 mm Hg, denoting a combined mild respiratory alkalosis (secondary to tachypnea) and mild metabolic alkalosis (secondary to alkalinization therapy).

Neurologic

Because of mental status and an opening pressure of 290 mm of H_2O, cerebral edema was suspected and a subarachnoid bolt was placed. Because pressure readings were between 8 and 11 cm of H_2O, peritoneal dialysis was deferred and fluids were kept as low as possible. After the salicylate level fell below 20 mg/dl, fluids and alkalinization were decreased appropriately and the bolt was removed.

Hepatic

The moderate elevation of the PTT was treated by the administration of fresh frozen plasma (FFP). Although the serum transaminases were elevated, a normal serum ammonia ruled out Reye's syndrome. Enzymes returned to normal over subsequent days.

Hematologic

Hematocrit decreased to 31 percent following hydration and then remained stable. PTT was corrected with FFP.

Metabolic

Serum glucose was maintained in the range of 80–120 mg/dl with IV D10W. Calcium chloride was given three times to maintain calcium above 7 mEq/L.

Hyperthermia

A hypothermia blanket was used to decrease body temperature.

Gastrointestinal Bleeding

NG aspirates and stools remained guaiac positive. Aluminum magnesium–based antacids were given on an alternating q2h regimen.

Following correction of the various metabolic disorders described, the child gradually improved, becoming alert and verbal within 47 hours of transfer. By 72 hours following admission, he was ready to be transferred from the ICU to the pediatric ward.

SUGGESTED READING

Done, A.K.: Aspirin overdose: incidence, diagnosis, and management. Pediatrics (Suppl) 62:890, 1978.

Done, A.K., Yaffe, S.J., and Clayton, J.M.: Aspirin dosage for infants and children. J. Pediatr. 95:617, 1979.

Gilman, A.G., Goodman, L.S., and Gilman, A.: The Pharmacological Basis of Therapeutics, 6th ed. New York, Macmillan, 1980, pp. 688–698.

Temple, A.R.: Pathophysiology of aspirin overdose toxicity with implications for management. Pediatrics (Suppl) 62:873, 1978.

Nursing Process for Patient Care:
Salicylate Ingestions

RESPIRATORY

Assess, Monitor, and Document

Respiratory rate
Depth
Color

Arterial blood gases
Heart rate

Anticipate

Combined respiratory alkalosis and metabolic
    acidosis

Pulmonary insufficiency with altered mental
    status

FLUID AND ELECTROLYTE BALANCE

Excessive salicylate ingestion severely disrupts fluid and electrolyte balance. There is significant water and sodium loss in response to the increased metabolic rate and heat production, tachypnea, and acidemia.

Assess, Monitor, and Document

Weight
State of hydration: thirst, mucous membranes,
    skin turgor, tears, blood pressure
Urine output, including specific gravity
Urine pH should be maintained above 7.5 (an
    alkaline urine promotes excretion of sali-
    cylates)

Laboratory data: serum electrolytes, espe-
    cially bicarbonate, BUN, creatinine, osmo-
    lality, and hematocrit
Urine electrolytes and osmolality
Fluid intake: accurate administration of pa-
    renteral fluids (use of infusion pump if avail-
    able)

Anticipate

Dehydration
Metabolic acidosis
Electrolyte abnormalities: hypokalemia, hy-
    pocalcemia (tetany), hyponatremia, hypo-
    glycemia

Shock
Renal failure

NEUROLOGIC

Assess, Monitor, and Document

Level of consciousness
Orientation

Pupillary response
Reflexes

Anticipate

Coma
Seizures

GASTROINTESTINAL

The gastric mucosa can be irritated directly by excessive ingestion of salicylates. Depending upon the quantity and duration of ingestion, significant upper gastrointestinal bleeding can occur.

Assess, Monitor, and Document

Nausea
Vomiting
Nasogastric (NG) drainage: amount, color,
   presence of blood

Stools: color, presence of blood

HEMATOLOGIC

Although rare, bleeding can be a problem owing to the effects of salicylates on prothrombin formation, Factor VII production, platelet aggregation, and capillary fragility.

Assess, Monitor, and Document

Bruises
Petechiae
PT and PTT
Hct
Bleeding

Puncture sites
Urine
Stools
Gastrointestinal drainage

Anticipate

Bleeding

RESPONSE OF CHILD

Assess, Monitor, and Document

Developmental level: fears, tasks
Degree of distress

Ability to cope
Strategies used to reduce emotional trauma

Anticipate

Emotional crisis

RESPONSE OF FAMILY

Assess, Monitor, and Document

Behavioral response: angry, guilty, fearful
Level of understanding of child's condition

Expected outcome
Ability to cope

Anticipate

Fear
Guilt
Family crisis

Inability to cope
Learning needs

MIND SET

Assess

Respiratory status
Fluid and electrolyte balance
Neurologic status

Gastrointestinal system
Hematologic status
Emotional response of child and family

Anticipate

Hyperthermia
Tachypnea
Hyperpnea
Vomiting
Metabolic acidosis
Altered level of consciousness
Seizures

Dehydration
Shock
Bleeding
Renal Failure
Emotional distress
Family crisis

Acetaminophen Intoxication

HARRIS E. BURSTIN, M.D.

With the increasing popularity of non-aspirin analgesic/antipyretic agents, acetaminophen intoxication has increased significantly.

Acetaminophen is metabolized in the liver by conjugation primarily with glucuronide and to a lesser degree with sulfuric acid. The resulting conjugated metabolites are biologically inactive. An additional, but minor, pathway for acetaminophen metabolism involves hydroxylation and deacetylation by cytochrome P_{450} mixed-function oxidase. The metabolites of this process are very biologically active until bound to glutathione and excreted in the urine.

When the usual dose and time interval recommendations of 10 to 15 mg per kg every 4 hours are followed, acetaminophen is a safe medication with minimal, if any, adverse effects. When large quantities of acetaminophen are ingested, however, the capacity to handle the reactive metabolites of the cytochrome P_{450} pathway may be exceeded, and it can bind to macromolecules in hepatocytes, causing centrilobular necrosis. With this pathophysiology in mind, it is easier to understand the clinical presentation of acetaminophen poisoning.

Within the first few hours of an acute ingestion, nonspecific symptoms of nausea, vomiting, and diaphoresis are evident (Phase I). Over the subsequent 48 to 72 hours, symptoms are absent or mild (Phase II). During this period, serum concentrations of transaminases and bilirubin begin to increase. It is not until 72 hours or more following ingestion that frank symptoms of acute hepatic failure present (Phase III). The patient now becomes jaundiced, is febrile, has changes in mental status, including encephalopathy, and may have bleeding problems.

Because clinical symptoms abate and are not again evident until 48 to 72 hours after a toxic ingestion, a high index of suspicion is required if appropriate care is to be delivered.

Patients commonly confuse analgesics, and many patients are unaware that brands other than Tylenol are acetaminophen and not aspirin. Acetaminophen is also commonly found in many combination-type cold medications. Therefore, the patient's history should include the exact amount of acetaminophen ingested. This information, plus a rapid reliable means of obtaining an acetaminophen level, can help identify patients who are at risk.

The nomogram shown in Figure 60–1, developed by Rumack and associates, predicts who will suffer possible hepatic toxicity based upon acetaminophen level and time elapsed since ingestion.

When a patient has ingested more than 7.5 gm or has a toxic level that falls within the toxic range of the nomogram, N-acetylcysteine is given. N-acetylcysteine, probably like glutathione, has the ability to bind the metabolic end-products of the cytochrome P_{450} system. When bound, they are no longer toxic and are safely excreted in the urine. N-acetylcysteine is most effective if given within the first 10 hours after ingestion. The usual dose is 140 mg per kg orally as a loading dose, followed by 70 mg per kg orally every 4 hours for 17 additional doses.

N-acetylcysteine has been found to be quite safe, with no major side effects. Owing to its taste, some patients will require it to be given by nasogastric (NG) tube. If an acetaminophen level cannot be obtained quickly and there is reason to suspect significant acetaminophen ingestion, N-acetylcysteine should be given pending results.

Blood work should also include bilirubin, transaminases, ammonia, glucose, electrolytes, complete blood count (CBC), and coagulation profile. A ferric chloride testing of the urine is helpful to rule out any combination aspirin ingestion.

If there is evidence of liver dysfunction, vigorous supportive care should be initiated (see Chapter 41). Follow-up is required to observe for possible sequelae.

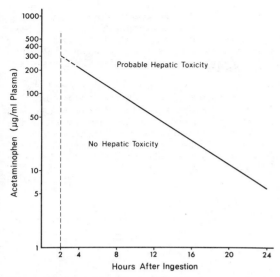

Figure 60-1. Semilogarithmic plot of plasma acetaminophen levels versus time. (From Rumack, B.H., and Matthew, H.: Acetaminophen poisoning and toxicity. Pediatrics, 55:871–876, with permission. Copyright American Academy of Pediatrics, 1975.)

A high index of suspicion, rapid analysis of acetaminophen level, and the use of N-acetylcysteine early in the course of treatment will spare many children from the morbidity and possible mortality of liver failure. Newer safety-capped bottles and public education are necessary to prevent ingestions.

CASE PRESENTATION

A 22-month-old male presented to the pediatric emergency service for the third time with a 7-day history of fevers and, now, with "spots" on his legs.

The child was first seen 6 days earlier and was sent home with a diagnosis of a viral upper respiratory infection. The mother was instructed to give the child 1 teaspoon of Tylenol elixir (160 mg of acetaminophen/5 ml) every 4–6 hours for temperature greater than 101°F.

The child returned to the emergency service 2 days later with temperature to 104°F. The same diagnosis was made, and the mother was instructed to alternate aspirin with the Tylenol. The mother began to alternate Tylenol with Tempra (160 mg of acetaminophen/5 ml), giving one or the other every 2 hours.

The patient began vomiting on the fifth day of illness. The mother called the emergency room and was told that the vomiting was probably a result of the child swallowing mucus; an over-the-counter decongestant/antihistamine was prescribed.

The following day, the patient seemed to improve. Though there was no temperature, the mother continued with Tylenol every 4 hours for the cold.

That night, the child began to spike temperature to 104°F and by early morning became unarousable with "spots" noted on his legs. The mother rushed him to the emergency room.

Physical Examination and Test Results

On physical examination, the patient was lethargic and irritable, with ecchymotic lesions over the legs and trunk. His vital signs were: T = 104.2°F, RR = 60 breaths/min, HR = 170 beats/min, BP = 80/55 mm Hg, and wt = 15 kg (33 lb).

The remainder of the examination was normal except for a liver palpable 3 cm below the right costal margin.

The working diagnosis became meningococcemia, and a spinal tap and blood cultures were performed. Ampicillin and chloramphenicol were given IV stat.

On further detailed history, the mother's use of acetaminophen every 2–4 hours for 7 days became evident and a stat acetaminophen level was ordered. Other requested laboratory studies included: CBCs, urinalysis, electrolytes, liver function tests (LFTs), and coagulation studies. It was estimated that as much as 8–10 gm of acetaminophen may have been ingested in 7 days.

Laboratory Evaluation

CBC: within normal limits; UA: normal; electrolytes: within normal limits. Results of LFTs were: SGOT: 199 mU/ml, SGPT: 105 mU/ml, total bilirubin: 2.5 mg/dl, ammonia: 30 μmol/L, PT: 20/11 sec, PTT: 67/33 sec. Acetaminophen level: 700 mg/ml. Hepatitis A and B screen were negative. The patient was transferred to the pediatric ICU and the following assessments were made.

Problem List

Intake and Output

The patient was made NPO. IV fluids of D2½/½/ normal saline (NS) at two thirds maintenance, because of the initial possibility of meningitis and subsequent cerebral edema, were started. Diuresis is of no benefit in the treatment of acetaminophen toxicity. Ten mEq of KCl/L was added after the patient voided.

Acetaminophen Toxicity

N-acetylcysteine was given via NG tube. Three gms were given stat, followed by 1.5 gms q4h for 17 doses.

Liver Failure

Fresh frozen plasma (FFP) was given stat and repeated three more times. One dose of vitamin K was given. Over the next 7 days, liver function slowly improved and the patient was treated by supportive means (see Chapter 41).

Infection

Ampicillin was discontinued after negative culture results. The chloramphenicol was not given again.

Two weeks after admission, the child was in stable condition and was sent to the ward and subsequently home.

SUGGESTED READING

Arena, J.M., et al.: Acetaminophen: report of an unusual poisoning. Pediatrics 61:68, 1978.

Atwood, S.: The laboratory in the diagnosis and management of acetaminophen and salicylate intoxications. Pediatr. Clin. North Am. 27 (4): 871, 1980.

Committee on Drugs, American Academy of Pediatrics: Commentary on acetaminophen. Pediatrics 61:108, 1978.

Committee on Drugs, American Academy of Pediatrics: Acetaminophen assay. Pediatrics, 67:303, 1981.

Piperno, E., Mosher, A. H., et al.: Pathophysiology of acetaminophen overdose toxicity: implications for management. Pediatrics (Suppl) ed.: 62:880, 1978.

Rumack, B., Peterson, R.: Acetaminophen overdose: incidence, diagnosis, and management in 416 patients. Pediatrics (Suppl) 62:898, 1978.

Nursing Process for Patient Care:

Acetaminophen Intoxication

The increasing use of acetaminophen rather than aspirin in the pediatric population has resulted in an increase in the number of children with acetaminophen intoxication. The target organ of excessive ingestion is the liver, because acetaminophen is metabolized in the liver. Excessive amounts of reactive metabolites can no longer be handled by the liver, and these metabolites bind to macromolecules in hepatocytes, causing necrosis. The nurse must be aware of the presentation of acetaminophen intoxication so that proper assessment can be made.

HEPATIC

Assess, Monitor, and Document

Phases of intoxication
    Nonspecific symptoms (I)
        Nausea
        Vomiting
        Diaphoresis
    Absent or mild symptoms (II)

Elevation of serum transaminases and bilirubin
Frank symptoms of liver failure (III)
    Altered level of consciousness
    Altered coagulation status
    Altered liver function tests

Anticipate

Acute liver failure

RESPONSE OF CHILD

Assess, Monitor, and Document

Developmental level: fears, tasks
Degree of distress

Ability to cope
Response to nursing interventions

Anticipate

Emotional crisis

RESPONSE OF FAMILY

Assess, Monitor, and Document

Behavioral response: angry, guilty, fearful
Level of understanding of child's condition

Expected outcome
Ability to cope

Anticipate

Guilt
Fear
Distress
Inability to cope

Learning needs related to administration of over-the-counter medication and environmental safety
Family crisis

MIND SET

Assess

Phase of intoxication
  Nonspecific symptoms
  Absent or mild symptoms

Frank symptoms of liver failure
Emotional response of child and family

Anticipate

Acute liver failure
  Abnormal liver function tests
  Encephalopathy

Bleeding
Emotional distress
Family crisis

Carbon Monoxide Poisoning

SOL S. ZIMMERMAN, M.D.

Among poisons, carbon monoxide (CO) has a unique status. Annually, it accounts for almost half the fatalities due to poisoning. Unlike most toxins, it is without color, taste, and odor and its intoxication is usually an unintentioned event. Its clinical presentation often consists of vague, general symptoms that are confused with illnesses of lesser consequence.

SOURCES

A colorless, odorless gas, carbon monoxide is present in the atmosphere at a concentration of less than 0.001 percent. Although small quantities are produced within man by the metabolism of hemoglobin, the major source of CO is the incomplete combustion of carbon-containing compounds. Such compounds include natural gas, coke oven gas, coal gas, and charcoal. The defective operation and inadequate venting of gas space heaters, hot water heaters, and stoves pose the threat of intoxication. The use of charcoal grills in confined spaces presents a similar hazard. CO is produced in fires, and among victims who die within the first few hours following the insult, it is a major cause of death. A very important source of carbon monoxide is the internal combustion engine; the exhaust contains CO in a concentration of 6 to 10 percent.

TOXICITY

The toxicity of CO depends upon three separate actions. First, it binds to hemoglobin with an affinity 250 times greater than that of oxygen. The result of that binding is carboxyhemoglobin (COHb). The partial pressure of oxygen will remain normal, but the saturation will be markedly reduced. Hemoglobin is 50 percent saturated with oxygen at a partial pressure of 30 mm Hg and with CO at a partial pressure of 0.10 mm Hg. Second, it binds to myoglobin and to intracellular cytochrome oxidases, primarily a_3 and P-450. The result is severe impairment of cellular oxidation and ensuing cellular anoxia. Third, CO causes a shift of the oxyhemoglobin dissociation curve to the left (Fig. 61–1).

Children appear to be more susceptible to the toxic effects of CO because of their lower hemoglobin concentrations and higher basal metabolic rates.

COHb levels in the blood are a function of both inspired concentration and duration of exposure. Inspired concentrations of 0.01 percent CO result in a COHb level of 15 percent. A concentration of 0.05 percent results in a COHb level of approximately 40 percent. In general, the anticipated level of a nonsmoking city dweller is 1 percent. Smokers will have COHb levels in the range 5 to 7 percent.

The acute presentation is that of toxic-metabolic encephalopathy (Table 61–1), often with concomitant involvement of the heart, lungs, kidneys, and skeletal muscles. The classic description of cherry red lips is variable and cannot be relied upon.

DIAGNOSIS

The diagnosis of CO poisoning is made from the history of exposure, physical examination, and laboratory determination of COHb level. Although most often the exposure is evident, the index of suspicion must remain high in any unexplained encephalopathy. With more and more older automobiles in operation, the inadvertent poisoning of passengers in moving cars has increased as a consequence of faulty exhaust systems.

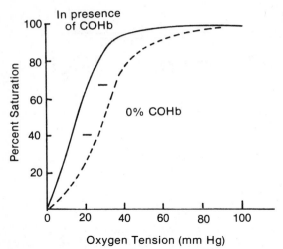

Figure 61–1. Oxygen saturation in a patient with carbon monoxide poisoning.

TREATMENT

The treatment of carbon monoxide poisoning rests upon termination of exposure and administration of oxygen to dissociate CO from hemoglobin. The half-life of COHb in room air is 5 hours; in 100 percent oxygen, it is 90 minutes; and in hyperbaric oxygen, it is less than 30 minutes. Hyperbaric oxygen is not only the most rapid means of dissociating COHb but also immediately corrects tissue hypoxia by increasing the amount of oxygen dissolved in plasma. Under normal condition of room air, the amount of dissolved plasma oxygen is 0.3 Vol%, a relatively insignificant fraction of the total oxygen content. Upon exposure to oxygen under 2.5 atmospheres of pressure, this dissolved plasma oxygen rises to a very significant 5.6 Vol%.

For levels of COHb greater than 25 percent, the treatment of choice is hyperbaric oxygen at 2 to 2.5 atmospheres for a duration of 1 to 2 hours. The availability of hyperbaric chambers is very limited; therefore, the therapy that is most often used is 100 percent oxygen until the COHb level falls to below 10 percent. Oxygen is administered by tight-fitting face mask or endotracheal tube, as determined by the child's level of consciousness.

The remaining therapy, like that of all poisonings, is supportive. If a mild metabolic acidosis exists, bicarbonate administration should be withheld, because acidosis shifts the oxyhemoglobin dissociation curve to the right. If a patient is being ventilated mechanically, hypercarbia should be avoided, because respiratory alkalosis compounds the effect of CO by further shifting the oxyhemoglobin dissociation curve to the left.

COMPLICATIONS

Cardiac

The heart is a common target organ for the hypoxia resulting from CO poisoning, particularly in adults. The EKG is a sensitive indicator of myocardial damage, and changes include ST-segment depression. T-wave inversions, atrial fibrillation, and intraventricular conduction defects. Although these findings may be present on admission, it is common to see them evolve over the first 24 hours.

Pulmonary

Pulmonary edema is a frequent complication found on autopsy in more than two thirds of patients who died following CO poisoning. There are multiple mechanisms by which this edema may occur. First, the toxic action of CO and its associated hypoxia result in increased capillary permeability. Second, prolonged hy-

Table 61–1. Carboxyhemoglobin (COHb) Levels and Resulting Symptoms

COHb Level in Blood (%)	Symptoms
10	Dyspnea upon vigorous exercise
20	Dyspnea upon moderate activity
30	Headache, irritability, altered judgment; throbbing at temples
40	More prominent headache, confusion, nausea, dizziness, weakness; dim vision
50	Syncope
60	Convulsions, obtundation
70	Coma (death upon prolonged exposure)
80	Fatal immediately

poxia may cause left ventricular dysfunction and congestive heart failure (CHF). Third, alteration in state of consciousness may be associated with aspiration and consequent edema.

Muscular

Muscle necrosis may be the result of tissue anoxia. In addition, compression and crush injuries occur in patients as they lose consciousness and fall. The positions in which they lie often result in venous obstruction and further tissue injury. Unconscious patients should be examined for evidence of soft-tissue injury and, if present, myonecrosis may be assumed and the possibility of renal complications should be indicated.

Renal

In the presence of significant myonecrosis, myoglobinemia and myoglobinuria may occur and result in acute renal failure. The early diagnosis of renal involvement is important, because forced diuresis and alkalinization of the urine may prevent progression to acute renal failure.

Neurologic

CO poisoning causes an anoxic encephalopathy. EEG is abnormal in more than 90 percent of patients; CAT scans may reveal decreased density in the area of the globus pallidus.

Clinical manifestations range from mild headache and irritability to coma. Severe involvement may be associated with decerebrate posturing, seizures, and trismus. Residual or delayed neurologic effects frequently include short-term memory deficits, speech impairment, cognitive change, personality alteration, and learning disability.

Because cerebral edema is a frequent occurrence, the management of the encephalopathy has included hyperventilation and the administration of steroids, but there have been no controlled studies as to efficacy. The role of intracranial pressure (ICP) monitoring is still being evaluated.

CASE PRESENTATION

J.S., a 4-year-old male, was found unconscious in the rear of the family station wagon after a 5-hour trip. Previously, he had been in excellent health.

Both parents and an older sibling were sitting in the front of the vehicle and complained of headaches and throbbing sensations at the temples.

Physical Examination

Upon arrival at the local hospital, physical examination revealed a well-developed, well-nourished 4-year-old, with irregular, slow, shallow respirations. Vital signs revealed a BP of 80/40 mm Hg, HR = 120 beats/min, RR = 12 breaths/min, and T = 38°C. Examination of the head, eyes, ears, nose, and throat was pertinent for bilateral retinal hemorrhage. Pupils were equal and reactive to light. There were roving eye movements, with no following of light. The lungs revealed poor aeration on auscultation but no adventitious sounds. He was unresponsive to verbal stimuli, but withdrew on painful stimulation. Deep tendon reflexes were depressed. The remainder of the examination was unremarkable.

Laboratory Evaluation

Laboratory values on admission included a WBC of 14,000 (55 percent segmented neutrophils, 20 percent band cells, 25 percent lymphocytes); platelets = 140,000/cu mm; hemoglobin = 13 gm/dl, hematocrit = 38 percent. Urinalysis revealed a specific gravity of 1.008 and no cellular material and was negative by dipstick. Arterial blood gas determination was: pH = 7.08, PO_2 = 69 mm Hg, PCO_2 = 61 mm Hg, and HCO_3 = 17. Serum chemistries showed: sodium = 136 mEq/L; potassium = 4.2 mEq/L; chloride = 101 mEq/L, bicarbonate = 18 mEq/L; chloride = 101 mEq/L, bicarbonate = 18 mEq/L; glucose = 92 mg/100 ml; calcium = 8.9 mg/100 ml; BUN = 16 mg/100 ml; creatinine = 0.4 mg/100 ml. COHb level was 54 percent. (Parents and sibling had levels ranging from 23–28 percent.) An EKG was within normal limits. An EEG revealed diffuse slow wave, low voltage α wave activity.

The impression on admission was CO poisoning with encephalopathy.

Problem List

Fluid and Electrolyte Balance

The patient has a urine of low specific gravity, normal serum electrolytes, and no clinical evidence of dehydration. Because of the encephalopathy and concern about the potential for pulmonary edema, fluids should be restricted to two thirds to three quarters of maintenance.

The metabolic component of the acidosis is mild and should not be treated, because acidosis shifts the oxyhemoglobin dissociation curve to the right and increases the delivery of oxygen to tissues.

Respiratory

Because of the irregular respirations and blood gas evidence of respiratory insufficiency, the child was intubated and 100 percent oxygen was administered in the absence of hyperbaric chamber. He would be hyperventilated to an arterial PCO_2 of 25 mm Hg because of concern about cerebral edema.

Toxic–Metabolic

Serial COHbs are to be followed every hour, and 100 percent oxygen should be administered until the COHb level falls to below 10 percent.

Neurologic

Cerebral edema frequently develops in patients with CO poisoning. Fluid restriction and hyperventilation have already been instituted. Oxygen is being administered to reverse the tissue hypoxia. Most often, steroids are added to the regimen. If the neurologic status deteriorates, diuretics should be used and strong consideration should be given to the placement of an ICP measuring device.

Observe for seizures, and institute anticonvulsants as necessary.

Ophthalmologic

Retinal hemorrhages are seen in CO poisoning, most often in circumstances of prolonged exposure. When hemorrhages are present in association with an unexplained encephalopathy, CO poisoning should be suspected. No specific treatment is required.

SUGGESTED READING

Bour, H., and Ledingham I.: Carbon Monoxide Poisoning. New York, Elsevier Science Publishing Co. Inc., 1967.

Boutros, A.R., and Hoyt, J.L.: Management of carbon monoxide poisoning in the absence of hyperbaric oxygen chamber. Crit. Care Med. 4:144, 1976.

Larkin, J.M., Brakos, B.J., and Moylan, J.A.: Treatment of carbon monoxide poisoning: prognostic factors. J. Trauma 16:111, 1976.

McBay, A.J.: Carbon monoxide poisoning, low-medicine notes, N. Engl. J. Med. 272:252, 1965.

Myers, R.A., Linberg, S.E., and Cowley, R.A.: Carbon monoxide poisoning: the injury and its treatment. JACEP 8:479, 1979.

Zimmerman, S.S., and Truxal, B.: Carbon monoxide poisoning. Pediatrics 68:215, 1981.

Nursing Process for Patient Care:

Carbon Monoxide Poisoning

RESPIRATORY

Assess, Monitor, and Document

Rate
Pattern
Breath sounds
Heart rate
Blood pressure
Color
Arterial blood gases
Endotracheal tube (post-intubation)
- Patency
- Position
- Breath sounds

Anticipate

Acute respiratory failure
- Altered level of consciousness
- Restlessness
- Agitation
- Cyanosis
- Decreased breath sounds
- Decreased rate
- Hypoxemia

Pulmonary edema
- Increased respiratory rate
- Rales and rhonchi
- Increased secretions

NEUROLOGIC

Assess, Monitor, and Document

Level of consciousness
Pupil size and reaction to light
Reflexes
Response to pain
Blood pressure
Temperature

Anticipate

Increased intracranial pressure (ICP)
- Altered level of consciousness
- Increased blood pressure
- Bradycardia
- Decreased respirations

Seizures

CARDIAC

Assess, Monitor, and Document

Heart rate
Rhythm
Blood pressure
Perfusion

Anticipate

EKG changes
- ST-segment depression
- T-wave inversions

Bradycardia
- Conduction defects

Premature ventricular contractions
Fibrillation: atrial, ventricular

FLUID AND ELECTROLYTE BALANCE

Assess, Monitor, and Document

Weight
State of hydration
Mucous membranes
Skin turgor
Tears
Blood pressure

Pulse
Breath sounds
Urine output including specific gravity
Laboratory data
    Serum electrolytes
    Hematocrit

Anticipate

Cerebral edema
    Altered level of consciousness
    Increased blood pressure (widening pulse
      pressure)
    Decreased pulse
    Decreased respiratory rate

Seizures
Pulmonary edema
    Increased respiratory rate
    Rales and rhonchi
    Increased secretions (may be frothy and/
      or pink tinged)

RESPONSE OF CHILD

Assess, Monitor, and Document

Developmental level: verbal, motor, psycho-
    social, cognitive
Perception of events surrounding intoxication

Behavioral response: fearful, anxious, tearful
Response to nursing interventions

Anticipate

Emotional distress
Educational needs related to environmental
    safety

RESPONSE OF FAMILY

Assess, Monitor, and Document

Behavioral response: angry, verbal, tearful
Level of understanding of child's condition
    and treatment

Expected outcome
Response to nursing interventions

Anticipate

Family crisis
Educational needs related to environmental
    safety

MIND SET

Assess

Respiratory status
Neurologic status
Cardiac status
Fluid and electrolyte balance

Renal status
Soft tissue for injury
Response of child and family

Anticipate

Alteration in respiratory status
  Hypoxia
  Pulmonary edema
Alteration in neurologic status
  Increased ICP
  Seizures
Alteration in cardiac status

Cardiac dysrhythmias
Alteration in fluid and electrolyte balance
Alteration in renal status
  Acute renal failure
Muscle necrosis
Emotional distress
Family crisis

Hydrocarbon Intoxication

ALAN G. KULBERG, M.D.

Distillation of petroleum for commercial usages produces a wide variety of compounds that may cause toxicity in humans (Table 62–1). The two major groups of compounds are the aliphatic (straight-chain) and the aromatic cyclic hydrocarbons. The aliphatic hydrocarbons are commonly found in charcoal lighter fluid, furniture polish, lacquer diluent, and varnish thinner and as a vehicle for unrelated compounds such as insecticides; they are most often implicated in cases of pulmonary aspiration. The low viscosity (the ease of flow over a surface) and low surface tension (spreadability) of these substances permit them to "migrate" into the tracheobroncial tree, even when they are swallowed into the gastrointestinal tract. In this sense, aspiration is usually an inadvertent consequence of ingestion.

Pulmonary aspiration of the low-viscosity hydrocarbons can produce a spectrum of clinical disease ranging from mild cough to extensive, devastating necrosis of parenchymal tissue. This chapter focuses primarily on the consequences of hydrocarbon *aspiration,* which is by far the most likely hydrocarbon–related clinical problem encountered in the pediatric intensive care unit (ICU).

PATHOGENESIS AND PATHOPHYSIOLOGY

The long-standing belief that pulmonary toxicity is the result of gastrointestinal absorption of the hydrocarbons with hematogenous spread to the lungs has not been supported by experimental or clinical evidence. Studies in animals have consistently shown poor absorption of hydrocarbons from the gastrointestinal tract, though in very high doses, histologic evidence of liver, but not lung, toxicity was noted. Furthermore, direct instillation of sublethal doses into the stomach of an animal whose esophagus has been ligated and divided, preventing aspiration, produced little or no pulmonary injury. In contrast, human suicide attempts by injection of hydrocarbons directly into an antecubital vein have resulted in rapid pulmonary toxicity, suggesting that hematogenous toxicity affects the first capillary bed that the substance encounters. In the esophageal ligature experiment, with rare exceptions, only the animals that developed pneumonitis developed a concomitant encephalopathy. The occasional minor CNS abnormalities may have been due to very large doses used with some systemic absorption or to the presence of aromatic impurities in the hydrocarbons. After hydrocarbon ingestion in children, chest x-rays are more consistent with aspiration than blood-borne toxicity, in which diffuse lung involvement is more likely. Gerarde demonstrated that the median lethal dose (LD_{50}) ratio of oral to intratracheal kerosene is 140:1, supporting the notion that very small amounts of aspirated hydrocarbons can effect toxicity and that it is unlikely that children will swallow large enough quantities to produce pulmonary lesions after gastrointestinal absorption. The average swallow in a small child is approximately 5 ml.

The high lipid solubility of the hydrocarbons permits their penetration of pulmonary tissues and disruption of surfactant, the phospholipid lining of the alveoli and distal bronchioles. Post mortem pathology of the lung reveals interstitial inflammation; vascular thromboses; hemorrhagic pulmonary edema; and necrosis of bronchial, bronchiolar, and alveolar tissue, with polymorphonuclear exudates, hyaline membrane formation, and atelectasis.

The pathophysiologic derangements that follow from such widespread tissue disruption include right-to-left shunts from atelectasis, alveolar fluid, and vascular thromboses, and diffusion and $\dot{V}/\dot{Q}$ abnormalities from interstitial edema, bronchospasm, and plugging of the airways with secretions and necrotic debris. The Pa_{O_2} is characteristically low, whereas the Pa_{CO_2} usually remains normal or low, secondary

Table 62–1. Biochemical and Clinical Properties of the Major Petroleum Distillates*

Product	Carbon Length	BP Range (°C)	Toxicities CNS	Toxicities Pulmonary	Uses
Gas	1 – 5	40	+	0	Fuel
Benzine (petroleum ether)	5 – 6	35 – 90	+	0	Rubber and industrial solvent
Gasoline	5 – 12	40 – 225	+	±	Fuel
Naphtha	7 – 10	94 – 175	+	±	Cigarette and charcoal lighter fluid, paint thinner, lacquer diluent
Mineral spirit	9 – 12	152 – 210	+	+	Dry cleaner, degreaser
Kerosene	10 – 16	175 – 325	±	+	Charcoal lighter fluid, space heater fuel, jet engine fuel, insecticide vehicle
Light gas oil	13 – 17	230 – 305	+	+	
Mineral seal oil	—	260 – 370	±	+	Furniture polish
Mineral oil	—	—	0	DA	Laxative, suntan and baby oils
Heavy gas oil	18 – 25	305 – 405	0	DA	Motor and household oils, transmission fluid
Petrolatum	26 – 38	405 – 515	0	0	Paraffin wax, petroleum jelly
Asphalt, tar	Final distillation residues—no toxicity			Paving, home construction	

*Toxicity key: + = major; ± = occasional/minor; 0 = generally absent; DA = toxicity only by direct aspiration; otherwise safe.

Table (with modifications) courtesy of Arnold Einhorn, M.D., with permission.

to tachypnea and hyperventilation. The early hypoxia sometimes seen even before the hydrocarbon has a chance to produce a pneumonitis may be due to replacement of alveolar gas by the highly volatile fumes of the lower molecular weight compounds (gasoline, naphtha, kerosene) that are inhaled during the ingestion process. This process may cause considerable central nervous system (CNS) depression as the toxin is absorbed through the alveolar-capillary membrane, with resultant hypoventilation and hypercarbia. Hypercarbia observed later in the clinical course should be interpreted as being caused by the patient's tiring, with decreased mechanical effort, resulting from the presence of an intrinsically sedating compound such as a chlorinated hydrocarbon or the concomitant ingestion of a sedative-hypnotic agent. One should also be alert to the presence in some hydrocarbon products of aniline dyes, which may cause methemoglobinemia; this should not be confused with the cyanosis of hypoxemia.

CLINICAL CONSIDERATIONS

Typically, children who aspirate a hydrocarbon product experience an immediate burning of the mouth and throat, followed by coughing, choking, gagging, and grunting respirations. When the substance enters the stomach and small bowel, nausea, bloating, and emesis may result. Approximately 50 percent of patients who develop early respiratory signs will have aspiration pneumonitis when observed six hours later. Special concern should be given to patients whose symptoms persist or worsen at the time of arrival at the hospital. Cyanosis may rapidly appear, with tachypnea, retractions of the accessory muscles of respiration, and tachycardia. Varying degrees of altered mental status, ranging from lethargy to coma, may be present, usually with concomitant clinical hypoxia. The most severely affected patients may develop hemoptysis, pulmonary edema, and frank respiratory insufficiency leading to death, usually within 36 hours.

Cardiovascular complications, though uncommon, have been reported and include pneumopericardium, cardiomegaly, and dysrhythmias with ST-segment and T-wave changes, as well as frank myocardial injury with depressed Q waves and ST-segment elevation on EKG.

Other clinical manifestations may include abdominal pain, diarrhea, and vomiting, which may compound the risk of further aspiration. Skin irritation may result if the hydrocarbon is spilled and is due to the lipophilic nature of the hydrocarbons.

Products such as organophosphate or chlorinated insecticides use petroleum distillates as a vehicle, and the resulting toxicity may be due to both components. Organophosphate toxicity is recognized by the typical cholinergic crisis of hypersalivation, urination, defecation, lacrimation, bronchorrhea, and skeletal muscle weakness, whereas the chlorinated and camphorated products may cause CNS excitation with seizures, and the nitrobenzene products may cause methemoglobinemia. It is imperative that clinicians dealing with ingestions of one of these additive-containing products not overlook the potential for hydrocarbon aspiration toxicity when evaluating for the specific toxicities of the additives.

The signs and symptoms of respiratory involvement may increase over the first 24 hours after aspiration, reach a plateau, then subside over the next week. Of all children who ingest hydrocarbon products, those who are symptomatic at the time of presentation to the hospital should be considered most at risk for pneumonitis. Patients who cough immediately upon exposure but improve quickly and are asymptomatic upon presentation are those most likely to have a favorable clinical course.

RADIOLOGIC EVALUATION

Chest x-rays may show evidence of aspiration within 30 minutes of ingestion, though in some cases it may be delayed 6 to 12 hours. Most, but not all, patients who present symptomatically have positive chest radiographs. On the other hand, a large percentage of patients with positive films may not have clinically significant disease. The clinical status should be regarded as the most important prognostic parameter in evaluating patients.

The most common radiographic pattern seen following aspiration is an increase in bronchovascular markings. Of the more organized patterns of pulmonic involvement on x-ray examination, bilateral basilar infiltrates, punctate, mottled perihilar densities, and bronchopneumonia are most commonly observed. Upper lobe involvement is not a frequent finding. A lateral view of the chest should be included in the evaluation to detect smaller retrocardiac infiltrates. Atelectasis may be widespread and sometimes indistinguishable from pneumonitis. Obstructive emphysema (air-trapping) may be seen in the lung periphery, and pleural effusion may develop. Though uncommon, pneumothorax or pneumomediastinum may evolve in the acute period. Mottled densities may become confluent over the first 2 to 3 days.

The most severely ill patients may show bilateral pulmonary edema and/or hemorrhage.

Late radiographic findings may include cysts and pneumatoceles and may occur long after the patient has improved. X-rays should be obtained 2 to 3 weeks after ingestion to document these changes; however, such findings usually resolve without incident.

LABORATORY STUDIES

The most important laboratory test with respect to patient management is the arterial blood gas (ABG), which is essential to the management of respiratory therapy. Hypoxemia and hypocapnia are the most common early ABG abnormalities; with progressive ventilatory insufficiency, hypercapnia may develop. A complete blood count (CBC) may initially reveal an acute leukocytosis secondary to the inflammatory response in the lung, but a persistence or a rise in the white blood cell (WBC) count beyond 48 hours, in conjunction with a compatible clinical picture, may reflect a secondary bacterial pneumonitis. A serum sample for type and crossmatch should be obtained if significant pulmonary hemorrhage or hemolysis occurs. The presence of nitrobenzene in the product may produce methemoglobinemia, which should be suspected when the patient has oxygen-refractory cyanosis. A drop of the patient's blood that appears brown compared with control blood in room air suggests a methemoglobin level of at least 10 percent. Ideally, direct measurement of methemoglobin should be done in order to more accurately guide therapy with intravenous (IV) methylene blue, mg/kg of a 1% solution. If the toxic additive is an organophosphate insecticide, determination of the red blood cell (RBC) cholinesterase activity may be useful in management. When indicated, heavy metal analysis should be performed.

There is no role for quantitative analysis for hydrocarbons in gastric contents, blood, or urine, and qualitative analysis is rarely of practical use in management.

THERAPY

The proper emergency management of hydrocarbon ingestions remains controversial. From the information presented thus far, a logical treatment strategy would call for basic supportive care for children who have hydrocarbon intoxication and a "leave-well-enough-alone" attitude toward those who present with no such signs or symptoms. In either case, inducing emesis with syrup of ipecac or gastric lavage with a nasogastric (NG) tube is probably not necessary and, moreover, may place the patient at further risk for aspiration beyond the damage that has already been incurred. The only situations in which induction of emesis is recommended are in alert, awake children who have ingested a hydrocarbon with a toxic additive or when a massive quantity has been swallowed. However, because the volume of a swallow in a small child is approximately 5 ml and there is a burning irritation felt on the mucous membranes upon contact, it is most unlikely that large volumes are ingested accidentally. Large ingested volumes are more likely to be encountered in older patients who ingest the substance intentionally, such as during a suicide attempt. Generally, the only situation that calls for gastric lavage is when an intubated child is believed to have ingested either a massive quantity or a product with a dangerous additive, and even then, only with ET tube protection of the airway. Whether or not to lavage the intubated child with aspiration pneumonitis when the quantity ingested is thought to be small, has not been resolved. The techniques for both methods of gastric evacuation, emesis and lavage, are discussed in detail in Chapter 58, Poisoning: General Principles of Management.

The major therapeutic goal for patients who ingest hydrocarbon products is to provide sound general respiratory support, thereby ensuring adequate oxygenation. Frequent ABG sampling is the keystone of clinical monitoring. Supplemental oxygen should be given as needed to maintain a Pa_{O_2} of at least 65 to 70 mm Hg. Awake patients or those with mild changes in mental status may require only nebulized oxygen by face mask or nasal cannula, whereas endotracheal intubation will often be necessary for more ill patients who require a very high Fi_{O_2} or who are hypercapneic secondary to pulmonary disease or hypoventilation due to loss of central respiratory drive or fatigue. Use of only a non-rebreathing mask with a reservoir attachment to deliver the oxygen may not be sufficient, because often, these patients also require vigorous pulmonary toilet. Endotracheal intubation also allows for the delivery of positive end–expiratory pressure (PEEP), which is a useful adjunct when high Fi_{O_2}s cannot maintain a satisfactory Pa_{O_2}. PEEP allows for use of a lower Fi_{O_2}, because of the effect of hydrocarbons on surfactant, PEEP may permit reexpansion of collapsed segments without surfactant and thus improve oxygenation.

Aminophylline is a useful adjunct to therapy when significant bronchospasm is present. Corticosteroids have no proven benefit and may, in fact, cause harm by impairing the normal inflammatory response in the lung. Antibiotics should not be used initially unless gross aspiration of gastric contents has occurred. The use of antibiotics later in the clinical course should be reserved for situations in which there is strong suspicion of secondary bacterial pneumonitis, as documented by a persistent or rising fever, an increased WBC count, and a worsening chest x-ray 48 hours or more after ingestion. When these indications occur, deep tracheal or bronchial cultures should be obtained, if possible, to identify the pathogen. Indiscriminate prophylactic use of broad-spectrum antibiotics may serve only to create a favorable environment for the emergence of resistant bacteria, particularly gram-negative organisms. IV fluids should be administered to maintain adequate hydration, but not overhydration.

Guidelines for treatment of specific toxicities from the different additives can be found in several current textbooks on clinical toxicology or from a regional poison control center.

CASE PRESENTATION

A 2-year-old boy was found with a soft-drink bottle filled with charcoal lighter fluid at a family picnic. Before the father could grab the bottle from him, the child took "one gulp" of the liquid, immediately started to cough violently and became cyanotic and progressively less responsive to verbal and tactile stimuli. In the emergency department, the father said the bottle contained "benzene."

Physical Examination

Physical examination revealed an extremely lethargic male child with cyanosis and respiratory distress. An orotracheal tube was inserted, and 50 percent oxygen was administered. An ABG revealed pH-7.38, PO_2 = 84 mm Hg, and PCO_2 = 30 mm Hg. He had a fever of 38.3°C (101°F). Within 2 hours of the beginning of therapy, the intubated child was awake, alert, and responding to verbal stimuli.

Problem List

Respiratory

The ABG is consistent with a V/Q mismatch commonly observed following hydrocarbon aspiration. With the child needing an Fi_{O_2} of 50 percent to achieve good oxygenation, the addition of a small amount of PEEP via the endotracheal tube might allow for a lower Fi_{O_2} while expanding lung segments collapsed owing to loss of surfactant.

Neurologic

The rapid reversal of the altered mental status with the institution of ventilatory support is consistent with the encephalopathy being secondary to hypoxia.

Toxicologic

The father stated that the bottle contained "benzene." Consultation with the poison control center revealed that "benzene" is available only in industry and not for home use. The father was asked to go home and bring back the bottle from which the child drank. The odor of the bottle was reminiscent of kerosene.

Because the child drank only a small quantity of the kerosene, gastric evacuation is not thought to be necessary; it is potentially a risk in this child who has a noncuffed endotracheal tube. Likewise, neither activated charcoal nor a cathartic is given.

After consultation with the local toxicology laboratory, it was believed that qualitative and quantitative analyses would not be helpful in the management; therefore no samples were sent. However, later questioning revealed that the child has pica and has been eating pieces of plaster that have been peeling from the living room wall; a lead level was sent. The parents are to be instructed about the principles of poison prevention and the hazards of storing toxic chemicals in familiar food containers without child-proof seals.

SUGGESTED READING

Anas, N., Mamasonthi, V., and Ginsberg, C.M.: Criteria for hospitalizing children who have ingested products containing hydrocarbons. JAMA 246:840, 1981.

Banner, W. and Watson, P.D.: Systemic toxicity following gasoline aspiration. Am. J. Emerg. Med. 3:292, 1983.

Beamon, R.F., Siegel, C.J., Landers, G., et al.: Hydrocarbon ingestion in children: A six-year retrospective study. JACEP 5:771, 1976.

Gerarde, H.W.: Toxicologic studies on hydrocarbons: IX. The aspiration hazard and toxicity of hydrocarbons and hydrocarbon mixtures. Arch. Environ. Health 6:35, 1963.

Giammona, S.T.: Effects of furniture polish on pulmonary surfactant. Am. J. Dis. Child. 113:658, 1967.

Nursing Process for Patient Care:
Hydrocarbon Intoxication

Ingestion of hydrocarbons results in pulmonary toxicity as a consequence of aspiration as opposed to absorption. Clinical manifestations range from mild cough to hemoptysis and pulmonary edema. Other organ systems are affected either directly or as the result of hypoxia.

RESPIRATORY

Assess, Monitor, and Document

Respiratory rate
Respiratory pattern, including depth
Work of breathing: retractions, nasal flaring, breath sounds
Secretions: amount, description
Level of consciousness
Color

Arterial blood gases
Response to therapy
    Supplemental oxygenation by mask
    Endotracheal intubation and assisted mechanical ventilation (PEEP)
    Aminophylline (if appropriate)

Anticipate

Alteration in respiratory status
Respiratory distress: tachypnea, retractions, nasal flaring
Atelectasis
Pulmonary edema

Change in level of consciousness
Respiratory insufficiency: hypoxia, hypercarbia, cyanosis
Respiratory arrest

NEUROLOGIC

Assess, Monitor, and Document

Behavior: agitated, restless
Level of consciousness: lethargy, stupor, coma
Blood pressure

Pulse
Pupillary response
Reflexes
Motor response

Anticipate

Alteration in neurologic function
    Increased intracranial pressure (ICP) secondary to cerebral edema
        Altered level of consciousness
        Increased blood pressure
        Decreased heart rate

Decreased respiratory rate
Altered reflex responses
Seizures
Coma
Posthypoxic encephalopathy

GASTROINTESTINAL

Assess, Monitor, and Document

Condition of mouth and throat: pain, redness, edema
Abdominal pain
Abdominal girth

Nausea
Emesis: amount, description
Bowel movements: description

Anticipate

Local irritation of mouth and throat
Alteration in gastrointestinal function
   Abdominal pain
   Abdominal distention

Nausea
Vomiting
Diarrhea

CARDIOVASCULAR

Assess, Monitor, and Document

Heart rate
Rhythm
Blood pressure: arterial, central venous

Perfusion: peripheral pulses, color and condition of skin, capillary filling

Anticipate

Alteration in cardiovascular status
   Decreased cardiac output
      Decreased arterial blood pressure
      Decreased peripheral perfusion: weak
   pulses, cool skin, poor capillary refill

Cardiac dysrhythmias
Pneumopericardium
Myocardial injury
   Depressed Q waves
   Elevated ST segment

HEMATOLOGIC

The hematologic status may be altered in response to the inflammatory process in the lung or a secondary bacterial pneumonitis. It is important to note that the presence of nitrobenzene in the product may produce methemoglobinemia.

Assess, Monitor, and Document

Complete blood count (CBC)

Anticipate

Alteration in hematologic status
   Increased white blood count (WBC)

Decreased hemoglobin
Methemoglobinemia

RESPONSE OF CHILD

Assess, Monitor, and Document

Developmental level: verbal, motor, psychosocial, cognitive
Perception of events surrounding ingestion and need for education

Behavioral response: fearful, anxious, tearful
Response to nursing interventions

Anticipate

Emotional trauma
Educational needs related to environmental
   safety

RESPONSE OF FAMILY

Assess, Monitor, and Document

Behavioral response: anxious, fearful, verbal, angry

Perception of events surrounding accidental ingestion

Feelings of guilt

Level of understanding of child's condition

Expected outcome

Response to nursing interventions

Anticipate

Emotional distress

Inability to cope

Family crisis

Educational needs related to environmental safety

MIND SET

Assess

Respiratory status

Neurologic status

Gastrointestinal status

Cardiovascular status

Hematologic status

Response of child and family

Anticipate

Alteration in respiratory status
  Respiratory distress
  Pulmonary edema
  Respiratory insufficiency
  Respiratory arrest
Alteration in neurologic status
  Change in level of consciousness

Alteration in gastrointestinal function
Alteration in cardiovascular status
  Dysrhythmias
Alteration in hematologic status
  Methemeglobinemia
Emotional trauma
Family crisis

INDEX

Page numbers in *italics* refer to illustrations; page numbers
followed by (t) refer to tables.